Cecil Review of

General Internal Medicine

Cecil Review of
General Internal Medicine

Sixth Edition

J. ALLEN D. COOPER, Jr., M.D.

Associate Professor, Department of Medicine
Division of Pulmonary and Critical Care Medicine
University of Alabama at Birmingham School of Medicine
Birmingham, Alabama

PETER G. PAPPAS, M.D.

Associate Professor, Department of Medicine
Division of Infectious Diseases
University of Alabama at Birmingham School of Medicine
Birmingham, Alabama

W. B. SAUNDERS COMPANY
A Division of Harcourt Brace & Company
Philadelphia, London, Toronto, Montreal, Sydney, Tokyo

W. B. SAUNDERS COMPANY
A Division of Harcourt Brace & Company

The Curtis Center
Independence Square West
Philadelphia, Pennsylvania 19106

Library of Congress Cataloging-in-Publication Data

Cecil review of general internal medicine / [edited by] J. Allen D.
    Cooper, Jr., Peter G. Pappas.—6th ed.
        p.   cm.
    Includes bibliographical references.
    ISBN 0-7216-6264-1
      1. Internal medicine—Examinations, questions, etc.   I. Cooper,
J. Allen D.   II. Pappas, Peter G.
RC46.C423   1995 Suppl.
616'.0076—dc20   95-49211

CECIL REVIEW OF GENERAL INTERNAL MEDICINE   ISBN 0-7216-6264-1

Printed in the United States of America

Last digit is the print number: 9   8   7   6   5   4   3   2   1

This book is dedicated to our children,
Thomas, Rebecca, Hayden, and Cameron.

CONTRIBUTORS

VERA A. BITTNER, M.D.

Associate Professor of Medicine, Division of Cardiovascular Disease, The University of Alabama at Birmingham, Birmingham, Alabama

Cardiology

GWENDOLYN C. CLAUSSEN, M.D.

Assistant Professor, The University of Alabama at Birmingham, Birmingham, Alabama

Dermatology

J. ALLEN D. COOPER, Jr., M.D.

Associate Professor of Medicine, The University of Alabama at Birmingham, Birmingham, Alabama

Pulmonary Diseases

ROBERT S. DIPAOLA, M.D.

Assistant Professor, Robert Wood Johnson Medical School, New Brunswick, New Jersey

Oncology

PETER F. ELLS, M.D.

Clinical Assistant Professor of Medicine, University Medical Center Stony Brook; Division Head (Acting), Division of Gastroenterology-Hepatology, SUNY at Stony Brook, New York

Gastrointestinal Disease

STUART J. FRANK, M.D.

Assistant Professor of Medicine, Division of Endocrinology and Metabolism, The University of Alabama at Birmingham; Chief, Endocrinology Section, Medicine Service, Birmingham Veterans Affairs Medical Center, Birmingham, Alabama

Diabetes Mellitus and Metabolism

R. BRUCE GAMMON, M.D.

Assistant Professor of Medicine, The University of Alabama at Birmingham; Medical Director, Medical Intensive Care Unit, Veterans Affairs Medical Center, Birmingham, Alabama

Critical Care

WILLIAM N. HAIT, M.D., Ph.D.

Professor of Medicine and Pharmacology, UMDNJ—Robert Wood Johnson Medical School; Director, The Cancer Institute of New Jersey, New Brunswick, New Jersey

Oncology

VAN B. HAYNE, Jr., M.D.

Associate Professor of Medicine, Division of Endocrinology and Metabolism, The University of Alabama School of Medicine, at Birmingham, Birmingham, Alabama

Endocrine/Reproductive Disease and Disease of Bone and Bone/Mineral Metabolism

LOUIS W. HECK, Jr., M.D.

Associate Professor of Medicine, The University of Alabama at Birmingham, Birmingham, Alabama

Rheumatology and Clinical Immunology

JOHN E. HUMPHRIES, M.D.

Assistant Professor, Departments of Internal Medicine and Pathology; Division of Hematology/Oncology; Associate Director, Special Coagulation Laboratory, University of Virginia School of Medicine, Charlottesville, Virginia

Hematology

ANN M. LINDGREN, M.D.

Assistant Professor of Dermatology, The University of Alabama at Birmingham, Birmingham, Alabama

Dermatology

PETER G. PAPPAS, M.D.

Associate Professor, Division of Infectious Diseases, The University of Alabama at Birmingham, Birmingham, Alabama

Infectious Diseases

DOUGLAS J. PEARCE, M.D.

Assistant Professor of Medicine, The University of Alabama at Birmingham; Director, Coronary Care Unit, University Hospital, Birmingham, Alabama

Cardiology

JOSEPH M. POLITO, III, M.D.

Clinical Instructor of Medicine, Division of Gastroenterology-Hepatology, University Medical Center Stony Brook, SUNY at Stony Brook, Stony Brook, New York

Gastrointestinal Disease

W. MITCHELL SAMS, M.D.

Professor of Dermatology; Chairman, Department of Dermatology, The University of Alabama at Birmingham, Birmingham, Alabama

Dermatology

PAUL W. SANDERS, M.D.

Associate Professor of Medicine, The University of Alabama at Birmingham; Chief, Nephrology Section, Veterans Administration Hospital, Birmingham, Alabama

Renal Disease

DAVID G. WARNOCK, M.D.

Professor of Medicine and Physiology; Director, Division of Nephrology Research and Training Center, The University of Alabama at Birmingham, Birmingham, Alabama

Renal Disease

AYMAN A. ZAYED, M.D.

Fellow, Division of Endocrinology and Metabolism, Department of Medicine, The University of Alabama at Birmingham, Birmingham, Alabama

Endocrine/Reproductive Disease and Disease of Bone and Bone Mineral Metabolism; Diabetes Mellitus and Metabolism

PREFACE

The practice of internal medicine becomes more complex each day. The unprecedented explosion in medical information has presented an enormous challenge to the practicing physician in making it more difficult to remain abreast of current information. Yet the need to remain up-to-date is essential, not only to provide the best care for our patients, but also because of current recertification requirements. Also, important non-scientific issues which face each physician, such as health care reform and medical-legal issues, have made it necessary for all physicians to keep up with developments in these areas as well. Given these circumstances, physicians must work even harder to maintain a current medical knowledge base. Therefore, an effective means of keeping up with the large amount of available new information is necessary. We believe that this book provides an efficient and relatively easy way of accompanying this formidable task.

This is the sixth edition of the *Cecil Review of General Internal Medicine*. This book is a companion to the *Cecil Textbook of Medicine,* and it is composed of questions pertaining to specific areas in internal medicine. It has been completely revised from the previous edition, but the format remains essentially the same. The questions are grouped according to subspecialty sections, and each section is written by authorities in their field. Questions are presented in a format similar to those used in American Board of Internal Medicine certification examinations. In addition, detailed answers to each of the questions are provided in a separate section and discussed with reference to chapters in *Cecil Textbook of Medicine*. Additional references are provided at each author's discretion. It is our hope that this book will be helpful to medical students, medical housestaff, physicians who are preparing to take internal medicine certification boards for the first time, and those who are eligible for recertification. We feel that the questions and answers presented herein are pertinent and sufficiently broad in their scope, that used together with *Cecil Textbook of Medicine*, provide a unique opportunity for reviewing the most current information in internal medicine.

ACKNOWLEDGMENTS

We would like to thank Mrs. Windell Ross and Ms. Beverly Jernigan whose many hours of technical assistance were essential in manuscript preparation. In addition, we would like to thank Mr. Ray Kersey of W. B. Saunders Company, whose efforts have led to the timely publication of the sixth edition of *Cecil Review of General Internal Medicine*.

CONTENTS

PART 1

CARDIOLOGY

Vera A. Bittner and Douglas J. Pearce

DIRECTIONS: For questions 1 to 56, choose the ONE BEST answer to each question.

1. All of the following are associated with an increased risk of coronary heart disease EXCEPT

- A. Short stature
- B. Diabetes mellitus
- C. High high-density lipoprotein (HDL) cholesterol level
- D. Hypertension
- E. Cigarette smoking

2. Sympathetic stimulation of the heart results in all of the following EXCEPT

- A. Increased force of contraction of ventricular muscle
- B. Increased conduction velocity through the atrioventricular (AV) node
- C. Increased velocity of ventricular muscle relaxation
- D. Decreased rate of phase IV depolarization in the sinus node, resulting in increased heart rate
- E. Increased velocity of ventricular muscle contraction

3. Major determinants of myocardial oxygen consumption are all of the following EXCEPT

- A. Systolic pressure
- B. Heart rate
- C. Myocardial contractility
- D. Basal oxygen requirement
- E. Force of atrial contraction

4. Activation of retronodal chemoreceptors during an inferior wall myocardial infarction (MI) may result in all of the following EXCEPT

- A. Hypotension
- B. Diaphoresis
- C. Tachycardia
- D. Nausea
- E. Salivation

5. Patients with asymptomatic ventricular premature contractions are best treated with which of the following?

- A. Propafenone
- B. Moricizine
- C. Mexiletine
- D. Amiodarone
- E. Reassurance

6. Appropriate treatments for wide QRS tachycardias of undetermined origin may include all of the following EXCEPT

- A. Intravenous lidocaine
- B. Cardioversion
- C. Intravenous verapamil
- D. Intravenous procainamide
- E. Carotid sinus massage

7. Multifocal atrial tachycardia is characterized by all of the following EXCEPT

- A. Difficult to treat, but responds best to digoxin at high doses
- B. Often seen in patients in the medical intensive care unit
- C. Therapy with catecholamines or theophylline may precipitate the arrhythmia
- D. Verapamil treatment may be helpful
- E. Treatment should be directed at the underlying illness

8. Which of the following statements about the epidemiology of hypertension is correct?

- A. Hypertension is more common in whites than in blacks.
- B. Over 10% of hypertensives have secondary hypertension.
- C. White coat hypertension increases in prevalence with increasing severity of blood pressure.
- D. Isolated systolic hypertension is especially common in hypertensives under the age of 30 years.
- E. More than half of the entire population over the age of 60 has hypertension.

9. Which of the following statements regarding the measurement of blood pressure is not correct?

- A. Mercury manometers are more accurate than aneroid manometers.
- B. Blood pressure should be measured after the patient has been seated comfortably for at least 5 minutes.
- C. Falsely low blood pressure readings occur when the cuff is too narrow or when the bladder is too short to encircle the arm.
- D. The blood pressure cuff should be inflated rapidly to 30 mm Hg above the palpated systolic

blood pressure to avoid a falsely low reading caused by an auscultatory gap.
  E. Blood pressure measurements by health care personnel tend to overestimate ambulatory blood pressures.

10. All of the following drugs and chemicals may cause or exacerbate hypertension EXCEPT
  A. Cyclosporine
  B. Licorice
  C. Calcium supplements
  D. Erythropoietin
  E. Nonsteroidal anti-inflammatory drugs

11. All of the following statements about renovascular hypertension are correct EXCEPT
  A. Renovascular hypertension is the most common curable cause of hypertension.
  B. Two thirds of patients with renovascular hypertension have atherosclerotic renal artery stenosis.
  C. Patients with fibromuscular dysplasia are less likely to develop cardiovascular complications than those with atherosclerotic disease.
  D. Percutaneous revascularization can often be performed at the time of diagnostic renal arteriography.
  E. Abdominal bruits are only present in a minority of patients with renovascular hypertension.

12. All of the following statements about severe hypertension are true EXCEPT
  A. In the absence of ongoing target organ damage, patients with severe hypertension do not require immediate blood pressure reduction.
  B. Severely elevated blood pressure is often discovered incidentally without symptoms or specific physical findings.
  C. Aortic dissection may be the presenting manifestation of a hypertensive emergency.
  D. In a hypertensive emergency, blood pressure should be lowered rapidly to normotensive levels.
  E. Patients receiving a continuous intravenous infusion of nipride must be carefully monitored for thiocyanate intoxication.

13. Congenital cardiac defects in which adult survival is expected include all of the following EXCEPT
  A. Bicuspid aortic valve
  B. Ostium secundum atrial septal defect
  C. Ventricular septal defect
  D. Ebstein's anomaly
  E. Tricuspid atresia

14. Patients with a bicuspid aortic valve often present to the physician with one or more of the following EXCEPT
  A. Infective endocarditis
  B. Aortic dissection
  C. Papillary muscle rupture
  D. Aortic stenosis
  E. Aortic insufficiency

15. Coarctation of the aorta may be associated with all of the following EXCEPT
  A. Aneurysm of the circle of Willis
  B. Central cyanosis
  C. Hypertension
  D. Rib notching
  E. Bicuspid aortic valve

16. Cyanosis is a characteristic feature of which of the following congenital anomalies?
  A. Secundum atrial septal defect
  B. Tetralogy of Fallot
  C. Pulmonary valve stenosis
  D. Coarctation of the aorta
  E. Patent ductus arteriosus

17. Medical complications of cyanotic congenital heart disease include all of the following EXCEPT
  A. Hyperuricemia
  B. Severe anemia
  C. Cholelithiasis
  D. Abnormal renal function
  E. Abnormal hemostasis

18. The following statements are true about cardiac tamponade EXCEPT
  A. Right heart catheterization characteristically reveals equalization of diastolic pressures.
  B. Tamponade occurs only when the effusion is large.
  C. Oliguria is often present.
  D. The jugular venous pulse manifests a prominent x descent.
  E. Pulsus paradoxus may be difficult to detect in hypotensive patients.

19. Features of constrictive pericarditis include all of the following EXCEPT
  A. Massive ascites may suggest end-stage liver disease.
  B. Hepatomegaly is due to passive congestion.
  C. Early diastolic ventricular filling is rapid.
  D. The y descent of the jugular venous pulse is diminished.
  E. Pericardial calcification may be visible on chest radiograph.

20. Which physical finding is NOT characteristic of dilated cardiomyopathy?
  A. S_3 gallop
  B. Pulmonary rales
  C. Diffuse, medially displaced left ventricular impulse
  D. Mitral regurgitation
  E. S_4 gallop

21. Endomyocardial biopsy may provide a definitive diagnosis in all of the following EXCEPT
  A. Amyloidosis
  B. Sarcoidosis
  C. Hypertrophic cardiomyopathy
  D. Hemochromatosis
  E. Myocarditis

22. Restrictive cardiomyopathy may be due to all of the following EXCEPT

    A. Carnitine deficiency
    B. Thiamine deficiency
    C. Glycogen storage disease
    D. Iron overload
    E. Amyloidosis

23. Carcinoid heart disease is commonly characterized by all of the following EXCEPT

    A. Median survival <2 years
    B. Aortic valve fibrosis with severe aortic regurgitation
    C. Tricuspid stenosis
    D. Symptoms of right heart failure
    E. Pulmonic valve stenosis or regurgitation

24. Raynaud's phenomenon has been associated with all of the following EXCEPT

    A. Vasospastic angina pectoris
    B. Scleroderma
    C. Occupational trauma in pianists
    D. Cryoglobulinemia
    E. Hyperthyroidism

25. Features of acrocyanosis include all of the following EXCEPT

    A. Female preponderance
    B. Arteriolar constriction and dilation of veins in the affected areas
    C. Hands are most often affected and are blue, cold to touch, and clammy
    D. Ulcerations and severe pain are common
    E. Acrocyanosis is more common among patients with psychiatric disorders

26. Features of thromboangiitis obliterans include all of the following EXCEPT

    A. Patients may develop ischemic bowel because of involvement of the visceral arteries.
    B. The disease occurs predominantly in men between the ages of 20 and 40 years.
    C. The disease affects predominantly large arteries of the lower extremities.
    D. Thromboangiitis obliterans is associated with superficial thrombophlebitis and Raynaud's phenomenon.
    E. Patients may complain of intermittent shocklike pain caused by ischemic neuropathy.

27. Which of the following abnormalities is NOT associated with an increased risk of venous thrombosis?

    A. Antithrombin III deficiency
    B. Protein S deficiency
    C. Protein C deficiency
    D. Alpha$_2$-antiplasmin deficiency
    E. Deficiency of heparin cofactor II

28. All of the following statements about the prophylaxis and treatment of venous thrombosis are correct EXCEPT

    A. Anticoagulation is not necessary in superficial thrombophlebitis.
    B. Low-dose heparin is the prophylactic treatment of choice in patients undergoing hip surgery.
    C. Monitoring of the activated partial thromboplastin time (aPTT) is not necessary during treatment with low-molecular-weight heparin fragments.
    D. Insertion of an inferior vena cava filter should be considered in patients with septic thromboembolic disease not controlled by antibiotics.
    E. Patients with iliofemoral thrombosis may benefit from thrombolytic therapy.

29. Which vessels are LEAST likely to develop atherosclerotic lesions?

    A. Abdominal aorta
    B. Intramural coronary arteries
    C. Carotid artery
    D. Superficial femoral artery
    E. Thoracic aorta

30. Characteristic physical findings in hypertrophic cardiomyopathy include all of the following EXCEPT

    A. Bisferiens carotid pulse
    B. Triple left ventricular impulse
    C. Mitral regurgitation
    D. Delayed carotid upstroke
    E. Systolic ejection murmur accentuated by Valsalva maneuver

31. All of the following statements are true regarding Doppler echocardiography EXCEPT

    A. Microbubbles in solution can be safely injected into the venous system to detect right-to-left intracardiac shunts.
    B. Microbubbles in solution can be safely injected into the coronary arteries to visualize coronary perfusion.
    C. It can be used to accurately calculate mitral and aortic valve areas.
    D. When tricuspid regurgitation is detected, it generally represents a pathologic finding.

32. Regarding the electrocardiogram (ECG), all of the following statements are true EXCEPT

    A. The normal QRS axis lies between 0 and +110 degrees.
    B. The normal P wave axis usually points in the same general direction as the normal QRS axis.
    C. The routine recording speed (paper speed) is 25 mm per second.
    D. At standard calibration, a 1-mV signal produces a 10-mm deflection on the ECG paper.
    E. With advancing age, the mean frontal plane QRS axis shifts rightward.

33. Regarding gated equilibrium radionuclide blood pool studies (MUGA scans), all of the following statements are correct EXCEPT

    A. ^{99m}Tc is bound to the patient's own erythrocytes.
    B. Data storage is gated to the cardiac cycle.
    C. Data are summed over several hundred cardiac cycles.

D. Global, but not regional, ventricular function can be assessed.

E. The rate of ventricular filling can be assessed, providing an index of diastolic function.

34. All of the following statements about radionuclide myocardial perfusion imaging are true EXCEPT

A. The myocardial distribution of thallium-201 is similar to that of potassium.

B. ^{99m}Tc sestamibi enters the myocardium according to the vascular distribution.

C. It is of the greatest diagnostic value in patients with low likelihood of coronary disease who have a normal resting ECG.

D. Thallium-201 is preferred to ^{99m}Tc sestamibi for assessing myocardial viability.

E. It requires heterogeneous myocardial blood flow to detect ischemia.

35. All of the following statements are true regarding cardiac catheterization EXCEPT

A. The incidence of death in patients with coronary artery disease is around 0.10%.

B. The incidence of MI is in the range of 0.05%.

C. The contrast agents used in cardiac angiography are negative inotropes.

D. The most accurate method to measure cardiac output in patients with low flow states is the Fick method.

E. In the United States, valvular heart disease is the most common diagnosis in patients undergoing cardiac catheterization.

36. Regarding heart failure, all of the following are independent predictors of survival EXCEPT

A. Left ventricular ejection fraction (LVEF)

B. Severity of mitral incompetence

C. New York Heart Association functional class

D. Occurrence of arrhythmias

E. Peak oxygen consumption

37. All of the following are causes of diastolic dysfunction EXCEPT

A. Paget's disease of bone

B. Hypertension

C. Hypertrophic cardiomyopathy

D. Myocardial ischemia

E. Infiltrative cardiomyopathy

38. Which of the following drugs has been demonstrated to improve symptoms and increase LVEF in patients with left ventricular systolic dysfunction?

A. Verapamil

B. Diltiazem

C. Nifedipine

D. Metoprolol

E. Disopyramide

39. Regarding the management of patients with heart failure resulting from diastolic dysfunction, all of the following statements are true EXCEPT

A. AV synchrony is particularly important.

B. Vigorous diuresis is critical to reduce left ventricular end-diastolic pressure (LVEDP).

C. Beta blockers are a good choice to lower heart rate and treat ischemia.

D. Heart rate–lowering calcium channel blockers may be helpful.

E. Sublingual nitroglycerin may be used to acutely treat ischemia and lower LVEDP.

40. Clinical signs of primary pulmonary hypertension include all of the following EXCEPT

A. Increased loudness of the pulmonic component of the second heart sound

B. Jugular venous distention

C. Right ventricular hypertrophy on ECG

D. Increased right heart border with prominent pulmonary venous pattern on chest radiograph

E. Ascites

41. All of the following statements are true regarding primary pulmonary hypertension EXCEPT

A. The etiology is unknown.

B. Most patients are responsive to pulmonary vasodilators.

C. It is more prevalent in woman.

D. Lung or heart-lung transplant is the only cure.

E. Chronic anticoagulation is advisable.

42. All of the following statements are true regarding myocardial ischemia EXCEPT

A. Ischemia typically begins in the subendocardium and spreads toward the epicardium.

B. As the ventricle becomes ischemic, systolic dysfunction occurs first, followed by diastolic dysfunction.

C. Variant (Prinzmetal's) angina is thought to be due coronary artery spasm.

D. Fifty per cent of patients presenting with unstable angina have multivessel coronary disease.

E. Twenty per cent of patients presenting with unstable angina progress to infarction unless treated.

43. All of the following are indicated in the initial management of unstable angina EXCEPT

A. Nifedipine

B. Intravenous heparin

C. Aspirin

D. Nitrates

E. Metoprolol

44. Which of the following beta blockers demonstrates intrinsic sympathomimetic activity?

A. Atenolol

B. Metoprolol

C. Nadolol

D. Propranolol

E. Acebutolol

45. Which of the following beta blockers are noncardio-selective (not beta$_1$ selective)?

A. Atenolol

B. Metoprolol

C. Betaxolol
D. Propranolol
E. Acebutolol

46. All of the following statements are true regarding peri-infarction arrhythmias EXCEPT

A. Bradyarrhythmias should be treated with atropine and temporary ventricular pacing if necessary.
B. Prophylactic lidocaine is not indicated.
C. Defibrillation is more successful if preceded by 1 to 2 minutes of chest compressions (cardiopulmonary resuscitation).
D. High-grade ventricular ectopy should be treated with lidocaine.
E. Recurrent Mobitz II block requires permanent pacing.

47. All of the following are consistent with the diagnosis of aortic stenosis EXCEPT

A. Delayed arterial pulse wave
B. Aortic thrill
C. Diamond-shaped systolic murmur
D. Syncope
E. Wide pulse pressure

48. All of the following are consistent with the diagnosis of mitral stenosis EXCEPT

A. Loud P_2
B. Opening snap
C. Diastolic rumble
D. Left ventricular strain pattern on ECG
E. Dyspnea

49. All of the following statements are true of aortic stenosis EXCEPT

A. Bicuspid valve is an uncommon etiology.
B. Chest pain, syncope, and heart failure are the typical symptoms.
C. Heart failure in aortic stenosis portends a poor prognosis.
D. Intestinal angiodysplasia has been associated with aortic stenosis.
E. Calcified aortic valves may destroy red cells and cause hemolytic anemia.

50. Antibiotic prophylaxis is recommended prior to dental, genitourinary, or gastrointestinal procedures in patients with the following valve lesions EXCEPT

A. Aortic stenosis
B. Aortic regurgitation
C. Mitral valve prolapse without regurgitation
D. Mitral regurgitation
E. Mitral stenosis

51. All of the following physical findings are consistent with the diagnosis of aortic insufficiency EXCEPT

A. Wide pulse pressure
B. Capillary pulsations in the nail beds
C. Delayed carotid upstroke
D. Austin Flint murmur
E. Head bobbing

52. All of the following are causes of aortic aneurysm EXCEPT

A. Atherosclerosis
B. Trauma
C. Takayasu's arteritis
D. Polyarteritis nodosa
E. Temporal arteritis

53. All of the following can be used to reliably exclude the diagnosis of aortic dissection EXCEPT

A. Aortography
B. Computed tomography scan
C. Magnetic resonance imaging (MRI) scan
D. Transesophageal echocardiography
E. Transthoracic echocardiography

54. All of the following statements are true regarding the treatment of aortic dissection EXCEPT

A. Nipride is used to lower blood pressure.
B. Beta blockers are begun to decrease *dp/dt*.
C. If the dissection involves a coronary artery, heparin is begun to limit clot propagation.
D. Types I and II dissections are treated surgically.
E. Type III dissections are managed medically.

55. All of the following significantly elevate cyclosporin levels EXCEPT

A. Phenobarbital
B. Diltiazem
C. Erythromycin
D. Ketoconazole
E. Fluconazole

56. The denervated, transplanted heart's response to common medications may be more or less than that normally seen. Regarding the postcardiac transplant patient, all of the following statements are true EXCEPT

A. Atropine has little effect on heart rate.
B. Ocular beta blockers profoundly lower heart rate.
C. To treat supraventricular tachycardias, adenosine doses should be doubled.
D. Isoproterenol can be used as an intravenous drip to treat bradycardia.
E. Atropine is used to treat vasovagal syncope.

DIRECTIONS: For questions 57 to 116, decide whether EACH statement is true or false. Any combination of answers, from all true to all false, may occur.

57. Which of the following statements correctly describe(s) cardiovascular disease epidemiology?

   A. Coronary heart disease incidence and mortality have declined dramatically in men and women in the United States since 1963.
   B. Mortality from coronary heart disease is increasing in several Eastern European countries.
   C. Women develop coronary heart disease 10 to 20 years later than their male counterparts with similar risk factor levels.
   D. Smoking cessation results in a rapid decline in the risk of developing lung cancer while coronary heart disease risk remains markedly elevated for many years.
   E. In all Western societies, women have lower HDL cholesterol levels than men.

58. Which of the following statements correctly characterize(s) major determinants of cardiac performance?

   A. Stroke volume increases with increasing afterload.
   B. Ventricular preload describes the load against which the ventricle must contract when it ejects blood.
   C. In normal hearts, ventricular inotropic state increases with increasing heart rate as a result of changes in Ca^{2+} availability.
   D. Hypoxia, ischemia, and acidosis decrease cardiac contractility.
   E. In failing hearts, right atrial pressure as assessed from the jugular venous pulse is a good indicator of left ventricular filling pressure.

59. Which of the following statements correctly describe(s) regulation of coronary blood flow?

   A. Increases in myocardial oxygen demand are chiefly met by increases in myocardial blood flow rather than enhanced myocardial oxygen extraction.
   B. Adenosine is a potent coronary vasodilator.
   C. Endothelium-dependent relaxing factor is an important endogenous regulator of coronary blood flow.
   D. Coronary perfusion pressure is an important determinant of coronary blood flow in individuals with normal hearts but not in patients with coronary stenoses.
   E. Alpha-adrenergic stimulation may cause coronary vasoconstriction.

60. Which of the following statements correctly describe(s) regulation of the peripheral circulation?

   A. Stimulation of carotid baroreceptors results in vagally mediated slowing of the heart rate.
   B. Marked stimulation of stretch receptors in the atria produces a depressor reflex that can result in syncope.
   C. Atrial natriuretic peptide is an endogenous vasodilator and causes renal sodium loss.
   D. Angiotensin II is a potent vasoconstrictor and inhibits aldosterone secretion.
   E. Venous return to the right heart decreases with inspiration.

61. Which of the following statements correctly describe(s) the mechanisms of drug-induced arrhythmias?

   A. Ventricular tachycardia mediated by digitalis is believed to be triggered by delayed after-depolarizations.
   B. Quinidine-induced torsades de pointes is believed to be triggered by early after-depolarizations.
   C. Verapamil slows AV conduction and can cause complete AV block.
   D. AV block caused by adenosine is vagally mediated and can be blocked by atropine.
   E. Hyperkalemia caused by amiloride enhances sinus node automaticity and causes sinus tachycardia.

62. Which of the following statements is/are true about digitalis?

   A. Side effects to digoxin may occur when digitalis serum levels are in the therapeutic range (1 to 2 ng per milliliter).
   B. Patients with pulmonary disease and cor pulmonale are at increased risk of digitalis toxicity.
   C. Verapamil, quinidine, amiodarone, and propafenone increase serum digoxin levels.
   D. Digitalis toxicity manifested as AV block is best treated with the infusion of potassium.
   E. Cholestyramine may decrease digoxin serum levels.

63. Which of the following conditions is/are definitive indications for pacemaker implantation?

   A. Complete heart block with a rate <40 beats per minute
   B. Mobitz I AV block with a heart rate of 44 per minute in a marathon runner
   C. Bifascicular block with intermittent symptomatic type II second-degree AV block
   D. Atrial fibrillation with a rate <40 beats per minute in the absence of drugs that impair AV conduction
   E. Complete heart block in a patient with inferior wall MI that resolves after 48 hours

64. Which of the following is/are predictors of thromboembolism in patients with atrial fibrillation?

   A. Previous thromboembolism
   B. History of hypertension
   C. Global left ventricular dysfunction
   D. Mitral stenosis
   E. Age <40 years

65. A 55-year-old woman presents with atrial fibrillation 3 years after a MI. She reports palpitations off and on for several months. She has a blood pressure of 134/78 mm Hg, a ventricular response of 146 beats per minute, and no evidence of congestive heart failure or valvular disease on exam. Appropriate initial therapy may include

    A. Immediate electrical cardioversion
    B. Intravenous quinidine
    C. Beta blocker
    D. Coumadin
    E. Digoxin

66. Which of the following statements correctly characterize(s) sudden cardiac death?

    A. The majority of autopsies in victims of sudden death reveal significant coronary artery disease.
    B. Sudden death occurs most commonly in the early morning hours.
    C. Resuscitation from sudden death is most likely when the presenting rhythm is a bradyarrhythmia.
    D. Excess alcohol consumption is a risk factor for sudden death.
    E. Social isolation predisposes to sudden death.

67. The acquired long QT syndrome can be due to

    A. Phenothiazines
    B. Terfenadine
    C. Hypokalemia
    D. Quinidine
    E. Erythromycin

68. Lifestyle changes that may reduce blood pressure and minimize the need for pharmacologic agents include

    A. Weight loss
    B. Reduction in alcohol consumption
    C. Aerobic exercise
    D. Supplementary dietary potassium
    E. Sodium restriction

69. Pregnancy in patients with congenital heart disease warrants special considerations, including which of the following?

    A. Cesarean section is the preferred mode of delivery.
    B. Early ambulation and use of elastic stockings are essential measures to minimize the risk of postpartum thromboembolism.
    C. Oxygen administration may predispose to epistaxis.
    D. The incidence of congenital heart disease in children born to mothers with congenital heart disease is significantly higher than in the general population.
    E. Patients with a secundum atrial septal defect should receive endocarditis prophylaxis.

70. Noncardiac surgery in patients with congenital heart disease warrants special considerations, including which of the following?

    A. Patients with congenital complete heart block may require temporary pacing.
    B. Patients with cyanotic congenital heart disease are at increased risk of paradoxical embolism from peripheral venous lines.
    C. Systemic hypotension increases the right-to-left shunt in cyanotic congenital heart disease.
    D. Bleeding risk is increased in cyanotic congenital heart disease.
    E. Patients with a bicuspid aortic valve are at increased risk of endocarditis.

71. Important causes of pericardial disease include

    A. Radiation
    B. Tuberculosis
    C. Dialysis
    D. MI
    E. Neoplastic disease

72. Characteristic features of chest pain in pericarditis include

    A. Worse with deep inspiration
    B. Better supine, worse when sitting up
    C. Characteristically radiates to the right trapezius ridge
    D. May be sharp or crushing
    E. May be located on the left side of the chest, suggesting pleurisy

73. Characteristic ECG findings in pericarditis (with or without associated pericardial effusion) include which of the following?

    A. The ECG may be normal.
    B. ST segment elevation and T wave inversion occur simultaneously.
    C. Depression of the PR segment is more common than ST segment elevation.
    D. The patient may present with new-onset atrial fibrillation.
    E. Electrical alternans may be present.

74. The systolic murmur of hypertrophic obstructive cardiomyopathy is accentuated by

    A. Administration of amyl nitrite
    B. Standing after squatting
    C. Handgrip
    D. Valsalva maneuver
    E. Rapid volume infusion

75. Which of the following statements about myocarditis is/are true?

    A. About 50% of patients with acute viral myocarditis experience spontaneous symptomatic improvement.
    B. Immunosuppressive therapy in acute viral myocarditis decreases mortality and improves left ventricular function.
    C. Echocardiographic abnormalities may be seen in up to 40% of patients infected with the human immunodeficiency virus.
    D. Lymphocytic myocardial infiltration is commonly observed in peripartum cardiomyopathy.
    E. Histologically, lymphocytic myocarditis is only rarely seen in cardiac transplant rejection.

76. Which of the following statements about dilated cardiomyopathies is/are true?

 A. Chagas' disease is caused by *Toxoplasma* and is a common cause of cardiomyopathy in South and Central America.
 B. Giant cell myocarditis is an unusual form of myocarditis that may be associated with pernicious anemia.
 C. Alcohol and acetaldehyde are direct myocardial toxins.
 D. Over half the pediatric patients who have received high doses of Adriamycin have evidence of impaired cardiac function 10 years later.
 E. Beriberi heart disease presents initially with profound depression in cardiac output.

77. Which of the following statements correctly characterize(s) hypertrophic cardiomyopathy?

 A. The disease is genetically transmitted as an autosomal recessive trait.
 B. Anginal-type chest pain may occur in the absence of epicardial coronary stenoses.
 C. Vasodilators are the antihypertensives of choice in obstructive hypertrophic cardiomyopathy because of their beneficial afterload reduction.
 D. Risk of sudden death is highest in young men with a family history of sudden death.
 E. Dual-chamber pacing may diminish the systolic gradient across the left ventricular outflow tract.

78. Which of the following statements correctly characterize(s) cardiac myxomas?

 A. Cardiac myxomas are usually located in the right atrium attached to the interventricular septum.
 B. Fever, malaise, and arthralgias may be presenting symptoms of myxoma.
 C. Left atrial myxoma may simulate mitral stenosis clinically and on physical exam.
 D. Myxomas may recur after surgical resection.
 E. Cardiac catheterization with pulmonary angiography is the diagnostic procedure of choice to image left atrial myxomas.

79. Drugs that are useful in the treatment of Raynaud's phenomenon include

 A. Ergotamine
 B. Calcium antagonists
 C. Beta blockers
 D. Reserpine
 E. Angiotensin-converting enzyme (ACE) inhibitors

80. Which of the following statements correctly characterize(s) arteriosclerosis obliterans?

 A. Women are more often affected than men.
 B. The superficial femoral artery is most commonly affected.
 C. Leriche's syndrome refers to isolated aortoiliac disease.

 D. Pentoxifylline increases walking distance by improving red cell deformability and reducing blood viscosity.
 E. Vasodilators improve perfusion in patients with ischemic pain at rest.

81. Which of the following statements correctly characterize(s) thrombophlebitis?

 A. Thrombi in veins consist mostly of platelets held together by fibrin.
 B. Thrombosis and inflammation of the venous wall generally coexist.
 C. Superficial thrombophlebitis is frequent after pregnancy.
 D. The three main factors leading to thrombosis are venous stasis, injury to the venous wall, and hypercoagulability.
 E. Deep venous thrombosis has a 3 : 1 male predominance.

82. Which of the following entities should be considered in the differential diagnosis of deep venous thrombosis?

 A. Ruptured Baker's cyst
 B. Ruptured calf muscle
 C. Lumbar disc pain
 D. Lymphedema
 E. Severe muscle cramp

83. Which of the following statements correctly describe(s) the pathology of atherosclerotic lesions?

 A. Fatty streaks contain foam cells and T lymphocytes (CD8- and CD4-positive cells).
 B. Fatty streaks may be present at birth.
 C. Rupture of an atherosclerotic plaque with superimposed thrombosis may cause sudden death.
 D. Foam cells derive from fibroblasts that migrate into the plaque from the adventitia and subsequently accumulate lipid.
 E. Areas of low shear stress at arterial bifurcations are common sites for atherosclerotic lesions.

84. Factors that predispose to atherosclerosis include

 A. Hypertension
 B. Cigarette smoking
 C. Diabetes mellitus
 D. Dysfunctional low-density lipoprotein (LDL) receptors
 E. A low LDL/HDL cholesterol ratio

85. The "response to injury" hypothesis of atherosclerosis is correctly described by which of the following statements?

 A. Endothelial injury may occur in the absence of morphologic changes in the endothelium.
 B. Early in atherosclerosis development, molecules are expressed at the endothelial cell surface that promote adherence of monocytes and lymphocytes.
 C. Growth factors that are important in atherogenesis include platelet-derived growth factor and tumor necrosis factor alpha.

D. Transforming growth factor beta induces the formation of connective tissue in atherosclerotic plaques.

E. Endothelial disruption exposes the underlying collagen matrix and serves as a nidus for platelet aggregation and mural thrombosis.

86. Angiographic regression studies in humans have shown that

A. Aggressive lipid-lowering therapy slows the progression of coronary atherosclerosis and may lead to plaque regression.

B. Lipid-lowering therapy may decrease the lipid content of plaques and diminish the risk of plaque rupture.

C. Angiographic regression can be achieved with lifestyle modifications.

D. Although significant angiographic benefit has been seen in most regression trials, reduction in clinical events has been disappointing.

E. Women do not seem to benefit from aggressive lipid-lowering therapy.

87. Regarding a frontal chest radiograph

A. The right heart border is formed by the superior vena cava and the right ventricle.

B. A portion of the inferior vena cava may be seen.

C. The uppermost bulge of the left border represents the aortic knob.

D. The frontal chest radiograph is highly sensitive at detecting chamber hypertrophy.

E. The heart appears larger on expiratory films.

88. The LVEF

A. Is the single best indicator of global left ventricular performance

B. Is the single best prognostic indicator in patients with ischemic heart disease

C. Increases with exercise in normal subjects

D. Usually equals the right ventricular ejection fraction in patients with ischemic heart disease

E. Should be assessed in all patients with congestive heart failure to differentiate systolic from diastolic dysfunction

89. Which of the following is/are established indications for MRI?

A. Diagnosis of thoracic aortic disease

B. Diagnosis of pericardial thickening resulting in constrictive pericardial disease

C. Evaluation of complex congenital heart disease

D. Evaluation for pericardiac mass

E. Noninvasive angiography of the intracranial carotid arteries

90. Which of the following is/are contraindications to MRI?

A. Sternal wires

B. Cardiac pacemakers and defibrillators

C. Cerebral aneurysm clips

D. Magnetically activated implants or foreign bodies

E. Mechanical ventilation

91. Regarding heart failure

A. Heart failure is the most common diagnosis-related group for patients age 65 or older in the United States.

B. Among patients with advanced heart disease, the 1-year mortality rate is 50%.

C. Antiarrhythmic drug therapy has been demonstrated to decrease mortality in patients with heart failure and arrhythmias.

D. LVEF is the single best prognosticator.

E. Of the patients who die of heart failure, 40 to 50% die suddenly.

92. Pertaining to valvular disease as an etiology of heart failure

A. Aortic insufficiency results in volume overload.

B. Aortic stenosis results in pressure overload.

C. Mitral insufficiency results in volume overload.

D. Pressure overload is better tolerated than volume overload.

E. Overloads that develop slowly are better tolerated than those that develop rapidly.

93. The principal determinants of cardiac output is/are

A. Heart rate

B. Preload

C. Afterload

D. Ejection fraction

E. Contractility

94. Regarding the clinical manifestations of heart failure

A. Impaired exercise tolerance is always present.

B. Orthopnea is due to an increase in pulmonary pressure caused by an increase in venous return from the lower extremities when the patient is supine.

C. Cheyne-Stokes respirations are common in advanced heart failure.

D. Pulsus alternans signifies severe ventricular dysfunction.

E. Clear lung fields generally exclude significant volume overload.

95. Regarding the management of patients with heart failure resulting from systolic ventricular dysfunction

A. Diuretics, vasodilators, and digoxin are the mainstays of pharmacologic therapy.

B. ACE inhibitors are the vasodilating drug of choice.

C. ACE inhibitor therapy should not be initiated until the patient with impaired systolic function is symptomatic.

D. Digoxin has been proven to decrease mortality.

E. In patients intolerant of ACE inhibitors, the combination of hydralazine and isosorbide may be beneficial.

96. Regarding angina pectoris

A. The most common etiology is coronary atherosclerosis.

B. Patients with aortic stenosis may develop angina despite angiographically normal coronary arteries.

C. The primary determinants of myocardial oxygen demand are heart rate, contractility, and blood pressure.

D. Even at rest, myocardial oxygen extraction is near maximal.

E. Coronary artery vasodilation is regulated by the vascular endothelium.

97. Which of the following statements regarding angina pectoris is/are true?

A. A normal baseline ECG effectively rules out angina as the diagnosis.

B. A normal cardiovascular exam rules out angina as the diagnosis.

C. The history is frequently the most powerful tool in making the diagnosis of angina pectoris.

D. ST segment changes occurring without pain are rare and less ominous.

E. A mitral regurgitation murmur may be heard.

98. Which of the following should be considered in the differential diagnosis of angina pectoris?

A. Gastroesophageal reflux
B. Chest wall pain
C. Peptic ulcer disease
D. Pulmonary embolism
E. Herpes zoster

99. Which of the following statements is/are true regarding the graded exercise test?

A. Horizontal or downsloping ST segment depression, ≥ 0.1 mV measured at 0.08 seconds after the J point, is considered positive.

B. The sensitivity and specificity of the test for detecting ischemia are in the 60% range.

C. False-positive tests are more likely in patients with a low probability of having ischemia.

D. False-negative tests are more likely in patients with a high probability of having ischemia.

E. The risk of death during a graded exercise test is about $1:10,000$.

100. Coronary artery bypass surgery has been demonstrated to reduce mortality in patients with

A. Left main stenosis of >50%
B. Three-vessel disease and impaired left ventricular systolic function
C. Multivessel disease with involvement of the proximal left anterior descending artery
D. Severe three-vessel disease
E. Severe impairment of systolic function with nonobstructive coronary disease

101. Which of the following statements is/are true regarding nitrates?

A. They are converted in the vasculature to nitric oxide.

B. They predominately relieve ischemia by increasing coronary blood flow.

C. Their effect at low doses is predominately on arterial beds.

D. They antagonize platelet activation.

E. Their use requires a nitrate-free interval to avoid tolerance in most patients.

102. Which of the following statements regarding cardiovascular disease is/are true?

A. Cardiovascular disease is the number one killer in America.

B. One-half million Americans die of acute MI annually.

C. Most deaths from MI occur after arrival at the hospital.

D. Most deaths from MI are sudden.

E. Age-adjusted rates of death from MI have declined in America since 1950.

103. Which of the following are recognized risk factors for ischemic heart disease?

A. Hypercholesterolemia
B. Isolated low HDL cholesterol level
C. Diabetes mellitus
D. Truncal obesity
E. Elevated plasma homocysteine level

104. Which of the following statements is/are true regarding right ventricular infarction?

A. It is generally seen in the setting of inferior wall infarction.

B. Elevated jugular venous pressure is seen on examination.

C. AV sequential pacing may improve cardiac output.

D. Dobutamine may improve hemodynamics.

E. Treatment includes volume loading and high-dose nitrates.

105. Which of the following statements regarding the diagnosis of MI is/are true?

A. A normal resting ECG excludes acute MI.

B. Creatine kinase, MB band (CK-MB) level is usually elevated in the plasma within 2 hours of symptom onset.

C. CK-MB plasma levels generally peak by 24 hours.

D. Elevated levels of lactate dehydrogenase (LDH)-1 typically persist in the plasma for 1 week.

E. Infarct-avid imaging (^{99m}Tc pyrophosphate) can aid in the diagnosis 24 to 72 hours postinfarction.

106. Which of the following statements regarding acute MI is/are true?

A. Approximately 65% of the deaths occur in the first hour.

B. Most death are due to ventricular fibrillation.

C. Coronary thrombolysis is the primary therapy unless contraindicated.

D. The incidence of stroke is increased with the thrombolytic therapy.

E. Primary angioplasty is an acceptable form of reperfusion therapy.

107. Which of the following statements is/are true regarding coronary artery bypass surgery?

A. Artificial conduits are replacing autografts.

B. The left internal mammary (thoracic) artery is the conduit of choice.

C. The long-term patency rate of the left internal mammary artery is superior to that of vein grafts.

D. The right gastroepiploic artery can be used as a conduit.

E. The radial artery has been successfully used as a conduit.

108. Which of the following statements regarding coronary artery bypass grafting is/are true?

A. Complete revascularization yields a better long-term outcome.

B. The operative mortality rate in patients <60 years of age with good ventricular function is 6 to 8%.

C. The operative mortality is increased in patients over age 70, in women, and in acute ischemia.

D. The incidence of perioperative infarction is 2 to 5%.

E. The incidence of perioperative stroke is 8 to 10%.

109. Which of the following statements regarding antibiotic prophylaxis is/are true?

A. The standard regimen for dental procedures consists of oral amoxicillin regardless of the valvular lesion.

B. The standard regimen for genitourinary and gastrointestinal procedures consists of intravenous or intramuscular ampicillin and gentamicin, followed by oral amoxicillin, regardless of valvular lesion.

C. Patients with permanent pacemakers should receive antibiotic prophylaxis.

D. Patients with a history of rheumatic fever without valvular lesions should receive prophylaxis.

E. Patients with valvular heart disease undergoing cardiac catheterization should receive antibiotic prophylaxis.

110. Which of the following statements pertaining to mitral stenosis is/are true?

A. Rheumatic fever is the primary etiology.

B. Longstanding mitral stenosis leads to right ventricular fibrosis.

C. Tachycardia is important to maintain cardiac output.

D. Dyspnea is the predominant symptom.

E. If atrial fibrillation develops, anticoagulants (except aspirin) should be avoided because of the increased risk of pulmonary hemorrhage.

111. Which of the following statements regarding mitral valve prolapse is/are true?

A. Five per cent of the population are afflicted.

B. There is a female preponderance.

C. Chest pain and palpitations are common.

D. Palpitations should be treated with type IA anti-arrhythmics.

E. Ruptured chordae results in acute pulmonary edema.

112. Which of the following statements regarding aortic aneurysms is/are true?

A. The abdominal aorta is the most common location.

B. Regurgitation of the aortic valve is a common finding.

C. Thoracic aneurysms are frequently complicated by thrombosis and embolism.

D. Abdominal aneurysms >5 cm in diameter should be referred for surgery.

E. The most common symptom of aneurysm is pain.

113. Which of the following statements regarding aortic dissection is/are true?

A. Type I dissections originate in the ascending aorta and involve the arch and descending aorta.

B. Type II dissections involve the ascending aorta only.

C. Type III dissections originate in the descending aorta.

D. The most common cause of aortic dissection is Marfan's syndrome.

E. The most common symptom of aortic dissection is pain.

114. Which of the following statements regarding the signs and symptoms of thoracic aortic dissection is/are true?

A. The pain may be primarily located in the anterior chest.

B. Each heartbeat may accentuate the pain.

C. Horner's syndrome may be seen on presentation.

D. MI may be the presenting finding.

E. Stroke may be the presenting finding.

115. Which of the following statements regarding cardiac transplant is/are true?

A. In the United States, the most common indication for transplant is ischemic heart disease, followed by idiopathic cardiomyopathy.

B. Presently, only 10 to 20% of potential donor hearts are harvested.

C. Up to 30% of patients die on the ''waiting list'' before they can get a heart.

D. Routine chronic immunosuppression consists of prednisone, azathioprine, and cyclosporin.

E. Hypertension is an uncommon side effect of cyclosporin.

116. Which of the following symptoms are consistent with rejection of a transplanted heart?

A. Malaise

B. Fatigue, lethargy

C. Low-grade fever

D. Supraventricular arrhythmia

E. Abdominal pain

DIRECTIONS: Questions 117 to 200 are matching questions. For each numbered item, choose the most likely associated lettered item from those provided. Each numbered item has ONLY ONE answer. Within each set of questions, each answer may be used once, more than once, or not at all.

QUESTIONS 117–120

Select from the list below the cardiac events that correspond most closely to the components of the jugular venous waveform.

A. Opening of the tricuspid valve and right ventricular relaxation
B. Right atrial relaxation
C. Pulmonic valve opening
D. Right atrial contraction
E. Passive right atrial filling with a competent tricuspid valve

117. *X* descent

118. *V* wave

119. *A* wave

120. *Y* descent

QUESTIONS 121–124

For each of the following adverse drug effects, select the most likely causative agent.

A. Amiodarone
B. Propranolol
C. Digoxin
D. Lidocaine
E. Procainamide

121. Convulsions

122. Hyperthyroidism

123. Atrial tachycardia with AV block

124. Arthralgias

QUESTIONS 125–128

For each of the following arrhythmias, select the most appropriate device therapy.

A. Implantable cardioverter-defibrillator
B. Temporary ventricular pacemaker
C. Rate-responsive ventricular pacemaker
D. Dual-chamber demand pacemaker
E. None

125. Asymptomatic sinus bradycardia at 40 beats per minute during sleep

126. Complete heart block in a patient with a VVI pacemaker who complains of fatigue and dizziness and who has retrograde P waves on a 12-lead ECG

127. Ventricular fibrillation remote from a MI in a patient who is noninducible in the electrophysiology laboratory

128. Complete heart block in a patient with a digoxin level of 3.5 ng per milliliter

QUESTIONS 129–132

Match the following antihypertensive agents with their therapeutic efficacy in specific patient subgroups.

A. ACE inhibitors
B. Diuretics
C. Beta blockers
D. Alpha-adrenergic receptor blockers
E. Centrally acting agents

129. Patients who have experienced a MI but have a normal LVEF

130. Patients with impaired LVEF

131. All patient subgroups, but particularly effective in black and the elderly

132. All patient subgroups, but especially useful in hypertensive men with concomitant benign prostatic hypertrophy

QUESTIONS 133–136

For each of the following adverse drug effects, select the most likely causative agent.

A. Pericardial effusion
B. Lupus-like syndrome
C. Coombs-positive hemolytic anemia
D. Dry cough
E. Gynecomastia and sexual dysfunction

133. Spironolactone

134. Minoxidil

135. Hydralazine

136. Methyldopa

QUESTIONS 137–140

Match the following pericardial diseases with their characteristic clinical findings.

A. Constrictive pericarditis
B. Cardiac tamponade
C. Both
D. Neither

137. Pericardial knock

138. Pulsus paradoxus

139. Kussmaul's sign

140. Decreased jugular venous pressure

QUESTIONS 141–144

Match the following cardiomyopathies with the clinical features listed below.

A. Dilated cardiomyopathy
B. Restrictive cardiomyopathy
C. Hypertrophic cardiomyopathy

141. May be difficult to distinguish from constrictive pericarditis

142. LVEF is often supranormal

143. Systolic anterior motion of the mitral valve may be seen echocardiographically

144. May be seen in patients with Duchenne's muscular dystrophy

QUESTIONS 145–148

Match the following cardiomyopathies with their characteristic ECG findings.
   A.   Chagas' disease
   B.   Hemochromatosis
   C.   Amyloidosis
   D.   Sarcoidosis
   E.   Hypertrophic cardiomyopathy

145. Low voltage

146. Right bundle-branch block

147. Advanced AV block

148. Pseudoinfarction pattern

QUESTIONS 149–152

Match the following cardiac abnormalities with the disorders listed below.
   A.   Floppy mitral valve
   B.   Tricuspid atresia
   C.   Congenital complete heart block
   D.   Ostium primum atrial septal defect
   E.   Patent ductus arteriosus

149. Down's syndrome

150. Marfan's syndrome

151. Maternal systemic lupus erythematosus

152. Congenital rubella

QUESTIONS 153–156

Match the following clinical features with the vascular diseases listed below.
   A.   Associated with idiopathic pulmonary hypertension
   B.   Anterior wall MI
   C.   Associated with Noonan's syndrome
   D.   Ulcers above the medial malleolus
   E.   Cutaneous hypersensitivity to tobacco products

153. Lymphedema

154. Embolic arterial occlusion of the lower extremity

155. Raynaud's phenomenon

156. Postphlebitic syndrome

QUESTIONS 157–160

Match the valve lesion with the appropriate chest radiograph finding.
   A.   Aortic stenosis
   B.   Aortic regurgitation
   C.   Mitral stenosis
   D.   Mitral regurgitation

157. Normal cardiac size, dilation and prominence of the ascending aorta

158. Marked cardiomegaly with pulmonary venous congestion

159. Enlarged left atrium and right ventricle

160. Enlarged left atrium

QUESTIONS 161–164

Match the following ECG intervals with the appropriate description.
   A.   RR interval
   B.   PR interval
   C.   QRS interval
   D.   QT interval

161. When the ventricular rhythm is regular, 60 divided by this interval (in seconds), equals the heart rate per minute

162. Represents the duration of electrical systole

163. Represents the ventricular depolarization time

164. Represents the AV conduction time

QUESTIONS 165–168

Match the following ECG segments or junctions with the appropriate description.
   A.   PR segment
   B.   ST segment
   C.   TP segment
   D.   J junction (point)

165. From the J point to the onset of the T wave

166. From the end of the T wave to the beginning of the next P wave

167. From the end of the P wave to the onset of the next QRS complex

168. Where the QRS complex ends and the ST segment begins

QUESTIONS 169–176

Match the form of heart failure with the most likely etiology. Each form of heart failure may be used more than once.
   A.   Low-output heart failure
   B.   High-output heart failure

169. Arteriosclerosis

170. Valvular disease

171. Hyperthyroid disease

172. Hypothyroid disease

173. Anemia

174. Pericardial disease

175. Beriberi

176. Paget's disease of bone

QUESTIONS 177–180

Match the terms regarding cardiac function with the appropriate description.

   A. Preload
   B. Afterload
   C. Inotropic state
   D. Lusitropic state

177. Refers to ventricular relaxation

178. Stretch of myocardial fibers at end-diastole

179. Resistance that the ventricle must overcome during systole in order to eject blood into the aorta

180. Refers to ventricular contractility

QUESTIONS 181–184

Match the mechanism of pulmonary hypertension to the most likely disease entity.

   A. Increased pulmonary blood flow
   B. Abnormalities in the pulmonary arteries
   C. Abnormalities in the pulmonary arterioles
   D. Abnormalities in the pulmonary veins or venules

181. Sickle cell anemia

182. Congenital heart disease with left-to-right shunt

183. Hypoxia

184. Scleroderma

QUESTIONS 185–192

Coronary atherosclerosis is the underlying disease in 90 to 95% of myocardial infarctions. For the remaining 5 to 10% of cases, match the pathology with the appropriate clinical situation or condition.

   A. Coronary emboli
   B. Thrombotic coronary artery disease
   C. Coronary vasculitis
   D. Coronary vasospasm
   E. Coronary ostial occlusion
   F. Congenital coronary anomalies
   G. Myocardial oxygen demand in excess of supply despite normal perfusion
   H. Trauma

185. Aortic dissection

186. Origin of left coronary artery from the pulmonary artery

187. Cocaine or amphetamine abuse

188. Polyarteritis nodosa

189. Street mugging

190. Prosthetic aortic valve

191. Oral contraceptive use

192. Carbon monoxide poisoning

QUESTIONS 193–196

Match the following adjunctive therapy for the treatment of MI with the appropriate desirable effect.

   A. Diltiazem
   B. ACE inhibitor
   C. Beta blockers
   D. Nitrates

193. Decreases the incidence of recurrent ischemia and infarction following non–Q wave infarction, but increases mortality if heart failure is present

194. Improves acute mortality in patients with pulmonary congestion

195. When used in the first 24 hours, lowers mortality by decreasing ventricular fibrillation and possibly myocardial rupture

196. When begun in the first 24 hours, lowers mortality at least partially by preventing ventricular remodeling

QUESTIONS 197–200

Match the following physical or laboratory finding with the appropriate valve lesion.

   A. Aortic stenosis
   B. Aortic regurgitation
   C. Mitral stenosis
   D. Mitral regurgitation

197. Harsh murmur transmitted to the carotids

198. Loud S_1

199. Apical holosystolic murmur with radiation to the axilla

200. Marfanoid body habitus

ANSWERS

1.(C) *Discussion:* Diabetes, hypertension, and cigarette smoking are strong independent risk factors for coronary heart disease. High HDL cholesterol decreases the risk of coronary heart disease. Men and women of short stature have an increased risk of coronary heart disease compared to their taller counterparts. (*Cecil, Ch. 31; Hebert et al*)

2.(D) *Discussion:* Sympathetic stimulation of the heart by sympathetic nerve stimulation or by circulating catecholamines increases heart rate, improves conduction velocity through the AV node, increases force and velocity of ventricular muscle contraction, and enhances ventricular muscle relaxation. Phase IV depolarization in the sinus node is enhanced. (*Cecil, Ch. 32*)

3.(E) *Discussion:* The relationship between heart rate, systolic blood pressure, and myocardial oxygen consumption is essentially linear. The product of heart rate and systolic pressure (rate-pressure product) is used clinically as a simplified index of myocardial oxygen requirement. Myocardial contractility and basal oxygen requirements to sustain cell maintenance processes are additional major determinants of myocardial oxygen consumption. The force of atrial contraction does not significantly influence myocardial oxygen requirements. (*Cecil, Ch. 32*)

4.(C) *Discussion:* The AV node is richly innervated by cholinergic fibers. Chemoreceptors located behind the AV node may be activated during ischemia of the inferior or posterior myocardium and may trigger vagally mediated responses, including nausea, hypotension, bradycardia, diaphoresis, and salivation. (*Cecil, Ch. 35*)

5.(E) *Discussion:* Premature ventricular contractions (PVCs) confer an adverse prognosis in patients with underlying structural heart disease, but treatment of PVCs does not improve prognosis in these patients. Among individuals with normal hearts, PVCs have no prognostic significance. If the patients are asymptomatic, the appropriate therapy in both settings is reassurance. Only very symptomatic PVCs should be treated pharmacologically, preferably with beta blockers unless otherwise contraindicated. (*Cecil, Ch. 35*)

6.(C) *Discussion:* Wide QRS tachycardias should be considered of ventricular origin unless proven otherwise. Intravenous lidocaine or procainamide and cardioversion are appropriate therapies. Carotid sinus massage only rarely converts ventricular tachycardia but is a fairly safe intervention in the absence of severe cerebrovascular disease. Verapamil characteristically causes cardiocirculatory collapse in patients with ventricular tachycardia and is thus contraindicated. In Wolff-Parkinson-White (WPW) syndrome, supraventricular impulses may conduct antegrade across the accessory pathway and cause a wide QRS tachycardia. Lidocaine, procainamide, and carotid sinus massage block conduction across the accessory pathway and may terminate the tachycardia. Atrial fibrillation commonly occurs after an episode of reciprocating tachycardia in WPW patients—verapamil and other agents that block the AV node may thus enhance conduction across the accessory pathway and may precipitate ventricular fibrillation. (*Cecil, Ch. 35*)

7.(A) *Discussion:* Multifocal atrial tachycardia is characterized by at least three different P wave morphologies, variable PP intervals, and ventricular rates above 100 beats per minute. It tends to occur in patients with multisystem and respiratory failure, and treatment should be directed at the underlying disturbances, including hypoxia, acidosis, and excessive catecholamine stimulation. Theophylline therapy may play a role, and serum levels may have to be reduced. Multifocal atrial tachycardia is resistant to digoxin but may respond to verapamil therapy. (*Cecil, Ch. 35*)

8.(E) *Discussion:* Hypertension is more common and more severe among blacks than among whites. Less than 5% of hypertension is due to secondary causes. White coat hypertension is more common among individuals with milder blood pressure elevations. Isolated systolic hypertension increases in prevalence with age. More than half of the entire population over the age of 60 has hypertension. (*Cecil, Ch. 37*)

9.(C) *Discussion:* Accurately measured blood pressures are paramount in the assessment and treatment of hypertension. Anaeroid manometers are less accurate than mercury manometers but are sufficient if frequently standardized against a mercury column. Blood pressure should be measured two or three times after the patient has been seated comfortably for at least 5 minutes, and the readings should be averaged. Falsely high blood pressure readings occur when the blood pressure cuff is too narrow or when the bladder is too short to encircle the arm. The auscultatory gap remains unexplained but can cause a significant underestimation of the true pressure unless systolic pressure is first determined by palpation and the blood pressure cuff is inflated 30 mm Hg above the palpated pressure. Blood pressures measured in the health care setting tend to be higher than ambulatory readings; the latter correlate better with target organ damage. (*Cecil, Ch. 37*)

10.(C) *Discussion:* Epidemiologic studies and some clinical studies suggest an inverse relationship between calcium intake and blood pressure, and calcium supplementation may be beneficial in the treatment of hypertension. Licorice causes a form of mineralocorticoid hypertension. Cyclosporine, erythropoietin, nonsteroidal anti-inflammatory agents, and many other drugs may cause or exacerbate hypertension. A careful diet and medication history is an important part of the evaluation of the hypertensive patient. (*Cecil, Ch. 37*)

11.(E) *Discussion:* High-pitched, systolic-diastolic or continuous abdominal bruits are strongly suggestive of renovascular obstruction and are found in one half to two thirds of patients with surgically proven renovascular hypertension. About one third of patients with renovascular hypertension have fibromuscular disease and two thirds have atherosclerotic disease. Those with atherosclerotic disease tend to be older, have higher systolic blood pressures, and develop more target organ damage than patients with essential hypertension. Patients with fibromuscular dysplasia are younger and less likely to develop cardiovascular complications. In patients with suitable lesions, percutaneous revascularization can often be performed at the time of diagnostic renal arteriography. (*Cecil, Ch. 37*)

12.(D) *Discussion:* Blood pressure lowering in a hypertensive emergency should be prompt but gradual, with a goal blood pressure slightly above normotensive levels. Precipitous blood pressure drops may cause target organ hypoperfusion. Patients receiving a continous intravenous infusion of nipride must be carefully monitored for thiocyanate intoxication. Patients with hypertensive emergencies may present with myocardial ischemia, acute left ventricular decompensation, aortic dissection, intracranial or subarachnoid hemorrhage, or ischemic stroke. However, severely elevated blood pressure is often discovered incidentally without symptoms or specific physical findings. In the absence of ongoing target organ damage, patients with severe hypertension do not require immediate blood pressure reduction with parenteral agents. (*Cecil, Ch. 37*)

13.(E) *Discussion:* A bicuspid aortic valve is the most common congenital anomaly of the heart. Patients generally come to attention because of progressive stenosis or aortic valve incompetence. Ostium secundum atrial septal defect may not be recognized during childhood. Adults may present with atrial arrhythmias, heart failure, or progressive pulmonary hypertension. Patients with ventricular septal defects generally survive to adulthood if the ventricular septal defect closes spontaneously or if a nonrestrictive defect is accompanied by elevated pulmonary vascular resistance, thus protecting the left ventricle from chronic volume overload. Ebstein's anomaly is an uncommon congenital defect. Accessory pathways are often present, and patients may present with tachyarrhythmias (WPW syndrome). Uncorrected tricuspid atresia is generally fatal in childhood, although rare instances of survival into adulthood and middle age have been documented. (*Cecil, Ch. 39*)

14.(C) *Discussion:* Patients with a bicuspid valve may develop progressive aortic stenosis or incompetence. They have an increased risk of endocarditis, and endocarditis prophylaxis is thus mandatory. Associated abnormalities of the aortic root may predispose them to aortic dissection. Papillary muscle rupture is not a feature of this anomaly. (*Cecil, Ch. 39*)

15.(B) *Discussion:* Cyanosis is not a feature of coarctation of the aorta unless coarctation occurs in association with a cyanotic congenital cardiac anomaly. Adults present with hypertension, and characteristic rib notching may be present on the chest radiograph. A bicuspid aortic valve is a common associated anomaly. A coexisting aneurysm of the circle of Willis is less common, but a fatal intracranial bleed may be the presenting manifestation in patients in their second or third decade of life. Patients are also at risk of aortic dissection distal to the coarctation site. (*Cecil, Ch. 39*)

16.(B) *Discussion:* Only tetralogy of Fallot is a cyanotic congenital defect. Patients with ostium secundum defect have a left-to-right shunt and are thus characteristically not cyanotic. Cyanosis may occur very late in the course when severe pulmonary hypertension supervenes and the shunt reverses (Eisenmenger's syndrome). (*Cecil, Ch. 39*)

17.(B) *Discussion:* Patients with cyanotic congenital heart disease have increased red cell mass. High hematocrits may lead to a hyperviscosity syndrome, further worsened by superimposed iron deficiency. Hyperuricemia is believed to be due to increased urate reabsorption resulting from renal hypoperfusion. Renal histology in congenital heart disease is abnormal, and patients are at increased risk of angiographic dye–induced renal failure. The risk of cholelithiasis is increased in cyanotic congenital heart disease (calcium bilirubinate stones). Patients with cyanotic congenital heart disease bruise easily, commonly have gingival bleeding, and may have severe and recurrent epistaxis and hemoptysis. (*Cecil, Ch. 39*)

18.(B) *Discussion:* The hemodynamic significance of a pericardial effusion depends on its rate of accumulation. Even small amounts of fluid that accumulate rapidly can significantly raise intrapericardial pressure and cause pericardial tamponade. Right heart catheterization characteristically reveals equalization of diastolic pressures (right atrial pressure, right ventricular diastolic pressure, pulmonary artery diastolic pressure, and pulmonary wedge pressure). As cardiac output diminishes, renal perfusion decreases, resulting in oliguria. The jugular venous pressure is elevated. The x descent is prominent and occurs simultaneously with the carotid pulse. Pulsus paradoxus is characteristic of pericardial tamponade but may be difficult to detect in hypotensive patients. (*Cecil, Ch. 44*)

19.(D) *Discussion:* Early diastolic ventricular filling is rapid. The y descent of the jugular venous pulse is prominent and coincides with the early diastolic dip of the ventricular pressure tracing. Venous filling pressures are high, resulting in chronic passive hepatic congestion, peripheral edema, and often massive ascites. Pericardial calcification on chest radiograph may be a valuable clue to the underlying diagnosis but is not commonly seen. (*Cecil, Ch. 44*)

20.(C) *Discussion:* The left ventricular impulse is diffuse and displaced laterally. S_3 and S_4 gallops are common. Mitral regurgitation is frequently present but may not always be audible. Basilar pulmonary rales are often present. In some individuals, right-sided manifestations such as right ventricular heave, jugular venous distention, hepatic congestion, and peripheral edema predominate. (*Cecil, Ch. 43*)

21.(C) *Discussion:* Endomyocardial biopsy may provide the definitive diagnosis in all the disorders listed except hypertrophic cardiomyopathy and may be essential in distinguishing restrictive cardiomyopathies from constrictive pericarditis. However, this procedure is limited by sampling error and is associated with significant risks. Because many disorders can be diagnosed by means other than endomyocardial biopsy, this procedure should not be routinely performed in all cardiomyopathy evaluations. (*Cecil, Ch. 43*)

22.(B) *Discussion:* Thiamine deficiency causes high-output cardiac failure (beriberi). Storage diseases such as glycogen storage disease and hemochromatosis, and infiltrative diseases such as amyloidosis, characteristically cause a restrictive cardiomyopathy. Hemochromatosis may also present as a dilated cardiomyopathy. Carnitine deficiency causes a restrictive picture. (*Cecil, Ch. 43*)

23.(B) *Discussion:* Carcinoid heart disease, seen in as many as 50% of patients with metastatic carcinoid, characteristically affects right-sided cardiac structures, with thickening and scarring of the endocardium and of the tricuspid and pulmonic valves, resulting in both stenosis and regurgitation. Symptoms of right heart failure are common, and median survival is <2 years. Involvement of left-sided cardiac structures has been described but is very rare. (*Cecil, Ch. 47*)

24.(E) *Discussion:* Raynaud's phenomenon is associated with a multitude of disorders, including occlusive arterial disease, connective tissue diseases, vascular injury from occupational trauma or cold exposure, neurogenic causes, disorders of intravascular coagulation or aggregation, and a variety of drugs. Supplementation with tri-iodothyronine to induce iatrogenic hyperthyroidism may be used to induce vasodilation in the digits and is particularly effective when used in conjunction with reserpine. (*Cecil, Ch. 46*)

25.(D) *Discussion:* Acrocyanosis occurs predominantly in women and is more common among patients with psychiatric disturbances. The hands are most often affected and are blue, cold to touch, and clammy. The precapillary arterioles are constricted while the veins are dilated. Patients complain of a cold feeling or numbness in the affected areas but do not have pain. Ulcerations are distinctly uncommon. (*Cecil, Ch. 46*)

26.(C) *Discussion:* Thromboangiitis obliterans is a disease of smokers and is probably autoimmune mediated. It occurs predominantly in young men and affects small and medium-sized arteries and veins. Visceral vessels may be affected in some patients. The disorder is associated with superficial thrombophlebitis and Raynaud's phenomenon. Patients may complain of rest pain in one or more digits, pain that is more severe at night, or paroxysmal shocklike pain with or without paresthesias. (*Cecil, Ch. 46*)

27.(D) *Discussion:* Alpha$_2$-antiplasmin deficiency is associated with a severe hemophilia-like bleeding tendency. Antithrombin III deficiency, protein S deficiency, protein C deficiency, and deficiency of heparin cofactor II are all associated with an increased risk of venous thrombosis and should be strongly suspected in younger individuals with recurrent thrombotic episodes. (*Cecil, Ch. 46*)

28.(B) *Discussion:* Low-dose heparin reduces the incidence of deep venous thrombosis in most surgical patients but is not effective prophylaxis in patients undergoing hip surgery. Anticoagulation with standard heparin preparations requires frequent monitoring of the aPTT. Monitoring of the aPTT is not necessary during treatment with low-molecular-weight heparin fragments. Patients with iliofemoral thrombosis and those with subclavian or axillary thrombosis may benefit from thrombolytic therapy. Insertion of an inferior vena cava filter should be considered in patients with contraindications to anticoagulation, in patients with recurrent emboli despite adequate anticoagulation, and in patients with septic thromboembolic disease not controlled by antibiotics. Anticoagulation is not necessary in superficial thrombophlebitis. (*Cecil, Ch. 46*)

29.(B) *Discussion:* The intramural coronary arteries are generally spared from atherosclerosis. Atherosclerosis of the pulmonary artery is rare and is associated with severe pulmonary hypertension. The aorta, the carotids, and the superficial femoral artery are commonly involved with atherosclerotic lesions. (*Cecil, Ch. 40*)

30.(D) *Discussion:* In hypertrophic obstructive cardiomyopathy, initial ventricular ejection is rapid. Sudden obstruction during ejection may result in a bisferiens carotid pulse in this disorder. The left ventricular impulse may be triple. The systolic murmur of hypertrophic obstructive cardiomyopathy is accentuated by maneuvers that decrease preload or afterload and thus gets louder during the Valsalva maneuver. Mitral regurgitation is often present. (*Cecil, Ch. 43*)

31.(D) *Discussion:* Microbubbles are an excellent echocontrast agent, are safe, and are used extensively to assess intracardiac and myocardial blood flow. Newer agents show promise in visualizing myocardial perfusion from a venous injection. Ninety per cent of normal subjects have Doppler echocardiographically detectable tricuspid regurgitation. (*Cecil, Ch. 33.3*)

32.(E) *Discussion:* The normal P and T wave axes point in the same general direction as the normal QRS axis. With advancing age, the frontal plane QRS axis frequently shifts left, which is not necessarily a pathologic finding. (*Cecil, Ch. 33.2*)

33.(D) *Discussion:* The gated equilibrium radionuclide blood pool study gates to the R wave, stores data based on the time of its occurrence in the cardiac cycle, and sums the data obtained over hundreds of cycles. Thus, markedly irregular RR intervals, such as seen in atrial fibrillation, compromise the data quality and results. Global systolic and diastolic function can be assessed by the time-activity curves. By dividing the left ventricular blood pool into discrete areas, regional ventricular function can be assessed. (*Cecil, Ch. 33.4*)

34.(C) *Discussion:* The most commonly used radionuclide perfusion agents are thallium-201 and ^{99m}Tc sestamibi. They enter the myocardium in proportion to regional blood flow. Thallium is taken up by the myocytes as a potassium analogue. They are most helpful at detecting ischemia when heterogeneity of blood flow is maximized by exercise or pharmacologic stress. Myocardial perfusion imaging is most helpful in the diagnosis of patients at intermediate risk for ischemic heart disease. (*Cecil, Ch. 33.4*)

35.(E) *Discussion:* Patients with a low flow state generally have a high atrial-ventricular oxygen (A-V O$_2$) content difference, allowing the Fick method of determining cardiac output to be very accurate:

$$\text{Fick cardiac output} = \frac{O_2 \text{ consumption}}{\text{A-V } O_2 \text{ difference}}$$

In patients with a high flow state, the thermodilution method may be superior. In the United States, coronary artery disease is the most common diagnosis in patients undergoing cardiac catheterization, followed by valvular disease and cardiomyopathy. (*Cecil, Ch. 33.6*)

36.(B) *Discussion:* Even when mitral regurgitation is the etiology for the heart failure, its severity does not predict mortality. LVEF remains the single best prognosticator. (*Cecil, Ch. 34*)

37.(A) *Discussion:* Diastolic dysfunction implies impaired relaxation of the ventricle. Hypertrophic and ischemic ventricles have impaired relaxation. If ischemia is severe, contractility is also impaired. In infiltrative cardiomyopathy (e.g., amyloidosis), relaxation is initially impaired, followed by contractile function. Paget's disease causes high-output failure. (*Cecil, Ch. 34*)

38.(D) *Discussion:* With the possible exception of the highly vasoselective agents (e.g., amlodipine, felodipine), all calcium channel blockers are detrimental in systolic dysfunction. Metoprolol and other beta blockers have paradoxically been shown to improve systolic function when used judiciously. Disopyramide is a potent negative inotrope. (*Braunwald*)

39.(B) *Discussion:* Heart failure resulting from diastolic dysfunction can be difficult to manage. Acutely, preload (LVEDP) should be lowered with nitroglycerin and diuresis. However, overdiuresis results in impaired ventricular filling (particularly when the ventricle is stiff) and a prerenal state develops. A slow heart rate and AV synchrony facilitate ventricular filling. Hypertension and ischemia should be treated vigorously. (*Cecil, Ch. 34*)

40.(D) *Discussion:* All are signs of right heart failure. However, pulmonary venous congestion seen on chest radiograph is more consistent with left heart failure as an etiology, not primary pulmonary hypertension. (*Cecil, Ch. 38*)

41.(B) *Discussion:* The cause of primary pulmonary hypertension is unknown. It has a female-male ratio of 3:1. Although early in the course the pulmonary vasculature may respond to vasodilators, most patients ultimately require lung or heart-lung transplant to survive. These patients are at high risk for pulmonary thrombosis and require chronic anticoagulation. (*Cecil, Ch. 38*)

42.(B) *Discussion:* As the ventricle becomes ischemic, diastolic dysfunction occurs first, followed by systolic dysfunction, then ECG changes, and finally chest pain. (*Cecil, Ch. 41.1*)

43.(A) *Discussion:* Calcium channel blockers should not be used as first-line agents in the management of unstable angina. If a calcium blocker is employed (i.e., beta blocker intolerance) a heart rate–lowering agent should be selected. An exception is patients with variant angina, who often benefit from the antispasmodic effect of calcium blockers. (*Cecil, Ch. 41.1*)

44.(E) *Discussion:* Acebutolol and pindolol are the beta blockers with intrinsic sympathomimetic activity that are available in the United States. (*Cecil, Ch. 41.1*)

45.(D) *Discussion:* Other noncardioselective beta blockers include timolol, nadolol, and penbutolol. (*Cecil, Ch. 41.1; Opie*)

46.(C) *Discussion:* Defibrillation is most successful if performed immediately and should not be delayed to obtain an airway, perform chest compressions, or insert intravenous lines. High-grade ventricular arrhythmias should be treated, but lidocaine prophylaxis is not indicated. Recurrent Mobitz II block implies damage below the AV node and requires pacing for fear of progression to complete heart block. (*Cecil, Ch. 41.2*)

47.(E) *Discussion:* A wide pulse pressure is seen with aortic regurgitation as a result of filling of the left ventricle during diastole. (*Cecil, Ch. 42*)

48.(D) *Discussion:* Mitral stenosis results in underfilling of the left ventricle and elevated pulmonary pressures, leading to dyspnea and a loud P_2. The thickened valve may open with a snap. Turbulence across it produces the diastolic rumble. Left ventricular strain pattern on ECG is seen in aortic valve disease. (*Cecil, Ch. 42*)

49.(A) *Discussion:* Over 50% of adults with aortic stenosis have a bicuspid aortic valve. The presence of heart failure reduces life expectancy to 2 years or less. (*Cecil, Ch. 42*)

50.(C) *Discussion:* Antibiotic prophylaxis is indicated in most valvular lesions, including mitral valve prolapse with regurgitation. Patients with mitral valve prolapse without regurgitation do not require prophylaxis. (*Cecil, Ch. 42*)

51.(C) *Discussion:* Delayed carotid upstroke is seen in aortic stenosis. Aortic insufficiency results in a vigorous carotid upstroke and wide pulse pressure, producing head bobbing and nail bed pulsations. The Austin Flint murmur is a diastolic rumble probably caused by the regurgitant jet striking the anterior mitral leaflet. (*Cecil, Ch. 42*)

52.(D) *Discussion:* Atherosclerosis is the most common cause of aortic aneurysm. Polyarteritis nodosa generally involves medium to small arteries. (*Cecil, Ch. 45*)

53.(E) *Discussion:* Transesophageal echocardiography and MRI are the best tests to exclude aortic dissection. The false-negative and false-positive rates for transthoracic echocardiography are unacceptably high. (*Cecil, Ch. 45*)

54.(C) *Discussion:* Heparin would result in further hemorrhage into the media and potentially increase the dissection. Indications for surgical management of type III dissections are persistent pain, bleeding, or neurologic or vascular compromise. (*Cecil, Ch. 45*)

55.(A) *Discussion:* A number of common drugs alter cyclosporin levels to a clinically significant extent. Among these, phenobarbital and phenytoin decrease cyclosporin levels. (*Cecil, Ch. 48*)

56.(C) *Discussion:* Adenosine, used at usual doses, can result in asystole in the transplanted heart. If used at all, the dose should be reduced by 75%. Although there will not be a chronotropic response to atropine, the vasodilatory response to vagal output is still attenuated. (*Cecil, Ch. 48*)

57.(A—True; B—True; C—True; D—False; E—False) *Discussion:* Coronary heart disease mortality rates peaked in the early 1960s in the United States and have steadily declined since in most Western societies. Rates have been increasing in several Eastern European countries, most prominently in Romania, where there has been an 85% increase between 1970 and 1988. Women develop coronary heart disease 10 to 20 years later than their male counterparts with similar risk factor levels. This difference in risk may in part be due to the higher HDL cholesterol levels in women. Smoking cessation rapidly decreases coronary heart disease risk in both men and women; cancer risk declines much more slowly. (*Cecil, Ch. 31*)

58.(A—False; B—False; C—True; D—True; E—False) *Discussion:* Afterload is the load against which the ventricle must contract when it ejects blood. Increases in afterload thus decrease stroke volume. Preload describes the loading condition of the heart at the end of diastole. Clinically, left ventricular filling pressure is often assessed by measuring pulmonary capillary wedge pressure with a balloon flotation catheter. Right atrial filling pressure is not a reliable estimate of left ventricular loading conditions. Increases in heart rate enhance the inotropic state of the myocardium via changes in Ca^{2+} availability, the so-called force-frequency relationship. Hypoxia, ischemia, and acidosis decrease cardiac contractility. (*Cecil, Ch. 32*)

59.(A—True; B—True; C—True; D—False; E—True) *Discussion:* Oxygen extraction in the heart is the highest of any organ under basal conditions; enhancement of oxygen extraction is thus not a major mechanism to increase myocardial oxygen delivery with stress. Adenosine is a potent vasodilator and is used clinically in nuclear perfusion imaging. Endothelium-dependent relaxing factor is released by intact endothelium in response to mechanical and metabolic stimuli and is an important endogenous regulator of coronary blood flow. Normal hearts have the ability to "autoregulate" perfusion pressure within certain limits, and coronary perfusion pressure does not become a limiting factor until mean perfusion pressure drops below 60 mm Hg. Coronary perfusion pressure is critical to maintain myocardial blood flow in patients with significant coronary stenoses, and great care should be taken not to induce systemic hypotension in these individuals. Alpha-adrenergic stimulation causes coronary vasoconstriction but is of relatively minor importance under normal conditions. (*Cecil, Ch. 32*)

60.(A—True; B—True; C—True; D—False; E—False) *Discussion:* The carotid baroreceptors increase their afferent impulses to the medulla in response to stretch of the wall of the arteries caused by increases in blood pressure. In turn, the vagal nerve is stimulated and heart rate slows. Vigorous stretching of the atrial receptors causes a vasodepressor response. This response may mediate syncopal episodes in patients with aortic stenosis. Atrial natriuretic peptide is released in response to atrial stretch. It is an endogenous vasodilator and causes renal sodium loss. Angiotensin II, produced from angiotensin I by renin, is a potent vasoconstrictor. It also stimulates aldosterone secretion and thus sodium and water retention. During inspiration, intrathoracic

pressure falls and venous return to the right heart is increased. (*Cecil, Ch. 32*)

61.(A—True; B—True; C—True; D—False; E—False) *Discussion:* Both early and late after-depolarizations can trigger arrhythmias. Digitalis-induced ventricular tachycardia is believed to be triggered by early after-depolarizations, whereas quinidine-induced torsades de pointes is believed to be triggered by late after-depolarizations. Verapamil slows atrioventricular conduction and can cause complete AV block. AV block caused by adenosine is due to direct depression of AV conduction and is not responsive to atropine. Potassium-sparing agents may cause severe hyperkalemia. Characteristic ECG findings in hyperkalemia include peaking of T waves, followed by PR prolongation, ST segment depression, QRS widening, eventually disappearance of the P waves, and ultimately ventricular fibrillation or asystole. (*Cecil, Ch. 35; Opie; Mariott*)

62.(A—True; B—True; C—True; D—False; E—True) *Discussion:* Although digitalis toxicity, including gastrointestinal symptoms, neurologic symptoms, and arrhythmias, is more likely to occur at levels of digoxin above the therapeutic range, side effects are not uncommon at levels below 2 ng per deciliter, especially among the elderly. Patients with pulmonary disease and cor pulmonale are at increased risk of digitalis toxicity. Verapamil, quinidine, amiodarone, and propafenone increase serum digoxin levels. Cholestyramine may decrease digoxin serum levels by binding digoxin to the resin. Digoxin should thus be given 1 hour before or 4 hours after cholestyramine administration. Potassium administration is contraindicated in digitalis-induced AV block because it may further impair AV conduction. (*Opie*)

63.(A—True; B—False; C—True; D—True; E—False) *Discussion:* Resting bradycardia and Mobitz I AV block in an athlete reflect increased vagal tone and are not an indication for permanent pacemaker placement. Reversible complete heart block in the setting of an inferior wall MI is not indicative of significant conduction system disease and is not an indication for permanent pacing. Joint statements by the American College of Cardiology and the American Heart Association provide detailed discussion of definitive and possible indications for permanent pacemaker placement. (*Cecil, Ch. 35; Frye et al*)

64.(A—True; B—True; C—True; D—True; E—False) *Discussion:* It has been known for many years that atrial fibrillation in patients with rheumatic heart disease carries a significant risk of thromboembolism. Predictors of thromoembolism in nonrheumatic atrial fibrillation have only recently been elucidated and include a history of previous thromboembolism, history of hypertension, global left ventricular dysfunction, recent congestive heart failure, and left atrial enlargement. Young age at onset of atrial fibrillation is not a risk factor for thromboembolism. (*SPAF Investigators, 1992a, 1992b*)

65.(A—False; B—False; C—True; D—True; E—True) *Discussion:* In this hemodynamically stable patient, immediate cardioversion is unnecessary and would be associated with increased risk of thromboembolism without prior anticoagulation. Quinidine may accelerate the ventricular response and should not be given prior to blocking the AV node. Either a beta blocker or digoxin would be appropriate for control of the ventricular response. Anticoagulation is appropriate treatment prior to cardioversion unless otherwise contraindicated. (*Cecil, Ch. 35*)

66.(A—True; B—True; C—False; D—True; E—True) *Discussion:* Over 90% of victims of sudden death who are autopsied have at least one significantly narrowed coronary artery, and more than 75% have three-vessel coronary artery disease. Acute thrombotic occlusion is noted in 60 to 75%. Platelet aggregability is highest in the early morning hours, when the incidence of sudden death peaks. Successful resuscitation is most likely when the patient is found to be in ventricular tachycardia or ventricular fibrillation and is immediately defibrillated. Only a few individuals with bradyarrhythmias or asystole at initial contact survive to leave the hospital. Both excess alcohol consumption and social isolation are recognized risk factors for sudden death. (*Cecil, Ch. 36*)

67.(All are True) *Discussion:* QT prolongation is common with many antiarrhythmic agents, but a number of noncardiac medications have also been implicated. The QT prolongation may be further magnified when multiple QT-prolonging drugs are used concurrently. (*Cecil, Ch. 35 and 36*)

68.(All are True) *Discussion:* The Treatment of Mild Hypertension Study has demonstrated that weight loss, reduced sodium and alcohol intake, and regular physical activity can result in substantial long-term blood pressure lowering in motivated individuals. In addition to the modalities listed, some authorities have suggested dietary calcium and magnesium supplementation as additional measures based on epidemiologic data and preliminary clinical studies. (*Cecil, Ch. 37; Neaton et al*)

69.(A—False; B—True; C—True; D—True; E—False) *Discussion:* Vaginal delivery is the preferred mode of delivery in patients with congenital heart disease unless there are clear obstetric indications for cesarean section. Early ambulation and use of elastic stockings are essential measures to minimize the risk of postpartum thromboembolism. This is even more important in patients with a right-to-left shunt, who are susceptible to paradoxical embolism. Oxygen administration may predispose to epistaxis as a result of drying of mucous membranes. The incidence of congenital heart disease in children born to mothers with congenital heart disease is significantly higher than in the general population. Patients with a secundum atrial septal defect are not at increased risk of endocarditis; antibiotic prophylaxis is not indicated. (*Cecil, Ch. 39*)

70.(All are True) *Discussion:* In patients with congenital complete heart block, vagal stimuli during surgery may significantly decrease heart rate. Those with slow heart rates at baseline, a wide QRS complex, inadequate responses to exercise, and a history of syncope are at increased risk of perioperative complications and should be paced perioperatively. Peripheral intravenous lines can present a significant hazard in patients with cyanotic congenital heart disease because of the increased risk of paradoxical embolism. Systemic hypotension increases the right-to-left shunt in cya-

notic congenital heart disease and may be fatal. Bleeding risk is increased in cyanotic congenital heart disease. Several congenital defects predispose to endocarditis. This consideration is particularly important in patients with a bicuspid aortic valve because this defect is the most common form of congenital heart disease among adults. (*Cecil, Ch. 39*)

71.(All are True) *Discussion:* Radiation injury to the pericardium may occur during the treatment of Hodgkin's disease, lung cancer, or breast cancer but may not become clinically apparent for many years after therapy. Tuberculous pericarditis is likely to become more important because the incidence of tuberculosis is increasing. Pericardial effusions are very common among patients with end-stage renal disease; the process of dialysis may be a contributing factor. A transient pericardial friction rub may be heard in up to one third of patients after MI; the incidence of pericarditis is even higher in autopsy series. Malignant pericardial effusions are not uncommon in patients with breast or lung cancer. (*Cecil, Ch. 44*)

72.(A—True; B—False; C—True; D—True; E—True) *Discussion:* Pericardial pain may be sharp or crushing and may be located precordially or on the left side of the chest. In contrast to pain caused by myocardial ischemia, pericardial pain worsens with deep inspiration and improves with sitting up. Radiation of pain to the right trapezius ridge is a specific sign for pericardial pain but is uncommon. (*Cecil, Ch. 44*)

73.(A—True; B—False; C—False; D—True; E—True) *Discussion:* In pericarditis, diffuse ST segment elevation occurs early and is followed by ST segment normalization. In contrast to typical ischemic changes, T waves in pericarditis do not invert until the ST segment has returned to baseline. When the patient is seen during the period of ST-segment normalization, the ECG may be normal. Depression of the PR segment is less common than ST elevation but is specific for pericarditis. Atrial arrhythmias are uncommon in acute pericarditis, but atrial fibrillation and flutter are seen in a minority of patients. Electrical alternans may be seen in patients with large pericardial effusions. (*Cecil, Ch. 44; Chou*)

74.(A—True; B—True; C—False; D—True; E—False) *Discussion:* The murmur of hypertrophic cardiomyopathy increases with maneuvers that diminish left ventricular cavity size and decreases with interventions that increase left ventricular cavity size. Administration of amyl nitrite, venous pooling in the standing position, and the Valsalva maneuver increase the loudness of the murmur; handgrip and rapid volume infusion make it softer. (*Cecil, Ch. 43*)

75.(A—True; B—False; C—True; D—True; E—False) *Discussion:* About 50% of patients with acute viral myocarditis improve spontaneous, 25% continue to deteriorate, and 25% stabilize with impaired left ventricular function. Controlled clinical trials of immunosuppressive therapy have not demonstrated any clinical benefit in acute viral myocarditis. Echocardiographic abnormalities are common in patients infected with the human immunodeficiency virus. Lymphocytic myocarditis has been found in 50% of autopsied hearts in infected patients. Lymphocytic myocardial infiltration also characterizes peripartum cardiomyopathy and cardiac transplant rejection. (*Cecil, Ch. 43*)

76.(A—False; B—True; C—True; D—True; E—False) *Discussion:* Chagas disease is caused by *Trypanosoma cruzi* and is a common cause of cardiomyopathy in South and Central America. *Toxoplasma* can cause a myocarditis that is likely to relapse even with appropriate therapy. Giant cell myocarditis is an unusual, often fulminant form of myocarditis that has been associated with pernicious anemia, thymoma, thyroiditis, and systemic lupus erythematosus. Alcohol may be responsible for or contributory to over 10% of heart failure cases in the United States. Alcohol and acetaldehyde are acute and chronic myocardial toxins and may cause irreversible injury. Over 60% of pediatric patients who have received at least 500 mg of Adriamycin per square meter have evidence of impaired cardiac function 10 years later. Beriberi heart disease is caused by thiamine deficiency and is initially characterized by a high cardiac output state. (*Cecil, Ch. 43*)

77.(A—False; B—True; C—False; D—True; E—True) *Discussion:* Hypertrophic cardiomyopathy is genetically transmitted as an autosomal dominant trait but also may occur sporadically as a result of single mutations. Oxygen demand in hypertrophic cardiomyopathy is high; anginal-type chest pain caused by relative myocardial ischemia may thus occur in the absence of epicardial coronary disease. Afterload reduction with vasodilators increases the gradient across the left ventricular outflow tract in obstructive hypertrophic cardiomyopathy and may lead to hemodynamic collapse. Risk of sudden death is highest in young men with a family history of sudden death. Additional predictors of sudden death include a history of syncope and nonsustained ventricular tachycardia on Holter monitoring. Dual-chamber pacing may diminish the systolic gradient across the left ventricular outflow tract by altering the sequence of ventricular activation. (*Cecil, Ch. 43*)

78.(A—False; B—True; C—True; D—True; E—False) *Discussion:* Cardiac myxomas are typically located in the left atrium attached to the interventricular septum but may occur in the right atrium as well. Myxomas are more common in women and may present with fever, malaise, and arthralgias, suggesting an underlying connective tissue disease. Left atrial myxomas may obstruct mitral inflow and cause symptoms suggestive of mitral stenosis. The diastolic tumor "plop" may be mistaken for the opening snap of mitral stenosis. Close follow-up after surgical resection is important because tumors may recur postoperatively. The diagnostic procedure of choice for the detection of myxomas is echocardiography. Cardiac catheterization is indicated preoperatively only if coexistent coronary artery disease is suspected. (*Cecil, Ch. 47*)

79.(A—False; B—True; C—False; D—True; E—True) *Discussion:* Both ergotamine and beta blockers have been associated with the development of Raynaud's phenomenon and should be avoided in patients with the disease. Calcium antagonists, and in particular nifedipine, have proven very useful in this disorder. Reserpine and ACE inhibitors have also proven effective. (*Cecil, Ch. 46*)

80.(A—False; B—True; C—True; D—True; E—False) *Discussion:* Arteriosclerosis obliterans refers to segmental atherosclerotic obstruction of arterial conduits predominantly in the lower limbs. It is more common in men than in women. The superficial femoral artery is most commonly affected. Leriche's syndrome refers to isolated aortoiliac disease. Smoking cessation and regular exercise are important components of therapy for arteriosclerosis obliterans. Pentoxifylline increases walking distance by improving red cell deformability and reducing blood viscosity. Vasodilators may be detrimental by diminishing perfusion pressure distal to the obstruction. (*Cecil, Ch. 46*)

81.(A—False; B—True; C—True; D—True; E—False) *Discussion:* Thrombi in veins consist mostly of red blood cells and a few platelets held together by fibrin. The three main factors leading to thrombosis are venous stasis, injury to the venous wall, and hypercoagulability. Thrombosis and inflammation of the venous wall generally coexist. Deep vein thrombosis is more common in women. Superficial thrombophlebitis is frequent after pregnancy. (*Cecil, Ch. 46*)

82.(All are True) *Discussion:* All conditions listed may mimic deep venous thrombosis. Differentiation of deep venous thrombosis from calf muscle rupture is particularly important because anticoagulation is contraindicated in the latter. (*Cecil, Ch. 46*)

83.(A—True; B—True; C—True; D—False; E—True) *Discussion:* Fatty streaks may be present at birth. They contain T lymphocytes (CD8 and CD4-positive cells) and foam cells. Foam cells are derived from circulating monocytes that migrate into the subintimal space, differentiate into macrophages, and become engorged with lipid droplets. Rupture of an atherosclerotic plaque with superimposed thrombosis may cause myocardial infarction and sudden death. Atherosclerotic lesions are often located in areas of low shear stress at arterial bifurcations. (*Cecil, Ch. 40*)

84.(A—True; B—True; C—True; D—True; E—False) *Discussion:* Hypertension, cigarette smoking, diabetes mellitus, and hypercholesterolemia are well-characterized risk factors for atherosclerosis. Familial hypercholesterolemia is characterized by absent or dysfunctional LDL receptors, and cholesterol levels may exceed 1000 mg per deciliter in homozygous individuals. High levels of HDL cholesterol are associated with a lower risk of atherosclerosis, as is a low ratio of LDL to HDL cholesterol. (*Cecil, Ch. 40*)

85.(A—True; B—True; C—False; D—True; E—True) *Discussion:* Endothelial injury may occur in the absence of morphologic changes in the endothelium. Functional abnormalities of the endothelium occur in the presence of hypercholesterolemia and are reversible with treatment of the lipid disorder. Early in atherosclerosis development, molecules are expressed at the endothelial cell surface that promote adherence of monocytes and lymphocytes. More severe endothelial injury may lead to endothelial disruption, which exposes the underlying collagen matrix and serves as a nidus for platelet aggregation and mural thrombosis. Growth factors that are important in atherogenesis include platelet-derived growth factor and transforming growth factor beta. The latter induces the formation of connective tissue in atherosclerotic plaques. Tumor necrosis factor alpha is not an important mediator in plaque development. (*Cecil, Ch. 40*)

86.(A—True;   B—True;   C—True;   D—False; E—False) *Discussion:* Angiographic regression trials have consistently shown decreased progression of coronary lesions, and plaque regression has been evident in some. Clinical events have been reduced to a greater degree than expected based on the small angiographic changes observed. This may be due to compositional changes in the atherosclerotic plaques that render them less susceptible to rupture. Angiographic regression can be achieved by dietary therapy and vigorous exercise. Both genders benefit equally from lipid-lowering therapy. (*Cecil, Ch. 40; Brown et al*)

87.(A—False;   B—True;   C—True;   D—False; E—True) *Discussion:* The normal right heart border on a chest radiograph is formed by the superior vena cava, the right atrium, and occasionally a portion of the inferior vena cava. Although fairly sensitive at detecting chamber enlargement, the chest radiograph is not a sensitive test for detecting chamber hypertrophy. (*Cecil, Ch. 33.1*)

88.(A—True;   B—True;   C—True;   D—False; E—True) *Discussion:* The LVEF is the single best indicator of overall ventricular function. As such, it is the best prognosticator for most forms of heart disease. The LVEF normally increases by about 5% with exercise. The left ventricle is frequently more impaired by ischemic heart disease, resulting in an LVEF less than the right ventricular ejection fraction. In patients presenting with heart failure, an index of LVEF is necessary to exclude diastolic dysfunction as an etiology. (*Cecil, Ch. 33.4*)

89.(A—True;   B—True;   C—True;   D—True; E—True) *Discussion:* MRI produces tomographic images in multiple planes without the necessity of intravascular contrast. By using different acquisition sequences, the blood pool or tissue structures can be enhanced. MRI is probably the imaging modality of choice in stable patients with aortic disease. (*Cecil, Ch. 33.5*)

90.(A—False;   B—True;   C—True;   D—True; E—False) *Discussion:* Cardiac pacemakers and defibrillators may be activated or deactivated by the strong magnetic field used in MRI. Cerebral aneurysm clips could rotate and result in hemorrhage. Sternal wires create image artifact but no danger. Mechanical ventilators, kept a safe distance from the magnet, can be used with long tubing to connect to the patient. (*Cecil, Ch. 33.5*)

91.(A—True;   B—True;   C—False;   D—True; E—True) *Discussion:* Heart failure is the number one diagnosis-related group in America for patients age 65 and older. Overall, 50% of the patients are dead within 5 years of diagnosis. In patients with severe heart failure, 50% are dead at 1 year. One half of the patients who die of heart failure die suddenly. Despite the presence of arrhythmias being a poor prognostic factor, antiarrhythmic drugs have not altered mortality. (*Cecil, Ch. 34*)

92.(A—True;   B—True;   C—True;   D—False; E—True) *Discussion:* Mitral and aortic insufficiency produce volume overload. Aortic and pulmonic stenosis result in pressure overload. Generally, volume overload is better tolerated and the heart may not decompensate for years. An exception is acute mitral regurgitation, wherein the heart has inadequate time to adapt. (*Cecil, Ch. 34*)

93.(A—True;   B—True;   C—True;   D—False; E—True) *Discussion:* The cardiac output is calculated by multiplying the heart rate by the stroke volume. The determinants of stroke volume are preload, afterload, and contractility. Ejection fraction is often used as a crude index of contractility. (*Cecil, Ch. 34*)

94.(A—True;   B—True;   C—True;   D—True; E—False) *Discussion:* Impaired exercise tolerance is the *sine qua non* of heart failure irrespective of etiology or ventricle involved. Pulsus alternans, thought to be due to impaired excitation-contraction coupling, is a sign of severe ventricular dysfunction. Clear lung fields do not exclude significant volume overload. As pulmonary pressures rise, lymphatic uptake of transudative fluid increases. (*Cecil, Ch. 34*)

95.(A—True;   B—True;   C—False;   D—False; E—True) *Discussion:* The prevention arm of SOLVD studied patients with a LVEF <0.35 and minimal to no symptoms, and observed a significant reduction in the combined endpoint of hospitalization or death in those treated with enalapril. Although no study to date has demonstrated a survival advantage from the use of digoxin, exercise tolerance is improved. (*Cecil, Ch. 34*)

96.(A—True;   B—True;   C—False;   D—True; E—True) *Discussion:* Angina pectoris is most commonly associated with coronary atherosclerosis, which can disrupt the endothelial regulation of vascular tone as well as cause mechanical obstruction to flow. The primary determinants of myocardial oxygen demand are heart rate, contractility, and wall stress. Wall stress is a function of intraventricular pressure, chamber size, and wall thickness. If wall stress is very high, as in aortic stenosis, ischemia can develop despite normal arteries. The myocardium extracts oxygen at near-maximal efficiency even at rest, so a decrease in supply can quickly result in ischemia. (*Cecil, Ch. 41.1*)

97.(A—False;   B—False;   C—True;   D—False; E—True) *Discussion:* The history is the most valuable tool in making the diagnosis of angina. Although physical findings of ischemia (intermittent mitral regurgitation, S₄, etc.) are helpful, they are frequently absent. A normal resting ECG does not exclude severe coronary atherosclerosis. Patients frequently have ischemic ST segment changes without symptoms. (*Cecil, Ch. 41.1*)

98.(All are True) *Discussion:* The differential diagnosis of angina includes most causes of chest pain. However, the astute clinician will be able to exclude most possibilities by obtaining a careful history. (*Cecil, Ch. 41.1*)

99.(All are True) *Discussion:* In general, the more severe the ST depression, the greater the likelihood of a true-positive graded exercise test. (*Cecil, Ch. 41.1*)

100.(A—True;   B—True;   C—True;   D—False; E—False) *Discussion:* There are a number of indications for coronary artery bypass surgery, including relief of angina. Only in conditions A to C and in patients with postinfarction ischemia has it been clearly demonstrated to alter mortality. (*Cecil, Ch. 41.1*)

101.(A—True;   B—False;   C—False;   D—True; E—True) *Discussion:* Nitrates are believed to be converted to nitric oxide in the vasculature. Nitric oxide is believed to be the same substance as endothelial-derived relaxing factor. At low doses, nitrates primarily act on the venous system. This results in venous pooling of blood, which lowers left ventricular filling pressure and thereby decreases wall stress and relieves ischemia. Nitrates at higher doses also dilate arterioles and antagonize platelet activation. (*Cecil, Ch. 41.1*)

102.(A—True; B—True; C—False; D—True; E—True) *Discussion:* The majority of patients who die from acute MI do so suddenly, whether hospitalized or not. Nonetheless, most MI deaths occur outside the hospital. (*Cecil, Ch. 41.2*)

103.(All are True) *Discussion:* Additional risk factors for ischemic heart disease include hypertriglyceridemia, smoking, elevated LDL cholesterol, and strong family history of premature cardiac disease. (*Cecil, Ch. 41.2*)

104.(A—True; B—True; C—True; D—True; E—False) *Discussion:* Right ventricular infarction is usually seen in the setting of inferior wall infarction and increases the risk of death. Physical findings include elevated jugular venous pressure with Kussmaul's sign, hypotension, and clear lung fields. Treatment includes volume loading, dobutamine, and AV sequential pacing to maintain AV synchrony. Nitrates should be used cautiously, if at all, to avoid preload reduction. (*Cecil, Ch. 41.2*)

105.(A—False; B—False; C—True; D—False; E—True) *Discussion:* The diagnosis of acute MI is generally made by the combination of history, ST segment changes, and an elevated plasma CK-MB level. However, a normal resting ECG does not exclude a significant infarction. CK-MB level generally is elevated in the plasma by 4 to 8 hours and peaks in 24 hours. LDH-1, which remains elevated for 72 hours, the troponins I and T, and infarct-avid imaging may help make the diagnosis when the patient arrives late. (*Cecil, Ch. 41.2*)

106.(A—True; B—True; C—True; D—False; E—True) *Discussion:* The vast majority of patients who die of MI die from ventricular fibrillation. Most succumb within the first hour. Reperfusion of the infarct-related artery is the primary form of therapy. Both thrombolysis and primary angioplasty are effective. Angioplasty offers the potential advantage of greater patency and less bleeding but has limited availability. The total incidence of stroke is the same, with or without thrombolytic therapy. However, a greater proportion of strokes are hemorrhagic if thrombolytics have been administered. (*Cecil, Ch. 41.2*)

107.(A—False; B—True; C—True; D—True; E—True) *Discussion:* No acceptable artificial conduits have been developed for coronary artery bypass grafting. The left internal mammary (thoracic) artery is the conduit of choice. (*Cecil, Ch. 41.3*)

108.(A—True; B—False; C—True; D—True; E—False) *Discussion:* It has become clear that patients who are completely revascularized have a better long-term survival and freedom from recurrent ischemia. The operative mortality rate in patients <60 years of age with good ventricles is 1%. The incidence of perioperative stroke is 2%. (*Cecil, Ch. 41.3*)

109.(A—True; B—True; C—False; D—False; E—False) *Discussion:* Alternative regimens and a complete description of the American Heart Association recommendations can be found in *JAMA* 264: 2919, 1990. (*Cecil, Ch. 42*)

110.(A—True; B—True; C—False; D—True; E—False) *Discussion:* AV synchrony and bradycardia are important to increase ventricular filling. Tachycardia decreases the ventricular filling time. Patients with mitral stenosis and atrial fibrillation are at high risk for thromboembolic events and require chronic anticoagulation. (*Cecil, Ch. 42*)

111.(A—True; B—True; C—True; D—False; E—True) *Discussion:* Palpitations should be managed with beta blockers or, occasionally, calcium channel blockers. It is a mistake to take a generally benign disease and increase the risk of mortality by beginning the patient on antiarrhythmics. Chordae rupture is one of the few serious complications of mitral valve prolapse. (*Cecil, Ch. 42*)

112.(A—True; B—True; C—False; D—True; E—True) *Discussion:* Abdominal aneurysms are frequently complicated by thrombosis and embolism, which are relatively uncommon with thoracic aneurysms. (*Cecil, Ch. 45*)

113.(A—True; B—True; C—True; D—False; E—True) *Discussion:* The most common cause of aortic dissection is hypertension. (*Cecil, Ch. 45*)

114.(All are True) *Discussion:* Patients frequently complain primarily or exclusively of anterior chest pain. The pain is often of maximal intensity from the onset, unlike ischemic pain, which often waxes and wanes. Compression of the superior cervical ganglion results in Horner's syndrome. Involvement of a coronary artery results in myocardial infarction. Involvement of a carotid artery may result in stroke. (*Cecil, Ch. 45*)

115.(A—True; B—True; C—True; D—True; E—False) *Discussion:* More than 90% of patients develop cyclosporin-induced hypertension. Diltiazem increases cyclosporin levels and can be used to treat hypertension and lower the necessary cyclosporin dosage. Beta blockers should be avoided because of the transplanted hearts' dependency on circulating catecholamines. (*Cecil, Ch. 48*)

116.(All are True) *Discussion:* The symptoms of transplant rejection are very nonspecific. Endomyocardial biopsy is necessary for a definitive diagnosis. (*Cecil, Ch. 48*)

117.(B); 118.(E); 119.(D); 120.(A) *Discussion:* The jugular venous pulse is best observed when the patient is positioned to allow observation of the venous column throughout the cardiac cycle. The *a* wave reflects right atrial contraction. The *x* descent reflects right atrial relaxation and continues with early right ventricular contraction. The *v* wave represents passive right atrial filling while the tricuspid valve is closed. The *y* descent reflects tricuspid valve opening and right ventricular relaxation. Pulmonic valve opening is not reflected in the jugular venous pulsation. (*Cecil, Ch. 30*)

121.(D); 122.(A); 123.(C); 124.(E) *Discussion:* Lidocaine accumulates in patients with hepatic insufficiency and heart failure and in the elderly. Neurologic adverse effects include drowsiness, confusion, visual disturbances, and convulsions. Serum levels should be monitored closely during prolonged infusions. Amiodarone causes a myriad of systemic side effects, among them hyper- or hypothroidism. Thyroid function tests should be monitored regularly. Atrial tachycardia with AV block is a "classic" digoxin-induced arrhythmia. Procainamide may cause a lupus-like syndrome. (*Cecil, Ch. 35*)

125.(E); 126.(D); 127.(A); 128.(B) *Discussion:* Asymptomatic sinus bradycardia during sleep does not require therapy. Retrograde P waves, fatigue, and dizziness in a patient with a VVI pacemaker indicate the "pacemaker syndrome," which is treated by upgrading to a DDD pacemaker to restore AV synchrony. An implantable defibrillator is the most appropriate device therapy in patients with ventricular fibrillation without underlying reversible cause and who are noninducible in the electrophysiology laboratory. Complete heart block caused by digitalis toxicity is reversible once the digoxin serum level declines. Temporary ventricular pacing is thus the treatment of choice. (*Cecil, Ch. 35*)

129.(C); 130.(A); 131.(B); 132.(D) *Discussion:* Beta blockers decrease morbidity and mortality after myocardial infarction and are the preferred antihypertensive agents in patients with preserved left ventricular function. Patients with hypertension and congestive heart failure, asymptomatic left ventricular dysfunction, or impaired ejection fraction after MI should be treated with an ACE inhibitor unless otherwise contraindicated. Low-dose diuretics have been shown to decrease morbidity and mortality in elderly patients with hypertension and are effective antihypertensives among blacks. Alpha blockers are effective antihypertensives in all major patient subgroups and are effective in the treatment of the obstructive symptoms of benign prostatic hypertrophy. (*Cecil, Ch. 37*)

133.(E); 134.(A); 135.(B); 136.(C) *Discussion:* Spironolactone may cause mastodynia, gynecomastia, and sexual dysfunction. Minoxidil may cause both pleural and pericardial effusions. Hydralazine frequently causes a positive antinuclear antibody test but only rarely causes a lupus-like syndrome at commonly used antihypertensive doses. Methyldopa may cause liver toxicity and rarely causes a Coombs-positive hemolytic anemia. Dry cough is a common side effect of ACE inhibitors. (*Cecil, Ch. 37*)

137.(A); 138.(B); 139.(A); 140.(D) *Discussion:* Jugular venous pressure is elevated in both pericardial tamponade and constrictive pericarditis. Pulsus paradoxus is an exaggerated decrease in systolic blood pressure during inspiration that is only seen in cardiac tamponade. In constrictive pericarditis, the negative intrathoracic pressure during inspiration is not transmitted to the heart: Pulsus paradoxus does not occur and jugular pressure may rise abnormally during inspiration (Kussmaul's sign). A pericardial knock is characteristic of pericardial constriction. (*Cecil, Ch. 44*)

141.(B); 142.(C); 143.(C); 144.(A) *Discussion:* Hemodynamically, restrictive cardiomyopathy and constrictive pericarditis may be difficult to distinguish. In selected cases, endomyocardial biopsy may be helpful. High LVEF and systolic anterior motion of the mitral valve on echocardiography are characteristic features of hypertrophic cardiomyopathy.

Patients with Duchenne's muscular dystrophy may develop a dilated cardiomyopathy. (*Cecil, Ch. 43*)

145.(C); 146.(A); 147.(D); 148.(E) *Discussion:* In the evaluation of cardiomyopathies, the ECG may provide important clues to the underlying etiology. Diffusely low QRS voltage on the ECG is a characteristic feature of cardiac amyloidosis. Right bundle-branch block is uncommon in dilated cardiomyopathy except in Chagas' disease. Sarcoidosis is often associated with significant conduction abnormalities. ECG patterns mimicking MI are seen in hypertrophic cardiomyopathy. (*Cecil, Ch. 43*)

149.(D); 150.(A); 151.(C); 152.(E) *Discussion:* Down's syndrome is frequently associated with congenital cardiac anomalies. Endocardial cushion defects are most common. Marfan's syndrome is a disorder of connective tissue and may be manifested by fusiform aortic aneurysms, aortic regurgitation, aortic dissection, or a floppy mitral valve. Maternal systemic lupus erythematosus is associated with complete heart block in the offspring. At times, the maternal lupus may not become symptomatic until years after the birth of an infant with congenital complete heart block. When mothers are infected with rubella during the first trimester, infants may be born with the congenital rubella syndrome. Patent ductus arteriosus is a characteristic congenital cardiac anomaly in this syndrome. (*Cecil, Ch. 39; Perloff*)

153.(C); 154.(B); 155.(A); 156.(D) *Discussion:* Lymphedema may be present at birth (simple congenital lymphedema). Other varieties are inherited (Milroy's disease and lymphedema associated with Noonan's syndrome). Secondary lymphedema may occur after surgical resection of lymph nodes or after radiation, or may be due to malignancy or infection (filariasis). Emboli in acute peripheral arterial occlusions are most commonly cardiac in origin and may include emboli from mural thrombi after myocardial infarction, emboli from valve vegetations, and emboli from atrial thrombi in patients with atrial fibrillation. Raynaud's phenomenon is seen in a variety of systemic illnesses, idiopathic pulmonary hypertension among them. Varicose veins or thrombophlebitis may give rise to the postphlebitic syndrome, with chronic venous stasis changes and, in severe cases, ulceration. The ulcers are characteristically located above the medial malleolus and arterial pulses are intact. Cutaneous hypersensitivity to tobacco products is present in many patients with thromboangiitis obliterans. (*Cecil, Ch. 46*)

157.(A); 158.(B); 159.(C); 160.(D) *Discussion:* The hypertrophic ventricle of aortic stenosis initially reduces the left ventricular cavity size without increasing heart size. However, poststenotic dilation of the aorta may be seen. The ventricle of aortic regurgitation is a dilated ventricle. The radiographic findings of mitral stenosis are left atrial enlargement, a prominent right ventricle, and pulmonary venous congestion. With mitral regurgitation, the left atrium may enlarge prior to enlargement of the left ventricle and pulmonary venous congestion. (*Cecil, Ch. 42*)

161.(A); 162.(D); 163.(C); 164.(B) *Discussion:* The RR interval is the interval between consecutive R waves and, if the heart rate is regular, can be divided into 60 to calculate the heart rate per minute. The PR interval measures the time from the onset of atrial depolarization to the onset of ventricular depolarization. It normally includes the time required for the electrical impulse to pass through the atria, AV node, His bundle, and bundle branches. In Wolff-Parkinson-White syndrome, the electrical impulse is conducted directly from the atria to the ventricle, bypassing the AV node, His bundle, and bundle branches and resulting in a short PR interval. The QT interval represents the duration of ventricular electrical systole and varies with heart rate. The QTc, the QT interval corrected for heart rate, may be calculated by dividing the QT interval by the square root of the RR interval. (*Cecil, Ch. 33.2*)

165.(B); 166.(C); 167.(A); 168.(D) *Discussion:* The ST segment is very important in the diagnosis of cardiac ischemia and pericarditis. Its level of elevation or depression is referenced to the TP segment. (*Cecil, Ch. 33.2*)

169.(A); 170.(A); 171.(B); 172.(A); 173.(B); 174.(A); 175.(B); 176.(B) *Discussion:* Most of the patients with heart failure seen in clinical practice have low to low-normal cardiac output. The most common forms of high-output heart failure are hyperthyroidism, Paget's disease, anemia, beriberi, and arteriovenous fistulas. Even then, it is very uncommon for adults to develop high-output failure without some underlying heart disease. (*Cecil, Ch. 34*)

177.(D); 178.(A); 179.(B); 180.(C) *Discussion:* In a practical sense, the preload is thought of as ventricular end-diastolic volume or pressure. Afterload, the resistance that the ventricle must overcome during systole in order to eject, is determined partially by the systemic vascular resistance. Lusitropy and inotropy refer to the relaxation and contractile states of the ventricle, respectively. (*Cecil, Ch. 34*)

181.(D); 182.(A); 183.(C); 184.(B) *Discussion:* Pathology at several sites in the cardiopulmonary system can result in increased pulmonary pressures. Increased pulmonary blood flow for any number of reasons results in pulmonary vasoconstriction and ultimately a permanent increase in pulmonary vascular resistance. A number of diseases (scleroderma, sarcoidosis, pulmonary emboli) can reduce the number of pulmonary arteries and increase vascular resistance. Hypoxia causes pulmonary arteriolar constriction. Sickle cell anemia may result in pulmonary venule obstruction. (*Cecil, Ch. 38*)

185.(E); 186.(F); 187.(D); 188.(C); 189.(H); 190.(A); 191.(B); 192.(G) *Discussion:* Coronary atherosclerosis is the underlying pathology in well the majority of cases of acute MI. However, 5 to 10% of infarctions are caused by a long list of less common pathologies. These include coronary emboli from valves and mural thrombi, thrombotic disease from hypercoagulable states, arterial obstruction from vasculitis, and degenerative vessel diseases such as pseudoxanthoma elasticum. The coronary ostia can be occluded by aortic dissection or aortitis. Several coronary anomalies can compromise coronary blood flow or perfuse the heart with venous blood. Rarely, oxygen demand can outstrip supply (carbon monoxide poisoning, thyrotoxicosis) despite normal perfusion. Finally, penetrating trauma can lacerate a coronary artery, impairing myocardial perfusion. (*Cecil, Ch. 41.2*)

193.(A); 194.(D); 195.(C); 196.(B) *Discussion:* Beta blockers, ACE inhibitors, and aspirin have all been clearly demonstrated to decrease mortality postinfarction. Diltiazem and verapamil decrease recurrent ischemic events but increase mortality if heart failure is present. Nitrates appear to decrease acute mortality in patients with pulmonary congestion. (*Cecil, Ch. 41.2*)

197.(A); 198.(C); 199.(D); 200.(B) *Discussion:* Although the murmurs of both aortic stenosis and mitral regurgitation can be loud at the apex and heard throughout the precordium, mitral murmurs do not radiate to the carotids. The classic physical findings of mitral stenosis are an opening snap, diastolic rumble, and loud S_1. Connective tissue disorders, such as Marfan's syndrome, can result in aortic regurgitation. (*Cecil, Ch. 42*)

BIBLIOGRAPHY

Bennett JC, Plum F (eds): Cecil Textbook of Medicine. 20th ed. Philadelphia, WB Saunders Company, 1996.

Braunwald E (ed): Heart Disease: A Textbook of Cardiovascular Disease. 4th ed. Philadelphia, WB Saunders Company, 1992.

Brown BG, Zhao XQ, Sacco DE, et al: Lipid lowering and plaque regression: New insights into prevention of plaque disruption and clinical events in coronary disease. Circulation 87:1781, 1993.

Chou TC: Electrocardiography in Clinical Practice. 3rd ed. Philadelphia, WB Saunders Company, 1991

Frye RL, Fisch C, Collins JJ, et al: Guidelines for permanent pacemaker implantation: A report of the Joint American College of Cardiology (AMA). J Am Coll Cardiol 4:434, 1984.

Hebert PR, Rich-Edwards JW, Manson JE, et al: Height and incidence of cardiovascular disease in male physicians. Circulation 88(part 1):1437, 1993.

Mariott HJL: Practical Electrocardiography. 8th ed. Chap. 30. Baltimore, Williams & Wilkins, 1988.

Opie LH: Drugs for the Heart. Philadelphia, WB Saunders Company, 1995.

Perloff JK: The Clinical Recognition of Congenital Heart Disease. 3rd ed. Philadelphia, WB Saunders Company, 1987.

Neaton JD, Grimm RH, Prineas RJ, et al: Treatment of Mild Hypertension Study: Final results. JAMA 270:713, 1993.

SPAF Investigators: Predictors of thromboembolism in atrial fibrillation: I. Clinical features of patients at risk. Ann Intern Med 116:1, 1992a.

SPAF Investigators: Predictors of thromboembolism in atrial fibrillation: II. Echocardiographic features of patients at risk. Ann Intern Med 116:6, 1992b.

PART 2

PULMONARY DISEASES

J. Allen D. Cooper, Jr.

DIRECTIONS: For questions 1 to 29, choose the ONE BEST answer to each question.

1. Which of the following are true about patients with obstructive sleep apnea?

- A. Females outnumber males
- B. Patients with the problem commonly awaken at night and have difficulty returning to sleep
- C. Mean age of onset is 40 to 50 years
- D. The majority of patients will improve with weight reduction
- E. All of the above
- F. B and D
- G. A, C, and D
- H. A and D

2. Which of the following disorders are associated with obstructive sleep apnea?

- A. Hypothyroidism
- B. Acromegaly
- C. Down's syndrome
- D. Chronic obstructive pulmonary disease
- E. All of the above
- F. B and D
- G. A, C, and D
- H. A and D

3. Nocturnal symptoms of obstructive sleep apnea include which of the following?

- A. Snoring
- B. Somnambulism
- C. Gastroesophageal reflux
- D. Enuresis
- E. All of the above
- F. B and D
- G. A, C, and D
- H. A and D

4. Daytime symptoms associated with obstructive sleep apnea include which of the following?

- A. Hypersomnolence
- B. Intermittent paralysis
- C. Automatic behavior
- D. Headaches
- E. All of the above
- F. B and D
- G. A, C, and D
- H. A and D

5. Which of the following disorders are associated with asbestos exposure?

- A. Mesothelioma
- B. Emphysema
- C. Bronchogenic carcinoma
- D. Pleural effusion
- E. All of the above
- F. B and D
- G. A, C, and D
- H. A and D

6. A 58-year-old man presents to you with symptoms of hemoptysis and fever. You order a chest radiograph, which is shown in the figure on page 27. What would be your next step(s)?

- A. Start intravenous antibiotics for treatment of pneumonia
- B. Collect sputum for cytology
- C. Have computed tomography (CT) scan of head and abdomen performed
- D. Consult a pulmonologist for possible bronchoscopy
- E. All of the above
- F. B and D
- G. A, C, and D
- H. A and D

7. Which of the following manifestations are contraindications to resection of a bronchogenic carcinoma?

- A. Hypercalcemia
- B. Pleural effusion
- C. Mediastinal adenopathy on CT scan
- D. Histologically documented hepatic metastases
- E. All of the above
- F. B and D
- G. A, C, and D
- H. A and D

8. Which of the following can cause a transudative pleural effusion?

- A. Congestive heart failure
- B. Ureteral obstruction
- C. Hypothyroidism
- D. Atelectasis
- E. All of the above
- F. B and D
- G. A, C, and D
- H. A and D

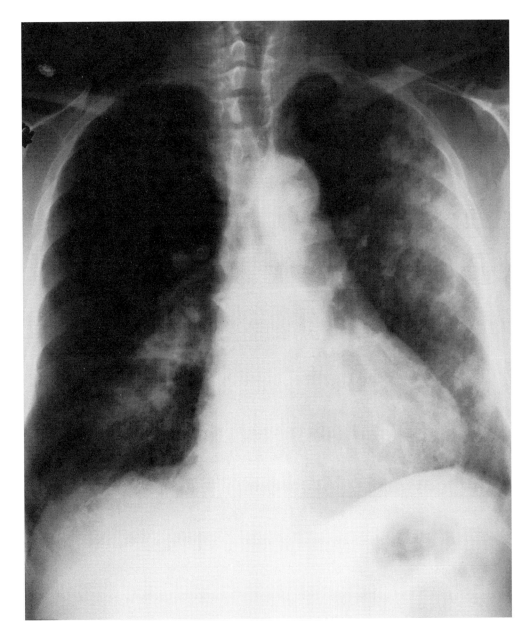

9. Which of the following is an indication for chest tube placement and drainage of a parapneumonic pleural effusion?

    A. pH <7.10
    B. Positive pleural fluid Gram's stain
    C. Lactate dehydrogenase (LDH) level >1000 units per ml
    D. Glucose ratio <0.5
    E. All of the above
    F. B and D
    G. A, C, and D
    H. A and D

10. Which of the following disorders can cause hemoptysis?

    A. Bronchiectasis
    B. Asthma
    C. Aspergilloma
    D. Pulmonary embolism

    E. All of the above
    F. B and D
    G. A, C, and D
    H. A and D

11. Which of the following factors help define asthma?

    A. Low diffusing capacity for carbon monoxide
    B. Airway hyperreactivity to methacholine
    C. Proximal bronchiectasis
    D. Reversible airflow obstruction
    E. All of the above
    F. B and D
    G. A, C, and D
    H. A and D

12. Which of the following chest radiographic abnormalities can be caused by rheumatoid arthritis?

    A. Pleural effusion
    B. Hyperexpansion

C. Multiple nodules
D. Reticulonodular infiltrates
E. All of the above
F. B and D
G. A, C, and D
H. A and D

13. A 30-year-old man presents to your clinic with symptoms of shortness of breath and nonproductive cough. Pulmonary function tests are shown in the table *below*. Which of the following other tests might be helpful in the *diagnosis* of his pulmonary disease?

Test	Actual Value	% Predicted
FVC	1.99 L	45
FEV$_1$	1.71 L	51
FEV$_1$/FVC	86%	
TLC	2.73	43
RV	0.74	40
D$_{LCO}$	4.2	14

A. Serum immunoglobulin precipitins to thermophilic fungi
B. Antinuclear antibody (ANA)
C. Gallium scan of the lungs
D. Open lung biopsy
E. All of the above
F. B and D
G. A, C, and D
H. A and D

14. Which of the following findings in patients with rheumatoid arthritis are associated with a higher incidence of pulmonary disease?

A. Female gender
B. High rheumatoid factor titer
C. History of smoking
D. Subcutaneous nodules
E. All of the above
F. B and D
G. A, C, and D
H. A and D

15. Which of the following collagen vascular diseases can cause pleural effusions?

A. Rheumatoid arthritis
B. Scleroderma
C. Polymyositis/dermatomyositis
D. Systemic lupus erythematosus (SLE)
E. All of the above
F. B and D
G. A, C, and D
H. A and D

16. Which of the following are risk factors for developing pulmonary side effects of bleomycin?

A. Total dose of the drug
B. Older age
C. Radiation therapy
D. Use of bleomycin in multidrug regimens

E. All of the above
F. B and D
G. A, C, and D
H. A and D

17. Which of the following can predispose to clot formation and subsequent pulmonary thromboembolism?

A. Immobilization
B. Obesity
C. Trauma
D. Malignancy
E. All of the above
F. B and D
G. A, C, and D
H. A and D

18. Which of the following are clinical syndromes that are associated with pulmonary embolism?

A. Pulmonary infarction
B. Diffuse wheezing
C. Acute right heart failure
D. Acute dyspnea, fever, elevated white blood cell count
E. All of the above
F. B and D
G. A, C, and D
H. A and D

19. Which of the following is an *absolute* contraindication to use of fibrinolytic agents for the treatment of pulmonary embolism?

A. Cerebrovascular accident within 2 months
B. Occult blood in the stool
C. Pregnancy
D. History of proliferative retinopathy
E. All of the above
F. B and D
G. A, C, and D
H. A and D

20. A patient has a 5-TU purified protein derivate (PPD) skin test that is reported as resulting in 6 mm of induration. Under which of the following situations would this be reported as a "positive" test?

A. The patient had recent close contact with an individual with active tuberculosis.
B. The patient is a nursing home resident.
C. A chest radiograph of the patient shows changes consistent with old tuberculosis.
D. The patient is human immunodeficiency virus (HIV) positive.
E. All of the above
F. B and D
G. A, C, and D
H. A and D

21. Which of the following are regimens used for prophylaxis to prevent deep venous thrombosis?

A. Heparin 5000 units subcutaneously every 12 hours
B. Streptokinase 25,000 units per h
C. Intermittent pneumatic compression
D. Heparin 5000 units every 8 h

E. All of the above
F. B and D
G. A, C, and D
H. A and D

22. Which of the following individuals should be treated with isoniazid for prevention of reactivation tuberculosis?

A. A 30-year-old with a 16-mm PPD and no other medical problems
B. A 45-year-old with an 18-mm PPD and no other medical problems
C. A 60-year-old with an 11-mm PPD and evidence of silicosis on chest radiograph
D. A 45-year-old nursing home resident with an 11-mm PPD
E. All of the above
F. B and D
G. A, C, and D
H. A and D

23. Which of the following are side effects of isoniazid therapy?

A. Hepatitis
B. Orange discoloration of secretions
C. Thrombocytopenia
D. Peripheral neuropathy
E. All of the above
F. B and D
G. A, C, and D
H. A and D

24. Which of the following can cause a pleural effusion with a glucose level of 10 mg per deciliter?

A. Rheumatoid arthritis
B. Pulmonary embolism
C. Esophageal perforation
D. Tuberculosis
E. All of the above

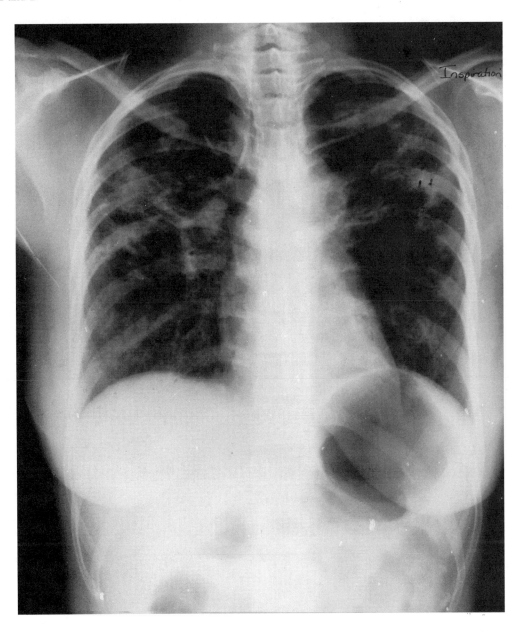

F. B and D
G. A, C, and D
H. A and D

25. A 65-year-old patient presents to the emergency room and a chest radiograph shows a right lower lobe posterior infiltrate. Which of the following would be important in the history for determining appropriate initial coverage?

A. The patient drinks 1 gallon of vodka per day.
B. The patient is a member of the American Legion.
C. The patient had an illness consistent with influenza infection starting 1 week ago.
D. The patient recently excavated a building site.
E. All of the above
F. B and D
G. A, C, and D
H. A and D

26. Which of the following are associated with *Mycoplasma pneumoniae* infection?

A. Erythema multiforme
B. Raynaud's phenomenon
C. Hemolytic anemia
D. Bullous myringitis
E. All of the above
F. B and D
G. A, C, and D
H. A and D

27. Which of the following pathogens more frequently cause nosocomial pneumonia than community-acquired pneumonia?

A. *Staphylococcus aureus*
B. *Streptococcus pneumoniae*
C. *Haemophilus influenzae*
D. *Pseudomonas aeruginosa*
E. All of the above
F. B and D
G. A, C, and D
H. A and D

28. A 65-year-old woman presents to your clinic with chronic cough. Which of the following problems might be contributing to this symptom?

A. Gastroesophageal reflux
B. Congestive heart failure
C. Asthma
D. Postnasal drip
E. All of the above
F. B and D
G. A, C, and D
H. A and D

29. A 24-year-old woman is referred to you because of an abnormal chest radiograph, shown in the figure on page 29. Which of the following studies should be performed for diagnosis or evaluation of this patient's problem?

A. Eye examination, including slit-lamp evaluation
B. Serum angiotensin-converting enzyme (ACE) level
C. Serum calcium level
D. Electrocardiogram
E. All of the above
F. B and D
G. A, C, and D
H. A and D

DIRECTIONS: Questions 30 to 54 are matching questions. For each numbered item, choose the most likely associated lettered item from those provided. With each set of questions, each lettered item may be used once, more than once, or not at all.

QUESTIONS 30–33

Match the following bronchogenic carcinoma cell types with associated findings.

    A. Squamous cell carcinoma
    B. Adenocarcinoma
    C. Small cell carcinoma
    D. Bronchoalveolar carcinoma

30. Cushing's syndrome

31. Hyercalcemia

32. Air bronchograms

33. Solitary brain metastasis

QUESTIONS 34–38

Match the following characteristics noted in pleural effusions with the associated disorders.

    A. Fluid LDH level of 120 IU per liter; fluid protein/serum protein ratio of 0.4
    B. Fluid values: pH 6.8, glucose level of 10 mg per deciliter, amylase level of 500
    C. Fluid values: pH 7.25, glucose level of 10 mg per deciliter, amylase level of 50
    D. Fluid values: LDH level of 120 IU per liter; creatinine level of 10 mg per deciliter
    E. Fluid values: pH 7.3, glucose level of 30 mg per deciliter amylase level of 500
    F. Fluid values: LDH level of 250 IU per liter; triglyceride level of 200 mg per deciliter
    G. Fluid value: ANA titer of 1:256 (peripheral 1:64)

34. Bronchogenic carcinoma

35. Esophageal perforation

36. Rheumatoid arthritis

37. Urinary obstruction

38. Cirrhosis

QUESTIONS 39–43

Match the following initial therapies with the most appropriate pulmonary pathogen

    A. Amantadine
    B. Doxycycline
    C. Erythromycin
    D. Cephotaxime
    E. Ciprofloxacin
    F. Piperacillin
    G. None of the above

39. *Mycoplasma pneumoniae*

40. Influenza B

41. *Chlamydia psittaci*

42. *Legionella pneumophila*

43. *Pseudomonas aeruginosa*

QUESTIONS 44–54

Match one or more of the following syndromes of obstructive pulmonary disease with one or more of the etiologies.

    A. Asthma
    B. Bronchiectasis
    C. Emphysema
    D. Bronchiolitis obliterans
    E. Bronchitis
    F. Upper airway obstruction caused by vocal cord paralysis

44. Bronchial hyperreactivity to inhalation of methacholine

45. Chlorine gas inhalation

46. Allergic bronchopulmonary aspergillosis

47. Textile mill work

48. Stridor

49. Tobacco smoke exposure

50. Low diffusing capacity for carbon monoxide

51. Clubbing

52. Flattened inspiratory flow-volume loop

53. Rheumatoid arthritis

54. Alpha$_1$-antiprotease (A1AP) deficiency

DIRECTIONS: For questions 55–58, you are to decide whether EACH statement is true or false. Any combination of answers, from all true to all false, may occur.

55. Which of the following statements is/are true regarding characteristics of genetically linked emphysema?

A. Emphysema caused by A1AP deficiency is commonly associated with cirrhosis in the same patient.

B. All patients with lower lobe bullae should have serum A1AP levels measured

C. Administration of intravenous recombinant A1AP results in a significant rise in lung concentrations of the protein.

D. Emphysema results from a single type of homozygous combination of the A1AP gene resulting in a specific amino acid substitution in the protein.

E. Patients with the ''null'' phenotype who have no detectable A1AP serum concentrations commonly develop cirrhosis at a very early age.

F. Lung transplantation results in normal pulmonary levels of A1AP.

56. Which of the following is/are true statements regarding patients with hemoptysis?

A. Melena is a sign that the blood produced originates from the gastrointestinal tract.

B. Hemoptysis in the setting of active pulmonary tuberculosis predicts that the sputum smear will be positive for acid-fast bacilli.

C. Patients with hemoptysis caused by aspergilloma commonly have positive serum precipitating antibodies to *Aspergillus.*

D. Lung abscess is a common cause of massive hemoptysis.

E. ''Gritty'' sputum noted in conjunction with hemoptysis suggests the presence of broncholithiasis.

F. Hemoptysis occurring after institution of anticoagulation therapy commonly occurs without an identifiable pulmonary lesion.

G. Hemoptysis preceded by a history of purulent phlegm production is strong evidence that bronchi-

tis is the cause of the bleeding and bronchoscopy is not indicated.

57. Which of the following is/are true statements regarding pulmonary thromboembolism?

A. Upper-extremity phlebitis does not result in embolism.

B. The most common chest radiograph abnormality is asymmetrical hypoperfusion (Westermark's sign).

C. A false-positive impedance plethysmography result can occur with any condition that impedes venous return.

D. An indication for placement of an inferior venocaval filter is a high risk of death from pulmonary embolism.

E. Intermittent pneumatic compression stockings are the method of choice for prevention of deep venous thrombosis after knee surgery.

F. Acute cor pulmonale caused by pulmonary thromboembolism occurs only when >50% of pulmonary arterial circulation is occluded by the embolism.

58. Which of the following is/are true statements about pulmonary manifestations of systemic diseases?

A. Scleroderma can cause isolated pulmonary hypertension.

B. The majority of patients with rheumatoid arthritis have some form of pulmonary disease.

C. Smoking increases the incidence of rheumatoid pulmonary nodules.

D. Pneumonitis may be the first manifestation of SLE.

E. A positive ANA titer in pleural fluid is diagnostic of pleural effusion caused by SLE.

F. Low diffusing capacity for carbon monoxide in the absence of altered lung volumes suggests isolated pulmonary hypertension in a patient with scleroderma

DIRECTIONS: For questions 59 to 79, choose the ONE BEST answer to each question.

59. A 28-year-old male nonsmoker presents with symptoms of intermittent shortness of breath. Pulmonary function tests are shown in the table *below*. Which one of the following medications is most important for initial use?

Test	Actual Value	% Predicted
FVC	2.43 L	84
FEV_1	1.93 L	73
FEV_1/FVC	75%	
MEF_{50}	1.85	59

    A. Ipatropium
    B. Inhaled corticosteroids
    C. Methotrexate
    D. Oral albuterol tablets
    E. Antihistamines

60. Which one of the following pharmacologic agents can precipitate bronchospasm in asthmatics?

    A. Oral captopril
    B. Timolol ophthalmic solution
    C. Intravenous nitroprusside
    D. Subcutaneous heparin
    E. Nicotine patches

61. Which one of the following occupations is associated with new-onset asthma with evidence of airway hyperreactivity?

    A. Paint sprayer
    B. Insulation installer
    C. Typist
    D. Truck driver
    E. Oceanographer

62. A 28-year-old HIV-positive woman presents to the emergency room with shortness of breath and a Po_2 of 62. A chemistry profile shows a serum LDH level of 1000. What is the most likely cause of the patient's respiratory complaints?

    A. Pulmonary alveolar proteinosis
    B. Pulmonary embolism
    C. *Pneumocystis carinii* pneumonia
    D. Congestive heart failure
    E. Pulmonary tuberculosis

63. Which of the following pulmonary function tests can be useful in the diagnosis of occult pulmonary hemorrhage?

    A. Forced expiratory volume in 1 second (FEV_1)
    B. Forced vital capacity (FVC)
    C. Total lung capacity
    D. Diffusing capacity for carbon monoxide
    E. Functional residual capacity

64. Which of the following is the most common malignancy associated with asbestos exposure?

    A. Pleural mesothelioma
    B. Non-Hodgkin's lymphoma of the lung

    C. Bronchogenic carcinoma
    D. Esophageal carcinoma
    E. Osteosarcoma

65. Which one of the following can be effectively diagnosed by bronchoscopy and transbronchial lung biopsy?

    A. Idiopathic pulmonary fibrosis
    B. Bronchiolitis obliterans with organizing pneumonia
    C. Pulmonary lymphangitic carcinomatosis
    D. Asbestosis
    E. Bleomycin pulmonary toxicity

66. Which of the following is the most common bacteria involved in pulmonary superinfection after influenza infection?

    A. *Staphylococcus aureus*
    B. *Nocardia asteroides*
    C. *Streptococcus pneumoniae*
    D. *Haemophilus influenzae*
    E. *Yersinia pestis*

67. Which one of the following is *not* a risk factor for developing pulmonary side effects from bleomycin administration?

    A. Cumulative drug dose
    B. Previous radiation therapy
    C. High inspired oxygen concentration
    D. Older age
    E. Concurrent administration with allopurinol

68. Which one of the following organisms more commonly infects the lungs of patients with pulmonary alveolar proteinosis than normal lungs?

    A. *Nocardia asteroides*
    B. Influenza A
    C. *Staphylococcus aureus*
    D. *Streptococcus pneumoniae*
    E. *Haemophilus influenzae*

69. Which one of the following is the most effective therapy for obstructive sleep apnea?

    A. Nasal continuous positive airway pressure
    B. Tracheostomy
    C. Uvulopalatopharyngoplasty
    D. Low-flow oxygen
    E. Oral prostaglandin E

70. Which of the following conditions or situations is *not* an indication for receiving a yearly influenza trivalent vaccine?

    A. Pregnancy
    B. Employment in a nursing home
    C. A 65-year-old man with no underlying medical condition
    D. A child with juvenile rheumatoid arthritis
    E. A 40-year-old woman with SLE

71. A 45-year-old man presents to your clinic for advice. As part of a routine physical, he was noted to have a 5-TU PPD that resulted in 6 mm of induration. He has no risk factors for HIV infection and does not know of any previous exposure to tuberculosis. What would be the next step in his evaluation?

    A. Place a ''second''-strength (25-TU) PPD
    B. Retest with a 5-TU PPD
    C. Order a chest radiograph
    D. Start isoniazid, 300 mg per day
    E. Advise him that the small amount of induration is insignificant and does not require treatment

72. A 24-year-old baker presents with symptoms of wheezing and shortness of breath that commonly occur after he has been at work for 1 to 2 hours. Pulmonary function tests show evidence of small airway obstruction. Which one of the following is the inhaled medication of choice for this problem?

    A. Ipatropium
    B. Cromolyn sodium
    C. Albuterol
    D. Beclomethasone
    E. Atropine

73. A 56-year-old woman neglects to tell you that she has a history of asthma. You have recently started her on propranolol for migraine headaches and she now presents to your clinic with severe wheezing and shortness of breath. Which of the following should be administered by inhalation immediately?

    A. Ipatropium
    B. Cromolyn sodium
    C. Albuterol
    D. Beclomethasone
    E. Epinephrine

74. Which of the following is *not* part of the diagnostic criteria for allergic bronchopulmonary aspergillosis?

    A. Proximal bronchiectasis
    B. History of asthma
    C. Eosinophilia
    D. Late-phase airway reaction to inhaled *Aspergillus* antigen
    E. Elevated serum immunoglobulin (Ig) E levels

75. Which one of the following serologies is helpful in distinguishing drug-induced SLE from the idiopathic form?

    A. Anti–histone H2A-H2B antibodies
    B. ANAs

    C. Anti–double stranded DNA antibodies
    D. Anti–extractable nuclear antigen antibodies
    E. Anti–neutrophil cytoplasmic antibodies

76. Appropriate treatment for Wegener's granulomatosis is which of the following?

    A. Prednisone alone
    B. Combined prednisone/cyclophosphamide followed by cyclophosphamide alone
    C. Colchicine
    D. Azathioprine
    E. Plasmapheresis

77. Which one of the following statements is true regarding patients with Langerhans' cell granulomatosis?

    A. The majority are females.
    B. Severe symptoms are almost always present when the chest radiograph is abnormal.
    C. Extrapulmonary involvement is common.
    D. The great majority are smokers.
    E. Improvement in disease rarely occurs without corticosteroid therapy.

78. Which of the following patients with pulmonary thromboembolism will benefit more from treatment with thrombolytic agents followed by heparin and coumadin instead of only heparin followed by coumadin?

    A. A 68-year-old with cor pulmonale caused by chronic pulmonary emboli
    B. A 25-year-old woman with hypotension caused by a massive pulmonary embolism
    C. A 50-year-old with chest pain and a pleural-based infiltrate on chest radiograph
    D. A 40-year-old with hemoptysis and chest pain
    E. An 80-year-old male who develops abrupt dyspnea 2 weeks after a cerebrovascular accident (CVA)

79. Which of the following laboratory values are elevated in 50% or more of patients with sarcoidosis?

    A. Calcium
    B. Gamma globulins
    C. Creatinine
    D. ANA
    E. Amylase

PULMONARY DISEASES

ANSWERS

1.(C) *Discussion:* The majority of patients with obstructive sleep apnea are men, by a 7:1 to 20:1 ratio. In general, patients with sleep apnea are not aware of arousal after episodes of apnea. Although sleep apnea can occur at any age, the usual age of onset is 40 to 50 years and the incidence increases with age from that point. Weight loss can improve symptoms of apnea, but the majority of affected patients need some other form of therapy. (*Kales et al*)

2.(E) *Discussion:* Patients with hypothyroidism have blunted respiratory drive responses to hypercapnea and hypoxia. In addition, goiters associated with this problem can add to upper airway obstruction. The association of acromegaly and Down's syndrome is probably due to redundant upper airway tissue that results in obstruction at night. Normal individuals demonstrate some evidence of mild airway obstruction at night; this is amplified by the presence of chronic obstructive pulmonary disease (COPD). Although the most common apnea associated with COPD is hyponea, intermittent upper airway obstruction with apnea also occurs. (*Kales et al*)

3.(E) *Discussion:* Virtually 100% of patients with obstructive sleep apnea are noted to snore. However, snoring does not necessarily imply the presence of apnea, and relief of snoring with upper airway surgery does not necessarily mean apnea has been adequately treated. Somnambulism occurs to a greater degree in patients with obstructive sleep apnea than in unaffected patients, but it is still relatively uncommon. Increased gastroesophageal reflux occurs, probably as a result of a marked decline in intrathoracic pressures during airway obstruction. Enurisis occurs in approximately 5% of patients affected with obstructive sleep apnea. (*Kales et al*)

4.(G) *Discussion:* In addition to night time symptoms, patients with obstructive sleep apnea can demonstrate abnormalities during the day as a result of the sleep disturbance that is associated with the syndrome. Hypersomnolence and automatic behavior probably occur as a result of loss of normal sleep architecture. Early morning headaches occur commonly, probably secondary to the hypercarbia that results from the intermittent apnea spells. Intermittent daytime paralysis does not occur in patients with obstructive sleep apnea; this is a symptom of narcolepsy. (*Kales et al*)

5.(G) *Discussion:* In general, all cases of mesothelioma are probably associated with some degree of asbestos exposure. In contrast to pleural plaques, the incidence of mesothelioma is not dose related; small amounts of inhaled asbestos can result in this malignancy. The incidence of bronchogenic carcinoma is mildly increased in subjects exposed to asbestos alone but is markedly increased in patients with both asbestos and tobacco smoke exposure. Pleural effusion caused by asbestos exposure can occur in the setting of malignancy caused by this material but can also be due to a benign pleurisy induced by very little asbestos exposure. Although a respiratory bronchiolitis can occur early after asbestos exposure, emphysema is not caused by this agent. (*Cecil, Ch. 54*)

6.(H) *Discussion:* The chest radiograph shows evidence of pneumonia with some volume loss. Because the patient presents with hemoptysis, bronchoscopy is indicated at some point during the patient's care. Other indications for bronchoscopy in this case would be a poorly resolving pneumonia or recurrence of the pneumonia in the same location. Sputum cytologies would not be of use in this patient because acute infection can affect cytopathologic examination. A CT scan of the head or abdomen would only be indicated if the patient has symptomatology or physical signs suggestive of abnormalities in these areas. (*Cecil, Ch. 55; American Thoracic Society*)

7.(D) *Discussion:* Resection of bronchogenic carcinoma is the best hope for cure of a patient. Therefore, thorough examination is needed to establish that a particular finding is definitely a contraindication to resection. Paraneoplastic hypercalcemia can be due to release of a parathyroid-like hormone that is not indicative of metastases; thus an elevated serum calcium level in the setting of bronchogenic carcinoma is not necessarily a contraindication to surgery. Pleural effusion can be caused by proximal obstruction resulting from the carcinoma and does not necessarily indicate pleural metastases. Mediastinal adenopathy on CT scan also does not necessarily indicate tumor involvement; tissue sampling by mediastinoscopy or thoracotomy is indicated prior to rejecting the patient for surgery. Documented hepatic metastases suggest metastatic disease and are a contraindication for resection. (*Cecil, Ch. 62; Bains*)

8.(E) *Discussion:* Transudative pleural effusions occur as a result of either a lowering of plasma oncotic pressure, an increase in the normal fluid flux through elevation of hydrostatic pressure, or impaired drainage of normal pleural fluid flux. Congestive heart failure causes a transudative effusion through elevation of pulmonary vascular pressures, with a subsequent increase in hydrostatic pressure. Hypothyroidism causes a transudative effusion through somewhat unclear mechanisms, although the cardiomyopathy associated with the syndrome may be the link between the two processes. Ureteral obstruction is a rare cause of transudative effusion, probably because of fluid leaking from the obstructed kidney through diaphragmatic pores into the pleural space. Elevated pleural fluid creatinine level is a hallmark of this problem. (*Cecil, Ch. 63; Sahn*)

9.(E) *Discussion:* Although the clinical situation must dictate the need for chest tube drainage in a particular patient, certain fluid characteristics suggest it may be necessary. All of the findings noted in the question suggest the fluid is an empyema with large numbers of inflammatory cells metabolizing glucose, resulting in a low pleural fluid glucose level, and producing carbon dioxide, resulting in a low pleural fluid pH. The markedly elevated pleural fluid LDH level suggests the normal filtration barrier has been markedly disrupted by the process. Although pleural effusions with some of these parameters might respond to conservative measures, a pleural effusion with a positive Gram's stain virtually never responds to anything less than chest tube drainage and antibiotic therapy. (*Cecil, Ch. 63; Sahn*)

10.(G) *Discussion:* Bronchitis secondary to infection or environmental exposures is the most common cause of hemoptysis. However, other causes must be considered when a patient presents with this syndrome. Bronchiectasis is a potential cause of massive hemoptysis; occasionally, vascular embolization or lung resection is needed to control hemorrhage in this setting. Aspergilloma within cavities can also cause massive hemoptysis. The diagnosis is suggested by a rounded opacity within the cavity that changes in location with position of the patient. Pulmonary embolism can cause hemoptysis, although this is rarely massive and is usually associated with an infiltrate/density on chest radiograph. Although asthma is a form of bronchitis, it does not cause hemoptysis, probably because of the species of inflammatory cells present in the bronchus in this condition. (*Cecil, Ch. 49; Winter and Ingbar*)

11.(F) *Discussion:* Asthma is a disease associated with bronchial edema, increased mucus production, and heightened bronchial reactivity to nonspecific agents such as histamine or methacholine. In general, tissue distruction does not occur in this syndrome until very late in its course, when subepithelial fibrosis may develop. Therefore, unlike emphysema, the diffusing capacity for carbon monoxide is normal in asthmatics and the airway obstruction is reversible to a variable degree. Proximal bronchiectasis can occur in the setting of allergic bronchopulmonary aspergillosis in the setting of asthma but does not occur in asthmatics without this syndrome. (*Cecil, Ch. 51*)

12.(E) *Discussion:* Rheumatoid arthritis can cause a variety of thoracic abnormalities. Risk factors for developing these abnormalities are the presence of (1) severe articular disease, (2) high rheumatoid factor titers, (3) subcutaneous nodules, and (4) systemic manifestations such as Felty's syndrome or myopericarditis. The most common thoracic abnormality associated with this disease is pleural effusion. Pulmonary nodules caused by rheumatoid arthritis are usually multiple and may cavitate. They usually are present in patients with concomitant subcutaneous nodules and are histologically indistinguishable. Hyperexpansion on chest radiograph may occur secondary to bronchiolitis obliterans associated with rheumatoid arthritis. In general, this problem is resistant to therapy. Reticulonodular infiltrates occur in conjunction with pulmonary fibrosis caused by rheumatoid arthritis as well as other collagen vascular diseases. (*Cecil, Ch. 54; Hunninghake and Fauci*)

13.(D) *Discussion:* The pulmonary function tests demonstrate a restrictive ventilatory defect with reduced lung volumes and increased FEV_1/FVC ratio. In addition, the diffusing capacity is decreased, suggesting a tissue-damaging process rather than simple respiratory muscle weakness. A number of diseases can cause this pulmonary function abnormality, which is indicative of an interstitial pulmonary process. These include hypersensitivity pneumonitis, collagen vascular diseases such as SLE, idiopathic pulmonary fibrosis, and sarcoidosis. Although serum precipitins are commonly elevated in patients with hypersensitivity pneumonitis, they are not diagnostic of this disorder because they may be elevated in subjects who have been exposed to thermophilic fungi but have no pulmonary disease. In addition, an elevated ANA titer is not diagnostic of a particular pulmonary process because it may be positive at low titer in patients with idiopathic pulmonary fibrosis as well as patients with SLE. Gallium scanning of the lungs is also nonspecific because it will be positive in lungs with virtually any type of inflammation from infectious or noninfectious causes. Of all the possible answers to this question, open lung biopsy is the only test that will commonly differentiate among all of the causes of restrictive ventilatory defects. (*Cecil, Ch. 54*)

14.(F) *Discussion:* More than 50% of patients with rheumatoid arthritis develop some degree of pulmonary disease. Specific syndromes, as noted previously, include (1) pleural disease, (2) pulmonary nodules, (3) bronchiolitis obliterans with or without organizing pneumonia, (4) upper airway obstruction, and (5) interstitial pneumonitis. In contrast to the overall population of patients with rheumatoid arthritis, men outnumber women who have pulmonary disease caused by this disease. In addition to male gender, high rheumatoid titer and subcutaneous nodules are risk factors for development of pulmonary disease in patients with rheumatoid arthritis. In contrast, smoking history appears to have no effect on development of pulmonary disease in this setting. (*Cecil, Ch. 54; Hunninghake and Fauci*)

15.(H) *Discussion:* Although pleural fibrosis is common in patients with scleroderma, pleural effusion is uncommon. Any form of pleural disease is uncommon in patients with polymyositis or dermatomyositis. Pleural effusion caused by rheumatoid arthritis is exudative, with low pH and low glucose level. A rheumatoid factor titer >1:320 is suggestive that a pleural effusion is due to rheumatoid arthritis. Pleural effusion in SLE is commonly associated with pleuritic pain. A pleural fluid ANA titer >1:160 is suggestive that the effusion is due to SLE. (*Cecil, Ch. 54; Hunninghake and Fauci*)

16.(E) *Discussion:* Overall, 4% of patients who receive bleomycin will develop pulmonary fibrosis as a result of use of the drug. However, certain risk factors markedly increase the chance of pulmonary side effects caused by this drug. In addition to the elements listed in the question, oxygen therapy can increase the risk of bleomycin pulmonary toxicity. (*Cecil, Ch. 54; Cooper et al*)

17.(E) *Discussion:* The three general factors that contribute to clot formation are stasis, trauma to blood vessels, and clotting abnormalities. Immobilization and obesity probably predispose to clot formation through venous stasis. Malignancy may predispose to clot formation through stasis resulting from obstruction by the malignancy or through paraneoplastic clotting abnormalities. Body trauma results in damage to blood vessels, with subsequent changes in endothelium that makes it more susceptible to clot formation. In addition to the factors listed, other factors that predispose to clot formation include surgery, particularly of the pelvis or hip area; excess estrogen states; advanced age; and primary hypercoagulable states. (*Cecil, Ch. 59; Moser*)

18.(G) *Discussion:* Although localized wheezing occurs rarely with pulmonary thromboembolism caused by pneumoconstriction, diffuse wheezing does not occur. Pulmonary infarction occurs as a result of occlusion of the pulmonary artery at a site distal to bronchial artery inflow, resulting in poor oxygenation of a segment of the lung. Acute right heart failure results from occlusion of greater than 50% of the pulmonary arterial circulation; presentation is generally associated with shock or syncope. Fever and elevated white blood cell count can occur with pulmonary embolism, although significant fever should not continue for more than 24 to 48 hours. (*Cecil, Ch. 59; Moser*)

19.(A) *Discussion:* Fibrinolytic agents are indicated in pulmonary embolic events that result in acute cor pulmonale with hypotension. Fibrinolytic agents have essentially replaced embolectomy and can be life saving in this setting. The major side effect of fibrinolytic agents is bleeding. If a patient has a potential site of bleeding that may be life threatening, such as a previous CVA, these are contraindicated. Although the other factors listed in the question are relative contraindications to the use of fibrinolytic agents, they are not absolute contraindications. (*Cecil, Ch. 59; Moser*)

20.(G) *Discussion:* Recent American Thoracic Society guidelines have changed the interpretation of PPD tests based on pretesting probability of tuberculosis infection. In the past, a cutoff of 10 mm of induration was used to determine positive versus negative reaction. However, currently 5 mm of induration constitutes a positive reaction in subjects with (1) a history of close contact with a patient with tuberculosis, (2) a chest radiograph suggestive of old tuberculosis, or (3) HIV-positive status. Patients in whom 10 mm of induration is currently considered to constitute a positive reaction are (1) patients with underlying diseases that predispose to reactivation of tuberculosis; (2) patients from foreign countries that have a high prevalence of tuberculosis; (3) low income, medically underserved patients; (4) alcohol and intravenous drug abusers; (5) nursing home residents; and (6) health care workers. PPD in all other subjects is not considered positive unless it is greater or equal to 15 mm of induration. (*Cecil, Ch. 311; American Thoracic Society/Centers for Disease Control*)

21.(G) *Discussion:* A number of different regimens have been devised to prevent thrombosis in high-risk situations. The benefits of these regimens must be balanced with the potential complications. A regimen containing heparin at 5000 units subcutaneously every 12 hours has been used in general surgery patients, as well as post–myocardial infarction (MI) and post-CVA patients. A regimen containing a similar dose of heparin on an every-8-hour schedule has been used with success in post-MI patients as well as general surgery patients with a higher risk than those given the every-12-hour regimen. A potential side effect of these regimens that must be kept in mind is heparin-induced thrombocytopenia. Intermittent pneumatic compression has the advantage of causing few side effects. This mode of prophylaxis has been used in a number of patient populations, including general surgery patients, post–knee surgery patients, trauma patients, and post-MI or -CVA patients. Streptokinase has not been used as prophylaxis against clot formation because (1) it is a fibrinolytic agent and dissolves clot rather than preventing it, and (2) it has serious potential side effects. (*Cecil, Ch. 59; Moser*)

22.(G) *Discussion:* Please refer to the comments associated with the answer to question 20. Because the risk of hepatitis caused by isoniazid increases with age, individuals with a positive PPD and no other risk factors are treated with this drug only if they are young (a cutoff of 35 years of age has been proposed). For this reason, the patient in A would be treated with isoniazid, whereas the patient in B would not. Because the patient in C suffers from an underlying disease (silicosis) that predisposes him to reactivation of tuberculosis, isoniazid prophylaxis is indicated. The patient in D would be treated because, despite his age, he is in an environment where he has the potential to spread tuberculosis to numerous individuals. (*Cecil, Ch. 311; American Thoracic Society/Centers for Disease Control*)

23.(H) *Discussion:* A number of antituberculosis medications are hepatotoxic, including rifampin, pyrazinamide, and isoniazid. In general, hepatitis induced by isoniazid is reversible unless there is underlying liver disease. Peripheral neuropathy induced by isoniazid is commonly responsive to thiamine; other antituberculosis medications do not cause a peripheral neuropathy. Orange discoloration of secretions is a complication of rifampin therapy; the discoloration is harmless. Thrombocytopenia is also a significant side effect of rifampin only. (*Cecil, Ch. 311; American Thoracic Society/Centers for Disease Control*)

24.(G) *Discussion:* Low glucose levels in pleural fluid can occur as a result of the presence of inflammatory cells that metabolize glucose or as a result of an alteration in glucose transport into the pleural space. It appears that a low pleural fluid glucose level in patients with rheumatoid arthritis is due to the latter mechanism. Studies have shown that administration of intravenous glucose does not increase the pleural fluid glucose level in these patients in a manner similar to that in control patients with pleural effusions. Although the cause of a low pleural glucose level in esophageal perforation or tuberculosis is not entirely clear, the low level is probably due to intense inflammatory reaction induced by these processes. Pulmonary embolism may induce a pleural effusion, but the glucose level is generally normal. (*Cecil, Ch. 63; Sahn*)

25.(G) *Discussion:* The most common location for aspiration pneumonia to occur is the lower lobe superior segment, followed by the lower lobe posterior basal segment. Aspiration pneumonias such as those that occur after passing out as a result of drinking alcohol or during a seizure are due commonly to anaerobic organisms. Therefore, an elicited history of excessive alcohol consumption would be important. Influenza infection also results in a shift in the type of organisms that cause pneumonia. Influenza predisposes an individual to bacterial pneumonias and, with *Staphylococcus aureus,* plays a greater role than in community-acquired pneumonias in the absence of previous influenza infection. Building excavation sites are a common source of certain pathologic fungi, particularly *Histoplasma capsulatum.* Therefore, although a localized lobar pneumonia would be atypical for this organism, this part of the history would be important. Conversely, although pneumonia caused by *Legionella pneumophila* was first reported at a convention for legionnaires, it has been shown to be a major cause of pneumonia in all patient groups. (*Cecil, Ch. 55; American Thoracic Society*)

26.(E) *Discussion: Mycoplasma pneumoniae* only exists in a human resevoir. Only 3 to 10% of infections result in pneumonia; the rest result in an upper respiratory illness. Bullous myringitis, when seen, should strongly suggest *Mycoplasma* infection. However, this manifestation, although relatively specific for the organism, is relatively rare. All of the other manifestations listed can be associated with *Mycoplasma* infection. The finding of cold agglutinin hemolytic anemia in a patient with pneumonia should strongly suggest *Mycoplasma* infection. (*Cecil, Ch. 55; American Thoracic Society*)

27.(H) *Discussion:* The most common causes of community-acquired pneumonia are *Mycoplasma pneumoniae, Streptococcus pneumoniae,* and *Haemophilis influenzae,* in that order. *Staphylococcus aureus* and *Pseudomonas aeruginosa* are relatively uncommon causes of community-acquired pneumonia except in the presence of other complicating factors such as COPD. In contrast, patients who are hospitalized more commonly develop pneumonias caused by other staphylococci or *Pseudomonas,* possibly because of the change in flora secondary to antibiotic therapy. (*Cecil, Ch. 55; American Thoracic Society*)

28.(E) *Discussion:* Chronic cough may be due to a variety of mechanisms. In cases in which the cause of chronic cough goes undiagnosed for several months, certain specific problems should be considered. Occult asthma with only mild reductions in flow rates is a common cause of this problem. Because inhaled beta-adrenergic agonists can sometimes precipitate the cough, the oral forms may be more effective. Chronic esophageal reflux is also a common cause of cough as a result of either aspiration of refluxed material or a reflex triggered by acid reflux into the lower esophagus. Patients with left ventricular dysfunction can also present with cough. This group of patients is hypersensitive to inhalation of methacholine, suggesting they have hyperactive airways similarly to patients with traditional asthma. Postnasal drip can be difficult to control and may cause chronic cough that does not diminish until sinus drainage is controlled. If cough persists despite efforts at treatment, bronchoscopy should be considered to rule out an endobronchial lesion as the cause of the cough. (*Cecil, Ch. 49*)

29.(G) *Discussion:* The chest radiograph shows bilateral hilar adenopathy and pulmonary infiltrates. These findings are most consistent with the diagnosis of sarcoidosis. However, diagnosis of sarcoidosis requires examination of involved tissue for findings of noncaseating granulomas. Although serum ACE levels can be elevated in patients with sarcoid, this is not 100% sensitive or specific. Other granulomatous diseases can result in a mild elevation in serum ACE levels. Three complications of sarcoidosis that are indications for corticosteroid therapy are (1) hypercalcemia, (2) uveitis, and (3) heart block. Appropriate tests for these complications are indicated in the evaluation of a patient with sarcoidosis. (*Cecil, Ch. 61*)

30.(C); 31.(A); 32.(D); 33.(B) *Discussion:* Secretion of hormone-like substances by bronchogenic carcinoma may result in a variety of paraneoplastic syndromes. Secretion of ectopic adrenocorticotrophic hormone (ACTH) occurs most commonly in the setting of small cell carcinoma of the lung. However, carcinoid tumors of the lung can also rarely produce ACTH. Hypercalcemia can occur via a number of mechanisms. However, the most common cause is a parathyroid-like peptide secreted by a number of tumor types, including nonbronchogenic carcinomas. Squamous cell carcinoma is the most common form of bronchogenic carcinoma that is associated with hypercalcemia. Bronchoalveolar carcinoma is a malignancy consisting of cells resembling airway lining cells. The chest radiograph manifestation of the malignancy is commonly an alveolar-like infiltrate that may contain air bronchograms. Adenocarcinoma of the lung is the bronchogenic carcinoma most likely to cause a single metastasis to the brain. In contrast, squamous cell carcinoma usually invades locally and small cell carcinoma metastasizes distally but usually in multiple sites. (*Cecil, Ch. 61*)

34.(E); 35.(B); 36.(C); 37.(D); 38.(A) *Discussion:* Pleural fluid exists in a balanced state between formation and absorption of fluid at the parietal surface. Excessive formation of pleural fluid results from an alteration in this balance. Increased formation may occur as a result of a reduction in plasma oncotic pressure (as in cirrhosis) or increased hydrostatic pressure (as in urinary obstruction or congestive heart failure), resulting in a transudation of plasma that is filtered through a relatively normal pleura, making the resultant transudate low in protein. Increased fluid formation can also occur as a result of involvement of the pleural surface with a process that alters the normal filtering process, and thus the resultant pleural fluid is relatively high in protein. One protein, LDH, is used to determine the amount of protein exudation into the pleural fluid. A value greater than 200 IU per liter or a ratio of pleural fluid LDH to serum LDH of greater 0.6 is strongly suggestive of an exudative pleural effusion. A ratio of total protein in the pleural fluid to serum total protein of greater than 0.5 is also suggestive of an exudative pleural effusion. Low glucose level or pH in pleural fluid is suggestive of an inflammatory process that results from metabolism of glucose, with formation of CO_2 and subsequent lowering of pH. A reduction in glucose can also occur as a result of impaired glucose transport into the pleural space, as in the case of pleural effusion caused by rheumatoid arthritis. Amylase may be elevated in pleural fluid for a variety of reasons, including carcinomatosis and pancreatitis. (*Cecil, Ch. 63; Sahn*)

39.(C); 40.(G); 41.(B); 42.(C); 43.(F) *Discussion:* "Atypical pneumonias" (i.e., pneumonias with no culturable organism) are commonly caused by *Mycoplasma* or *Legionella* infection. Both of these organisms are susceptible to erythromycin therapy. *Chlamydia psittaci* can also cause an atypical pneumonia. Although this organism may be partially responsive to erythromycin, doxycycline is currently the drug of choice. *Pseudomonas aeruginosa,* a major cause of nosocomial pneumonia, has developed resistance patterns over the years, making use of certain agents, such as ampicillin, ineffective against this organism. In addition, although ciprofloxacin is an effective antibiotic against *Pseudomonas,* the development of resistance can be rapid, so ciprofloxacin is indicated only in infections caused by strains of *Pseudomonas* that are documented to be resistant to other agents. Although influenza A infection is responsive to amantadine, influenza B is resistant. In fact, no currently available agents are effective against influenza B infection. (*Cecil, Ch. 55; American Thoracic Society*)

44.(A); 45.(D); 46.(A,B); 47.(E); 48.(F); 49.(C,E); 50.(B,C); 51.(B); 52.(F); 53.(D); 54.(B,C) *Discussion:* Airway obstruction, occurring in either large proximal airways or smaller peripheral airways, can be due to a number of processes. Bronchial obstruction occurs in the setting of bronchitis caused by bronchial edema and mucus impaction. Bronchitis may occur as a result of environmental exposures, such as tobacco abuse, or occupational exposure, as in byssinosis caused by cotton dust exposure in textile mills. Asthma is a form of bronchitis that is associated with influx of eosinophils into the airway. All asthmatics have hyper-responsiveness to inhalation of certain agents such as methacholine or histamine. Asthmatics are also the patient population who are susceptible to allergic bronchopulmonary aspergillosis, a syndrome in which *Aspergillus* colonization of the bronchus results in an immediate hypersensitivity reaction to the organism, with resultant increased IgE levels and exacerbation of asthma. It appears that this syndrome results from development of specific IgE antibodies to *Aspergillus.* Physical examination findings can help in differentiation of forms of airway obstruction. Of all of the disorders listed, only bronchiectasis has conclusively been shown to cause clubbing. Stridor (inspiratory wheezing) is also suggestive of upper airway obstruction at an extrathoracic site; this may be associated with flattening of the inspiratory flow-volume loop. Bronchiolitis obliterans, a process in which bronchioles are gradually obliterated by either intraluminal or extraluminal processes, may occur secondary to a number of disorders, including rheumatoid arthritis and chlorine gas exposure, as well as other problems such as drug exposure or viral infections. Emphysema, most commonly caused by tobacco abuse, can also occur as a result of deficiency of AlAP, a protein that protects the lung against protease digestion. Emphysema, in contrast to asthma, is commonly associated with a reduction in the diffusing capacity for carbon monoxide. (*Cecil, Ch. 51 and 52*)

55.(A—False; B—True; C—True; D—False; E—False; F—True) *Discussion:* A number of phenotypes of the AlAP gene can cause deficiency and subsequent disease syndromes. Major disease syndromes that are caused by deficiency of this protein are emphysema and cirrhosis. Patients with emphysema caused by this deficiency commonly present at early ages and have lower lobe bullous lung disease,

in contrast to the bullous lung disease induced by smoking, which is usually upper lobe. Interestingly, liver and lung disease caused by AlAP deficiency are generally independent and rarely occur in the same patient. Administration of recombinant AlAP either intravenously or by aerosol can result in raised alveolar levels of this protein. Lung transplantation can also result in normal alveolar levels of this protein, which is produced by the transplanted lung. (*Cecil, Ch. 51 and 52*)

56.(A—False; B—True; C—True; D—True; E—True; F—False; G—False) *Discussion:* Hemoptysis can occur as a result of a number of disorders, the most common of which are bronchitis, bronchiectasis, infection, and malignancy. Massive hemoptysis (>200 to 500 ml per 24 hours) can be due to a number of processes, including lung abscess and even simple bronchitis. In general, even when a patient is receiving anticoagulant therapy, hemoptysis is due to a pathologic process. In addition, although onset of purulent phlegm preceding hemoptysis may suggest bronchitis is the cause of the bleeding, other causes should be ruled out, especially in smokers. A history of expectorating sputum with hard material ("gritty sputum") should suggest broncholithiasis caused by a calcified lymph node eroding into a bronchus, causing hemoptysis and occasionally atelectasis. Active or inactive tuberculosis can cause hemoptysis. When it is due to active infection, the chance of a positive sputum smear for acid-fast bacilli is higher. Serum precipitins for *Aspergillus* are commonly elevated in patients with aspergilloma but they are not specific; patients without aspergilloma may also show positive precipitins. (*Cecil, Ch. 49; Winter and Ingbar*)

57.(A—False; B—False; C—True; D—True; E—True; F—True) *Discussion:* Pulmonary thromboembolism most commonly results from embolism of clots originating in the large pelvic or lower extremity veins. However, pulmonary embolism can also originate from upper extremity thrombophlebitis. Acute cor pulmonale can occur after pulmonary embolism but only when at least 50 to 66% of the pulmonary vasculature has been obstructed. Chest radiograph findings are usually very nonspecific in pulmonary embolism. Although asymmetrical hypoperfusion may be present, it is a rare phenomenon. Impedance plethysmography is more specific for identification of clot in lower extremity veins, but it can be obscured by venous stasis. Intermittent pneumatic compression prevents clot formation, probably through stimulation of endothelium prostacyclin production, and is the method of choice for prophylaxis against post–knee surgery clot formation. (*Cecil, Ch. 59; Moser*)

58.(A—True; B—True; C—False; D—True; E—False; F—True) *Discussion:* All collagen vascular diseases can result in a variable degree of pulmonary side effects. These side effects can result in a number of disease syndromes that may overlap between specific collagen vascular diseases. At autopsy, >50% of patients with rheumatoid arthritis have some evidence of pulmonary disease, which may manifest as (1) pleural effusion, (2) necrobiotic nodules, (3) bronchiolitis obliterans with organizing pneumonia, (4) upper airway obstruction caused by cricoarytenoid arthritis, or (5) interstitial pneumonitis. Smoking does not increase the risk of developing any of these complications of rheumatoid arthritis. Scleroderma also can cause a variety of pulmonary complications, including (1) isolated pulmonary hypertension, (2) pulmonary fibrosis, and (3) aspiration resulting from esophageal abnormalities. An isolated reduction in diffusing capacity for carbon monoxide without reductions in lung volumes in a patient with scleroderma should raise the suspicion of pulmonary vascular disease. SLE can also cause a variety of pulmonary complications. Pleurisy caused by SLE is usually painful. The presence of lupus cells in the pleural fluid is diagnostic of lupus pleuritis. Although an ANA titer that is greater in pleural fluid than serum is suggestive of lupus pleuritis, an ANA titer that is equal to or less than the serum titer is not specific for lupus pleuritis. (*Cecil, Ch. 54; Hunninghake and Fauci*)

59.(B) *Discussion:* The patient has mild airway obstruction on pulmonary function testing. Because the patient is a nonsmoker and relatively young, the most likely diagnosis is asthma. The current recommendations for the treatment of asthma include early use of inhaled corticosteroids to reduce bronchial inflammation. Although inhaled beta-adrenergic agonists might be helpful in this patient to relieve symptoms, they should only be used as needed, while inhaled corticosteroids should be used on a regular basis. (*Cecil, Ch. 51*)

60.(B) *Discussion:* Airway tone is maintained by a balance between cholinergic and adrenergic tone. Increased cholinergic activity tends to produce bronchospasm, whereas enhanced adrenergic tone will produce bronchodilation. Any pharmacologic agents that can alter this balance may precipitate bronchospasm. Timolol, a beta-adrenergic antagonist, can precipitate bronchospasm by inhibiting normal adrenergic-modulated airway bronchodilation. ACE inhibitors such as captopril can induce cough in 10% of patients but have not been shown to induce bronchospasm in asthmatics. (*Cecil, Ch. 51*)

61.(A) *Discussion:* A large number of occupations have been associated with new-onset asthma. Agents that induce asthma in these settings range from low-molecular-weight compounds to larger molecular-weight substances such as proteins that induce specific allergic responses. Isocyanates are examples of low-molecular-weight substances that induce asthma. These compounds are found in spray paint and plastics. Although insulation installers may be exposed to significant amounts of asbestos, this would result in fibrosis rather than bronchospasm. (*Cecil, Ch. 54*)

62.(C) *Discussion:* The clinical scenario shows an HIV-positive patient with significant hypoxemia and elevated LDH. This combination should strongly suggest infection with *Pneumocystis carinii* pneumonia because serum LDH will be elevated, commonly to high levels, in a significant number of HIV antibody–positive patients with this infection. Serum LDH can also be useful to follow the treatment and outcome of patients with this infection. Commonly, serum LDH will diminish with treatment but elevate once again if there is a relapse of the infection. (*Cecil, Ch. 365*)

63.(D) *Discussion:* The diffusing capacity for carbon monoxide attempts to measure the surface area of alveolar capillary membrane by determining the amount of hemoglobin

in the thorax using the avid hemoglobin that binds carbon monoxide. Because hemoglobin that binds carbon monoxide can be intravascular or extravascular, as in the case of pulmonary hemorrhage, the diffusing capacity can quantitate the degree of pulmonary hemorrhage. This may be useful in certain disorders such as Goodpasture's syndrome, in which new hemorrhage can be relatively occult. (*Cecil, Ch. 50*)

64.(C) *Discussion:* Although malignant mesothelioma is essentially always associated with a history of exposure to asbestos, it is a relatively uncommon malignancy. In contrast, the risk of bronchogenic carcinoma, a common malignancy, increases markedly in the setting of combined asbestos and tobacco smoke exposure. Asbestos exposure alone also results in a two- to threefold increase in bronchogenic carcinoma. (*Cecil, Ch. 54*)

65.(C) *Discussion:* In contrast to pulmonary lymphangitic carcinomatosis, the other disorders listed in the question are associated with nonspecific or segmental histologic manifestations, making the diagnosis difficult from the amount of tissue obtained by transbronchial lung biopsy. In contrast, lymphangitic spread of tumor is generally diffuse and biopsy findings are specific. (*Cecil, Ch. 62*)

66.(C) *Discussion:* Influenza infection is associated with an increased risk of bacterial pneumonia. Although the relative makeup of pathogens that cause bacterial pneumonia after influenza infection is different than that in overall community-acquired pneumonia, *Pneumococcus* is still the most frequent pathogen. Interestingly, *Haemophilus influenzae* received its name because it was thought to cause influenza; this has since been disproven, and *H. influenzae* has been shown to frequently cause pneumonia even in the absence of influenza. Although it does cause postinfluenza pneumonia, the relative incidence in that setting is not particularly increased. Pneumonia caused by *Staphylococcus aureus* is increased in incidence after influenza infection, but the absolute incidence is still less than that of pneumococcal or *Hemophilus* infection. (*Cecil, Ch. 332*)

67.(E) *Discussion:* Bleomycin causes pulmonary side effects in approximately 4% of all patients who receive the drug. However, certain risk factors are associated with increased incidence of these reactions. Bleomycin forms reactive oxygen species as a mechanism of its action; this is probably why radiation and oxygen therapy synergize with bleomycin to cause pulmonary disease. Older age may predispose to bleomycin toxicity because of the natural loss in antioxidants associated with aging; however, this is not proven. To date, no studies have demonstrated synergistic toxicity between bleomycin and allopurinol. (*Cecil, Ch. 54; Cooper et al*)

68.(A) *Discussion:* For unclear reasons, the incidence of pulmonary nocardiosis is increased in patients with pulmonary alveolar proteinosis. One possibility is that some component in the phospholipid-laden fluid present in the alveoli of patients with this disorder may enhance growth of the organism; however, this has not been proven. The other organisms listed in the question can infect patients with pulmonary alveolar proteinosis but not to a greater degree than normal patients. (*Cecil, Ch. 307*)

69.(B) *Discussion:* Although other forms of therapy are less invasive, tracheostomy is the most effective therapy. Uvulopalatopharyngoplasty will be successful in approximately 45% of cases overall and is 75 to 80% successful if the level of obstruction is documented to be at the soft palate. The efficacy of low-flow oxygen is minimal, and intermittent apnea is certainly not reversed. Nasal continuous positive airway pressure is the preferred therapy for the majority of patients because of the noninvasive nature and efficacy of this therapy. Oral prostaglandin E has not been studied for the treatment of obstructive sleep apnea. (*Kales et al*)

70.(A) *Discussion:* Target groups for influenza vaccination include (1) persons 65 years of age or older; (2) residents of nursing homes; (3) adults or children with chronic disorders especially those receiving immunosuppressives; (4) children and teenagers who are receiving long-term aspirin therapy, such as those with juvenile rheumatoid arthritis; (5) health care workers, including nursing home workers; and (6) family members of patients with any of the above risk factors. (*Cecil, Ch. 332*)

71.(C) *Discussion:* As noted in the discussion of question 20, a PPD showing greater than 5 mm of induration is interpreted as positive if (1) the patient is HIV antibody positive, (2) a chest radiograph of the patient is consistent with tuberculosis infection, or (3) the patient has a history of close contact with a patient with tuberculosis. Because this patient has no evidence of HIV infection or history of tuberculosis exposure, a chest radiograph is needed to determine whether tuberculosis therapy is indicated. Although a repeat 5-TU PPD might be indicated to establish whether there is a booster response, this would not be needed if the chest radiograph is consistent with tuberculosis infection. A 25-TU PPD is generally no longer used in the clinical setting. (*Cecil, Ch. 311; American Thoracic Society/Centers for Disease Control*)

72.(B) *Discussion:* Asthma caused by allergens in flour dust is relatively common in bakers. A large percentage of bakers develop antibodies to flour, and a subset of these will develop asthma. Baker's asthma is probably associated with release of inflammatory mediators such as leukotrienes that are important in other forms of allergen-induced asthma, such as that caused by pollen inhalation. Cromolyn, an agent that blunts release of these mediators, can be effective in this situation. Alternatively, filter masks can be used to reduce exposure to allergen; this may be highly effective, although somewhat cumbersome. (*Cecil, Ch. 54*)

73.(A) *Discussion:* As noted in question number 60, airway tone is maintained by a balance between cholinergic and adrenergic stimulation. Ablation of adrenergic tone, as in the patient presented, can result in bronchospasm via blockage of adrenergic receptors by propranolol. Because the adrenergic receptors are blocked, treatment with adrenergic agonists such as albuterol or epinephrine would be ineffective. In addition, treatment with anti-inflammatory agents such as cromolyn or beclomethasone would also be ineffective in this patient because the onset of action of these agents is slow. Therefore, ipatropium, an agent that increases cho-

linergic tone, is the agent of choice in this patient. (*Cecil, Ch. 51*)

74.(D) *Discussion:* Allergic bronchopulmonary aspergillosis is a disorder that occurs in asthmatics who develop specific IgE antibodies to *Aspergillus*, with resultant worsening of their asthma and subsequent proximal bronchiectasis. These patients appear to develop immediate hypersensitivity reactions to the fungus, with subsequent eosinophilia and greatly elevated (usually >1000 IU per ml) IgE levels. Treatment with corticosteroids is monitored by measuring sequential serum IgE levels and tapering the corticosteroids when they return toward normal. (*Cecil, Ch. 51*)

75.(A) *Discussion:* Drug-induced SLE is more commonly associated with pulmonary disease than native SLE but less commonly associated with renal disease. Antihistone antibodies are the only test that reliably distinguishes the two different forms of SLE. Anti–neutrophil cytoplasmic antibodies are useful in the diagnosis of Wegener's granulomatosis, not in the diagnosis of SLE. (*Cecil, Ch. 240*)

76.(B) *Discussion:* Wegener's granulomatosis is a vasculitis that can involve the lungs, sinuses, and kidneys as well as multiple other organs. Lung biopsy in involved areas shows necrotizing granulomatous vasculitis. The mean age of onset is 41 years, and common presenting symptoms are hemoptysis or renal failure. Cytoplasmic pattern anti–neutrophil cytoplasmic antibody titer is 93% sensitive and 97% specific for diagnosis of the disease. Because the disease appears to be immunologic in nature, immunosuppressives have been effective. In fact, the combination of prednisone and cyclophosphamide therapy results in a complete remission in 93% of patients. Prednisone therapy alone is also partially effective, but azathioprine and plasmapheresis have not been studied systematically. (*Cecil, Ch. 245*)

77.(D) *Discussion:* Langerhan's cell granulomatosis is a disease characterized by destructive granulomatous lesions in a variety of tissues, with the presence of a specific cell, the Langerhans cell, that can best be identified by electron microscopy. The mean age of onset is 20 to 40 years, and it is rarely seen in blacks. Of note, 90 to 100% of patients with the syndrome are smokers. Chest radiograph changes include infiltrates and cystic changes in the middle and upper lung zones; spontaneous pneumothorax may occur. Overall, the prognosis of the disease when it involves the lung is good; spontaneous resolution occurs in the majority of patients. (*Cecil, Ch. 54*)

78.(B) *Discussion:* Thrombolytic agents have replaced pulmonary embolectomy in the setting of massive central embolism with hypotension. To date, no studies have convincingly demonstrated any advantage for use of thrombolytic agents in other presentations of pulmonary embolism, although there may be a mild late benefit in reducing residual symptoms. However, because thrombolytic agents do have significant morbidity, they should not be used in the majority of patients with pulmonary embolism. Absolute contraindications to use of thrombolytic agents include (1) active bleeding, (2) history of CVA in the last 2 months, and (3) active intracranial disease, including neoplasm. (*Cecil, Ch. 59; Moser*)

79.(B) *Discussion:* Only 2% of patients with sarcoidosis have hypercalcemia; this rises to 15% in patients with disseminated disease. Elevated levels of ACE occur in patients with sarcoidosis, especially those with disseminated disease. However, less than 50% of patients overall develop this laboratory abnormality. An elevated ACE level is not particularly useful in diagnosing sarcoidosis because other granulomatous diseases may rarely cause an elevation in this enzyme. However, the ACE level may be useful in following the treatment of sarcoidosis because it tends to mirror the granuloma load. In contrast to elevated ACE levels, over 50% of patients with sarcoidosis will develop hypergammaglobulinemia. Although this is a nonspecific finding, it probably reflects the immunologic nature of this disorder. (*Cecil, Ch. 61*)

BIBLIOGRAPHY

American Thoracic Society: Guidelines for the initial management of adults with community acquired pneumonia. Am Rev Respir Dis 148:1418, 1993.

American Thoracic Society/Centers for Disease Control: Diagnostic standards and classification of tuberculosis. Am Rev Respir Dis 142:725, 1990.

Bains MS: Surgical treatment of lung cancer. Chest 100:826, 1991.

Bennett JC, Plum F (eds): Cecil Textbook of Medicine. 20th ed. Philadelphia, WB Saunders Company, 1996.

Cooper Jr JAD, White DA, Matthay RA: State of the art: Drug-induced pulmonary disease. Am Rev Respir Dis 133:321, 488, 1986.

Hunninghake GW, Fauci AS: State of the art: Pulmonary involvement in the collagen vascular diseases. Am Rev Respir Dis 119:471, 1979.

Kales A, Vela-Bueno A, Kales JD et al: Sleep disorders: Sleep apnea and narcolepsy. Ann Intern Med 106:434, 1987.

Moser KM: Venous thromboembolism. Am Rev Respir Dis 141:235, 1990.

Sahn SA: State of the art: The pleura. Am Rev Respir Dis 138:184, 1988.

Winter SM, Ingbar DH: Massive hemoptysis: Pathogenesis and management. J Intens Care Med 3:171, 1988.

PART 3

CRITICAL CARE MEDICINE

R. Bruce Gammon

DIRECTIONS: For questions 1 to 22, choose the ONE BEST answer to each question.

QUESTIONS 1-3

A 30-year-old woman is admitted to the hospital with fever and back pain. Laboratory tests reveal a profound leukocytosis. The urine contains numerous leukocytes and gram-negative rods. A presumptive diagnosis of pyelonephritis is made. She is admitted to the hospital and broad-spectrum antibiotics are instituted. Eight hours after admission, her blood pressure falls to 70 mm Hg systolic and the urine output falls to 10 ml per hour.

1. Which of the following is the MOST appropriate initial intervention?

   A. Administration of high-dose bolus steroids
   B. Administration of normal saline, 500-ml bolus
   C. Administration of an antiendotoxin monoclonal antibody
   D. Infusion of dopamine at 3 μg per kilogram per minute
   E. Infusion of dobutamine at 5 μg per kilogram per minute

Resuscitative efforts are successful at stabilizing the blood pressure. However, she develops progressive dyspnea and hypoxemia and requires intubation. After review of all clinical and laboratory data, you make a diagnosis of the acute respiratory distress syndrome (ARDS).

2. What is the appropriate basis for making this diagnosis?

   A. Elevated protein in tracheal secretions
   B. Elevated serum levels of von Willebrand factor
   C. Severe hypoxia accompanying septic shock
   D. A transbronchial biopsy revealing hyaline membranes
   E. Hypoxia, diffuse pulmonary infiltrates, absence of another etiology

3. Which of the following statements about ARDS is correct?

   A. The lung injury score provides a means of assessing severity.
   B. Detailed study of the lungs with computed tomography reveals homogeneous involvement of all lung regions.
   C. Ninety per cent of ARDS patients will not survive.
   D. Most survivors of ARDS will have permanent, severe impairment of lung function.
   E. ARDS does not develop in neutropenic patients.

4. Which of the following monitoring devices provides evidence of organ ischemia in septic patients?

   A. Swan-Ganz catheter
   B. Gastric tonometer
   C. Arterial catheter
   D. Esophageal balloon
   E. Pulse oximeter

5. A 48-year-old man develops respiratory failure secondary to sepsis, and mechanical ventilation is initiated. One morning, his gas exchange deteriorates and his peak pressures rise. The plateau pressure has also risen. The chest radiograph is shown in the figure on page 44, *top*. What is the diagnosis?

   A. Pneumothorax
   B. Mainstem intubation
   C. Atelectasis
   D. Pulmonary edema
   E. Endotracheal tube obstruction

6. A 70-year-old woman develops congestive heart failure and oliguria, and you elect to insert a pulmonary artery catheter. During insertion of the catheter, the patient suddenly becomes pulseless. The rhythm strip is shown in the figure on page 44, *bottom*. What has happened?

   A. Ventricular perforation
   B. Complete heart block
   C. Ventricular tachycardia
   D. Ventricular fibrillation
   E. Pneumothorax

7. The mortality of ARDS is

   A. 10%
   B. 25%
   C. 40%
   D. 80%
   E. 100%

QUESTIONS 8-11

A 50-year-old man presents with respiratory failure from pneumonia, and mechanical ventilation is initiated using assist-control ventilation. The following ventilator settings are used: tidal volume = 800 cc, respiratory rate = 16, fraction of inspired oxygen (FIO_2) = 0.50, positive end-expiratory pressure (PEEP) = 5 cm H_2O, sensitivity = 2 cm H_2O, inspiratory flow rate = 80 liters per minute. On these settings, the peak inspiratory pressure

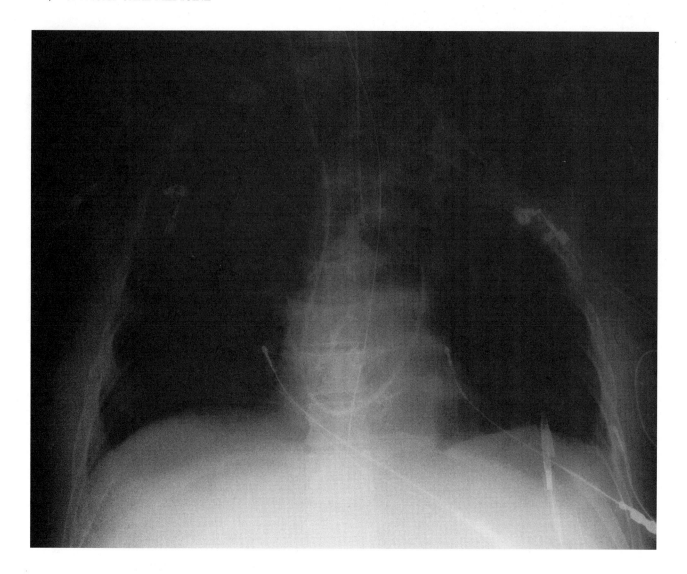

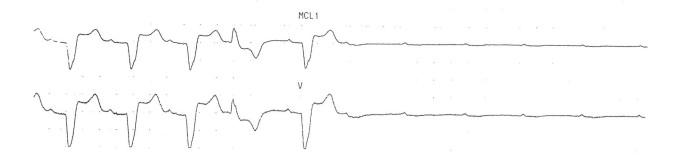

is 45 cm H_2O and the plateau inspiratory pressure is 32 cm H_2O.

8. What is the static compliance (ml per centimeter of H_2O)?

   A. 10
   B. 18
   C. 20
   D. 25
   E. 30

9. What is the effective (dynamic) compliance (ml per centimeter of H_2O)?

   A. 10
   B. 18
   C. 20
   D. 25
   E. 30

Later in the day, the ventilator settings are changed. Following the change, the peak inspiratory pressure is 40 cm H_2O and the plateau pressure is 32 cm H_2O. Lung mechanics are unchanged.

10. Which of the following ventilator changes could lead to these pressures?

   A. A reduction in inspiratory flow to 50 liters per minute
   B. A decrease in tidal volume to 650 cc
   C. An increase in PEEP to 10 cm H_2O
   D. A decrease in PEEP to 0 cm H_2O
   E. An increase in sensitivity to 5 cm H_2O

You elect to continue ventilation on these settings. The next morning the patient is agitated and in respiratory distress, and oximetric saturations have dropped. The plateau pressure has increased from 32 to 44 cm H_2O and the peak pressure has increased from 40 to 52 cm H_2O. The ventilator settings have not changed.

11. Which of the following is the most likely cause of the patient's deterioration?

   A. Occlusion of the endotracheal tube
   B. Bronchospasm
   C. Endotracheal tube cuff leak
   D. Mucus plugging
   E. Pneumothorax

12. Which of the following patients would be the most likely to be successfully ventilated with a negative-pressure ventilator?

   A. An 18-year-old man with ARDS
   B. A 53-year-old woman with amyotrophic lateral sclerosis
   C. A 22-year-old woman with an acute exacerbation of asthma and respiratory failure
   D. A 72-year-old man with advanced interstitial lung disease
   E. A 44-year-old man with severe sleep apnea syndrome

13. What is the most common disorder associated with development of the adult respiratory distress syndrome?

   A. Fat embolism
   B. Pancreatitis
   C. Pneumonia
   D. Sepsis
   E. Severe burns

14. A 44-year-old woman is admitted with septic shock and develops ARDS. She is intubated and treated with broad-spectrum antibiotics. After 10 days of antibiotics, she is improved; ventilator weaning is initiated. Because of a persistent low-grade fever, multiple cultures are obtained. The sputum culture returns positive for *Candida albicans*. The chest radiograph continues to slowly improve. Which of the following statements is true?

   A. Treatment should be initiated with intravenous amphotericin B.
   B. Treatment should be initiated with intravenous fluconazole.
   C. The *Candida* is most likely only a colonizing organism and should not be treated.
   D. An open lung biopsy should be performed.
   E. *Candida albicans* is never a pathogen in critically ill patients.

QUESTIONS 15 AND 16

An 18-year-old woman is admitted to you after suffering a grand mal seizure. She required intubation in the emergency room for airway protection; however, the emergency room physician noted that a large amount of vomitus was present in her posterior oropharynx at the time of intubation. Twelve hours later, she develops diffuse infiltrates and hypoxemia consistent with ARDS.

15. Which of the following is characteristic of aspiration of gastric contents?

   A. The extent of lung injury depends primarily on the volume and acidity of aspirated material.
   B. Seventy per cent of patients with gastric aspiration will develop ARDS.
   C. High-dose corticosteroids are indicated for witnessed aspiration.
   D. Clindamycin should be started immediately.
   E. Immediate bronchoscopy is indicated.

On the second hospital day, crepitance is noted on the upper chest. The radiologist notes mediastinal emphysema on the morning radiograph but does not see a pneumothorax. Her clinical status has not changed.

16. Which of the following is true?

   A. Placement of bilateral chest tubes is indicated.
   B. Pneumothorax always follows the development of mediastinal emphysema.
   C. Mediastinal drainage should be performed.
   D. The patient is at increased risk of pneumothorax and should be closely monitored.
   E. High-frequency ventilation should be initiated.

17. A 73-year-old man is admitted with dyspnea that has developed over several days. He has a 100-pack-year smoking history and known chronic obstructive pulmonary disease (COPD) and coronary artery disease. Following admission, he becomes hypotensive and a Swan-Ganz catheter is placed. The following hemodynamic profile is obtained:

right atrial pressure = 22 mm Hg, pulmonary artery pressure = 44/22 mm Hg, pulmonary capillary wedge pressure = 22 mm Hg, cardiac index = 1.9 liters per minute per square meter, systemic vascular resistance = 2100 dyne/sec/cm^{-5}. What is the most likely diagnosis?

    A. Congestive heart failure
    B. Septic shock
    C. Hypovolemia
    D. Massive pulmonary embolism
    E. Cardiac tamponade

18. A 22-year-old man with known human immunodeficiency virus infection is admitted to the hospital with progressive dyspnea and fever. He has been on Dapsone for prophylaxis against *Pneumocystis carinii* pneumonia. The chest radiograph reveals lobar pneumonia in the right lower lobe, and a cephalosporin is administered. An oximetric saturation of 85% is obtained on 6 liters per minute oxygen by nasal cannula. However, an arterial blood gas reveals a Po_2 of 150 mm Hg at the same time as the oximetry reading. What is the most likely diagnosis?

    A. Elevated methemoglobin
    B. Elevated carboxyhemoglobin
    C. Oximeter probe malfunction
    D. Hyperbilirubinemia
    E. Shock with digital hypoperfusion

19. A 55-year-old woman is mechanically ventilated for an exacerbation of COPD, and a central venous catheter is placed for intravenous access. Seven days after admission, she develops fevers to 38.9°C. Blood cultures are obtained, and 2 days later the lab informs you that they are growing *Candida albicans*. The patient is hemodynamically stable and is clinically improving. Which of the following is the optimal management strategy?

    A. Removal of the central venous catheter
    B. Removal of the central venous catheter and initiation of fluconazole, 400 mg daily
    C. Initiation of fluconazole, 400 mg daily; the catheter is left in place

    D. Initiation of intravenous amphotericin B, 30 mg daily; the catheter is left in place
    E. Removal of the central venous catheter and discontinuation of all antibacterial therapy

20. A 66-year-old man with advanced COPD presents to the emergency room with 2 days of increasing dyspnea. Diffuse end-expiratory wheezing is noted. The chest radiograph is clear; arterial blood gases reveal a pH of 7.33, a Pco_2 of 55 mm Hg, and a Po_2 of 49 mm Hg. Aggressive bronchodilators are instituted, and oxygen 1 liter per minute by nasal cannula is administered. A blood gas 30 minutes later reveals a pH of 7.30, a Pco_2 of 62 mm Hg, and a Po_2 of 61 mm Hg. Which of the following is the most appropriate intervention?

    A. Remove supplemental oxygen
    B. Increase oxygen to 4 liters per minute
    C. Continue oxygen at 1 liter per minute
    D. Proceed with intubation and initiation of mechanical ventilation
    E. Administer sodium bicarbonate, 2 ampules

21. Which of the following is the preferred treatment for severe lithium overdose (serum level >3.5 mEq per liter)?

    A. Hemodialysis
    B. Activated charcoal by nasogastric tube
    C. Normal saline infusion
    D. Normal saline infusion plus furosemide
    E. Intravenous sodium bicarbonate

22. A 53-year-old man is admitted to the intensive care unit with a history of increasing angina. Nitroglycerin and heparin infusions are started. Two hours later he develops severe chest pain and diaphoresis. As you examine him, he becomes unresponsive and no pulse can be obtained. The monitor shows fine ventricular fibrillation. Which of the following is the BEST initial intervention?

    A. Intubation and bag ventilation
    B. Synchronized countershock, 100 J
    C. Lidocaine, 100-mg intravenous bolus
    D. Unsynchronized countershock, 200 J
    E. Epinephrine, 1-mg intravenous bolus

DIRECTIONS: For questions 23 to 40, decide whether EACH choice is true or false. Any combination of answers, from all true to all false, may occur.

23. A 56-year-old man is admitted with pneumonia and respiratory failure requiring mechanical ventilation. On the third hospital day, the respiratory therapist notes that the patient's peak airway pressure has increased by 20 cm H_2O over the past 24 hours. You determine that the ventilator settings and plateau airway pressure have not changed. Which of the following are possible causes of the elevation in airway pressure?

A. Worsening pneumonia
B. Kinking of the endotracheal tube
C. Partial endotracheal tube obstruction with dried secretions
D. Pneumothorax
E. Pulmonary edema

24. Which of the following significantly affect the arterial P_{CO_2} in a patient receiving mechanical ventilation?

A. Arterial P_{O_2}
B. Physiologic dead space
C. Respiratory rate
D. Body CO_2 production
E. Tidal volume

25. A 70-year-old white man with advanced COPD presents to you in the emergency room with pneumonia and an exacerbation of COPD. He is awake and alert, with acceptable work of breathing, and arterial blood gases reveal a pH of 7.30, a P_{CO_2} of 65 mm Hg, and a P_{O_2} of 48 mm Hg. He is visiting relatives, and his private physician near his hometown 300 miles away tells you he has advanced disease and should not be intubated. He and his family state that they wish mechanical ventilation if it has a chance of helping him. Aggressive bronchodilator therapy and antibiotics are initiated. Which of the following is/are appropriate therapeutic plans?

A. Begin oxygen at 1 liter per minute by nasal cannula
B. Write a "Do Not Intubate" order on the chart
C. Intubate the patient
D. Begin oxygen 40% by face mask
E. Administer sodium bicarbonate

26. Which of the following is/are characteristic of cardiovascular function in volume-resuscitated septic shock?

A. Normal or increased cardiac output
B. Decreased left ventricular ejection fraction
C. Reduced systemic vascular resistance (SVR)
D. Increased tissue oxygen extraction
E. Increased end-diastolic volume

27. Which of the following statements is/are characteristic of sepsis?

A. Eighty per cent of cases of gram-negative bacteremia are accompanied by the manifestations of septic shock.
B. The incidence of sepsis has been declining over time.
C. Any site of infection can result in sepsis.

D. Fungal infections are not associated with development of sepsis.
E. Sepsis is the most common cause of death in intensive care units.

28. A 75-year-old man with hypertension and a previous cerebrovascular accident is brought to the emergency room in August after being found at home comatose. The skin and mucus membranes are dry, and his core temperature is 41.5°C. Which of the following increases the patient's likelihood of developing heat stroke?

A. Lack of acclimatization
B. Impaired awareness of the environment
C. Inability to leave the environment
D. Intoxication
E. Lack of air conditioning

29. Which of the following statements is/are characteristic of hypercapnic respiratory failure?

A. Hypoxia is not corrected with 100% oxygen.
B. It is often associated with airflow obstruction.
C. The need for mechanical ventilation is determined by the level of P_{CO_2}.
D. Most patients do not require supplemental oxygen.
E. Lethargy and somnolence often occur.

30. The end-tidal CO_2 tension will closely approximate the arterial P_{CO_2} in which of the following situations?

A. A 26-year-old man ventilated for central nervous system depression from tricyclic overdose
B. A 30-year-old woman with ARDS
C. A 65-year-old man with an acute exacerbation of COPD
D. A 40-year-old woman with no known pulmonary disease undergoing an elective cholecystectomy
E. A 77-year-old man with advanced interstitial lung disease and respiratory failure

31. Which of the following is/are important steps in the measurement of intrinsic PEEP?

A. Performance of an inspiratory hold maneuver
B. Performance of an expiratory hold maneuver
C. Equilibration of pressure in airways and ventilator tubing
D. Coaching the patient to give a maximal inspiratory effort
E. Coaching the patient to give a maximal expiratory effort

32. Which of the following physiologic variables are needed to calculate oxygen consumption (V_{O_2})?

A. FI_{O_2}
B. Pulmonary capillary wedge pressure
C. Arterial oxygen content
D. Cardiac output
E. Mixed venous oxygen content

33. Which of the following may reduce CO_2 production (V_{CO_2})?

   A. Reduction in fever with antipyretics
   B. Nutritional support with a high-fat, low-carbohydrate formula
   C. Overfeeding
   D. Hyperventilation
   E. Nutritional support with a low-fat, high-carbohydrate formula

34. Which of the following is/are characteristics of breaths delivered by pressure-support ventilation?

   A. Patient initiated
   B. Fixed tidal volume
   C. Preset airway pressure
   D. Variable inspiratory flow rate
   E. Fixed inspiratory time

35. Which of the following are major risk factors for gastrointestinal hemorrhage in the intensive care unit?

   A. Head injury
   B. Mechanical ventilation
   C. Coagulopathy
   D. Ileus
   E. Renal failure

36. You are counseling a family regarding the advisability of tracheostomy for a patient who has received mechanical ventilation for 2 weeks. They ask what benefits may be achieved by this procedure. Which of the following are advantages of tracheostomy over endotracheal intubation?

   A. Patient comfort is increased.
   B. The risk of tracheal stenosis is substantially reduced.
   C. The risk of laryngeal trauma is reduced.
   D. Secretion clearance is facilitated.
   E. Endotracheal tubes deteriorate after 3 weeks.

37. Which of the following should be part of a comprehensive ventilatory strategy for patients with ARDS?

   A. Limitation of the plateau pressure to 35 cm H_2O
   B. Maintenance of a normal arterial P_{CO_2}
   C. Use of moderate levels of PEEP for improvement in oxygenation

   D. Use of early high-frequency ventilation
   E. Use of short inspiratory time to maximize exhalation time

38. Which of the following statements is/are true regarding intermittent mandatory ventilation (IMV)?

   A. The set respiratory rate indicates the exact number of full machine breaths per minute.
   B. Patients can initiate full machine breaths above the set rate.
   C. The set tidal volume indicates the volume of all breaths received by the patient.
   D. The patient can breath spontaneously above the set machine rate.
   E. PEEP cannot be used with IMV.

39. A 24-year-old woman is referred to you from the psychiatry department for the evaluation of drug overdose. The patient refuses to give any history but was found with an empty bottle of acetaminophen. She is awake and alert. Nasogastric lavage reveals no pill fragments. Which of the following statements is/are true regarding acetaminophen toxicity?

   A. A timed serum level is needed to determine the potential for toxicity.
   B. *N*-acetylcysteine is ineffective if given more than 12 hours after ingestion.
   C. Hepatic coma from acetaminophen toxicity usually occurs 48 to 96 hours after ingestion.
   D. Tinnitus is a common complaint.
   E. The absence of pill fragments eliminates significant acetaminophen ingestion.

40. Which of the following statements is/are true regarding theophylline toxicity?

   A. Toxicity occurs at lower serum levels in acute overdose than in chronic intoxication.
   B. Activated charcoal administration will reduce the serum half-life of theophylline.
   C. Severe toxicity should be treated with charcoal hemoperfusion.
   D. Urine alkalinization will increase drug clearance.
   E. Seizures should be treated with physostigmine.

DIRECTIONS: Questions 41 to 65 are matching questions. For each numbered item, choose the most likely associated lettered item from those provided. Each numbered item has ONLY ONE answer. Within each set of questions, each answer may be used once, more than once, or not at all.

QUESTIONS 41–45

Match the following receptor stimulation data with their appropriate vasopressors, as shown in the figure, *below*.

41. Norepinephrine

42. Dopamine

43. Epinephrine

44. Phenylephrine

45. Dobutamine

QUESTIONS 46–50

Match the following causative diseases to their associated types of respiratory failure.

    A. Carbon monoxide poisoning
    B. Cardiac tamponade
    C. Adult respiratory distress syndrome
    D. Amyotrophic lateral sclerosis
    E. Cyanide poisoning

46. Hypercarbic respiratory failure

47. Hypoxic respiratory failure

48. Failure of oxygen extraction

49. Reduced arterial oxygen content

50. Reduced tissue oxygen delivery

QUESTIONS 51–54

Match the following causative diseases to their associated types of shock.

    A. Acute myocardial infarction
    B. Left atrial myxoma
    C. Bowel ischemia with sepsis
    D. Gastrointestinal hemorrhage

51. Obstructive shock

52. Cardiogenic shock

53. Distributive shock

54. Hypovolemic shock

QUESTIONS 55–60

Match the following agents (they are not all poisons) to the appropriate clinical syndrome of toxicity.

    A. Theophylline
    B. Verapamil
    C. Scopolamine
    D. Amitriptyline
    E. Insecticide
    F. Wood alcohol

55. Delirium, dry mucous membranes, urinary retention

56. Abdominal pain, convulsions, fasciculations, headache

57. Abdominal pain, blurred vision, altered mental status, anion-gap acidosis

58. Cardiac arrhythmias, vomiting, seizures

59. Seizures, hypotension, prolonged QT interval

60. Hypotension, bradycardia, coma

	α Stimulation	β_1 Stimulation	β_2 Stimulation	Specific Renal and Splanchnic Receptors
A.	+ + +	–	–	–
B.	+ + +	+ + +	+ + +	–
C.	–	+ + +	–	–
D.	+ + +	+ + +	–	–
E.	+ +	+ +	–	+

QUESTIONS 61–65

You are given the following compliance and gas exchange data obtained from a patient with acute respiratory failure. Match each data set with the most likely etiology of respiratory failure. In each case, assume the patient weighs 70 kg and that the following ventilator settings are used: assist control, tidal volume = 700 cc, respiratory rate = 14, PEEP = 0, see figure, *below*.

61. Adult respiratory distress syndrome

62. Chronic obstructive pulmonary disease

63. Status asthmaticus

64. Drug overdose

65. Massive pulmonary embolism

	pH	P_{CO_2} (mm Hg)	P_{O_2} (mm Hg)	FIO_2	Peak Inspiratory Pressure (cm H_2O)	Plateau Pressure (cm H_2O)
A.	7.12	55	76	0.6	30	26
B.	7.35	47	82	0.4	56	34
C.	7.46	33	94	0.3	26	22
D.	7.38	54	65	0.35	38	26
E.	7.42	38	68	1.0	48	45

PART 3

CRITICAL CARE MEDICINE

ANSWERS

1.(B) *Discussion:* This patient has developed sepsis with hypotension and acute renal failure. Unless there is a strong suspicion of volume overload, volume resuscitation is the initial therapy of choice. Pressor agents such as dopamine and dobutamine may be useful to increase systemic vascular resistance and improve cardiac output but should be initiated after fluids have been given. To date, no anti-inflammatory agent (including high-dose steroids and antiendotoxin antibodies) has been shown to improve outcome in sepsis. (*Cecil, Ch. 70*)

2.(E) *Discussion:* ARDS is defined clinically as a combination of severe hypoxia and bilateral pulmonary infiltrates in the absence of another etiology such as congestive heart failure. Because ARDS is characterized by increased pulmonary capillary permeability, markers of endothelial injury, such as von Willebrand factor, have been investigated as early markers of ARDS but remain research tools at present. Hyaline membranes and high-protein edema fluid are characteristic of ARDS but are not used currently to define the disorder. (*Cecil, Ch. 68; Matthay*)

3.(A) *Discussion:* It is now recognized that ARDS occurs with varying degrees of severity, and the lung injury score, which factors lung compliance, gas exchange, PEEP level, and radiographic involvement, is often used to quantify the severity. Computed tomography studies reveal that the distribution of consolidation in ARDS is *heterogeneous*, involving the most dependent areas of the lung most severely. The published mortality of ARDS varies but is approximately 40 to 50%; the majority of survivors will have little residual pulmonary dysfunction. ARDS does occur in neutropenic patients; this evidence indicates that, although the neutrophil plays a major role in mediating the endothelial injury that occurs in ARDS, other factors are also involved. (*Cecil, Ch. 65; Matthay*)

4.(B) *Discussion:* The gastric tonometer is a gas-permeable balloon that is placed into the stomach, usually attached to a conventional nasogastric tube. Saline is placed into the balloon and allowed to equilibrate with stomach gases for several hours; the CO_2 tension of the saline is then measured and an "intramucosal pH" of the stomach is calculated from the Henderson-Hasselbalch equation using arterial bicarbonate concentrations. Clinical studies indicate that a fall in intramucosal pH is an early indicator of organ ischemia in sepsis. The Swan-Ganz catheter, arterial catheter, and pulse oximeter are important monitoring devices for septic patients but do not provide information on end-organ function. Esophageal manometry is useful for calculating work of breathing but does not monitor end-organ function. (*Cecil, Ch. 68*)

5.(B) *Discussion:* This patient has a left mainstem intubation, which leads to a fall in static compliance. This is seen as a rise in both peak and plateau pressures. Pneumothorax, atelectasis, and pulmonary edema also lead to a reduction in static compliance. An endotracheal tube obstruction will lead to a fall in dynamic compliance, which is accompanied by a rise in peak pressure but no change in static pressure. (*Cecil, Ch. 68*)

6.(B) *Discussion:* This patient has developed complete heart block without ventricular escape. During passage through the right ventricle, transient right bundle-branch block may occur, leading to complete heart block if the patient has pre-existent left bundle-branch block, as is the case with this patient. Although in the past temporary pacing was recommended for patients with left bundle-branch block who required Swan-Ganz catheter placement, the complication of complete heart block is so uncommon that this is no longer recommended. (*Pingleton*)

7.(C) *Discussion:* The mortality of ARDS varies from series to series, with recent reports indicating a mortality of 40 to 50%. The mortality of ARDS seems to be slowly declining over time, but the precise reason for this decline is unclear. (*Cecil, Ch. 65*)

8.(E) *Discussion:* Static compliance is calculated by the following formula:

$$C_{stat} = \frac{\text{Tidal volume}}{(\text{Plateau pressure} - \text{PEEP})}$$

For this patient, the static compliance = $(800)/(32 - 5)$ = 29.6 ml per centimeter of H_2O. (*Cecil, Ch. 68*)

9.(C) *Discussion:* Effective (dynamic) compliance is calculated by the following formula:

$$C_{dyn} = \frac{\text{Tidal volume}}{(\text{Peak pressure} - \text{PEEP})}$$

For this patient, the effective compliance = $(800)/(45 - 5)$ = 20 ml per centimeter of H_2O. (*Cecil, Ch. 68*)

10.(A) *Discussion:* The peak pressure has fallen without a change in the plateau pressure. This indicates that the ventilator change must have affected flow-resistive work, which would alter peak pressure without altering static pressure. The only listed intervention that affects flow-resistive work is the reduction in inspiratory flow rate. Answers B, C, and D would all have led to changes in the plateau pressure. Answer E would not have directly affected the peak or plateau pressure. (*Cecil, Ch. 68*)

11.(E) *Discussion:* The peak and plateau pressures have both increased, indicating a reduction in both static and dynamic compliance. The only choice that would affect both is pneumothorax. Choices A, B, and D would lead to increased airway resistance and an increase in flow-resistive work. This would cause a reduction in dynamic compliance (reflected by an increased peak airway pressure) but would not affect static compliance. A system leak (C) will usually lead to reduced airway pressures. (*Cecil, Ch. 68*)

12.(B) *Discussion:* In negative-pressure ventilation, negative pressure is placed around the chest to effect ventilation. In the past, this was performed using large tanks that enclosed the entire body except the head (iron lungs), but, currently, rigid shells that encase the thorax (cuirass ventilators) are used. Negative-pressure ventilation is rarely performed and is useful only in selected patients with near-normal lung mechanics, as is seen in neuromuscular disease. It should not be used in critically ill patients. (*Cecil, Ch. 68*)

13.(D) *Discussion:* A large number of diseases may lead to ARDS, including all of the listed entities. However, the greatest risk for development of ARDS is seen in patients with sepsis. (*Cecil, Ch. 65*)

14.(C) *Discussion:* Fungi, particularly *Candida* species, are an important cause of intensive care unit morbidity and mortality and may cause line, bloodstream, or disseminated infections. However, they frequently colonize without causing disease, particularly in patients receiving broad-spectrum antibiotics. *Candida albicans* is an infrequent cause of pneumonia and, in the setting of a patient who is clinically improving with a stable radiograph, the presence of *Candida* in the sputum should not lead to initiation of antifungal therapy. (*Edwards and Filler*)

15.(A) *Discussion:* The severity of lung injury following the aspiration of gastric contents depends primarily on the acidity of the contents and the volume of aspirate. Approximately one third of patients will develop ARDS; there are no data to support the use of high-dose corticosteroids. Initially, chemical pneumonitis is present and antibiotics are not indicated; the presence of increased fever or worsening gas exchange 48 to 72 hours later should prompt concern for a bacterial process and initiation of antibiotics. Bronchoscopy would be indicated to evaluate for the presence of a foreign body if localized atelectasis develops. (*Cecil, Ch. 54.2*)

16.(D) *Discussion:* Pneumothorax follows the development of mediastinal emphysema in approximately 40 to 50% of ventilated patients. Most clinicians believe that, in such high-risk situations, the optimum approach is to follow closely, with a high suspicion for pneumothorax if deterioration occurs. Chest tube placement is not indicated for "prophylaxis" against pneumothorax because this would lead to placement of a large number of unnecessary tubes. High-frequency ventilation would not be of benefit. Drainage of mediastinal gas in this setting is not indicated. (*Marcy*)

17.(E) *Discussion:* The hemodynamic profile reveals a low cardiac index, elevated SVR, and elevated right atrial, pulmonary artery, and pulmonary capillary wedge pressures. This profile could be seen with either cardiogenic shock or cardiac tamponade; however, the equalization of diastolic pressures is most consistent with cardiac tamponade. Septic shock usually causes an elevated cardiac index and low SVR, whereas hypovolemia would be associated with reduced filling pressures. Obstructive shock from massive pulmonary embolism would cause an elevation in right-sided pressures, low cardiac index, and high SVR but would not be associated with a high pulmonary capillary wedge pressure. (*Cecil, Ch. 69*)

18.(A) *Discussion:* Methemoglobinemia can be caused by a large number of medications, including Dapsone. Methemoglobinemia drives the oximeter saturation to 85%, and is the most likely diagnosis in this patient. Carboxyhemoglobinemia would cause an elevated oximeter saturation. All of the other listed entities may cause inaccurate oximeter readings, but the saturation of 85% makes methemoglobinemia the most likely diagnosis. (*Wahr and Tremper*)

19.(B) *Discussion:* Candidemia is a common complication with indwelling catheters, and most studies agree that the culprit line should be removed if this occurs. This should be accompanied by institution of antifungal therapy. A recent controlled trial has shown that fluconazole is an effective as amphotericin B for candidemia in non-neutropenic patients and, given its lower toxicity, should be used for therapy in this case. (*Edwards and Filler; Rex et al*)

20.(C) *Discussion:* The primary goal of oxygen administration in this setting is to increase oxygen saturations to >90% using the lowest flow available. Hypercarbia often results when the Po_2 is increased but, if reasonably tolerated (absence of lethargy, pH >7.20), mechanical ventilation should not be instituted. In this case, the Po_2 of 61 mm Hg should be adequate to obtain saturations of 90%, and therefore higher flows are not indicated. Removal of oxygen would lead to the return of unacceptable hypoxia. Sodium bicarbonate should not be given as therapy for a respiratory acidosis in this setting. (*Cecil, Ch. 65*)

21.(A) *Discussion:* For mild lithium overdose, normal saline alone may be given. However, for severe overdoses, hemodialysis is indicated. There is no role for forced diuresis or alkalinization, and activated charcoal will not speed removal of absorbed lithium. (*Cecil, Ch. 72*)

22.(D) *Discussion:* Early defibrillation is critical in patients with ventricular fibrillation and should be the initial intervention. The initial countershock should be 200 J, increasing to 300 and then 360 J if unsuccessful. Lidocaine, epinephrine, and airway control are important in managing patients who do not respond to defibrillation. Synchronized cardioversion has no role in the resuscitation of ventricular fibrillation. (*Cecil, Ch. 69*)

23.(A—False; B—True; C—True; D—False; E—False) *Discussion:* Elevations in peak airway pressure can be caused by an increase in airway resistance, decreased compliance of the respiratory system, or changes in ventilatory settings (increased flow, tidal volume, or PEEP). The plateau airway pressure is measured by holding inspiration until gas flow ceases and is affected by changes in respiratory system compliance or in ventilator settings (tidal volume or PEEP). However, as a static measurement, the plateau pressure is not affected by changes in airway resistance. In this patient, the plateau pressure has not changed, indicating that there is no change in compliance; the ventilator settings also have not changed. Therefore, the increased peak airway pressure must be due to increased airway resistance, which could be caused by kinking of the endotracheal tube or partial occlusion by secretions. Pneumothorax, worsening pneumonia, and pulmonary edema would all reduce static compliance and lead to elevations in plateau airway pressure as well as peak airway pressure. (*Cecil, Ch. 68*)

24.(A—False; B—True; C—True; D—True; E—True) *Discussion:* The arterial P_{CO_2} is determined by the following relationship:

$$P_{CO_2} \propto \frac{V_{CO_2}}{V_A}$$

where V_{CO_2} = body CO_2 production and V_A = alveolar ventilation. Alveolar ventilation, in turn, is equal to the minute ventilation minus wasted ventilation (dead space ventilation). Therefore, physiologic dead space, respiratory rate, body CO_2 production, and tidal volume are all important determinants of the P_{CO_2}. (*Cecil, Ch. 68*)

25.(A—True; B—False; C—False; D—False; E—False) *Discussion:* This patient has acute respiratory failure caused by an exacerbation of COPD in the setting of preexistent chronic respiratory failure. Initial therapy should include aggressive administration of bronchodilators and administration of oxygen to raise the P_{O_2} to the level of 55 to 60 mm Hg, which is best done by careful administration of low-flow oxygen. High inspired oxygen concentrations may reduce respiratory drive and alter ventilation-perfusion relationships, leading to worsened hypercarbia. In a situation in which the patient has clearly stated wishes regarding life support, these wishes should be followed. However, because the patient is awake with a blood pH of >7.20, mechanical ventilation should not be instituted at the present time. Sodium bicarbonate should not be used as therapy of a respiratory acidosis in this setting. (*Cecil, Ch. 65; Gammon et al*)

26.(A—True; B—True; C—True; D—False; E—True) *Discussion:* After volume resuscitation, most patients with sepsis will have an elevated cardiac output and reduced SVR. However, this is associated with a reduction in left ventricular ejection fraction. The cardiac output is maintained by increasing the left ventricular end-diastolic volume and by increasing heart rate. Tissue oxygen extraction is usually impaired in sepsis. (*Cecil, Ch. 70*)

27.(A—False; B—False; C—True; D—False; E—True) *Discussion:* Approximately 50% of cases of gram-negative bacteremia result in septic shock. The incidence of sepsis has been increasing, and sepsis is currently the most common cause of death in intensive care units. Sepsis is a systemic inflammatory response to infection and may result from infection at any site. Although most commonly caused by bacterial infections, sepsis may also result from fungal infections. (*Cecil, Ch. 70*)

28.(All are True) *Discussion:* Nonexertional heat stroke usually occurs in debilitated patients exposed to high heat and humidity. Poor awareness of the surroundings, intoxication, and immobility may render the patient unable to leave the environment. Lack of acclimatization increases suscepti-

bility to heat, and lack of air conditioning can lead to hazardous temperatures in hot summer conditions. (*Cecil, Ch. 71*)

29.(A—False; B—True; C—False; D—False; E—True) *Discussion:* Hypercapnic respiratory failure describes conditions characterized by failure to eliminate carbon dioxide. This leads to elevations in P_{CO_2} as well as some degree of hypoxia. Most patients will require oxygen supplementation, but it is usually much less than 100%. Common conditions leading to hypercapnic respiratory failure include COPD, neuromuscular diseases, and drug overdose. Because many of these patients have *chronic* hypercapnia, the decision to institute mechanical ventilation should not be based on the absolute level of P_{CO_2} but on the adverse consequences of hypercarbia, including acidosis (pH <7.20) or altered mental status (lethargy, somnolence), or an excessive work of breathing. (*Cecil, Ch. 65; Gammon et al*)

30.(A—True; B—False; C—False; D—True; E—False) *Discussion:* The end-tidal CO_2 tension approximates the arterial CO_2 tension when ventilation-perfusion relationships in the lung are normal. In situations in which there are areas of lung that are ventilated but poorly perfused (dead space ventilation), the CO_2 content present in expired gas from these regions will be reduced and will dilute the CO_2 content from other regions, leading to a fall in end-tidal CO_2. Therefore, in diseases that alter ventilation-perfusion relationships, the end-tidal CO_2 tension will usually be lower than the arterial CO_2 tension. This holds true for patients with COPD, interstitial lung disease, and ARDS. Cases A and D represent cases without underlying pulmonary disease, and the end-tidal CO_2 should closely approximate the arterial P_{CO_2}. (*Cecil, Ch. 68*)

31.(A—False; B—True; C—True; D—False; E—False) *Discussion:* Intrinsic PEEP ("auto-PEEP") occurs when exhalation is incomplete, which happens most commonly in ventilated patients with obstructive lung diseases. In such cases, positive pressure exists at the alveolar level but may not be detected at the ventilator pressure port during the exhalation phase. Auto-PEEP is measured by performing an expiratory hold maneuver on the ventilator (in which neither inspiration or further exhalation is allowed) and allowing the pressure to equilibrate between lung and ventilator tubing. A rise in pressure during this maneuver indicates the presence of auto-PEEP. Reliable readings are only obtained in periods devoid of patient activity, and therefore the patient should not be coached during the maneuver. (*Gammon et al*)

32.(A—False; B—False; C—True; D—True; E—True) *Discussion:* Total body oxygen consumption (V_{O_2}) can be measured by indirect calorimetry or can be calculated using parameters determined with a Swan-Ganz catheter. The equation for calculating the oxygen consumption is as follows:

$$V_{O_2} = \text{Cardiac output} \times (C_aO_2 - C_vO_2)$$

where C_aO_2 = arterial oxygen content and C_vO_2 = mixed venous oxygen content. (*Cecil, Ch. 68*)

33.(A—True; B—True; C—False; D—False; E—False) *Discussion:* CO_2 production is determined by the metabolic rate of the body and substrate utilization. Fever will increase the metabolic rate, and reduction of fever will lead to a decrease in CO_2 production. The respiratory quotient (RQ) is the ratio of CO_2 production to oxygen consumption. Fat is metabolized with an RQ of 0.7, and carbohydrates are metabolized with an RQ of 1.0. Therefore, high-fat, low-carbohydrate nutrients will reduce CO_2 production. Overfeeding will lead to an increase in CO_2 production. (*Weissman and Kemper*)

34.(A—True; B—False; C—True; D—True; E—False) *Discussion:* Pressure support is a mode of ventilation that delivers a preset airway boost to spontaneous patient breaths. The patient initiates each breath, and tidal volume and inspiratory flow are patient determined, depending on respiratory mechanics and patient effort. Pressure support is often more comfortable for patients and is commonly used in ventilator weaning. (*Cecil, Ch. 68; Gammon et al*)

35.(A—True; B—True; C—True; D—False; E—True) *Discussion:* A large number of factors place a patient at risk for stress ulceration and gastrointestinal hemorrhages. These include head injury, mechanical ventilation, renal failure, coagulopathy, burns, sepsis, shock, and major trauma. The risk of bleeding is increased when multiple risk factors are present. (*Fisher et al*)

36.(A—True; B—False; C—True; D—True; E—False) *Discussion:* The major advantages of tracheostomy include patient comfort and improved secretion clearance. Removal of the endotracheal tube may also reduce the risk of vocal cord injury. Tracheal stenosis may occur after either tracheostomy or endotracheal intubation, and reduction in this risk by early tracheostomy has not been shown. Modern endotracheal tubes are quite durable, although they may become plugged with secretions or develop cuff leaks. (*Pingleton*)

37.(A—True; B—False; C—True; D—False; E—False) *Discussion:* The current recommendations for mechanical ventilation in ARDS center on limiting airway pressures. This strategy is based on numerous animal studies that demonstrate that high-pressure, high-volume ventilation is injurious to the lung. Important parts of this strategy include a limitation in plateau airway pressure to 35 cm H_2O, the use of moderate levels of PEEP to include gas exchange, and acceptance of increased arterial CO_2 tensions. High-frequency ventilation has not been shown to offer advantages over more conventional ventilation. In patients with severe gas exchange derangement, the use of *prolonged* inspiratory times may improve oxygenation; short inspiratory times may be useful in patients with airflow obstruction but are not useful in ARDS. (*Cecil, Ch. 65; Gammon et al*)

38.(A—True; B—False; C—False; D—True; E—False) *Discussion:* In IMV, the ventilator delivers breaths at the preset tidal volume and at the preset respiratory rate. Between these breaths, patients are allowed to breath spontaneously without machine assist. The patient determines the volume of the spontaneous breaths. IMV is often combined with pressure support, which allows the spontaneous patient breaths to be accompanied by a pressure boost. PEEP is commonly used with IMV. (*Cecil, Ch. 68; Gammon et al*)

39.(A—True; B—False; C—True; D—False; E—False) *Discussion:* The most severe complication of acetaminophen toxicity is fulminant hepatic failure, which occurs 48 to 96 hours after ingestion. The serum level of acetaminophen that indicates risk of hepatic toxicity varies as a function of time after ingestion, and a nomogram is available to allow determination of risk based on a timed serum level. *N*-acetylcysteine is effective if administered within 24 hours of ingestion. Tinnitus is seen with salicylate toxicity, not acetaminophen toxicity. (*Cecil, Ch. 72*)

40.(A—False; B—True; C—True; D—False; E—False) *Discussion:* Manifestations of theophylline toxicity include nausea, vomiting, cardiac arrhythmias, and seizures. Toxicity occurs at lower serum levels in patients who use theophylline chronically. Treatment includes activated charcoal, which reduces the enterohepatic circulation of theophylline, and charcoal hemoperfusion if the toxicity is severe. Urine alkalinization will not speed elimination. Seizures should be treated with benzodiazepines; physostigmine has no role. (*Cecil, Ch. 72*)

41.(D); 42.(E); 43.(B); 44.(A); 45.(C) *Discussion:* Phenylephrine is an isolated alpha-stimulatory agent that is sometimes used to treat hypotension caused by low SVR. Norepinephrine is a powerful alpha and beta$_1$ stimulant commonly used in cases of sepsis and refractory shock. Dopamine has less potent alpha and beta$_1$ effects than norepinephrine but has renal and splanchnic vasodilatory effects at lower doses. Dobutamine has isolated beta$_1$ effects and is used primarily for inotropic support in patients with cardiac dysfunction. Epinephrine has powerful alpha, beta$_1$, and beta$_2$ effects. (*Cecil, Ch. 69*)

46.(D); 47.(C); 48.(E); 49.(A); 50.(B) *Discussion:* Hypercarbic respiratory failure, characterized by inability to achieve adequate CO_2 removal, is commonly seen in obstructive diseases and neuromuscular diseases, in this case amyotrophic lateral sclerosis. ARDS is the prototype of hypoxic respiratory failure, with shunt physiology and the requirement for a high concentration of inspired oxygen. Although hypercarbic and hypoxic respiratory failure are the classic forms, the term "respiratory failure" also is used to describe any process that interferes with tissue oxygen delivery or utilization. In cyanide poisoning, adequate oxygen is delivered to tissues but cannot be used because of blockade of mitochondrial cytochrome oxidase. Carbon monoxide binds to hemoglobin with a much greater affinity than oxygen, leading to a reduced arterial oxygen content. The low output state of cardiac tamponade leads to reduced tissue oxygen delivery. (*Cecil, Ch. 65*)

51.(B); 52.(A); 53.(C); 54.(D) *Discussion:* Obstructive shock is caused by lesions that occlude vascular beds or channels, in this case left atrial myxoma. Acute myocardial infarction is a common cause of cardiogenic shock, characterized by a low output state caused by pump failure or valvular disease. Distributive shock, seen in sepsis, is characterized by a normal to high cardiac output with a reduced SVR and a redistribution of blood flow away from critical tissues. Acute hemorrhage is a common cause of hypovolemic shock. (*Cecil, Ch. 69*)

55.(C); 56.(E); 57.(F); 58.(A); 59.(D); 60.(B) *Discussion:* The primary manifestations of scopolamine toxicity relate to anticholinergic properties, leading to altered mental status, dry mucous membranes, and urinary retention. Organophosphates, common components of insecticides, irreversibly inhibit acetylcholinesterase, leading to cholinergic manifestations of abdominal pain, vomiting, fasciculations, and convulsions. Methanol (wood alcohol) is converted to formic acid in the body, with classic symptoms including blurred vision and anion-gap acidosis. Permanent blindness may result. Theophylline toxicity causes nausea and vomiting early, which can be followed by cardiac arrhythmias and seizures. Severe tricyclic overdose causes prolongation of the QT interval, with the potential for ventricular arrhythmias, seizures, and hypotension. Calcium channel blocker overdoses cause bradycardia, hypotension, and coma; intravenous calcium may be life saving in such instances. (*Cecil, Ch. 72*)

61.(E); 62.(D); 63.(B); 64.(C); 65.(A) *Discussion:* This question requires knowledge of the expected changes in gas exchange, hemodynamics, and compliance in the listed diseases. Data set A reveals a combined metabolic and respiratory acidosis, abnormal oxygenation with an increased FIO_2 requirement, and near-normal lung compliance. Massive pulmonary embolism, which leads to high dead space ventilation, hypoxia, and obstructive shock, would be the most likely diagnosis to lead to this picture. Data set B reveals an acute respiratory acidosis, mildly impaired oxygenation, and a pronounced elevation in peak inspiratory pressure out of proportion to plateau pressure, indicating elevated inspiratory resistance. This is most characteristic of status asthmaticus. Data set C reveals a mild respiratory alkalosis, near-normal oxygenation, and normal compliance, most consistent with a disease that does not affect lung parenchyma, such as drug overdose. Data set D reveals a compensated respiratory acidosis with impaired oxygenation, associated with a mildly elevated peak airway pressure. This is most consistent with an exacerbation of COPD. Data set E reveals profound hypoxia with elevated peak and plateau pressures, indicating a reduced static and dynamic compliance. This is characteristic of ARDS. (*Cecil, Ch. 65; Gammon et al*)

BIBLIOGRAPHY

Bennett JC, Plum F (eds): Cecil Textbook of Medicine. 20th ed. Philadelphia, WB Saunders Company, 1996.

Edwards JE, Filler SG: Current strategies for treating invasive candidiasis: Emphasis on infections in nonneutropenic patients. Clin Infect Dis 14(Suppl 1):S106, 1992.

Fisher RL, Pipkin GA, Wood JR: Stress-related mucosal disease: Pathophysiology, prevention, and treatment. Crit Care Clin 11:323, 1995.

Gammon RB, Strickland JH, Kennedy JI, Young KR: Mechanical ventilation: A review for the internist. Am J Med 99:553, 1995.

Marcy TW: Barotrauma: Detection, recognition, and management. Chest 104:578, 1993.

Matthay MA: The adult respiratory distress syndrome: Definition and prognosis. Clin Chest Med 11:575, 1990.

Pingleton SK: Complications of acute respiratory failure. Am Rev Respir Dis 137:1463, 1988.

Rex JH, Bennett JE, Sugar AM, et al: A randomized trial comparing fluconazole with amphotericin B for the treatment of candidemia in patients without neutropenia. N Engl J Med 331:1325, 1994.

Wahr JA, Tremper KK: Noninvasive oxygen monitoring techniques. Crit Care Clin 11:199, 1995.

Weissman C, Kemper M: Metabolic measurements in the critically ill. Crit Care Clin 11:169, 1995.

PART 4

RENAL DISEASE

Paul W. Sanders and David G. Warnock

DIRECTIONS: For questions 1 to 57, Choose the ONE BEST answer to each question.

QUESTIONS 1 AND 2

A 45-year-old black man presents with hilar adenopathy, pulmonary infiltrates, and erythema nodosa. On transbronchial biopsy, he is found to have noncaseating granulomata. Special stains of the tissue reveal no organisms.

1. Potential clinical renal manifestations in this patient may include

    A. Hypercalcemic nephropathy
    B. Hyposthenuria
    C. Granulomatous infiltration of the renal interstitium
    D. Immune complex–mediated glomerulonephritis
    E. All of the above
    F. None of the above

2. The hypercalcemia of sarcoidosis

    A. Reflects extrarenal 1-alpha-hydroxylation of 25-hydroxyvitamin D
    B. Rarely produces nephrocalcinosis
    C. Responds well to prednisone
    D. A and C
    E. A, B, and C

QUESTIONS 3 AND 4

A 60-year-old man with end-stage renal failure from chronic glomerulonephritis presents with acute onset of gross hematuria and mild flank pain. He has been on dialysis for 4 years and his course has otherwise been uneventful. He was afebrile and the hematuria resolved without intervention.

3. Which of the following is the most sensitive imaging method in this setting?

    A. Renal ultrasound
    B. Computed tomography
    C. Angiography
    D. Intravenous pyelogram
    E. None of the above

4. True statements about acquired cystic kidney disease (ACKD) include all of the following EXCEPT

    A. ACKD occurs exclusively in hemodialysis patients and not in patients receiving peritoneal dialysis.
    B. ACKD is rare in patients without renal failure.

    C. ACKD is frequently asymptomatic but can produce pain, fever, and hematuria.
    D. ACKD is associated with renal cell carcinoma.
    E. ACKD has a male predominance.

5. Renal neoplasms in dialysis patients

    A. Respond well to chemotherapy
    B. Are rarely bilateral
    C. Do not occur in renal transplant recipients
    D. Infrequently metastasize unless the tumor size is >3 cm
    E. None of the above

QUESTIONS 6–9

A 43-year-old man developed cellulitis of his left lower extremity but resisted medical evaluation for nearly 10 days. However, when the condition did not improve, he saw his physician, who admitted him to the hospital. His admission serum creatinine level was 1.2 mg per deciliter. He was treated with a 2-week course of intravenous antibiotics that consisted of nafcillin, clindamycin, and gentamicin. Ten days into this treatment, a serum creatinine level is obtained and is 3.5 mg per deciliter. Renal ultrasound shows normal-sized kidneys without hydronephrosis.

6. Possible causes of this patient's acute renal failure include

    A. Acute tubular necrosis
    B. Acute glomerulonephritis
    C. Allergic interstitial nephritis
    D. A, B, and C
    E. A and C

On further evaluation, he was found to have a blood pressure of 160/95 mm Hg, a decrease in urine output to less than 30 ml per hour, and a urinalysis that showed 2+ protein, 2+ hemoglobin, red blood cells (RBCs), and RBC and tubule epithelial cell casts.

7. Based on these findings, the most likely diagnosis is

    A. Gentamicin nephrotoxicity
    B. Postinfectious glomerulonephritis
    C. Hypersensitivity reaction to a beta-lactam antibiotic
    D. Cannot determine from information available
    E. None of the above

8. True statements regarding poststreptococcal glomerulonephritis include

    A. Serum complement, C3, and total hemolytic complement are usually low.

    B. Poststreptococcal acute glomerulonephritis has an excellent prognosis for recovery.

    C. Glomerulonephritis can develop after either skin or pharyngeal streptococcal infections.

    D. A, B, and C

    E. A and C

9. The most common intrinsic (primary) glomerular lesion is

    A. Anti–glomerular basement membrane (GBM) glomerulonephritis

    B. Idiopathic membranoproliferative glomerulonephritis

    C. Amyloidosis

    D. Immunoglobulin (Ig) A nephropathy

    E. Idiopathic focal and segmental glomerulosclerosis

QUESTIONS 10–13

A 67-year-old white man is referred to you for evaluation of renal failure. Evaluation includes the following laboratory values:

Serum chemistries

Sodium	135 mEq/L
Potassium	4.2 mEq/L
Chloride	109 mEq/L
Bicarbonate	24 mEq/L
Glucose	101 mg/dl
Calcium	11.9 mg/dl
Phosphorus	4.3 mg/dl
Albumin	4.0 g/dl

Urine chemistries

Creatinine clearance	55 ml/min
protein	6.2 g/day
Hematocrit	29%

10. Based on the data presented, the patient appears to have

    A. Acute glomerulonephritis

    B. Acute vasculitic lesion

    C. Reflux nephropathy

    D. Atheroembolic renal disease

    E. Nephrotic syndrome

    F. None of the above

11. Tests to perform at this point to make a diagnosis might include

    A. Urine immunoelectrophoresis

    B. Bone marrow aspiration and biopsy

    C. Serum immunoelectrophoresis

    D. Radiographic survey of the bones

    E. All of the above

    F. None of the above

12. The low anion gap in this patient most likely reflects

    A. The presence of lithium

    B. Acidosis

    C. A low serum albumin

    D. A high circulating level of IgG

    E. None of the above

13. Deposition of monoclonal immunoglobulin light chains in the kidney can produce all of the following, EXCEPT

    A. Casts in the lumen of the tubules

    B. Amyloidosis, type AL

    C. Granular deposits with glomerular injury

    D. Vasculitis

    E. Acute tubular necrosis

QUESTIONS 14–16

A 50-year-old woman presents with an abrupt decline in urine output and renal failure. Her past medical history is significant only for hysterectomy 1 month earlier and chronic migraine headaches controlled with methysergide. She takes no other medications. The following data were obtained:

Serum chemistries

Sodium	130	mEq/L
Potassium	6.2	mEq/L
Chloride	99	mEq/L
Bicarbonate	16	mEq/L
Glucose	101	mg/dl
Calcium	7.9	mg/dl
Phosphorus	6.3	mg/dl
Creatinine	3.2	mg/dl

Urinalysis

pH	5.5
Specific gravity	1.010
Protein	trace
Hemoglobin	trace
Sediment	unremarkable

Urine output over the past 12 hours was 60 ml.

14. Which study do you perform now to assist with the diagnosis?

    A. Renal ultrasound

    B. Kidney biopsy

    C. Selective renal arteriograms

    D. 24-hour urine collection for protein and immunofixation electrophoresis

    E. None of the above

The patient receives treatment for the hyperkalemia. The fractional excretion of sodium was 1.3%. Repeat urinalysis was unchanged and renal function did not improve with gentle hydration. A renal ultrasound demonstrated echogenic, normal-sized kidneys with minimal hydronephrosis bilaterally. No stones were evident.

15. Possible etiologies of the renal failure include

    A. Acute tubular necrosis

    B. Urinary tract obstruction

    C. Acute glomerulonephritis

    D. Allergic interstitial nephritis

    E. Cannot determine from the data given

16. A computed tomogram of the abdomen demonstrated mild hydronephrosis of both kidneys with mildly dilated proximal ureters that were deviated medially and appeared to be extrinsically compressed at the level of the mid to lower ureter. The most likely diagnosis is

    A. Obstruction related to kidney stones bilaterally

B. Obstruction secondary to retroperitoneal adenopathy
C. Retroperitoneal fibrosis
D. Obstruction secondary to adenocarcinoma
E. Acute tubular necrosis
F. Cannot determine from the data given

QUESTIONS 17–19

A 25-year-old man presents with a history of upper respiratory symptoms, followed by streaky hemoptysis and malaise. His blood pressure is 140/90 mm Hg and he has trace lower extremity edema. Pertinent laboratory data include a serum urea nitrogen level of 86 mg per deciliter and creatinine level of 3.5 mg per deciliter. Urinalysis shows 2+ protein, 3+ blood, 5 to 10 RBCs per high-power field, and rare red cell casts. Chest roentgenogram demonstrates opacities in both lung fields.

17. The most likely diagnosis at this point is

A. Wegener's granulomatosis
B. Anti-GBM disease
C. Postinfectious glomerulonephritis
D. Allergic interstitial nephritis
E. None of the above

18. The most appropriate initial diagnostic study should be

A. Bronchoscopy with biopsy
B. Open lung biopsy
C. Biopsy of the nasal mucosa
D. Computed tomogram of the chest and abdomen
E. Percutaneous renal biopsy with immunofluorescence microscopic examination

19. The clinical course of this lesion

A. Depends on how rapidly treatment is initiated
B. Can be predicted by the amount of urine output
C. Can be predicted by the serum creatinine concentration at presentation
D. All of the above
E. A and C

QUESTIONS 20–23

A 50-year-old woman with a 10-year history of non–insulin-dependent diabetes mellitus complains of low back pain and is prescribed indomethacin, 25 mg three times per day. She returns for evaluation 4 weeks later with the following laboratory abnormalities:

Serum electrolytes	
Sodium	136.0 mEq/L
Potassium	6.2 mEq/L
Chloride	106.0 mEq/L
Bicarbonate	18.0 mEq/L
Serum urea nitrogen	55 mg/dl
Serum creatinine	5.3 mg/dl

Her serum creatinine level was 2.2 mg per deciliter both 1 and 6 months previously.

20. Potential causes of the deterioration in this patient's renal function include

A. Renal ischemia secondary to reduced renal blood flow from prostaglandin inhibition

B. Urinary tract obstruction
C. Allergic interstitial nephritis
D. A, B, and C
E. A and C

21. True statements about allergic interstitial nephritis secondary to nonsteroidal anti-inflammatory agents include

A. Hematuria is frequently present.
B. Eosinophilia is frequently present.
C. The presence of eosinophils in the urine supports the diagnosis.
D. A, B, and C
E. A and C

Further review of the patient's record revealed a history of use of acetaminophen and aspirin over the past 20 years for low back pain and headache. Urinalysis showed 1+ protein, 10 to 20 white blood cells (WBCs) per low-power field, and four to six white blood cell casts per low-power field. Renal ultrasound demonstrated small kidneys with hydronephrosis bilaterally. On the second hospital day, small fragments of tissue were identified in the urine.

22. Given this information, the most likely diagnoses should now include

A. Chronic interstitial nephropathy
B. Allergic interstitial nephritis
C. Papillary necrosis
D. A, B, and C
E. A and C

23. Potential causes of this patient's hyperkalemia include

A. Hyporeninemia from prostacyclin inhibition
B. Renal tubular acidosis from urinary tract obstruction
C. Renal failure
D. A, B, and C
E. A and C

QUESTIONS 24–27

A 39-year-old, 50-kg man presents to the emergency department with a history of alcoholism and recent onset of obtundation. He lives alone and can provide no other information. On presentation, he has a grand mal seizure that lasts for 2 minutes. Routine physical exam findings include a blood pressure of 120/70 mm Hg, heart rate of 110 per minute, and no evidence of head trauma, papilledema, or focal neurologic findings. His mental status does not change with intravenous injections of thiamine and 50% dextrose. Laboratory evaluation includes

Serum electrolytes	
Sodium	136 mEq/L
Potassium	5.0 mEq/L
Chloride	99 mEq/L
Bicarbonate	12 mmol/L
Serum urea nitrogen	42 mg/dl
Serum creatinine	4.2 mg/dl
Arterial pH	7.10
Arterial P_{CO_2}	40 mm Hg
Arterial O_2	85 mm Hg

24. This patient has which of the following acid-base disorder(s)?

    A. Simple metabolic acidosis

    B. Simple respiratory acidosis

    C. Mixed metabolic and respiratory acidosis

    D. Combined metabolic acidosis, respiratory acidosis, and metabolic alkalosis

    E. None of the above

25. Potential causes of this patient's problem might include

    A. Methanol ingestion

    B. Uremia

    C. Ethylene glycol ingestion

    D. A, B, and C

    E. A and C

26. Ethylene glycol overdose

    A. Produces an anion-gap metabolic acidosis

    B. Is associated with the presence of octahedral crystals typical of calcium oxalate in the urine

    C. Can cause oliguric acute renal failure

    D. A, B, and C

    E. A and C

27. Initial emergency management of ethylene glycol overdose includes

    A. Creation of an alkaline diuresis

    B. Intravenous infusion of ethyl alcohol

    C. Hemodialysis

    D. A, B, and C

    E. A and C

QUESTIONS 28–31

A 56-year-old white man presented to his physician with complaints of headache and fatigue and no prior history of medical problems. He reportedly had a blood pressure of 196/115 mm Hg and a ''normal'' laboratory evaluation. His physician prescribed captopril, 25 mg twice daily, and instructed the patient to return in 2 weeks. The patient is brought into the emergency department 5 days later with severe proximal muscle weakness, extreme fatigue, nausea, and vomiting.

28. Without other information available, which of the following is/are possible?

    A. The patient has symptomatic renal failure related to converting enzyme inhibition.

    B. Life-threatening hyperkalemia is present.

    C. This patient probably has renovascular hypertension.

    D. A, B, and C

    E. A and C

29. If the serum potassium level was 7.2 mEq per liter and his electrocardiogram revealed absent P waves and markedly prolonged QRS duration suggestive of a ''sine wave'' pattern, appropriate initial management could include

    A. Calcium gluconate, 10%, 10 ml administered intravenously

    B. Albuterol, 10 mg, via nebulized inhaler

    C. Intravenous regular insulin, 5 units, plus 50 ml of 50% dextrose

    D. A, B, and C

    E. A and C

30. The patient's serum creatinine concentration was 6.7 mg per deciliter. After stopping the captopril, this fell to 1.5 mg deciliter. Which of the following statements is/are correct?

    A. The patient probably had hemodynamically significant bilateral renal artery stenosis.

    B. The patient probably had a glomerulonephritis related to the captopril therapy.

    C. If another converting enzyme inhibitor is used, this complication should not recur.

    D. A, B, and C

    E. A and C

31. Potential complications of converting enzyme inhibitors include

    A. Acute renal failure

    B. Persistent cough

    C. Acute severe hypotension

    D. Hyperkalemia

    E. All of the above

    F. A and C

QUESTIONS 32–35

An 18-year-old man presents to the emergency department with dysuria and fever. On further questioning, he relates two prior episodes of a urinary tract infection successfully treated with oral antibiotics. His evaluation is unremarkable except for a blood pressure of 160/105 mm Hg. Urinalysis reveals 3+ protein, a specific gravity of 1.012, and a pH 5.5, and a microscopic examination shows two to five RBCs and 5 to 10 WBCs per high-power field. The serum creatinine level was 4.9 mg deciliter. He is referred to a urologist, who performs a voiding cystourethrogram that demonstrates vesicoureteral reflux bilaterally.

32. Which of the following is the *most* likely cause of this clinical syndrome?

    A. Obstructive uropathy at the level of the prostate

    B. Chronic tubulointerstitial nephritis

    C. Chronic glomerulonephritis

    D. Reflux nephropathy

    E. Acute glomerulonephritis

33. The cause of this patient's renal failure

    A. Will likely progress to end-stage renal disease

    B. Will stabilize and cause no further problems

    C. Is producing the hypertension

    D. A and C

    E. None of the above

34. The patient's 24-hour urine protein excretion rate is 2.9 grams per 24 hours. This suggests

    A. The patient has focal and segmental glomerulosclerosis

    B. The patient has membranoproliferative glomerulonephritis

C. The patient will eventually progress to end-stage renal failure
D. A and C
E. None of the above

35. The initial renal lesion in this patient

A. Could be prevented by surgical intervention now
B. Is most likely associated with a renal cortical scar
C. Is an uncommon cause of end-stage renal failure
D. A and C
E. None of the above

QUESTIONS 36–39

A 24-year-old woman is admitted for abnormal uterine bleeding and a uterine mass. A preoperative ultrasound demonstrates mild bilateral hydronephrosis and normal-sized kidneys. She undergoes general anesthesia with resection of a large uterine leiomyoma. Her postoperative course is complicated with confusion, followed by obtundation. Her blood pressure is 120/80 mm Hg supine and upright and her resting heart rate is 90 beats per minute. Her weight is now 55 kg. The following laboratory values were obtained the morning after operation:

Serum electrolytes
Sodium	170.0 mEq/L
Potassium	4.0 mEq/L
Chloride	136.0 mEq/L
Bicarbonate	22.0 mmol/L
Serum urea nitrogen	24 mg/dl
Serum creatinine	0.9 mg/dl
Serum glucose	90 mg/dl
Urine osmolality	80 mOsm/kg
Urine sodium	25 mEq/L

36. The most appropriate initial choice of intravenous fluids is

A. 5% dextrose in water
B. 5% dextrose in 0.25% sodium chloride
C. 5% dextrose in 0.45% sodium chloride
D. 5% dextrose in 0.9% sodium chloride
E. None of the above

37. If one assumes no loss of solute, what is the calculated water deficit?

A. 3 liters
B. 5 liters
C. 7 liters
D. 9 liters
E. 11 liters

38. Factors that control serum osmolality include

A. Thirst
B. Atrial natriuretic hormone
C. Antidiuretic hormone (ADH)
D. A, B, and C
E. A and C

39. The patient is given aqueous vasopressin, 10 mU per kilogram body weight, intravenously, and her urine osmolality 2 hours later is 520 mOsm per kilogram. The most likely diagnosis of this patient's hypernatremia is

A. Nephrogenic diabetes insipidus secondary to relief of urinary tract obstruction

B. Central diabetes insipidus
C. Osmotic diuresis secondary to retention of nitrogenous waste products
D. Sodium chloride retention
E. None of the above

QUESTIONS 40 AND 41

A 67-year-old man is brought to the emergency room with fever, nausea, and vomiting. For the past 10 days he has taken ampicillin for an upper respiratory infection. Temperature is 38.1°C. Blood pressure is 125/70 mm Hg (supine) and 90/56 mm Hg (standing). Pulse rate is 92 per minute (supine) and 122 per minute (standing). Physical findings include rare basilar rales and wheezes, a faint macular rash on the trunk and legs, and a moderately enlarged prostate. A roentgenogram of the chest shows a faint right lower lobe infiltrate. Urinalysis shows 1+ proteinuria, 10 to 20 WBCs and 20 to 30 RBCs per high-power field, and several white cell casts. A Wright's stain of spun urinary sediment reveals many eosinophils. Other laboratory data include

Serum electrolytes
Sodium	134 mEq/L
Potassium	5.8 mEq/L
Chloride	110 mEq/L
Bicarbonate	14 mEq/L
Blood urea nitrogen	88 mg/dl
Serum creatinine	2.8 mg/dl
WBC count	13,200/cu mm
Eosinophils	12%
Polymorphonuclear leukocytes	68%
Lymphocytes	12%
Monocytes	8%
Arterial pH	7.24

Urine chemistries
Sodium	58 mEq/L
Chloride	34 mEq/L
Potassium	17 mEq/L
pH	5.7

40. Which of the following is the MOST likely cause of this clinical syndrome?

A. Obstructive uropathy at the level of the prostate
B. Acute glomerulonephritis
C. Tubulointerstitial nephritis
D. Volume depletion
E. Mild chronic renal insufficiency

41. Which of the following is LEAST likely to contribute to hypotension in this patient?

A. Vomiting
B. Decreased glomerular filtration rate (GFR)
C. Salt-losing nephropathy
D. Pneumonia
E. Fever

QUESTIONS 42 AND 43

A 59-year-old male truck driver comes to the emergency room because of lethargy, nausea, and vomiting over the preceding 5 days and markedly decreased urinary volume. He has a history of mild hypertension treated with dietary salt restriction. For the past several months he has had urinary hesitancy and nocturia. Blood pressure is 105/60 mm Hg; pulse rate is 125 per minute. There is a 20-mm Hg orthostatic drop in blood pressure. Physical examination shows prostatic enlargement. The patient is unable to produce a urine specimen. The bladder is not distended by percussion. Plain film of the abdomen shows two renal outlines of normal size. Ultrasound examination of the kidneys shows normal renal size; there is no dilation of the renal pelvis or ureters. Laboratory studies show

Serum electrolytes
Sodium	132 mEq/L
Potassium	5.2 mEq/L
Chloride	90 mEq/L
Bicarbonate	22 mEq/L
Blood urea nitrogen	110 mg/dl
Serum creatinine	13 mg/dl
Calcium	8.1 mg/dl
Phosphate	6.2 mg/dl
Hemoglobin	13.5 g/dl

After rehydration with 5 liters of normal saline, the patient remains anuric. The next morning, repeat ultrasound examination of the kidneys shows bilateral distention of the renal pelvis. Placement of a bladder catheter yields 2000 ml of clear urine, and urine production continues at 1000 ml per hour over the next 5 hours.

42. Which of the following is the MOST likely explanation of the abnormalities of renal function seen in this patient?

A. Chronic renal failure
B. High circulating levels of vasopressin
C. Obstructive uropathy at the level of the prostate
D. Renal artery stenosis
E. A toxic nephropathy

43. Which of the following BEST explains the initially normal ultrasound examination?

A. Improper interpretation of the examination
B. Extracellular fluid (ECF) volume depletion
C. Acute glomerulonephritis
D. Bilateral ureteral obstruction
E. Uric acid nephropathy

QUESTIONS 44 AND 45

A 66-year-old man with recently diagnosed small cell carcinoma of the lung, without apparent central nervous system metastases, comes to the hospital with confusion. There is no history of vomiting and he takes no medicine. Physical examination reveals a blood pressure of 116/80 mm Hg, jugular venous pressure of 6 cm H_2O, and obtundation without any localizing findings. There is no clinical evidence of ECF depletion. Laboratory tests include

Serum electrolytes
Sodium	108 mEq/L
Potassium	4.4 mEq/L
Chloride	82 mEq/L
Bicarbonate	20 mEq/L

Blood urea nitrogen	6	mg/dl
Serum creatinine	0.7	mg/dl
Serum uric acid	3.8	mg/dl
Serum osmolality	222	mOsm/kg

Urine
Sodium	50	mEq/L
Potassium	12	mEq/L
pH		5.0
Osmolality	860	mOsm/kg

44. What is the major mechanism contributing to this patient's hyponatremia?

A. Osmotic diuresis
B. Impaired free water clearance
C. Laboratory artifact in the measurement of serum sodium
D. ADH effect based on a physiologic nonosmotic stimulus
E. Decreased total body water with a larger decrease in total body sodium

45. Which mechanism explains the measured level of urine sodium?

A. Osmotic diuresis
B. Salt-losing nephropathy
C. Impaired free water clearance
D. Increased distal delivery of an impermeant anion
E. The patient is in sodium balance and the ECF compartment is not depleted

QUESTIONS 46 AND 47

A 68-year-old man has increasing hypertension 3 weeks after an aortic angiogram and subsequent repair of an abdominal aortic aneurysm. In the hospital, he received brief courses of several drugs, including cephalosporin, cimetidine, and heparin. He is currently receiving aspirin and dipyridamole. Physical examination now shows a blood pressure of 170/110 mm Hg. Bruits are heard in both femoral arteries. There is some mottling of the lower extremities and subungual petechiae on a lower extremity nail bed. Laboratory data include

Serum electrolytes
Sodium	142 mEq/L
Potassium	5.1 mEq/L
Chloride	104 mEq/L
Bicarbonate	20 mEq/L
Blood urea nitrogen	60 mg/dl
Serum creatinine	3.2 mg/dl

Complete blood count
Hematocrit	35%
WBC count	10,500/cu mm
Polymorphonuclear leukocytes	80%
Lymphocytes	12%
Eosinophils	8%

Urinalysis shows a pH of 5.0, 2+ protein, and one to three WBCs and 10 to 15 RBCs per high-power field. Wright's stain of the urine is positive for eosinophils.

46. Choose the diagnosis MOST likely to explain the azotemia and hypertension in this patient.

    A. Nephrosclerosis
    B. Atheroembolic disease
    C. Drug-induced interstitial nephritis
    D. Radiocontrast-induced renal disease
    E. Postoperative acute tubular necrosis

47. Which is the MOST likely prognosis for the renal disease?

    A. Complete recovery in 2 to 3 days
    B. Complete recovery in 10 to 14 days
    C. Stabilization of the renal function at the current level
    D. Progressive deterioration of renal function over months
    E. The disorder has no characteristic course

QUESTIONS 48 AND 49

A 49-year-old woman with known polycystic renal disease and a serum creatinine level of 3.0 mg/dl comes to the emergency room because of abdominal and flank pain. She states that she noted some blood-tinged urine the preceding day. Physical examination shows a blood pressure of 180/105 mm Hg, pulse of 92 per minute, and temperature of 38°C. There is no orthostasis. Large bilateral upper quadrant masses are palpated; the right is somewhat tender. Bowel sounds are normal. A plain film of the abdomen reveals large upper quadrant masses bilaterally. An abdominal sonogram shows large polycystic kidneys with multiple overlapping echoes. A few areas in the upper pole of the right kidney have complex echoes; no solid masses are seen. Urinalysis shows 1+ protein and >100 RBCs and 5 to 10 WBCs per high-power field.

48. Which of the following is the most likely cause of the patient's condition?

    A. Renal infarction
    B. Urinary infection
    C. Renal cell carcinoma
    D. Hemorrhage into a renal cyst
    E. Arteriovenous malformation of the kidney

49. Which procedure is most reasonably indicated at this time?

    A. Observation and bed rest
    B. Surgical exploration
    C. Renal angiography
    D. Intravenous pyelogram
    E. Computed tomography scan of the abdomen

QUESTIONS 50 AND 51

A 40-year-old woman was evaluated for edema of some months' duration and was found to have the nephrotic syndrome. The 24-hour urinary protein excretion was 11 grams. Serum creatinine level was 0.9 mg per deciliter, and creatinine clearance was 88 ml per minute. A percutaneous renal biopsy obtained a small piece of cortex that revealed only four glomeruli with a normal light microscopic pattern. Immunofluorescence was negative, and electron microscopy revealed fusion of the glomerular foot processes without evidence of immune deposits. After an 8-week course of prednisone, 60 mg daily, the edema was slightly improved, although the patient noted cushingoid appearance. The 24-hour urinary protein excretion was 5 grams. Prednisone was discontinued and she was managed with diuretics and sodium restriction, with an improvement of the edema. Two years later, the patient is found to have persistent edema and a serum creatinine of 3.7 mg per deciliter, with 14 grams of protein in a 24-hour collection of urine.

50. If a renal biopsy were to be performed now, the most likely histologic diagnosis would be

    A. IgA nephropathy
    B. Minimal change glomerulopathy
    C. Membranous glomerulonephritis
    D. Focal and segmental glomerulosclerosis
    E. Membranoproliferative glomerulonephritis

51. Which of the following should be used to treat the recurrent nephrotic syndrome in this patient?

    A. Aspirin plus dipyridamole
    B. Prednisone, 60 mg orally daily
    C. Prednisone plus cyclophosphamide
    D. Methylprednisolone, 1 gram daily for 3 days
    E. None of the above

QUESTIONS 52 AND 53

A 78-year-old man is brought to the emergency room by a neighbor who was alarmed after not hearing from him for 3 days. The patient is barely conscious and has an obvious left hemiparesis. Blood pressure is 90/60 mm Hg with a pulse rate of 120 per minute. He is afebrile. The mucous membranes are dry, and there is tenting of the skin over the forehead. There is early skin breakdown on the left hip. The remainder of the physical examination is consistent with a cerebrovascular accident. There is no sign of heart failure or pulmonary infiltrates. Weight is 70 kg. Laboratory studies show

Serum electrolytes	
Sodium	162 mEq/L
Potassium	5.0 mEq/L
Chloride	120 mEq/L
Bicarbonate	24 mEq/L
Serum glucose	181 mg/dl

52. This patient's total body sodium content is

    A. High because the serum sodium concentration is high
    B. Low
    C. Normal
    D. Cannot be determined from the information given

53. In planning fluid therapy, which of the following is appropriate?

    A. Half of the calculated water deficit should be administered as hypotonic fluid immediately and the remainder over 8 to 12 hours.
    B. Initial ECF volume repletion should be made with isotonic saline, followed by correction of the free water deficit with hypotonic fluids over 48 hours.

C. Furosemide should be administered and the measured urinary sodium loss should be replaced with hypotonic saline.
D. The calculated free water deficit should be administered as half-normal saline over the next 24 hours.
E. The calculated free water deficit should be administered as half-normal saline over the next 48 hours.

QUESTIONS 54 AND 55

A 78-year-old woman is evaluated in the emergency room because of a 4-day history of vomiting, muscle cramps, and low-grade fever. She has been unable to eat anything and has drunk only tea, water, and carbonated drinks. The previous history is unremarkable.

54. Which of the following would be the most likely electrolyte disturbance?

A. Hyponatremia
B. Hyperkalemia
C. Hypokalemia
D. Anion-gap acidosis
E. Hyperchloremic metabolic acidosis

55. The most likely urinary electrolyte findings would be

A. Urine sodium = 30 mEq per liter; urine potassium = 60 mEq per liter
B. Urine sodium = 30 mEq per liter; urine chloride = 90 mEq per liter
C. Urine sodium = 30 mEq per liter; urine chloride = 30 mEq per liter
D. Urine sodium = 3 mEq per liter; urine potassium = 20 mEq per liter
E. Urine sodium = 3 mEq per liter; urine chloride = 50 mEq per liter

QUESTIONS 56 AND 57

A 60-year-old man is seen in the emergency room because of muscle cramps and paresthesias. He has a history of recurrent squamous cell carcinoma of the head and neck and finished a course of *cis*-platinum 3 weeks before admission to the emergency room. Local radiation therapy is planned for the immediate future. He has also noted frequent watery diarrhea over the past month and has not been able to eat or drink well. Physical examination does not show significant volume depletion. There is a positive Chvostek's sign, serum calcium level of 5.8 mg per deciliter, and serum magnesium level of 0.7 mEq per liter. The urinary magnesium concentration on a random urine sample is 20 mEq per liter.

56. Which factor is LEAST likely to have contributed to the hypomagnesemia in this patient?

A. Diarrhea
B. Hypocalcemia
C. Poor oral intake
D. *Cis*-platinum therapy
E. A paraneoplastic syndrome from a squamous cell carcinoma

57. Which factor is MOST likely to have contributed to the hypocalcemia?

A. Diarrhea
B. Hypomagnesemia
C. Poor oral intake
D. *Cis*-platinum therapy
E. A paraneoplastic syndrome from a squamous cell carcinoma

DIRECTIONS: For questions 58 to 79, decide whether EACH choice is true or false. Any combination of answers, from all true to all false, may occur.

58. Which of the following statements is/are true about the renal hypoperfusion syndromes?
   A. Salt avidity and increased renin secretion are usually observed.
   B. Effective circulating volume has a greater effect on systemic blood pressure than does renin secretion in the setting of renal hypoperfusion.
   C. Occlusive disease causes renal hypoperfusion, elevated renin secretion, and hypertension in the setting of a normal effective circulating volume.
   D. Unilateral renal occlusive disease is not associated with azotemia if the contralateral kidney maintains normal function.
   E. Nephrotoxic agents (cyclosporine, amphotericin B, radiocontrast dyes) can cause acute renal vasoconstriction with renal hypoperfusion, increased salt avidity, and azotemia.

59. Which of the following findings is/are characteristic of the mild acute glomerulonephritis syndrome?
   A. Hematuria
   B. Hypertension
   C. Dependent edema
   D. Persistent proteinuria >3.0 grams per day
   E. Minimal azotemia

60. Which of the following statements is/are true concerning creatinine clearance?
   A. Creatinine clearance normally exceeds "true" measurements of GFR in chronic renal failure.
   B. Cimetidine and trimethoprim can block the secretory component of creatinine clearance.
   C. Urinary creatinine excretion is primarily influenced by the muscle mass in the steady state.
   D. The secretory component of creatinine excretion may become more apparent when serum creatinine concentrations are elevated.
   E. Creatinine clearance is linearly related to the serum creatinine concentration.

61. Which of the following statements is/are true concerning calcium/phosphate balance in chronic renal failure?
   A. Increased circulating levels of parathyroid hormone (PTH) are observed because of reduced renal catabolism and increased secretion.
   B. Hyperphosphatemia reduces PTH secretion.
   C. Extrarenal production of 25-hydroxy-vitamin D_3 is increased in chronic renal failure.
   D. 1,25-Dihidroxy-vitamin D_3 increases gut absorption of calcium and phosphorus.
   E. A normal calcemic response to PTH is not observed in chronic renal failure with 1,25-dihydroxy-vitamin D_3 deficiency.

62. Which of the following statements is/are true concerning "uremic" pericarditis?
   A. A friction rub, pleuritic chest pain, and enlarged cardiac size are typical findings in uremic pericarditis.
   B. Hypertension, tachycardia, and raised jugular venous pressures are the hallmarks of cardiac tamponade.
   C. Aggressive dialysis can worsen "uremic" pericarditis.
   D. Volume overload can be improved by ultrafiltration in the setting of tamponade.
   E. Emergent surgical intervention is indicated if the pericardial effusion causes hemodynamic compromise.

63. Which of the following statements is/are true concerning the anemia of chronic renal failure?
   A. Erythropoietin deficiency is primarily related to the loss of renal mass.
   B. Iron deficiency and hyperparathyroidism are important causes of resistance to erythropoietin response.
   C. Overcorrecting the hematocrit (i.e., above 35%) can cause hypertension, headaches, and occasional seizures.
   D. Increased release of oxygen from hemoglobin is an important factor in the adaptation to anemia in chronic renal failure.
   E. Erythropoietin reduces blood transfusion requirements and will reduce the incidence of iron overload– and transfusion-related infections in the end-stage renal disease population

64. Which of the following statements is/are true concerning chronic ambulatory peritoneal dialysis?
   A. Relatively reduced peritoneal surface limits the usefulness of this approach in children.
   B. Insulin-dependent diabetics have severe problems with glycemic control because of the large amounts of glucose absorbed from the peritoneal dialysate.
   C. Dialysis clearance of large molecules (>800 kD) is enhanced with peritoneal dialysis.
   D. The overall dialysis efficiency is similar for hemodialysis and peritoneal dialysis if the duration of dialysis is considered (12 hr per week for hemodialysis versus continuous dialysis with the peritoneal approach).
   E. Peritonitis is a common problem with chronic ambulatory peritoneal dialysis and is usually caused by gram-negative organisms.

65. Which of the following statements is/are true concerning tissue typing and renal transplantation?
   A. Siblings with the same biologic parents have a 25% chance of being human leukocyte antigen (HLA) incompatible
   B. By definition, a true biologic parent shares 1 HLA haplotype with each child.
   C. In vitro cytotoxicity tests do not predict rejection in the transplant setting.

D. Major histocompatibility complex class II antigens, expressed on B lymphocytes and vascular endothelial cells, are pivotal in the rejection process.

E. Mandatory sharing of six-antigen-matched cadaver kidneys with the best matched recipient will dramatically improve graft survival for nearly all transplant recipients.

66. Which of the following statements is/are true concerning cyclosporine?

A. This agent has dramatically improved renal allograft survival.

B. The use of more specific, targeted immunosuppressants (cyclosporine, OKT3) has reduced the incidence of opportunistic infections.

C. Cyclosporine markedly slows the recovery from acute tubular necrosis and potentiates the adverse effects of other nephrotoxic agents.

D. Toxicities of cyclosporine include nephrotoxicity, tremor, hyperglycemia, hypertension, and hyperkalemia.

E. Close monitoring of dosing and serum levels can eliminate the clinical toxicity of cyclosporine.

67. Which of the following statements about membranoproliferative glomerulonephritis (MPGN) is/are true?

A. MPGN does not reoccur after renal transplantation.

B. This clinicopathologic entity occurs primarily in young adults.

C. Hypocomplementemia may be severe.

D. MPGN may be a primary (idiopathic) renal lesion or may occur in systemic illnesses, including hepatitis B antigenemia and other infections and systemic lupus erythematosus.

E. The clinical course is typically benign.

68. Which of the following statements about hemolytic-uremic syndrome (HUS) is/are true?

A. HUS may occur after gastroenteritis, especially following *Escherichia coli* 0157:H7 infections.

B. HUS has a particularly poor renal prognosis in children.

C. A HUS syndrome may occur with pregnancy or the use of oral contraceptive agents.

D. Important features of HUS include microangiopathic hemolytic anemia, thrombocytopenia, reduced haptoglobin levels, and minimal evidence of disseminated intravascular coagulation.

E. Relapse of HUS does not occur.

69. Which of the following statements is/are true of the nephrotic syndrome?

A. Plasma volume is usually increased.

B. It is usually associated with renal sodium wasting.

C. It occurs with either diffuse or focal forms of glomerulonephritis.

D. The incidence of infection is increased.

E. Albumin infusions are of significant benefit for treatment of hypoalbuminemia and edema.

70. Which of the following is/are the direct results of chronic, but rarely acute, renal failure?

A. Elevated alkaline phosphatase level from bone

B. Radiographic signs of renal osteodystrophy

C. Bilaterally small kidneys

D. Dilute urine with a high urine sodium concentration

E. Hypertension

71. Which of the following is/are characteristic of analgesic-associated nephropathy?

A. Equal gender distribution

B. Normal-sized kidneys

C. Anemia out of proportion to azotemia

D. Sterile pyuria

E. Papillary necrosis

72. A 47-year-old man has an excretory urogram for investigation of microscopic hematuria discovered on a routine urinalysis. He is apparently healthy and entirely without complaints. Kidneys are of normal size, with calcification of and collection of dye in dilated medullary structures. Serum electrolytes, blood urea nitrogen, creatinine, calcium, phosphorus, and uric acid levels are normal. Creatinine clearance is 103 ml per minute. Urinalysis reveals rare RBCs and no protein. Which of the following is/are true of this patient?

A. There is a significant chance that he will develop symptomatic renal stones.

B. There is a significant chance that he has hypercalciuria.

C. He is likely to have impaired maximal urine concentration.

D. His condition is likely to progress gradually to chronic end-stage renal disease.

E. His children each have a 1:2 chance of developing the same condition.

QUESTIONS 73 AND 74

A 57-year-old woman comes to the emergency room because of malaise and edema. She has been previously healthy and takes no medicines. A comprehensive physical examination, including routine laboratory tests, was performed 3 months ago and was entirely normal. The patient reports these symptoms for a few weeks. She has noted no change in her urine volume but does note nocturia. Physical examination shows a mildly ill woman with hypertension and pedal edema. No other remarkable physical findings are noted. Laboratory studies show

Serum electrolytes	
Sodium	138 mEq/L
Potassium	5.3 mEq/L
Chloride	100 mEq/L
Bicarbonate	18 mEq/L
Blood urea nitrogen	62 mg/dl
Serum creatinine	4.8 mg/dl
Hematocrit	31%
WBC count	9700/cu mm
Erythrocyte sedimentation rate	40 mm/hr

Urinalysis shows a pH of 5.5, 2+ protein, 10 to 20 RBCs per high-power field, and rare RBC casts. Antinuclear antibodies, complement (CH_{50}), antistreptolysin-O (ASO) titer, and rheumatoid antibodies were normal. A percutaneous renal biopsy is performed. Light microscopy reveals that about 80% of the glomeruli seen are affected with proliferating epithelial crescents. Immunofluorescence shows nonspecific trapping of low levels of IgG and IgA, complement, and fibrin.

73. Which of the following renal syndromes is/are likely to appear with this clinical and histologic picture?

    A. IgA nephropathy
    B. Polyarteritis nodosa
    C. Wegener's granulomatosis
    D. Poststreptococcal glomerulonephritis
    E. Idiopathic rapidly progressive glomerulonephritis

74. Which of the following therapies is/are appropriate at this time?

    A. Hemodialysis
    B. Plasmapheresis
    C. Cyclophosphamide
    D. Intravenous methylprednisolone
    E. Warfarin and dipyridamole

75. Which of the following statements is/are true of uremic acidosis?

    A. Urine pH is usually greater than 6.0.
    B. Hypokalemia worsens the acidosis by suppressing ammonia production.
    C. Anion-gap acidosis develops only when the GFR falls below 20 ml per minute.
    D. Renal ammonia production and excretion are low, considering the degree of acidosis.
    E. Bicarbonate wasting is observed when isotonic bicarbonate is infused to restore the serum bicarbonate to normal levels.

76. Which of the following statements about aminoglycoside-induced tubule damage is/are true?

    A. Functional abnormalities of tubule function may cause hypokalemia and hypomagnesemia.
    B. Severe oliguric acute renal failure is the rule.
    C. Toxicity is related to the dose of aminoglycoside and the duration of therapy.
    D. Risk factors include the age of the patient, the baseline serum creatinine concentration, and ECF volume depletion.
    E. All aminoglycosides are equally nephrotoxic.

77. Which of the following statements about pregnancy-induced hypertension (preeclampsia) is/are true?

    A. Onset is associated with elevation of the serum uric acid level.
    B. Nephrotic-range (>3.5 grams per day) proteinuria can occur.
    C. This syndrome typically occurs between 12 and 24 weeks of gestation.
    D. GFR and renal blood flow are usually unchanged in preeclampsia.
    E. Clinical manifestations of preeclampsia generally resolve within 6 weeks after delivery.

78. Which of the following statements about renal calculi is/are true?

    A. Crystals seen on urinalysis confirm their formation in the kidney.
    B. Treatment of all patients with renal calculi should include a high fluid intake (minimum 2 liters) if tolerated.
    C. Hexagonal-shaped crystals in the urine are always pathologic.
    D. Magnesium ammonium phosphate crystals (struvite) are associated with urinary tract infections with urea-splitting organisms.
    E. Alkalinization of the urine with potassium citrate may be effective in preventing the formation of both uric acid and calcium stones.

79. Which of the following statements about autosomal dominant polycystic kidney disease (ADPKD) is/are true?

    A. ADPKD is the most common hereditary disease in the United States.
    B. Hepatic cysts support the diagnosis of ADPKD.
    C. Although half of the offspring of one affected parent will inherit the gene that produces ADPKD, expression of the disease is variable.
    D. Renal calculi are uncommon in ADPKD.
    E. Microscopic and macroscopic hematuria can occur.
    F. The incidence of intracranial aneurysms is higher in patients with ADPKD than the general population.

DIRECTIONS: Questions 80 to 91 are matching questions. For each numbered item, choose the most likely associated lettered item from those provided. Each numbered item has ONLY ONE answer. Within each set of questions, each answer may be used once, more than once, or not at all.

QUESTIONS 80–87

For each of the complications listed below, select the most likely associated therapeutic agent.

A. Impaired free water excretion
B. Nephrogenic diabetes insipidus
C. Secondary nephrotic syndrome
D. Hypokalemia
E. Hyperkalemia

80. Gold

81. Chlorpropamide

82. Lithium

83. Carbenicillin

84. Succinylcholine

85. D-Penicillamine

86. Spironolactone

	A	B	C	D	E
Sodium	142	138	138	138	122
Potassium	5.7	2.2	3.7	5.7	5.7
Chloride	100	112	112	112	76
Bicarbonate	16	16	16	16	16

QUESTIONS 87–91

For each of the following serum electrolyte determinations, select the most appropriate clinical diagnoses.

87. Diabetic ketoacidosis

88. Type IV renal tubular acidosis (RTA)

89. Distal (type I) RTA

90. Proximal (type II) RTA

91. Uremic acidosis

PART 4

RENAL DISEASE

ANSWERS

1.(E); 2.(D) *Discussion:* This patient has sarcoidosis with systemic manifestations that included pulmonary and skin involvement. Renal lesions in sarcoidosis are variable but may involve glomeruli and the tubulointerstitium. Immune complex–mediated glomerulonephritis may be more common in those patients who have erythema nodosa. Granulomatous infiltration of the kidney may produce a variety of tubular abnormalities that include inability to concentrate the urine, nephrogenic diabetes insipidus, and renal tubular acidification defects. The hypercalcemia that occurs with sarcoidosis results from the presence in the macrophages of 25-hydroxy-vitamin D 1-alpha-hydroxylase, which produces 1,25-dihydroxy-vitamin D_3(calcitriol) and thereby facilitates gastrointestinal absorption of calcium. Prolonged hypercalcemia produces renal failure from nephrocalcinosis. Typically, hypercalcemia responds very well to prednisone. (*Cecil, Ch. 61 and 80*)

3.(B); 4.(A); 5.(D) *Discussion:* One of the challenges in the management of the patient with end-stage renal failure is ACKD. ACKD has a male predominance and occurs in patients who have received any form of renal replacement therapy, including hemodialysis and peritoneal dialysis. ACKD can also develop in any patient who has chronic renal failure (serum creatinine level >3 mg per deciliter) but is not yet on dialysis. Although successful renal transplantation retards or reverses ACKD, the associated renal cell carcinoma accounts for nearly 2% of deaths in renal transplant patients. Most patients with ACKD are asymptomatic, even when renal cell carcinoma develops. When symptomatic, a common manifestation is hematuria. Although ultrasound is convenient and relatively inexpensive, computed tomography appears to be the best imaging tool to identify small tumors. Generally, tumors <3 cm do not metastasize but should be followed closely if elective nephrectomy is not performed. In almost 10% of patients, the tumors are bilateral, and some have advocated elective bilateral nephrectomy even in those individuals with unilateral disease. Metastatic disease has a variable course, but some patients survive for several years despite metastases. Results of use of adjuvant chemotherapy have been disappointing. (*Cecil, Ch. 89*)

6.(D); 7.(B); 8.(D) *Discussion:* This patient's acute renal failure is due to an intrinsic renal lesion. The differential diagnosis includes immune complex–mediated acute glomerulonephritis from a cutaneous bacterial infection, aminoglycoside-induced acute tubular necrosis, and allergic interstitial nephritis from beta-lactam antibiotics. However, the clinical presentation, which consisted of hypertension, oliguria, and hematuria with RBC casts, is classic for the syndrome of acute glomerulonephritis. Acute glomerulonephri-

tis may occur after pharyngeal or cutaneous streptococcal infections. The latent period between the onset of a streptococcal pharyngeal infection and clinically apparent acute nephritis is 6 to 20 days (average 10 days), whereas for impetigo the latent period has been more difficult to determine but is probably longer. Postinfectious glomerulonephritis is generally associated with low serum complement levels. The prognosis for complete recovery from poststreptococcal glomerulonephritis is excellent in pediatric patients. The prognosis for renal recovery in adults is somewhat less predictable, although probably fewer than 5% of adult patients may have clinical evidence of persistent renal disease at follow-up. (*Cecil, Ch. 79*)

9.(D) *Discussion:* IgA nephropathy is an intrinsic renal disease of undetermined cause. It represents the most common cause of primary glomerular disease in Europe, Australia, and the United States. The lesion is characterized by mesangial immune deposits composed of IgA that are predominantly polymeric and of mucosal origin. (*Cecil, Ch. 79*)

10.(F); 11.(E); 12.(D); 13.(D) *Discussion:* This patient has multiple myeloma, and his renal failure most likely is related to overproduction of immunoglobulin light chains. He has anemia, a reduced anion gap, and reduction in creatinine clearance. In addition, he has significant proteinuria and hypercalcemia. Ordinarily, proteinuria in that range strongly suggests a glomerular lesion, but the patient has a normal serum albumin. Thus, the presence of a low-molecular-weight protein that is readily filtered at the glomerulus, such as immunoglobulin light chain, could explain the proteinuria. Immunoelectrophoresis or immunofixation electrophoresis of the serum and urine serve to sort out the proteinuria and establish the diagnosis. The diagnosis is then confirmed using bone marrow aspiration and biopsy and bone survey. The most common renal lesion of multiple myeloma is cast nephropathy, which results from precipitation of the immunoglobulin light chain in the tubule lumen. Other renal lesions include amyloidosis (type AL), monoclonal immunoglobulin light chain deposition disease, acute tubular necrosis, and tubulointerstitial nephritis. Although deposition of light chains also occurs in arterioles, a true vasculitis has not been described. (*Cecil, Ch. 79*)

14.(A); 15.(B); 16.(C) *Discussion:* This patient has a classic presentation of retroperitoneal fibrosis. These patients often present with diminished urine output, and, despite careful evaluation, it is difficult to show significant obstruction because the kidneys and ureters are encased in fibrotic material in the retroperitoneal space. The computed tomogram generally confirms the diagnosis by showing medial deviation and extrinsic compression of the ureters (lateral deviation suggests retroperitoneal adenopathy). Retroperitoneal fibrosis is usually idiopathic, but radiation therapy, aortic aneurysm, and malignancy are other causes. Finally, a small percentage of patients develop retroperitoneal fibrosis from drugs, especially methysergide, an ergot alkaloid. (*Cecil, Ch. 81*)

17.(B); 18.(E); 19.(D) *Discussion:* Anti-GBM glomerulonephritis is a disease typically of young men. Patients often present after an upper respiratory infection with pulmonary hemorrhage and renal failure from glomerulonephritis. Because success of treatment is dependent on how early in the course it is initiated, the most appropriate initial study is percutaneous renal biopsy with indirect immunofluorescence staining, which demonstrates the characteristic linear deposits of IgG in glomerular capillary loops. Although antibody to GBM may be diagnostic of anti-GBM disease, this test may take weeks to complete. Sampling lung tissue may not provide diagnostic results and therefore delay treatment, and this patient had evidence of significant renal involvement. Response to treatment is poor in patients who are oliguric on presentation or who have serum creatinine concentrations greater than 6 mg per deciliter. (*Cecil, Ch. 79*)

20.(D); 21.(E); 22.(E); 23.(D) *Discussion:* This patient has chronic renal failure with superimposed acute renal failure. Prerenal and postrenal factors as well as intrinsic renal diseases are possible causes of the acute renal failure, and further studies are needed to make the diagnosis. Because the patient was taking indomethacin, renal syndromes associated with nonsteroidal anti-inflammatory drugs (NSAIDs) are major considerations. One of these syndromes producing acute renal failure is renal ischemia from a hemodynamically mediated reduction in renal blood flow. This syndrome most often occurs in those conditions in which the renin-angiotensin system is activated, such as cirrhosis, severe congestive heart failure, and volume depletion. It also occurs in patients with pre-existing intrinsic renal disease. NSAID-induced allergic interstitial nephritis can occur after 2 weeks to 18 months of therapy. Hematuria, pyuria, and proteinuria are frequently seen and serve to differentiate such interstitial nephritis from the hemodynamically mediated renal failure from NSAIDs described above. Occasionally, nephrotic-range proteinuria from a concomitant minimal change glomerulopathy is seen. Unlike antibiotic-associated allergic interstitial nephritis, eosinophilia, fever, and rash are generally not present. Although eosinophilia is also infrequent in this syndrome, when it is found it supports the diagnosis. A third syndrome is hyperkalemia, which usually occurs in patients with antecedent renal impairment. Prostacyclin inhibition decreases renin release by the kidney and aldosterone secretion by the adrenal gland through a decrease in angiotensin II formation and directly inhibiting potassium-mediated aldosterone secretion. This patient's hyperkalemia may have been due partially to decreased aldosterone activity, although urinary tract obstruction also produces a renal tubular acidosis with hyperkalemia. A fourth renal complication of NSAID use is chronic interstitial nephropathy, often with papillary necrosis, probably the result of medullary ischemia from decreased medullary blood flow. This diagnosis is associated with a longstanding use of >3 kg of combinations

of analgesics. Along with a compatible history, this patient has small kidneys with hydronephrosis and demonstrates fragments of tissue in the urine. The findings support the diagnosis of chronic interstitial nephropathy from analgesic abuse and now superimposed urinary tract obstruction presumably from sloughing of the papillary tip into the ureters bilaterally. (*Cecil, Ch. 80*)

24.(C); 25.(E); 26.(D); 27.(D) *Discussion:* This description represents the classic presentation of ethylene glycol ingestion. The typical patient is usually an alcoholic who elects to substitute ethanol for antifreeze, which is another available alcohol-containing solution. Symptoms of acute poisoning resemble those of alcoholic intoxication but they progress to stupor, obtundation, coma, and seizures. In addition, a characteristic severe anion-gap metabolic acidosis develops as the ethylene glycol is metabolized to glycolic acid and oxalate. The metabolic acidosis is also aggravated by increased production of lactic acid as a result of alteration of the intracellular redox state. Acute renal failure develops early in the course of ethylene glycol overdose and is probably related to intratubular obstruction from oxalate deposition. Characteristic calcium oxalate crystals are present in the urine. If treatment is not instituted early in the course, renal failure can be permanent. Thus, it is important to recognize this significant clinical presentation. Treatment consists of creating an alkaline diuresis, intravenous infusion of ethanol to prevent the conversion of ethylene glycol to its toxic metabolites (glycolic acid and oxalate), and hemodialysis to remove the toxic metabolites. The patient presented with a mixed metabolic and respiratory acidosis. This conclusion is evident when the P_{CO_2} is examined because, in a simple metabolic acidosis, the respiratory compensation is rapid and obeys the following relationship: for every 1-mEq per liter decrease in $[HCO_3^-]$ the P_{CO_2} will fall 1.25 mm Hg. In this example, the P_{CO_2} should have been 25 mm Hg and instead was inappropriately elevated at 40 mm Hg. Most likely, the seizure produced this respiratory depression. The patient has a marked increase in his anion gap, suggesting the addition of unmeasured anions, in this case glycolic acid and lactic acid. Uremia is an unlikely cause of this degree of an elevated anion gap. (*Cecil, Ch. 76 and 80*)

28.(D); 29.(D); 30.(A); 31.(E) *Discussion:* The age of onset of hypertension and the patient's race make the diagnosis of essential hypertension very unlikely and the most plausible cause renal artery stenosis. Because converting enzyme inhibition produced reversible acute renal failure, hemodynamically significant bilateral renal artery stenosis is probably present. Converting enzyme inhibitors have revolutionized the management of hypertension and left ventricular failure, but the physician prescribing these agents should be aware of their potential side effects. The first widely recognized complication is acute severe hypertension, which occurs when the blood pressure is dependent on the renin-angiotensin system, as in those patients who have volume depletion or renal artery stenosis. When renal perfusion pressure is decreased, as in bilateral renal artery stenosis, the intrinsic renin-angiotensin system of the kidney functions to maintain filtration fraction and thus GFR. Inhibition of this system can produce hemodynamically mediated depression of glomerular filtration and subsequent acute renal failure.

This complication may occur more readily with the long-acting converting enzyme inhibitors. By preventing aldosterone release by the adrenal gland, hyperkalemia can develop independently of alteration in renal function. Other complications of captopril include granulocytopenia, a glomerulopathy with proteinuria and rarely nephrotic syndrome, and angioneurotic edema. Views on the emergent management of hyperkalemia have changed. Calcium and insulin are still recommended to antagonize the effects of hyperkalemia on the cardiac conduction system and to shift potassium into cells, respectively. Recently, selective beta agonists have been shown to shift effectively potassium into cells; beta agonists also potentiate the effect of insulin to lower the serum potassium concentration. The efficacy of bicarbonate administration to decrease the serum potassium level has been questioned. Although most authorities still recommend the use of bicarbonate to treat hyperkalemia, it should not be the sole agent utilized and should not interfere with other more definitive therapies. (*Cecil, Ch. 75.3 and 80*)

32.(D); 33.(D); 34.(D); 35.(B) *Discussion:* This patient has reflux nephropathy, which is a preventable common cause of end-stage renal failure throughout the world. Estimates of the prevalence of reflux nephropathy among end-stage renal failure patients range from 9 to 21%. The pathophysiologic mechanisms of reflux nephropathy are thought to center on a defect in the vesicoureteral junction that allows transmission of a high intravesical pressure to the ureter and kidney. With severe vesicoureteral reflux, urine may actually reflux into the kidney (so-called intrarenal reflux). When the urine becomes infected, the intrarenal reflux of infected urine results in cortical scarring of the kidney. Thus, in the management of reflux nephropathy, early surgical correction of the abnormal vesicoureteral junction and prevention of recurrent urinary tract infections remains the mainstay of prevention of this lesion. As nephrons become damaged, hypertension results. Reflux nephropathy is the most common cause of hypertension in children and adolescents. Finally, proteinuria develops and often can result in nephrotic syndrome. Renal biopsy at that time demonstrates focal segmental glomerulosclerosis with associated IgM and C3 deposition. Typically, renal failure then ensues. Renal failure is therefore due to the anatomic injury to the kidney, hypertension, and the glomerulopathy. As mentioned, reflux nephropathy is a preventable lesion, and for this reason it is suggested that all patients who have a urinary tract infection within the first 5 years of life be evaluated for vesicoureteral reflux. About 1.6% of children will have at least one urinary tract infection during the first 5 years of life and between 30 and 50% of these will have vesicoureteral reflux. Of these patients who have vesicoureteral reflux, 19% have or will develop some renal scarring and half of these patients will also have hypertension before the age of 30. Approximately 1% of these children develop chronic renal failure and eventually require treatment for end-stage renal disease. (*Cecil, Ch. 81*)

36.(A); 37.(C); 38.(E); 39.(B) *Discussion:* This patient has a disorder of osmoregulation resulting in acute hypernatremia. The inappropriately low urine osmolality in the face of severe hypernatremia with an estimated serum osmolality of 352 mOsm per kilogram supports a diagnosis of diabetes insipidus, either central (absent ADH) or nephrogenic. The

increase in urine osmolality with vasopressin confirms a central diabetes insipidus. Ordinarily, patients with diabetes insipidus do not manifest hypernatremia because of an intact thirst mechanism that allows repletion of excreted water losses. Thus, these patients usually present with symptoms of polydipsia and polyuria. With general anesthesia, this patient's thirst mechanism became impaired and she was unable to replete urinary losses of water; severe hypernatremia resulted. To calculate the deficit in free water (x) one assumes that total body water is 60% of body weight and there has been no loss of solute. That is,

Total body solute now = Total body solute at baseline

$[Na]_{now} \times$ (total body water)$_{now}$

$$= [Na]_{baseline} \times \text{(total body water)}_{baseline}$$

170 mEq/L $\times$ (55 kg $\times$ 0.6)

$$= 140 \text{ mEq/L} \times [(55 \text{ kg} \times 0.6) + x]$$

Rearranging this equation to solve for x

$$x = (170 - 140)(33)/140 = 7 \text{ liters}$$

Because the hypernatremia developed acutely, this severe water deficit, which was over 21% of her total body water, can be safely repaired rapidly. The most appropriate management is free water because there was no apparent significant loss of solute, which would manifest clinically as intravascular volume depletion. (*Cecil, Ch. 75.2*)

40.(C); 41.(B) *Discussion:* The most likely diagnosis is acute tubulointerstitial nephritis. The presence of fever, rash, and eosinophilia is highly suggestive of but not essential to the diagnosis. Pyuria with eosinophiluria is very common in this disorder. Although most commonly associated with methicillin, it may occur as a consequence of other penicillin derivatives as well as many other drugs. Tubulointerstitial nephritis is often associated with mild proteinuria and renal tubular dysfunction out of proportion to the decrement in the GFR. These defects often include hyperchloremic acidosis with a normal anion gap, hyperkalemia, inappropriate renal salt loss, and inability to form a concentrated urine. (*Cecil, Ch. 80*)

42.(C); 43.(B) *Discussion:* The most likely diagnosis is obstructive uropathy. The well-preserved hemoglobin concentration and only slightly depressed calcium concentration suggest that the renal failure is of recent onset. The history of urinary hesitancy suggests that the patient has prostatism. The ultrasound examination that was normal initially, then showed signs of obstruction the next day, was caused by severe volume depletion resulting in inadequate urine flow and inadequate pressure to distend the renal pelvis. In the presence of anuria, bladder catheterization must be performed to eliminate lower urinary tract obstruction, a potentially reversible cause of acute renal failure. (*Cecil, Ch. 81*)

44.(B); 45.(E) *Discussion:* The patient's clinical and laboratory data are highly suggestive of the syndrome of inappropriate antidiuretic hormone secretion (SIADH), a common consequence of oat cell carcinoma of the lung. He has hyponatremia with a high urine osmolality. To make the diagnosis of SIADH, there must be no evidence of ECF concentration. Associated findings that support the notion of ECF *expansion* are blood urea nitrogen and serum creatinine and uric acid concentrations. The ADH elaborated by the tumor represents a nonphysiologic stimulus for continued urinary concentration in the face of hypo-osmolality. Thus, the patient has an impaired free water clearance and continues to retain free water despite hyponatremia. The presence of a high urine sodium concentration despite hyponatremia and hypo-osmolality underscores the fact that in SIADH there is *expansion* of the ECF. Therefore, the major physiologic stimulus to sodium retention—ECF volume depletion—is not present. In SIADH, sodium excretion reflects sodium intake and not plasma osmolality. (*Cecil, Ch. 75.2*)

46.(B); 47.(D) *Discussion:* The patient has renal atheroembolic disease. In this disorder, cholesterol microemboli from ragged atherosclerotic plaques in the major vessels are showered distally. They lodge in the kidney as well as other organs, where their effects may be silent or may produce cutaneous lesions, pancreatitis, or central nervous system manifestations. In the kidney, cholesterol crystals may lodge in the small arterioles and produce an inflammatory perivascular reaction that ultimately leads to sclerosis of the blood vessel. This sclerosis, accompanied by varying degrees of inflammation, is often accompanied by the pathologic hallmark of the disease: the cholesterol cleft, a cleftlike area that was occupied by the cholesterol crystal. These clefts may be found in many organs. The precipitating events of cholesterol embolization may be major trauma, major vessel angiography, or vascular surgery; it may occasionally occur spontaneously. The renal manifestations include hypertension, eosinophilia, and progressive renal impairment developing over weeks to months after the precipitating event. The azotemia is usually not reversible (although exceptions have been reported). Although not treatable, this disorder should be considered as an explanation for progressive azotemia and hypertension that develop weeks to months after an aortic angiogram or aortic surgery. (*Cecil, Ch. 85*)

48.(D); 49.(A) *Discussion:* In polycystic kidney disease, the kidneys are massively enlarged with tubular cysts—dilations of tubules that continue to enlarge over years. Among the complications of this disorder are bleeding and infection of the cysts. The typical presentation of cyst bleeding is flank or abdominal pain and hematuria, although blood loss is not usually severe and stops spontaneously. Because bacteriuria and urinary infection are also very common in polycystic kidney disease, the index of suspicion for urinary tract infection should be high. Renal ultrasound examination of polycystic kidneys usually shows masses of large, overlapping cysts. The presence of cysts with complex echoes in this case is consistent with bleeding into a cyst. However, because there may be an increased incidence of renal cell carcinoma in polycystic renal disease, and bleeding or complex sonographic echoes may be a manifestation of this, a computed tomography scan with contrast may be useful in ruling out renal cell carcinoma. (*Cecil, Ch. 89*)

50.(D); 51.(E) *Discussion:* This is an example of focal sclerosing glomerulonephritis that was initially diagnosed as minimal change disease—an occurrence that is not uncommon. The initial renal biopsy diagnosis was minimal change or nil disease based on the absence of any specific light microscopic and immunofluorescence findings, along with the absence of any electron microscopic findings other than fusion of the glomerular epithelial foot processes. The treat-

ment, prednisone, was appropriate for this diagnosis. However, the development of azotemia is not characteristic of minimal change disease. Focal sclerosing glomerulonephritis is a common cause of nephrotic syndrome. It is most often idiopathic, although it can be associated with heroin abuse as well as long-term vesicoureteral reflux. It begins with the juxtamedullary nephrons and causes focal and segmental sclerosis of the glomerular tuft without immune deposits. It is therefore not uncommon to miss this diagnosis on an initial renal biopsy and to diagnose minimal change disease—a diagnosis of exclusion. Focal sclerosing glomerulonephritis is not generally believed to be responsive to steroid therapy. (*Cecil, Ch. 79*)

52.(B); 53.(B) *Discussion:* The patient's presentation is not unusual. Hypernatremia in adults, with rare exceptions of hypothalamic function, is a serious disorder with considerable mortality precisely because, in order for the patient to become hypernatremic, considerable other pathology must be present. Although there may be an impairment of thirst sensation in the elderly, the urge to drink when plasma sodium is elevated is strong. It is usually the patient with significant sensory impairment and inability to seek water who becomes hypernatremic. This patient's free water deficit is about 6 liters. In addition, however, his physical exam shows that his total body sodium content is decreased. Depletion of sodium manifests clinically because of ECF volume depletion. Intravascular volume depletion produces hypotension with hypoperfusion of vital organs. Therefore, isotonic saline should be started to repair the sodium content deficit. At the same time, correction of the water deficit will also be initiated because isotonic saline is dilute with respect to the serum sodium concentration of 162 mEq per liter. In the treatment of hypernatremia, it is important to consider that the brain is a major target of disorders of water metabolism. In hypernatremia, in order to avoid brain shrinkage, the brain generates intracellular solute, often termed "idiogenic osmoles," to offset plasma hyperosmolality. These osmotically active substances are generated in hypernatremia after several hours. Rapid reduction of plasma sodium will result in swelling of a brain in which intracellular solute has been generated. Therefore, correction of hypernatremia of more than a few hours' duration should be undertaken slowly. It has been suggested that the plasma sodium concentration be decreased no more than about 2 mEq per liter. This generally translates to correction over about 48 hours. Seizures are the clinical manifestation of cerebral edema in over-rapid correction of hypernatremia. (*Cecil, Ch. 75.1 and 75.2*)

54.(A); 55.(D) *Discussion:* This patient is losing gastric contents—sodium, chloride, and acid—and replacing them with fluids that are essentially free water. Although a normal individual will excrete free water to maintain plasma osmolality, volume depletion (as well as pain) is a potent nonosmotic stimulus to the release of ADH. ADH impairs free water clearance by preventing the formation of dilute urine. The final result in this patient will be loss of NaCl and HCl and retention of free water, producing hyponatremia and metabolic alkalosis. ECF volume depletion will cause renin and aldosterone production. This favors avid distal sodium reabsorption as well as potassium and proton secretion by the distal tubule. In addition, the incremental elevation of plasma bicarbonate after each episode of vomiting may obligate further potassium loss. Hypokalemia and metabolic alkalosis will eventually result as well. (*Cecil, Ch. 75.3 and 75.4*)

56.(D); 57.(B) *Discussion:* The two major routes of magnesium loss are the urine and gastrointestinal tract. A normal individual placed on a magnesium-free diet will rapidly lower urinary magnesium losses to an almost negligible level. Hypomagnesemia will ensue because of persistent gastrointestinal losses. Renal magnesium wasting is seen in a variety of disorders, including diuretic use, Bartter's syndrome, hyperparathyroidism, hyperaldosteronism, and hyperthyroidism, and as a result of toxic injury by a variety of drugs, including aminoglycosides and *cis*-platinum. Although the magnesium loss with *cis*-platinum may be profound, it probably abates within 1 to 2 months. The patient in question has hypomagnesemia because of continued diarrheal gastrointestinal loss with poor oral intake. The contribution of *cis*-platinum–induced renal magnesium wasting is highlighted by the elevated urinary magnesium concentration. When extrarenal magnesium loss is present, the normal renal response is avid magnesium conservation; 24-hour urinary magnesium excretion falls to a few milliequivalents per day within 1 week of extrarenal hypomagnesemia. Pure hypomagnesemia can cause hypocalcemia by impairment of PTH release and action. (*Cecil, Ch. 80*)

58.(All are True) *Discussion:* Renal hypoperfusion can be caused by a primary reduction in effective circulating volume, or by unilateral renal occlusive disease, or by bilateral acute renal vasoconstriction. Increased renal salt avidity and renin secretion are constant findings. Azotemia and hypertension depend on the volume status and whether or not the hypoperfusion is a unilateral (i.e., occlusion) or bilateral (i.e., vasoconstriction, hypovolemia) process. (*Cecil, Ch. 73*)

59.(A—True; B—False; C—False; D—False; E—True) *Discussion:* In this case of glomerular inflammation, glomerular blood flow is sufficient to maintain the glomerular filtration at normal or near-normal levels. Typical findings include hematuria, red cell casts, modest proteinuria (<2 grams per 24 hours), minimal azotemia, and minimal or no edema. Because renal perfusion is well maintained, hypertension and salt retention are generally absent. (*Cecil, Ch. 79*)

60.(A—True; B—True; C—True; D—True; E—False) *Discussion:* Creatinine is an end-product of muscle creatinine metabolism. The creatinine production rate correlates with muscle rather than whole body mass and is reasonably constant from day to day in the same individual. Urinary creatinine excretion is the sum of filtration and secretion. Creatinine secretion normally accounts for only 20% of creatinine excretion but can increase if glomerular filtration is impaired out of proportion to impairments of renal plasma flow. Organic bases such as cimetidine can block creatinine secretion but do not affect the filtration component of creatinine excretion. Thus, cimetidine can increase serum creatinine and decrease creatinine clearance rate but, in the steady state, will not change the absolute excretion of creatinine. Because of the nonlinear relationship between creatinine clearance and the serum creatinine concentration, changes in serum creatinine level can be an insensitive indi-

cator of reductions in the glomerular filtration rate in the 60- to 100-ml per minute range. (*Cecil, Ch. 73*)

61.(A—True; B—False; C—False; D—True; E—True) *Discussion:* Renal production of 1,25-dihydroxy-vitamin D_3 is impaired very early in the course of chronic renal failure. As a primary consequence of reduced gut calcium absorption, hypocalcemia ensues, which stimulates PTH secretion. In this setting of secondary hyperparathyroidism and reduced calcium absorption, the development of renal osteodystrophy is a near certainty. The renal metabolism of 1,25-dihydroxy-vitamin D_3 to its active 1-alpha-hydroxy metabolite is a central aspect of the disordered calcium/phosphate homeostasis in chronic renal failure. (*Cecil, Ch. 77*)

62.(A—True; B—True; C—False; D—False; E—True) *Discussion:* Inadequate dialysis is the most common cause of uremic pericarditis. Because of the development of extensive pericardial capillaries and the bleeding tendency in uremia, the pericardial fluid is usually hemorrhagic and may accumulate quite rapidly. Any evidence of hemodynamic compromise becomes a surgical emergency. Right-sided filling pressures are critical in maintaining cardiac output in the setting of pericarditis, so volume depletion should be avoided. (*Cecil, Ch. 77 and 78.1*)

63.(All are True) *Discussion:* The availability of erythropoietin has changed the clinical features of end-stage renal disease. Cardiac performance, appetite, and general sense of well-being are augmented by maintenance of the hematocrit in a reasonable range (approximately 30%). (*Cecil, Ch. 77*)

64.(A—False; B—False; C—True; D—True; E—False) *Discussion:* Children do quite well with peritoneal dialysis because of a relative increase in peritoneal surface area. Diabetics do quite well with minimal hemodynamic instability on peritoneal dialysis. Hyperglycemia is easily controlled by adding insulin to the dialysate. Infections are not all uncommon and in the great majority of instances are caused by gram-positive organisms from the skin. (*Cecil, Ch. 78.1*)

65.(A—True; B—True; C—False; D—True; E—False) *Discussion:* Tissue typing and proper matching have a tremendously beneficial effect on graft survival. *In vitro* cytotoxicity testing between donor cells and recipient serum has nearly eliminated "hyperacute" rejection. Despite these advances, it is unusual to find the "perfect" six-antigen match for a cadaver kidney because of the tremendous polymorphism of the HLA system. In the meantime, advances in immunotherapy have dramatically improved graft survival in the usual setting when the HLA matching is less than perfect. (*Cecil, Ch. 78.2*)

66.(A—True; B—True; C—True; D—True; E—False) *Discussion:* Cyclosporine has revolutionized organ transplantation, and represents the first generation of targeted immunosuppressants. It is currently being used in combination with conventional immunosuppressants (glucocorticoids, azathioprine) and other target immunosuppressants such as OKT3 and antilymphocyte globulin. Cyclosporine toxicity remains a constant problem despite careful monitoring of blood levels. The therapeutic window has not been established because a number of cyclosporine metabolites have undefined therapeutic and toxic profiles. (*Cecil, Ch. 78.2*)

67.(A—False; B—True; C—True; D—True; E—True) *Discussion:* MPGN refers to a clinicopathologic entity that occurs primarily in young adults. Activation of the complement pathway is a typical feature of this lesion, and hypocomplementemia may be severe, especially in type II MPGN. Most of these patients have a circulating IgG autoantibody (so-called C3 nephritic factor) that binds to C3 convertase of the alternative complement pathway, protecting it from inactivation. About 70% of patients will have a depressed serum C3. MPGN may occur in association with several infectious conditions (such as hepatitis B or infective endocarditis), systemic lupus erythematosus, mixed essential cryoglobulinemia, sickle cell disease, scleroderma, and alpha$_1$-antitrypsin deficiency. MPGN can occur after renal transplantation. (*Cecil, Ch. 79*)

68.(A—True; B—False; C—True; D—True; E—False) *Discussion:* HUS is a form of thrombotic microangiopathy characterized clinically by microangiopathic hemolytic anemia, thrombocytopenia, reduced haptoglobin levels, and minimal evidence of disseminated intravascular coagulation. HUS may occur in children 3 to 10 days after a bout of gastroenteritis, particularly one caused by O157:H7 *E. coli* strains. HUS occurs less frequently in adults, frequently in association with pregnancy or oral contraceptives. The renal prognosis in children is good: Although renal failure may occur in 60% of children, it usually resolves spontaneously within about 2 weeks. However, about 14% will develop chronic renal failure. Those patients who present with a diarrheal prodrome tend to have the most favorable outcome. (*Cecil, Ch. 79*)

69.(A—False; B—False; C—True; D—True; E—False) *Discussion:* The nephrotic syndrome—heavy proteinuria, edema, and hypoalbuminemia—is a common consequence of a variety of glomerular diseases of both focal and diffuse pathology. It is characterized by an often decreased plasma volume and avid sodium retention. Management of nephrotic edema includes salt restriction and diuretics. Although albumin infusions are of transient benefit, the added albumin is rapidly lost from the circulation. There is an increased infection rate in the nephrotic syndrome, a finding attributed to loss of circulating immunoglobulins. (*Cecil, Ch. 79*)

70.(A—True; B—True; C—True; D—False; E—False) *Discussion:* Although hypocalcemia, hyperphosphatemia, and disorders of PTH are present in both acute and chronic renal failure, elevation of bone alkaline phosphatase and radiographic signs of osteodystrophy are present only in established renal disease. Bilaterally small kidneys are a characteristic of the chronic disease. Hypertension may occur in either form. A dilute urine with a high urine sodium concentration does not distinguish acute from chronic renal disease. (*Cecil, Ch. 76 and 77*)

71.(A—False; B—False; C—True; D—True; E—True) *Discussion:* The diagnosis of analgesic-associated nephropathy, which is often difficult to establish, has been made with increasing frequency in this country. It has been estimated to account for at least 20% of cases of chronic interstitial nephropathy. It is believed to arise from toxic effects of analgesics or their metabolites on the deep renal interstitium. Although phenacetin has been suggested as the most nephropathic analgesic compound, there is strong indication that aspirin, especially in combination with phenacetin, is also significant. The incidence is predominantly in women. There is usually a history of consumption of >3 kg of analgesic, although this history is characteristically difficult to elicit. In the late stages, excretory urography usually shows small kidneys with cortical scarring and evidence of papillary necrosis. Anemia out of proportion to the degree of azotemia is common and is attributed to chronic gastrointestinal blood loss. (*Cecil, Ch. 80*)

72.(A—True; B—True; C—True; D—False; E—False) *Discussion:* Medullary sponge kidney is a disorder characterized by ectasia and calcification of medullary collecting tubules. It is most often diagnosed by its characteristic appearance on excretory urogram in an asymptomatic patient. It is probably a congenital rather than a hereditary disorder, although it occurs in several systemic diseases, including the Ehlers-Danlos syndrome. Renal calculi, hypercalciuria, and urinary tract infection are common. A decreased urine concentrating ability is frequent, but other functional tubular abnormalities and renal insufficiency are not common in this disorder. (*Cecil, Ch. 83*)

73.(A—False; B—False; C—False; D—False; E—True); 74.(A—False; B—True; C—False; D—True; E—False) *Discussion:* Rapidly progressive glomerulonephritis is a clinical syndrome that includes a heterogeneous group of disorders characterized by a rapid deterioration of renal function and proliferation of epithelial crescents affecting more than 80% of glomeruli. Etiologic disorders include Goodpasture's syndrome, Henoch-Schönlein purpura, poststreptococcal acute glomerulonephritis, a variety of immune complex diseases, and idiopathic rapidly progressive glomerulonephritis. Poststreptococcal acute glomerulonephritis usually appears with a recent history of a streptococcal infection and is associated usually with an elevated ASO titer. IgA nephropathy is characterized by prominent deposition of IgA in glomeruli. Because idiopathic crescentic glomerulonephritis is relatively uncommon, there are few large studies on treatment. Plasmapheresis, pulse steroids, and low-dose heparin have proven effective in some patients, primarily those with significant immune deposits visible on immunofluorescence staining of renal biopsy tissue. Goodpasture's syndrome appears to be responsive to the removal of anti-GBM antibodies with plasmapheresis and immunosuppression. The prognosis for this disorder is variable. (*Cecil, Ch. 79*)

75.(A—False; B—False; C—True; D—True; E—True) *Discussion:* The acidosis of advanced uremia is a state in which renal compensatory mechanisms are inadequate to maintain external acid-base balance. Even before acidosis appears in uremia, careful balance studies indicate that there is a net positive acid balance (i.e., acid is buffered by body tissues, including bone). The normal renal compensatory mechanisms in acidosis include an increased in renal ammoniagenesis; ammonia is the major urinary buffer responsible for the increment in acid excretion. In addition, there is an increased fractional proximal reabsorption of bicarbonate. When uremic acidosis supervenes, the reduction in renal mass prevents an appropriate increment in urinary ammonia. When the GFR is below about 20 to 25% of normal, there is an absolute retention of organic and inorganic acid anions, leading to an increased anion gap. At this point, although the urine is normally acid, a bicarbonate load cannot be adequately reabsorbed and bicarbonaturia will result on alkali loading. Hyperkalemia inhibits and hypokalemia stimulates renal ammoniagenesis. (*Cecil, Ch. 75.4 and 77*)

76.(A—True; B—False; C—True; D—True; E—False) *Discussion:* Aminoglycoside-induced nephrotoxicity is a common cause of acute renal failure, accounting for 10 to 15% of all cases in the United States. Functional tubule abnormalities may produce potassium and magnesium wasting and symptomatic hypokalemia and hypomagnesemia. Risk factors include an elderly age, pre-existing renal failure, ECF volume depletion, administration of high doses of aminoglycosides, and prolonged duration of therapy. Generally, a nonoliguric type of acute renal failure occurs and the prognosis is excellent. Aminoglycosides are not equally nephrotoxic, although all can cause acute renal failure. (*Cecil, Ch. 76 and 80*)

77.(A—True; B—True; C—False; D—False; E—True) *Discussion:* Pregnancy-induced hypertension (preclampsia) typically occurs in the third trimester, although it can rarely occur as early as the twenty-fourth week of gestation. The syndrome is characterized by hypertension, proteinuria (which can be in the nephrotic range), edema, and reductions in GFR and renal blood flow. Uric acid levels increase because of decreased renal clearance. The clinical manifestations of preeclampsia generally resolve spontaneously within 12 weeks after delivery; persistence of renal abnormalities suggest an underlying primary renal disease. (*Cecil, Ch. 86*)

78.(A—False; B—True; C—True; D—True; E—True) *Discussion:* Most crystals seen on routine urinalysis are formed after voiding, when the urine cools and becomes alkaline. To demonstrate that crystals are formed in the kidney, examine a freshly voided urine sample. Hexagonal-shaped crystals are seen in cystinuria, a common aminoaciduria affecting about 1:7000 individuals. Cystine is the least soluble of the naturally occurring amino acids, especially in acidic solutions; hence the tendency toward renal stone formation in these patients. Magnesium ammonium phosphate crystals (struvite) are associated with urinary tract infections with urea-splitting organisms. Treatment of all patients with renal calculi should include a high fluid intake (minimum 2 liters) if tolerated. Successful therapy should produce at least one bout of nocturia, because the urine tends to become acidic and concentrated. Alkalinization of the urine with potassium citrate may be effective in preventing the formation of both uric acid and calcium stones; alkalinization will also help patients with cystinuria, but a urine pH of >7.5 is necessary to produce the desired effect. (*Cecil, Ch. 82 and 88*)

79.(A—True; B—True; C—True; D—False; E—True; F—True) *Discussion:* ADPKD is the most common hereditary disease in the United States, affecting 500,000 people. Although half of the offspring of one affected parent will inherit the gene that produces ADPKD, expression of the disease is variable. Renal failure, for example, can occur as early as the first decade of life in some patients; in others renal function can remain well preserved throughout life. Patients can present with microscopic and macroscopic hematuria, renal calculi, hypertension, or subarachnoid bleeding from intracranial aneurysms, which may be found in 10 to 40% of patients with ADPKD. The presence of hepatic cysts on ultrasound supports the diagnosis of ADPKD. (*Cecil, Ch. 89*)

80.(C); 81.(A); 82.(B); 83.(D); 84.(E); 85.(C); 86.(E) *Discussion:* Impaired free water excretion is characteristic both of drugs causing true SIADH, such as vincristine, cyclophosphamide, and chlorpropamide, and of drugs with intrarenal effects, such as the thiazide diuretics. Nephrogenic diabetes insipidus, unresponsive to vasopressin and leading to polyuria and pure water loss, may be a side effect of such drugs as lithium, demethylchlortetracycline, and vinblastine. The nephrotic syndrome can result from the administration of heavy metals, penicillamine, and anticonvulsants. Recently the syndrome has been associated with the use of NSAIDs, especially fenoprofen. Hypokalemia based on renal potassium loss can result from administration of both thiazides and loop diuretics. In addition, depolarizing muscle relaxants such as succinylcholine can produce sudden hyperkalemia based on rapid shifts of potassium from muscle cells to ECF. (*Cecil, Ch. 75, 75.2, 75.3*)

87.(E); 88.(D); 89.(B); 90.(C); 91.(A) *Discussion:* Type IV RTA is characterized by hyperkalemia and hyperchloremic acidosis with a normal anion gap. Distal (type I) RTA is also characterized by hyperchloremic acidosis with a normal anion gap, but hypokalemia is often a feature because bicarbonate present in the distal tubule acts as a nonreabsorbable anion and can obligate continued potassium loss. Proximal (type II) RTA is again characterized by normal anion-gap hyperchloremic acidosis. In the steady state, however, there is no bicarbonaturia and no hypokalemia. Uremic acidosis is caused both by a failure of ammoniagenesis and by renal net acid secretion (as in type IV RTA) but also by a net retention of nonmetabolizable acids, producing an elevated anion gap. Finally, in diabetic ketoacidosis, the clue is the elevated anion gap, as well as hyponatremia caused by hyperglycemia. (*Cecil, Ch. 75.4*)

BIBLIOGRAPHY

Bennett JC, Plum F (eds): Cecil Textbook of Medicine. 20th ed. Philadelphia, WB Saunders Company, 1996.

PART 5

ONCOLOGY

Robert S. DiPaola and William N. Hait

DIRECTIONS: For questions 1 to 35, choose the ONE BEST answer to each question.

1. A 34-year-old woman has two sisters and a mother who have had cancer of the breast. All of the following statements are true EXCEPT

- A. Cancer of the breast can be inherited in an autosomal dominant fashion.
- B. Carcinoma of the ovary and breast may be inherited in association.
- C. Her brother has little chance of acquiring cancer of the breast because it is not known to be inherited in males.
- D. If the patient has a *BRCA-1* gene abnormality, the risk of breast cancer can be greater than 80% by age 65.

QUESTIONS 2 AND 3

A 56-year-old male shipyard worker is found to have a 2-cm mass (T_1) in the right middle lobe of the lung on a chest radiograph. A fine-needle aspirate reveals adenocarcinoma.

2. The following statements about non–small cell lung carcinoma are true EXCEPT

- A. Risk factors include smoking and radon exposure.
- B. Asbestos increases the risk of mesothelioma without increasing the risk of non–small cell lung carcinoma.
- C. Bronchoalveolar carcinoma can present as a diffuse pneumonitis.
- D. Adrenal metastasis occurs in approximately 40% of patients.

3. If a preoperative computed tomography (CT) scan reveals no mediastinal lymphadenopathy (N_{0-1}), proper management of the mass should be

- A. Radiation therapy
- B. Surgical resection, if mediastinoscopy also reveals no involved mediastinal lymph nodes
- C. Initial chemotherapy prior to further surgical procedures
- D. Combined chemotherapy and radiation

4. Which of the following chemotherapy drugs is most likely to cause renal failure?

- A. Vincristine
- B. Cyclophosphamide
- C. Cisplatin
- D. Carboplatin
- E. Mesna (sodium 2-mercaptoethanesulfonate)

QUESTIONS 5 AND 6

A 55-year-old man is diagnosed as having acute myelogenous leukemia. Four days after he is induced with idarubicin and cytarabine chemotherapy, the following laboratory values return: prothrombin time = 16 seconds (normal: <13), fibrinogen = 80 (normal: >120), platelets = 50,000 (normal: 120,000), and uric acid level = 14 mg per deciliter (normal: <9.0).

5. All of the following statements regarding the management of this patient are true EXCEPT

- A. Allopurinol should be continued.
- B. Intravenous fluids with bicarbonate should be initiated.
- C. The chemotherapy should be discontinued immediately.
- D. Fresh frozen plasma and cryoprecipitate could be given.

6. The most likely type of leukemia to be diagnosed in this patient is

- A. M_0
- B. M_3 (promyelocytic leukemia)
- C. M_7 (megakaryocytic)
- D. M_2

7. A 56-year-old man was evaluated in your office after a recent surgery diagnosed carcinoma of the ascending colon. The pathology report stated that the tumor was through the bowel wall and involved three lymph nodes (Duke's stage C). You advise the patient about adjuvant therapy. You should recommend

- A. No further treatment
- B. Treatment with only radiation therapy to the region of resection
- C. Treatment with combined radiation and chemotherapy
- D. Treatment with chemotherapy such as 5-fluorouracil (5-FU) and levamasole

8. A 50-year-old woman was diagnosed as having a stage I (T_1, N_0, M_0) infiltrating ductal carcinoma of the breast and was treated with a modified radical mastectomy. A bone scan is obtained and reveals increased uptake in the lumbar spine. Proper management would be to

- A. Initiate chemotherapy for metastatic disease
- B. Administer radiation therapy to the spine

C. Perform further radiologic studies to better define this lesion

D. Treat the back pain medically if symptoms occur, and do not repeat further studies

9. Which of the following statements regarding ovarian carcinoma is true?

A. Use of oral contraceptive agents is a risk factor.

B. The CA-125 tumor-specific antigen test is a good screening test.

C. Those patients with complete primary surgical debulking have improved survival.

D. All patients should undergo a surgical re-exploration (second-look surgery) after chemotherapy.

10. All of the following statements regarding carcinoma of the stomach are true EXCEPT

A. In the United States, the incidence of proximal gastric and esophagogastric junction adenocarcinoma is increasing.

B. Factors that increase the risk of carcinoma of the stomach include pernicious anemia, *Helicobacter pylori,* and blood group A.

C. A palpable left supraclavicular lymph node (Virchow's node) usually represents metastatic disease.

D. Adjuvant chemotherapy definitely improves survival.

11. A 23-year-old man was evaluated by a gastroenterologist secondary to rectal bleeding. The colonoscopy reveals more than 100 polyps throughout the colon. A biopsy of one reveals a villous adenoma. Which of the following statements is true?

A. He may have a family history of colon cancer inherited in what appears to be an autosomal dominant fashion.

B. He has no increased risk of colon carcinoma and requires no further follow-up.

C. He likely has gastric polps that are of high malignant potential.

D. The gene for this syndrome has not been located to a specific chromosome.

12. All of the following statements are true concerning the hereditary nonpolyposis colon carcinoma (HNPCC) syndrome EXCEPT

A. This disorder is inherited as an autosomal dominant disorder.

B. HNPCC is more common than familial adenomatous polyposis.

C. This disorder tends to predispose to left-sided colon carcinoma.

D. Some patients can present with extraintestinal tumors.

13. Which of the following statements is true regarding carcinoma of the rectum?

A. Adjuvant radiation and chemotherapy do not improve survival.

B. The most common site of distant recurrence is the brain.

C. Local recurrence is not usually a problem.

D. Rectal bleeding is a frequent presentation.

QUESTIONS 14–16

On a mammogram, a 50-year-old woman has a single small cluster of suspicious microcalcifications in the upper outer quadrant of the right breast that is clinically nonpalpable.

14. Initial management should include

A. A fine-needle aspirate

B. A mastectomy

C. A needle-localized excisional biopsy

D. No further evaluation

15. The pathologic evaluation revealed tumor cells contained within ducts, without invasion (see the figure on page 77). The surgical margins of the specimen were involved with disease. The next step should be

A. Mastectomy, because the surgical margins were involved.

B. The choice of mastectomy or a re-excision (lumpectomy) without axillary lymph node dissection.

C. Chemotherapy followed by mastectomy.

D. Radiation therapy.

16. A second surgical procedure showed that the tumor was infiltrating beyond the ducts (infiltrating ductal carcinoma). You would now inform the patient that

A. She still has an option of re-excision (lumpectomy), in contrast to mastectomy, but additionally requires an axillary lymph node dissection.

B. She will require a mastectomy.

C. She will not require radiation therapy if she undergoes lumpectomy.

D. Chemotherapy should be given prior to further surgery.

17. Which of the following statements is true regarding gastric carcinoma?

A. Presenting features may include Trousseau's syndrome, perirectal wall metastasis (Blumer's shelf), acanthosis nigricans, and a mass at the umbilicus (Sister Mary Joseph node).

B. Usual distant sites of metastasis include the liver and lungs.

C. Local recurrence, with or without distant recurrence, occurs in most patients with recurrence after initial surgery.

D. All of the above.

18. All of the following statements regarding the biology and treatment of pancreatic carcinoma are true EXCEPT

A. The only intervention that offers a chance for cure is surgical resection.

B. A palpable gallbladder (Courvoisier's sign) is present in most patients.

C. Cystadenocarcinoma histology indicates a favorable prognosis.

D. Jaundice is a presenting symptom in most patients with a tumor at the head of the pancreas.

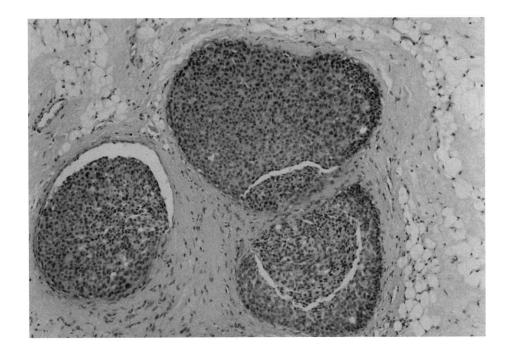

19. Which of the following statements regarding treatment of pancreatic carcinoma is true?

   A. Adjuvant chemotherapy plus radiation therapy does not improve survival compared to radiation or chemotherapy alone.
   B. Most patients with pancreatic carcinoma are resectable.
   C. Most patients with metastatic pancreatic carcinoma have an initial response to 5-FU chemotherapy.
   D. Pancreaticoduodenectomy (Whipple procedure) is the surgical procedure of choice.

20. Which one of the following chemotherapy agents can cause myocardial damage?

   A. Vincristine
   B. Adriamycin (doxorubicin)
   C. Methotrexate
   D. 5-FU

21. Which of the following is a reasonable treatment for the management of inflammatory breast cancer?

   A. Preoperative chemotherapy followed by surgery and radiation
   B. High-dose chemotherapy followed by stem cell or bone marrow rescue
   C. Hormonal therapy
   D. All of the above

22. Following surgical resection, adjuvant chemotherapy is MOST reasonable for which of the following malignancies?

   A. Gastric carcinoma
   B. Stage I non–small cell lung cancer
   C. Soft tissue sarcoma
   D. Duke's stage C (involvement of the bowel wall and lymph nodes) colon carcinoma

QUESTIONS 23 AND 24

A 47-year-old woman undergoes complete resection of a retroperitoneal sarcoma. The pathology report is a high-grade malignant fibrous histiocytoma.

23. The appropriate management would be

   A. Adjuvant chemotherapy with methotrexate, Adriamycin, and dacarbazine
   B. Radiation therapy combined with chemotherapy
   C. No additional therapy
   D. Consideration of bone marrow transplant

24. The patient returns 1 year later with a single pulmonary nodule noted on CT scan. The next appropriate option would be

   A. Chemotherapy
   B. Radiation to the pulmonary lesion
   C. Surgical resection of the pulmonary nodule
   D. Close follow-up without further therapy

25. A 58-year-old man with a diagnosis of squamous cell carcinoma of the lung develops altered mental status. His calcium is noted to be 14 mg per deciliter (normal: 8.6 to 10.4). Which of the following statements is true?

   A. The tumor most likely to cause hypercalcemia is colon carcinoma.
   B. Common symptoms include diarrhea and fever.
   C. Treatment should include hydration.
   D. Elevated parathyroid hormone itself is the most common cause.

26. Which of the following statements regarding non-Hodgkin's lymphoma is true?

   A. Treatment for low-grade lymphomas can include watching and waiting without initiating chemotherapy until symptoms arise.
   B. Patients with stage I follicular small cleaved cell lymphomas (limited to one nodal site, on one side

of the diaphragm) should be treated with chemotherapy.

C. Patients with stage I intermediate-grade non-
Hodgkin's lymphoma should be treated with surgery only.

D. CHOP chemotherapy should be used initially in
all grades and stages of lymphoma.

27. Which of the following statements regarding bladder
carcinoma is true?

A. Risk factors include smoking and prior treatment
with cyclophosphamide.

B. Hematuria is an uncommon presenting symptom.

C. Transurethral resection is the standard treatment
used in patients with deep muscle invasion.

D. Patients with metastatic disease are generally
treated with combined radiation and chemotherapy.

QUESTIONS 28 AND 29

A 59-year-old man is diagnosed as having renal cell carcinoma after nephrectomy. The pathology reveals tumor
involving the kidney with extension through Gerota's fascia (Robson stage II).

28. All of the following statements are true EXCEPT

A. Patients with von Hippel–Lindau syndrome have
an increased risk of bilateral renal tumors.

B. Risk factors for renal cell carcinoma include
smoking.

C. This patient should be treated with adjuvant
chemotherapy.

D. The classic presenting triad of abdominal mass,
pain, and hematuria occurs in only about 10% of
patients.

29. One year later, he is found to have multiple bilateral
pulmonary nodules. Appropriate treatment is

A. High-dose chemotherapy and stem cell rescue
B. Radiation therapy
C. Interleukin-2 biologic therapy
D. Resection of all pulmonary nodules

QUESTIONS 30–32

A 60-year-old man is found to have an elevated prostate-
specific antigen (PSA) value of 7 ng per milliliter (normal: <4.0).

30. A transrectal biopsy reveals adenocarcinoma. Which
of the following statements is true?

A. PSA values increase with age.

B. Cigarette smoking is a risk factor for prostate
cancer.

C. Using PSA to screen has definitely improved survival.

D. PSA is a more specific test than prostatic acid
phosphatase.

31. Which of the following statements regarding the next
most appropriate management is true?

A. Because tumor is confined to the prostate, antiandrogen therapy should be used.

B. If it appears that tumor involves the seminal vesicles (stage C), radical prostatectomy should be the
next step.

C. Radical prostatectomy is superior to radiation therapy if the tumor appears to be limited to the prostate (stage B).

D. Options include radiation or radical prostatectomy.

32. A bone scan is obtained and reveals metastatic disease. All of the following statements are true EXCEPT

A. Chemotherapy is a standard primary treatment option.

B. Strontium-89 is useful in decreasing bone pain
from metastasis.

C. Increased bone pain (flare) can occur after the initiation of a luteinizing hormone–releasing hormone (LHRH) agonist.

D. Patients could be treated with a LHRH agonist or
orchiectomy.

33. A 56-year-old woman with a history of smoking
comes to the office 2 years after the diagnosis of Duke's
stage B colorectal cancer with a carcinoembryonic antigen
(CEA) level that is five times normal. The BEST approach
to this patient should be

A. No further evaluation because the elevation of
CEA is likely secondary to smoking

B. Evaluate for potentially curable lesions with a liver
scan and colonoscopy

C. Obtain tests with other tumor markers, such as CA-
125, prior to further evaluation

D. No further evaluation if the preoperative CEA
level was also elevated

34. The MOST correct statement regarding tumor markers is

A. The CA-125 value is normal in some patients with
early-stage ovarian cancer.

B. Patients with seminoma usually have elevated
alpha-fetoprotein (AFP) levels.

C. The AFP level is not useful as a screening test for
any malignancy.

D. Most tumor markers are useful as a screening test;
few markers are of use to follow for a treatment
response.

35. A 60-year-old man who chews tobacco and smokes
cigarettes noted whitish patches on his tongue and came to
the office for evaluation. You notice a large white patch on
his tongue (leukoplakia) and a reddened patch inside his left
cheek. You discuss recommendations with the patient and
his family. Which of the following statements is true?

A. No further evaluation is needed.

B. Biopsy of both lesions should be obtained because
they can be malignant.

C. Cigarette smoking increases the risk of prostate
carcinoma.

D. The environmental tobacco smoke is not a risk to
the nonsmoking family members.

DIRECTIONS: For questions 36 to 64, decide whether EACH choice is true or false. Any combination of answers, from all true to all false, may occur.

QUESTIONS 36–39

A 30-year-old woman with red hair and fair skin, who has history of resection of a 2.5-mm nodular melanoma 1 year ago, presents with pancytopenia and abnormal liver function studies. A micrograph of a bone marrow biopsy is shown in the figure *below*. The cells stained positive for S-100 and HMB-45 immunostains. Magnetic resonance imaging (MRI) of the liver and spleen is shown in the figure, *top*. Her laboratory studies reveal an elevated lactate dehydrogenose (LDH) level.

36. Which of the following statements is/are true regarding the treatment of this patient?

   A. Resection of the liver lesions should be considered.

   B. Bone marrow transplantation should be performed.

   C. Chemotherapy should be considered.

   D. Biologic agents such as interferon and interleukin-2 have activity against this tumor.

37. Factors that may have increased her risk of melanoma include

   A. Red hair

   B. Fair skin

   C. Alcohol

   D. Family history

38. Which of the following statements is/are true?

   A. The HMB-45 and S-100 immunostaining was helpful in documenting this recurrence as melanoma.

   B. Most tumors arise in a pre-existing nevus.

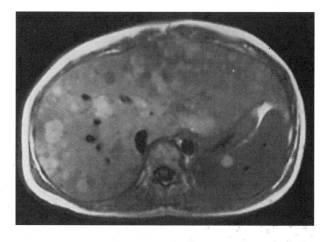

   C. The most common type seen is superficial spreading melanoma.

   D. Nodular melanoma has the worse prognosis.

39. Which of the following statements is/are true?

   A. Adjuvant therapy (treatment after the initial resection) is of proven benefit.

   B. Elective lymph node dissection was not a reasonable option at the time of her initial lesion.

   C. Serum LDH is often elevated in metastatic melanoma.

   D. Survival is worse for superficial spreading melanoma.

40. A 47-year-old woman underwent a biopsy of a mammographic abnormality. The pathology report reveals lobu-

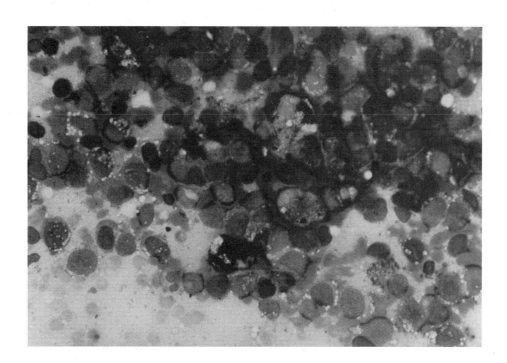

lar carcinoma in situ (LCIS). Which of the following statements is/are true?

A. A mastectomy is the standard treatment for LCIS.
B. LCIS is a marker of increased risk of breast carcinoma.
C. Standard therapy for LCIS includes tamoxifen.
D. The risk of future breast cancer is equal in the affected and contralateral breast.

41. A 30-year-old man comes for evaluation of a small left testicular mass. An orchiectomy reveals pure seminoma. Which of the following statements regarding the diagnostic evaluation is/are true?

A. Seminoma is the most common single germ cell neoplasm.
B. Most patients with nonseminomatous germ cell tumors have elevated AFP or beta-human chorionic gonadotropin (beta-hCG) levels.
C. Patients with pure seminoma often have an elevated AFP level.
D. Beta-hCG may be elevated in pregnancy, hypogonadism with increased luteinizing hormone levels, marijuana use, and other neoplasms such as lung and bladder cancer.

42. Which of the following statements regarding the treatment of seminoma is/are true?

A. Seminoma is sensitive to radiotherapy.
B. Patients with stage II tumors (involved retroperitoneal lymph nodes) with extensive retroperitoneal disease could be treated with chemotherapy.
C. Most patients with seminoma will be stage I, with a greater than 90% survival rate.
D. Stage I seminoma (confined to the testis) is usually treated with adjuvant chemotherapy after surgical resection.

43. A 63-year-old woman is admitted to the emergency room 10 days after adjuvant therapy for breast cancer with a fever of 38.9°C and a white blood cell count of 500 cells per cu mm. Which of the following is/are the most appropriate next step(s)?

A. If fever persists for 2 days, antifungal therapy should be initiated.
B. Granulocyte colony-stimulating factor (G-CSF) should always be started at the time of neutropenia.
C. Antibiotics started should cover gram-negative organisms.
D. G-CSF could reasonably be started after the next cycle of chemotherapy.

44. A 63-year-old man with metastatic lung carcinoma notes the onset of intense back pain and leg weakness over the last few days. Which of the following is/are the most appropriate management?

A. He should be treated with analgesics only.
B. Further evaluation should include MRI of the spine.
C. A plain radiograph is likely to demonstrate abnormalities.
D. Surgery is the usual initial treatment.

45. Which of the following statements is/are true with regard to cancer epidemiology?

A. Breast cancer is the most common cancer in women.
B. Prostate cancer is the most common cancer found in men.
C. More women die from breast cancer each year than from lung carcinoma.
D. The incidence of gastric tumors is decreasing.

QUESTIONS 46 AND 47

A 50-year-old woman presents with multiple liver nodules. Biopsy reveals moderately differentiated adenocarcinoma of unknown primary.

46. Which of the following statements is/are true regarding unknown-primary tumors?

A. The most common etiology is lymphoma
B. Unknown-primary cancers occur in 50% of all cancer cases.
C. Unknown-primary poorly differentiated tumors occur more commonly than squamous tumors.
D. Moderately differentiated tumors are found to be of lung or pancreas primary in 40% of patients at autopsy.

47. Which of the following is/are true regarding treatment of unknown-primary tumors?

A. Patients with poorly differentiated midline tumors should be treated with a cisplatin chemotherapy regimen.
B. Women who present with peritoneal carcinomatous involvement should be treated with a lymphoma-type regimen.
C. Because breast cancer is a common cause of moderately differentiated tumor, all patients should be started on tamoxifen.
D. A regimen that includes 5-FU is often used in patients with moderately differentiated adenocarcinoma.

48. Which of the following statements regarding drug resistance is/are true?

A. P glycoprotein is a transporter protein that can actively pump out drugs.
B. Substrates for P glycoprotein include anthracyclines and taxol.
C. Expression of P glycoprotein can increase with treatment.
D. Verapamil analogues may be useful in altering multidrug resistance.

49. A 60-year-old man with a diagnosis of small cell lung cancer is found to have hyponatremia. His urine has a high sodium concentration. Which of the following statements is/are true?

A. The cause of this abnormality is likely the production of antidiuretic hormone.
B. This can also occur with severe pulmonary infections.

C. Cyclophosphamide and vincristine are used to treat this syndrome.
D. Treatment should be focused on treating the underlying malignancy.

50. Which of the following is/are true regarding chemotherapy pharmacokinetics?

A. Leucovorin enhances the effect of 5-FU.
B. Resistance to methotrexate usually occurs through overexpression of P glycoprotein.
C. Methotrexate inhibits dihydrofolate reductase.
D. 5-FU acts to inhibit thymidine synthetase via a metabolite.

QUESTIONS 51–53

A 30-year-old man presents with a palpable cervical lymph node. A biopsy reveals nodular sclerosing Hodgkin's disease.

51. Which of the following statements is/are true regarding Hodgkin's disease?

A. The Reed-Sternberg cell is pathognomonic.
B. The most common subtype is nodular sclerosing.
C. The lymphocyte-depleted subtype has a worse prognosis.
D. Most cells in the pathology specimen are malignant.

52. After a staging laparotomy, this patient is classified as stage II. Which of the following is/are true?

A. If this patient has pruritis, he would be considered a stage IIb.
B. Stage II represents only one lymph node site of disease.
C. A staging laparotomy is usually important in patients considered for radiation therapy.
D. If he does not have b symptoms radiation is an option.

53. Which of the following statements is/are true about treatment of Hodgkin's disease?

A. Patients with stage IV disease should be treated with combination chemotherapy.
B. Patients with large mediastinal masses could be treated with both chemotherapy and radiation.
C. Stage Ib patients should not be treated with radiation therapy alone.
D. Fever is considered an a symptom.

54. Which of the following statements is/are true regarding brain metastasis?

A. The common sources include lung and breast cancer.
B. Melanoma is the tumor most likely to have brain metastasis.
C. Surgical resection should be considered in patients with solitary metastasis.
D. Chemotherapy is the primary treatment for most patients.

55. Which of the following statements is/are true regarding superior vena cava syndrome?

A. Infection is the most common cause.
B. The most common malignancy causing superior vena cava syndrome is gastric cancer.
C. Dyspnea is a common symptom.
D. Treatment should always include surgical resection.

56. Which of the following statements is/are true regarding esophageal carcinoma?

A. Risk factors include tylosis and Barrett's esophagitis.
B. Most adenocarcinomas are associated with Barrett's esophagitis.
C. The incidence is higher in blacks than in whites.
D. Squamous cell carcinoma is the most common histology.

57. Which of the following statements is/are true regarding the treatment of esophageal carcinoma?

A. Chemotherapy alone should always be used prior to surgery.
B. Combined chemotherapy and radiation is used in patients with local but unresectable disease.
C. Most patients are cured with surgery.
D. The most common reason for inoperability is invasion of the tracheobronchus.

58. Which of the following statements is/are true regarding clinical trials?

A. A phase I clinical trial evaluates an agent for response.
B. Phase II clinical trials usually require a site of measurable disease.
C. A randomized trial usually requires large numbers of patients.
D. The maximum tolerated dose of a novel agent is best evaluated in a phase III trial.

59. Which of the following statements is/are true regarding multiple myeloma?

A. Bone scans are usually normal.
B. $Beta_2$-microglobulin levels can be prognostic.
C. Treatment for hyperviscosity includes plasmapheresis.
D. The serum or urine protein electrophoresis is abnormal in $<50\%$ of patients.

60. Which of the following statements is/are true regarding chemotherapy drug resistance?

A. Resistance to etoposide can be due to altered topoisomerase II.
B. Resistance to doxorubicin occurs only through the expression of P glycoprotein.
C. Topotecan acts through effects on topoisomerase I.
D. Vincristine is a substrate to P glycoprotein.

61. A 62-year-old man is diagnosed as having advanced lung carcinoma. He is noted to have proximal muscle weakness. Electromyographic studies reveal an abnormal Tensilon test. Which of the following statements is/are true?

A. He most likely has small cell histology.
B. He will likely have ocular and bulbar muscle dysfunction.
C. The electromyographic findings can distinguish this condition from myasthenia gravis.
D. Treatment mainly consists of treating the malignancy.

62. Which of the following statements is/are true with regard to interferon?

A. Interferon is used for the treatment of hairy cell leukemia.
B. Its toxicities include fever.
C. Interferon should never used in combination with chemotherapy.
D. Interferon is active in Kaposi's sarcoma.

63. Which of the following statements is/are true with regard to malignant pericardial effusions?

A. The most common etiologies include lung and breast cancer.
B. Dyspnea is a common symptom.
C. Most patients present with jugular venous distention.
D. Cytology is usually negative.

64. Which of the following statements is/are true regarding tumor resistance?

A. Tumor cell death by apoptosis is an active process.
B. The *p53* tumor suppressor gene blocks tumor cell death.
C. The *bcl-2* oncogene induces tumor cell death by apoptosis.
D. Tumor resistance can be mediated by failure to undergo apoptosis.

DIRECTIONS: Questions 65 to 101 are matching questions. For each numbered item, choose the most likely associated lettered item from those provided. Each numbered item has ONLY ONE answer. Within each set of questions, each lettered item may be used once, more than once, or not at all.

QUESTIONS 65–70

Match the following chemotherapy combinations to each appropriate tumor type.

    A. 5-FU and leucovorin
    B. Cytoxan, methotrexate, and 5-FU
    C. 5-FU and levamisole
    D. Cisplatin and cytoxan
    E. Taxol
    F. Tamoxifen

65. Duke's stage C colon carcinoma

66. Stage II estrogen receptor–positive breast cancer in a postmenopausal woman

67. Metastatic colon carcinoma

68. Treatment for stage IIIc ovarian carcinoma

69. Metastatic breast cancer after progression on CMF and CAF chemotherapy

70. Stage II estrogen receptor–negative breast cancer in a premenopausal woman

QUESTIONS 71–75

Match the following signs and symptoms with the most appropriate disorder.

    A. Hyperkeratosis and pigmentation of the axilla and neck (acanthosis nigricans) and the sudden development of seborrheic keratosis
    B. Painful red papules on the upper extremities along with fever and neutrophilia (Sweet's syndrome)
    C. Necrolytic migratory erythema
    D. "Moon facies" and a "buffalo hump"
    E. Tylosis (hyperkeratosis of the palms)

71. Acute leukemia

72. Gastric carcinoma

73. Esophageal squamous cell carcinoma

74. Glucagonoma

75. Small cell lung carcinoma

QUESTIONS 76–81

Select the most likely genetic abnormality to be associated with the following malignancies.

    A. *HER-2* overexpression
    B. t(15;17)
    C. Del 17p (*p53* gene)
    D. t(14;18)
    E. *BRCA-1*
    F. *bcr-abl*

76. Bilateral breast cancer with a strong family history of breast and ovarian cancer

77. Infiltrating ductal carcinoma of the breast

78. Low-grade follicular lymphoma

79. Acute promyelocytic leukemia

80. Li-Fraumeni multicancer syndrome

81. Chronic myelogenous leukemia

QUESTIONS 82–86

Match the following chemotherapy agents with the appropriate accompanying toxicity.

    A. Tamoxifen
    B. Vincristine
    C. Idarubicin
    D. Cyclophosphamide
    E. Cytarabine (cytosine-arabinoside)

82. Hemorrhagic cystitis

83. Peripheral neuropathy

84. Endometrial carcinoma

85. Congestive heart failure

86. Cerebellar dysfunction and conjunctivitis

QUESTIONS 87–91

A 25-year-old man presents with a testicular mass. An orchiectomy is performed and the pathologic evaluation reveals an embryonal carcinoma. Match the appropriate management based on the extent of disease. (*Note:* Answers may be used more than once.)

    A. Retroperitoneal lymph node dissection
    B. Bleomycin, etoposide, and cisplatin (BEP) chemotherapy
    C. Radiation therapy
    D. Close surveillance without further therapy
    E. A or D
    F. B or D

87. Clinical stage I (involvement of the testis only by CT scan)

88. Metastatic disease to the lungs (stage III)

89. Pathologic involvement of the retroperitoneal lymph nodes (stage II)

90. Lymph node recurrence after surveillance for clinical stage II disease

91. Pathologic stage I (involvement of the testicle only with negative retroperitoneal lymph node dissection)

QUESTIONS 92–97

Match the carcinogen with the most appropriate carcinoma.

    A. Benzene
    B. Vinyl chloride
    C. Estrogens

D. Phenacetin analgesics
E. Arsenic
F. Beta-naphthylamine
G. Progesterone combined with estrogen

92. Endometrial cancer

93. Hepatic angiosarcoma

94. Leukemia

95. Renal carcinoma

96. Squamous cell skin cancer

97. Bladder carcinoma

QUESTIONS 98–101

A 55-year-old man has a biopsy of a pulmonary nodule. Match the following initial management plan to the listed disease evaluations.

A. Pamidronate
B. Combined radiation and chemotherapy
C. Systemic chemotherapy
D. Surgical resection

98. Both a lung and a bone marrow biopsy reveal small cell lung cancer.

99. A lung biopsy reveals squamous cell carcinoma and laboratory studies a calcium level of 15 mg per deciliter (normal: 8 to 10).

100. Biopsy reveals adenocarcinoma and mediastinoscopy reveals no involved mediastinal lymph nodes.

101. Biopsy reveals adenocarcinoma. CT scan shows involvement of the mediastinal lymph nodes and the patient is not considered resectable.

PART 5

ONCOLOGY

ANSWERS

1.(C) *Discussion:* Genetic factors account for about 5% or more of women with cancer of the breast. Recently, a gene responsible for inherited breast cancer was identified. This gene, called *BRCA-1,* appears to code for a tumor suppressor protein (a protein that acts as a negative regulator of tumor growth), and the predisposition to cancer is inherited in an autosomal dominant fashion. Abnormalities of this gene are linked to cancer of both the breast and ovary. Another gene called *BRCA-2* is also linked to breast cancer. Additionally, *BRCA-2* is associated with male breast cancer and does not appear to be associated with ovarian cancer, in contrast to *BRCA-1.* Therefore, male members of families with a *BRCA-2* abnormality are at risk for inheriting breast cancer. Other inherited predispositions to breast cancer exist. One example is the Li-Fraumeni syndrome, which is caused by an abnormality in the *p53* gene, a common tumor suppressor gene. Families with this syndrome have a high rate of female breast cancer along with other tumors. In fact, about 1% of women diagnosed as having breast cancer before the age of 30 years have germline mutations in *p53*. Given these possible genetic factors, the risk of breast cancer in some women is extremely high (women inheriting *BRCA-1* have a greater than 50% chance of developing it before age 50, and an 80% chance by the age of 65). Clinical trials analyzing the role of serologic studies to identify these gene abnormalities are warranted. (*Cecil, Ch. 156; Miki et al*)

2.(B); 3.(B) *Discussion:* Risk factors for lung carcinoma include smoking, radon, and asbestos exposure. Asbestos exposure, prevalent in shipyard workers, also increases the risk of mesothelioma. The most common histologies in lung carcinoma include squamous cell, small cell, adenocarcinoma, and large cell. Bronchoalveolar histology, as one category of adenocarcinoma, is unique in that it can present as a rapidly progressive pneumonic form. Adrenal metastasis occurs in about 40% of patients with non–small cell lung carcinoma, and a staging evaluation should include a CT scan of this region. In stages I and II disease (which represents tumor within the lung, without extension, 2 cm or more from the carina and at most involving the hilar or bronchopulmonary lymph nodes [N_1]), complete excision gives a chance of cure. Therefore, in this patient, without mediastinal lymphadenopathy (N_2) and with a tumor <3 cm (T_1), the proper management should be surgery, with a 5-year survival rate of greater than 50%. If the mediastinal lymph node involvement is minimal (N_2), surgical resection could still be possible. Some have been evaluating the role of chemotherapy prior to surgical resection (neoadjuvant) in this group. Patients with more extensive mediastinal involvement or tumors extending to the pleura, chest wall, or pericardium (T_3) may be treated with chemotherapy and

radiation therapy, because surgical resection may not be possible. (*DeVita et al; Dillman et al*)

4.(C) *Discussion:* Many chemotherapy agents are cleared from the body through the kidney. Specifically, carboplatin is eliminated by glomerular filtration and tubular secretion. Because 65% of a carboplatin dose is excreted in the urine, significant dose adjustments are needed for patients with abnormal renal function. Although eliminated by the renal route, carboplatin is not as renally toxic as cisplatin. Cisplatin has a dose-related nephrotoxicity that is usually reversible. This nephrotoxicity is enhanced with the use of nephrotoxic agents such as aminoglycoside antibiotics. Vincristine is an alkaloid that is eliminated by the hepatobiliary system. Its major toxicity is a peripheral neuropathy. Cyclophosphamide is an alkylating agent with potential bladder toxicity, causing hemorrhagic cystitis. This toxicity can be reduced with adequate hydration or the use of the protectant agent sodium 2-mercaptoethane sulfonate (mesna). The protectant mesna, on hydrolysis to mercaptan in the urine, inactivates acrolein, the bladder-toxic metabolite of cyclophosphamide. (*Cecil, Ch. 162; DeVita et al*)

5.(C); 6.(B) *Discussion:* The French-American-British Cooperative Group established a classification system for acute leukemia. Acute myelogenous leukemia is categorized as M_1 through M_7. Recently, an additional category called M_0 (an undifferentiated subtype) was added. M_3, or promyelocytic leukemia, is characterized by numerous promyelocytes (with heavily granulated cells). This subtype often manifests with disseminated intervascular coagulation (DIC), especially after the initiation of treatment. DIC usually presents with elevated fibrin split products and reduced fibrinogen, as in this patient. This can be treated with blood product support (transfusing platelets, cyopreciptate, and fresh frozen plasma to correct the thrombocytopenia, hypofibrinogenemia, and coagulation factors, respectively). Alternatively, some will start patients with M_3 acute myelogenous leukemia on a low dose of heparin to prevent the development of DIC. Because chemotherapy is the only chance for possible cure, this must be continued. Other complications of induction chemotherapy include tumor lysis syndrome. This is characterized by the elevation of uric acid and phosphate, and ultimately can result in renal failure. In an effort to reduce tumor lysis, allopurinol and hydration are started prior to treatment. Additionally, alkalization of the urine with intravenous bicarbonate will decrease the precipitation of uric acid stones. (*Cecil, Ch. 163; DeVita et al*)

7.(D) *Discussion:* The benefit of adjuvant treatment for patients with colon carcinoma has been clearly demonstrated for some subgroups of patients. Currently, it is standard to treat patients with Dukes' stage C (stage III) with adjuvant chemotherapy. A landmark study evaluated treatment of stage II patients (with tumor invading the muscularis propria but not the lymph nodes) and stage III patients (with tumor involving the lymph nodes). Patients with stage III disease had a significantly reduced rate of death (by 33%) with treatment using 5-FU and levamisole compared to no adjuvant treatment. This survival benefit was not seen in patients with stage II disease. Therefore, it has become standard to treat patients with stage III colon carcinoma with adjuvant therapy. Although a survival benefit has not been demonstrated in patients with stage II disease, some would consider treating patients with stage II disease if they have poor prognostic factors. Factors indicating poor prognosis include patients presenting with obstruction, perforation, and T_4 lesions (tumor that has invaded through the serosa). Because further clinical trials have been ongoing to assess the benefit of adjuvant chemotherapy in patients with stage II disease, we may eventually find a survival benefit in certain patients within this group.

Radiation therapy has been shown to be of benefit in patients with rectal carcinoma. However, no randomized trial has demonstrated a benefit in the adjuvant setting in colon cancer. By reviewing series of patients in a retrospective manner, some have demonstrated a decrease in local recurrence with radiation therapy without any significant improvement in total survival. Therefore, radiation to the local region after surgery could be considered in some cases. It is not reasonable, however, to give only radiation therapy, because standard treatment with systemic therapy demonstrates a survival benefit to patients receiving chemotherapy. (*DeVita et al; Moertel; Moertel et al*)

8.(C) *Discussion:* Bone scans are often used as a preoperative screening test to identify patients with metastatic disease. However, a positive bone scan is found in less than 5% of patients with stage I and II breast cancer. Given the low likelihood of positive scans in this early-stage group of patients, it is reasonable not to obtain them as part of a routine metastatic evaluation. Additionally, the false-positive rate is high, particularly for older patients. Patients with stage III disease, in contrast, have positive bone scans 20 to 25% of the time. Because this patient has an abnormal bone scan, it should not be ignored. However, given the high rate of false-positive results with bone scans, it should be evaluated further. Plain radiographs of the bone or MRI may be helpful studies to further evaluate these lesions. If a lesion appears to be suspicious for metastatic disease, a biopsy should be considered to document metastatic disease. (*Cecil, Ch. 162; DeVita et al*)

9.(C) *Discussion:* Risk factors for ovarian carcinoma have included a lower mean number of pregnancies and a history of infertility. Oral contraceptives may actually reduce the risk of ovarian cancer. The risk of ovarian cancer is also increased in women who have had breast cancer. The CA-125 test is useful to follow patients undergoing or completing treatment for ovarian carcinoma. In fact, most studies show that failure of the CA-125 levels to return to normal by the fourth treatment course is a bad prognostic sign. The usefulness of CA-125 as a screening test, however, has not been proven. In fact, only 50% of patients with clinically detectable ovarian cancer have elevated CA-125 levels. Patients with residual disease after initial surgery have decreased survival. However, some have argued that patients who can be optimally cytoreduced represent a different population of patients with improved survival related to the tumor biology and not the technique of cytoreduction. Although initial (primary) cytoreduction appears to be important, the importance of a second-look surgical reassessment and cytoreduction in patients who have completed a planned course of treatment is not clear. It is true, however, that the second-look operation can yield more accurate information about the disease status. Approximately 50% of patients who are clinically without evidence of disease still have residual disease on surgical re-exploration. A second exploration and cytoreduction may be important as new second-line therapies are tested. Therefore, it is reasonable to perform a second-look surgery in various clinical trials testing new agents. (*Cecil, Ch. 208; DeVita et al*)

10.(D) *Discussion:* Gastric carcinoma has decreased in incidence in the United States. However, the number of patients with proximal gastric and gastroesophageal adenocarcinoma has increased over the last 15 years. This is troubling because, stage for stage, these proximal tumors have a poorer prognosis. Potential risk factors for gastric cancer have included nutritional, environmental, and medical factors. Specifically, smoked food, smoking, high nitrate consumption, subtotal gastric resection, *Helicobacter pylori* infection, and blood type A have been implicated. Pernicious anemia also seems to be associated. In contrast, there are no consistent data to support that alcohol consumption affects the incidence. Although there has been some concern that histamine receptor antagonists suppress gastric acid secretion and predispose to gastric carcinoma, this is not proven. Indeed, gastric cancer seen in cases described with this association is usually found within 5 years of treatment, suggesting that it was not causal; instead, the gastric cancer may have been already present at the time the histamine receptor antagonist was initiated. Disease that has spread beyond the perigastric, common hepatic, splenic, or celiac lymph nodes is metastatic. One common site is the left supraclavicular lymph node (Virchow's node), which is at the site where the thoracic duct empties into the venous system. Many studies have been conducted to assess the role of adjuvant therapy in gastric carcinoma. Although the Gastrointestinal Tumor Study Group found a survival benefit with the use of adjuvant chemotherapy, many other randomized trials did not. Therefore, outside of a clinical trial, it is not standard to give adjuvant therapy. A current intergroup trial is addressing this issue, but it is still without final results at this time. (*Cecil, Ch. 100; Gastrointestinal Tumor Study Group; DeVita et al*)

11.(A) *Discussion:* Several inheritable syndromes are associated with a high risk for colon carcinoma. Familial adenomatous polyposis (FAP) is inherited in an autosomal dominant fashion. This syndrome is caused by an abnormality of the long arm of chromosome 5 (the adenomatous polyposis coli [*APC*] gene). Its incidence is approximately 1:8000 births. Affected individuals almost always have colorectal polyps by the age of 35. Patients with FAP have an increased risk of gastric polyps. However, in contrast to the colon polyps, the gastric polyps do not have much malignant potential. Gardner's syndrome also is an autosomal dominant disorder with extraintestinal manifestations, including osteomas and desmoid tumors. Turcot's syndrome is a variant of Gardner's syndrome with central nervous system tumors. Recommendations for all first-degree relatives of individuals with FAP or Gardner's syndrome can include flexible proctosigmoidoscopy beginning between the ages of 10 and 12, yearly until age 40 and every 3 years thereafter. (*Cecil, Ch. 156; Toribara and Sleisenger; DeVita et al*)

12.(C) *Discussion:* HNPCC includes a colorectal site-specific cancer syndrome (Lynch type I) and the cancer-family syndrome (Lynch type II). These account for approximately 6% of inherited colorectal carcinoma cases and are more common than FAP. Both are transmitted as an autosomal dominant trait. The *MSH2* gene, a DNA repair gene on chromosome 2p, has been identified as causing HNPCC. The HNPCC syndromes mostly affect the right colon, and the average age of onset is 45 years. Women who have the Lynch type II variety have an increased incidence of endometrial, ovarian, and breast cancer. Families and individuals with HNPCC should receive yearly fecal occult blood testing and colonoscopy every 2 years beginning at age 25, or at an age of 5 years younger that the age of the youngest patient diagnosed with colorectal cancer in the family, whichever comes first. (*Cecil, Ch. 156; Toribara and Sleisenger*)

13.(D) *Discussion:* Patients with rectal carcinoma often present with gross red blood from the rectum. Indeed, patients who present with hematochezia should be evaluated with endoscopy, and hemorrhoidal bleeding should be diagnosed only by exclusion. After initial surgery, the incidence of local recurrence can be significant. In fact, patients with positive lymph nodes have up to a 65% chance of local recurrence. Radiation therapy with and without chemotherapy has been evaluated in patients after complete surgical resection. A trial performed by the Gastrointestinal Tumor Study Group demonstrated a survival advantage to radiation therapy combined with 5-FU chemotherapy. Although this study additionally used another agent called methyl-CCNU, a follow-up study demonstrated that the 5-FU chemotherapy with radiation was just as effective as therapy with both methyl-CCNU and 5-FU. Therefore, standard therapy for patients with resected rectal cancer of stage B2 and C includes 5-FU chemotherapy and radiation therapy. Common distant sites of recurrence include the liver and lungs. (*Cecil, Ch. 162; DeVita et al*)

14.(C); 15.(B); 16.(A) *Discussion:* Options for patients with a palpable mass in the breast include a fine-needle aspirate, excisional biopsy, or tru-cut biopsy. However, if the abnormality is only defined by a mammogram, the biopsy must be performed by a needle localization of the abnormality. Ductal carcinoma in situ is defined by demonstrating carcinoma within breast ducts (see figure with question 15), not penetrating the basement membrane. After an initial biopsy finding of ductal carcinoma in situ, most patients have the option of a conservative approach or mastectomy. The conservative approach includes removal of the tumor (lumpectomy) with clear surgical margins. In patients with pure in situ cancer, the likelihood of axillary lymph node involve-

ment is low and, therefore, an axillary lymph node dissection is not recommended. In contrast, patients with invasive tumor (defined as tumor penetrating through the basement membrane of the mammary ducts) should undergo an axillary dissection. Patients who elect to undergo a lumpectomy should also receive a course of radiation therapy, because it has been demonstrated to decrease the risk of in-breast recurrence in both in situ and invasive cancer.

Most patients with invasive carcinoma also have the option of lumpectomy or mastectomy, with equal survival. Therefore, in appropriately selected patients, the option of lumpectomy with radiation is a reasonable alternative to mastectomy. Additional radiation therapy to patients who undergo lumpectomy is important because studies comparing lumpectomy alone to lumpectomy with radiation reveal a significant decrease in local recurrence for those who receive radiation. In fact, 90% of the women treated with breast irradiation after lumpectomy remained free of ipsilateral breast tumor, as compared with 61% of those not treated with irradiation after lumpectomy. Chemotherapy has been given in the preoperative setting (neoadjuvant) for patients with locally advanced breast cancer, but has not, outside of a clinical trial, been considered standard in patients with stage I or II disease. However, chemotherapy is often given to appropriate patients with stage I and II breast cancer in the adjuvant setting, resulting in an improved disease-free and overall survival. (*Cecil, Ch. Fisher et al; 1989, 1993; Silverstein et al; DeVita et al*)

17.(D) *Discussion:* Most patients with gastric cancer have a combination of symptoms such as weight loss, anorexia, and abdominal pain. On examination, a large peritoneal implant in the pelvis (Blumer's shelf), a large ovarian mass (Krukenberg's tumor), a left supraclavicular lymph node (Virchow's node), a left anterior axillary lymph node (Irish's), or a lymph node at the umbilicus (Sister Mary Joseph node) may be palpable. Distant sites of recurrence include the liver, lungs, omentum, peritoneum, spleen, and adrenals. Local recurrence is common. In fact, one group found that, in patients having curative gastic resection and subsequent second-look operations, 29% of those with tumor recurrence had locoregional failure alone and 88% had locoregional failure as some component of failure. (*Cecil, Ch. 100; DeVita et al*)

18.(B); 19.(D) *Discussion:* Risk factors for pancreatic cancer include smoking and chronic pancreatitis. Most are ductal adenocarcinomas (80%). Although 5-year survival in these patients is about 17% with surgical resection, those with cystadenocarcinoma have a better prognosis and are cured with surgery about 50% of the time. At presentation, fewer than 33% have a palpable gallbladder, and jaundice is common for tumors at the head of the pancreas, where most occur. Surgical excision is the only chance for cure, and the Whipple procedure is the procedure of choice. Most patients are not resectable. In fact, only 25% of those explored are resected. In patients who undergo surgical resection, survival is improved with combined chemotherapy and radiation after surgery. Only about 15% of patients with metastatic disease respond to standard chemotherapy. (*Cecil, Ch. 108; Kalser and Ellenberg; DeVita et al*)

20.(B) *Discussion:* Adriamycin is an anthracycline antibiotic. The mechanism of tumor cytotoxicity includes intercalation into DNA and poisoning of topoisomerase II, resulting in DNA strand breaks. Both doxorubicin and daunorubicin (a second anthracycline) can cause a cumulative, dose-dependent cardiomyopathy that can lead to congestive heart failure. This occurs in about 1 to 10% of patients with a total dose of 550 mg per square meter of Adriamycin. Adriamycin can also cause bone marrow suppression, mucositis, and alopecia. Extravasation of anthracyclines can lead to a severe skin reaction. (*Cecil, Ch. 162*)

21.(D) *Discussion:* Inflammatory breast cancer is accounts for 1 to 4% of all breast carcinomas. The prognosis is extremely poor with local therapy alone (surgery or radiation therapy). Therefore, a combined-modality approach using preoperative chemotherapy (neoadjuvant) followed by surgery, if possible, and radiation therapy has been pursued, with an improved 5-year survival rate. Hormonal therapy using the antiestrogen agent tamoxifen is often included in such a combined-modality approach and may be important. Finally, recent clinical trials have been initiated evaluating the role of high-dose chemotherapy with stem cell rescue. (*Cecil, Ch. 208; DeVita et al*)

22.(D) *Discussion:* Although it is the subject of ongoing clinical trials, it is not clear that adjuvant chemotherapy confers a survival benefit after complete resection for gastric carcinoma, early stage lung cancer, or soft tissue sarcoma. In contrast, survival after resection of Duke's stage C colon carcinoma is improved with adjuvant therapy. Indeed, 5-FU with levamisole improved survival by 33% in a well-conducted randomized trial. This benefit, however, was not demonstrated for Duke's stage B colon carcinoma. (*Cecil, Ch. 100; DeVita et al; Moertel et al*)

23.(C); 24.(C) *Discussion:* Sarcomas represent a diverse category of tumors. Histologically there are three categories of sarcoma: spindle cell (which tend to be radiation and chemotherapy resistant); small or round cell (which are radiation sensitive and chemotherapy sensitive); and pleomorphic (which is a variant histologically between the other two). Both the small cell and pleomorphic variants are always high grade, whereas the spindle cell variant can be of low or high grade (such as fibrosarcoma or malignant fibrous histiocytoma, as in this case). High-grade soft tissue sarcomas such as malignant fibrous histiocytoma are treated by complete surgical excision. Although almost half of the patients will develop metastatic disease, the use of adjuvant chemotherapy has not been shown to improve survival in patients with soft tissue sarcoma of the retroperitoneum. Patients with sarcoma of the extremities, in contrast, may benefit with adjuvant chemotherapy, although this is controversial. The treatment of low-grade malignant spindle cell sarcomas also involves wide surgical excision. Preoperative radiation is sometimes used to improve the ability to resect. Small cell sarcomas, such as osteosarcoma, are treated with combined chemotherapy, radiation, and surgical excision, with improved survival compared to surgery alone. The lung is the most frequent site of distant metastases, followed by the bone and liver. Resection of isolated pulmonary recurrences are important. In some series, about a third of patients with isolated metastasis were disease free at 3 years after surgical resection. (*DeVita et al*)

25.(C) *Discussion:* Hypercalcemia of malignancy is a life-threatening metabolic disorder. It is most common in myeloma, breast cancer, and non–small cell lung cancer. It is uncommon in colon and small cell lung cancer. Symptoms usually include pruritus, dehydration, constipation, lethargy, and coma. Mechanisms of hypercalcemia include the production of a parathyroid hormone–related protein, prostaglandins, and cytokines. Treatment of hypercalcemia includes fluid hydration, diuretics, corticosteroids (which inhibit gastrointestinal calcium resorption and osteoclast-mediated resorption), an antitumor antibiotic such as plicamycin (mithramycin), and bis-phosphonates such as etidronate and pamidronate. (*Cecil, Ch. 163; DeVita et al*)

26.(A) *Discussion:* Non-Hodgkin's lymphoma is classified by histologic grade. Those with low grade (follicular small cleaved cell, small lymphocytic, and follicular mixed) can grow slowly over years. This group of lymphomas can be treated by local measures such as radiation or surgery if localized (stage I or II). However, if the disease is more advanced (stage III or IV), a reasonable approach is to follow and treat with chemotherapy when symptomatic. In fact, a randomized trial conducted at Stanford University has not demonstrated a survival advantage to the immediate institution of chemotherapy in this group of patients. Intermediate- and high-grade lymphomas are treated with chemotherapy combinations such as CHOP (cytoxan, Adriamycin, vincristine, and prednisone). (*DeVita et al*)

27.(A) *Discussion:* Etiologic agents implicated in bladder carcinoma include smoking, occupational exposures (chemicals, dyes, leather, paints, rubber, and plastics), pelvic irradiation, and cylophosphamide chemotherapy. Smoking is responsible for about 45% of male and 37% of female bladder carcinoma deaths. The most common presenting symptom is hematuria, which occurs in approximately 80% of patients. The standard treatment for superficial bladder carcinoma is transurethral resection; in patients at high risk of recurrence, adjuvant intravesicular treatment (with agents such as BCG) is often added. Most patients with deep muscle invasion should be treated with cystectomy. Patients with metastatic disease are treated with combination chemotherapy agents such as MVAC (methotrexate, vincristine, Adriamycin, and cisplatin). (*DeVita et al*)

28.(C); 29.(C) *Discussion:* Renal cell carcinoma occurs in sporadic and familial forms. Patients can have familial renal cell carcinoma inherited in an autosomal dominant fashion or associated with von Hippel–Lindau syndrome. In the latter, as many as 35% of patients develop renal cell carcinoma. In inherited renal cell carcinoma, the tumor is often bilateral. Possible etiologic factors include cigarette smoking and use of phenacetin-containing analgesics. The usual presenting symptoms include hematuria, abdominal mass, and pain. The classic triad of all three occurs in only 9% of patients. The Robson staging system includes stage I (limited to the kidney), stage II (confined to Gerota's fascia), stage III (involvement of the renal vein or inferior vena cava or local hilar lymph nodes), and stage IV (renal cell carcinoma that has spread to the local adjacent organs or to distant sites).

Metastases usually occur in the bone, lung, and brain. The 5-year survival for stage I is 66%, for stage II is 64%, for stage III is 42%, and for stage IV is 11%. After surgical excision of early-stage patients, adjuvant chemotherapy or radiation therapy has not been conclusively shown to benefit. Although some advocate resection of the involved kidney in those patients with metastatic disease who have not undergone nephrectomy, this has not been shown to improve survival. Nephrectomy in this setting is performed to decrease symptoms such as pain and hemorrhage. Patients with a solitary metastasis can have a good 5-year survival rate following surgical resection. Success of systemic treatment for metastatic disease has been limited. Renal cell carcinoma is chemotherapy resistant. Vinblastine has been used but is associated with only a 7% response rate. Alternative therapies have been used, including biologic agents. Interferon has had response rates of 15 to 20%. Interleukin-2 in combination with lymphokine-activated killer cell therapy has had a response rate similar to that of its use as a single agent (15 to 20%). (*DeVita et al*)

30.(A) *Discussion:* Prostate carcinoma is the most common cancer in men. It is second only to lung carcinoma as a cause of cancer death in men. Studies have failed to demonstrate socioeconomic status, alcohol, cigarette smoking, or occupational exposure as risk factors. Currently, PSA and rectal examination have been used to screen for prostate cancer in patients over the age of 50, although survival has not been shown to be improved with the addition of PSA to the screening. PSA is a serine protease secreted into the seminal fluid. It has a half-life of about 2 to 4 days. PSA has greater sensitivity, although less specificity, compared to prostatic acid phosphatase. A PSA value above 10 ng per milliliter has a positive predictive value of 65%. A certain level of PSA density (PSA per prostate weight measured by ultrasound) may be more predictive of cancer. PSA increases with age and should be adjusted to age. In patients with cancer who undergo prostatectomy, detectable levels present 6 to 8 weeks after surgery represent persistent disease. A PSA value that does not fall after radiation therapy also predicts persistent disease. (*Cecil, Ch. 158; DeVita et al*)

31.(D) *Discussion:* In the American Urologic Association staging, patients with stage B cancer represent those with tumor clinically limited to the prostate. Stage A represents tumor that is found during a non–cancer-related procedure such as a transurethral prostate resection. Stage C represents invasion of the seminal vesicles, prostatic apex, or bladder neck. Stage D1 represents lymph node involvement and D2 metastatic disease. Patients with early disease (stage B) are usually considered for treatment with radiation or radical prostatectomy. Both approaches appear equally successful, and a decision is made on the basis of the various risks involved in each approach and the patient's ability to undergo surgery. New nerve-sparing techniques cause impotence in less than 50% of patients, incontinence in 5%, and a 0.3% mortality rate. If the tumor is more extensive (stage C), radiotherapy is often given. Chemotherapy outside of a clinical trial is not standard. (*DeVita et al*)

32.(A) *Discussion:* Patients with metastatic disease can be treated with antiandrogen therapy. However, it is not clear when to initiate therapy or if therapy should include a second antiandrogen for a combined therapy to attempt total androgen blockade. In one trial, 603 men with stage D2 disease were randomized to leuprolide (a LHRH agonist), which will inhibit testosterone levels, or leuprolide and flutamide (a nonsteroidal pure antiandrogen). The progression-free response was increased by 3 months and survival by 7 months (36 versus 28) by total androgen blockade. The benefit was not seen in patients with poor performance status and severe osseous disease. In patients who progress after attempts at antiandrogen therapy, agents such as ketoconazole, steroids, and aminoglutethemide have been tried with minimal response. Currently, chemotherapy has little role in the treatment of metastatic prostate cancer outside of a clinical trial. Cytotoxic agents such as estramustine and vinblastine have been used with some response, but it is unclear if survival is improved. Alternative therapies include strontium-89, which can reduce the need for analgesics and prolong the period before pain progression. (*Crawford et al; Porter et al; DeVita et al*)

33.(B) *Discussion:* CEA levels are elevated in many types of carcinoma and can be elevated in smokers, although not to such an extreme as in this case. Because both limited recurrence of colorectal cancer in the liver and local recurrence can be curable, and elevated CEA levels might precede other evidence of recurrence, patients like this should undergo further evaluation. However, there is no evidence that following CEA levels postoperatively identifies a salvageable group. High preoperative levels in patients with colorectal cancers correlate with a worse prognosis. (*Cecil, Ch. 158; DeVita et al*)

34.(A) *Discussion:* Tumor markers are measured in the blood and often represent products secreted by malignant cells. Most have not been useful as a screening test but can be useful to follow treatment. CA-125 recognizes an antigen secreted by ovarian cancer. This test is not specific and, therefore, is of little use as a screening test. For example, the CA-125 value is normal in up to 50% of patients with stage I ovarian cancers. The CA-125 value can be used to follow response to chemotherapy. In patients with testicular cancer, high levels of hCG or any elevation of AFP indicates a nonseminomatous tumor, because patients with seminoma do not have elevated AFP and have only modest elevations of hCG. Either marker is elevated in most patients with nonseminomatous tumors and can be used to follow response of treatment. AFP is useful as a screening test for hepatoma in patients at high risk in Asian countries. (*Cecil, Ch. 208; DeVita et al*)

35.(B) *Discussion:* Premalignant lesions found in the aerodigestive tract include leukoplakia and erythoplakia. Each has a propensity for malignant transformation. Leukoplakia is often found on the mucous membranes of the oral cavity, tongue, oropharynx, and larynx. It consists of white patches. If biopsied, the pathology specimen can reveal hyperkeratosis, hyperplasia, carcinoma in situ, or invasive carcinoma. Erythroplakia is characterized by red superficial patches. It is even more commonly associated with dysplasia and carcinoma in situ or malignancy than is leukoplakia (up to 40%). Leukoplakia is found in up to 50% of people who chew tobacco. Smoking cigarettes is the primary cause of cancer of the lung, larynx, oral cavity, and esophagus. It is not a known risk factor for prostate carcinoma. Environmental smoke increases the risk of lung carcinoma in nonsmokers. (*Cecil, Ch. 155; DeVita et al*)

36.(A—False; B—False; C—True; D—True); **37.**(A—True; B—True; C—False; D—True); **38.**(All are True); **39.**(A—False; B—False; C—True; D—False) *Discussion:* This patient has recurrent metastatic disease to the liver and bone marrow. Metastasis occurs, from most common to least found clinically, in the skin and subcutaneous tissue, lungs, liver, brain, and bone. Serum LDH is a useful marker of metastatic disease. Treatment includes surgical excision in superficial lesions and solitary brain metastasis. No initial therapy may be an option in patients with favorable sites such as the lung or bone but not the liver. Therapy for metastatic disease may consist of combination chemotherapy with agents such as dacarbazine, cisplatin, BCNU, and tamoxifen. Biologic agents such as interleukin-2 and interferon have activity. The incidence of melanoma has increased. The cause of this increase is unclear, but may be secondary to increased sun exposure. Risk factors include red hair, with a threefold risk, fair skin, and family history. The four major growth patterns are superficial spreading melanoma (70%), nodular melanoma, lentigo maligna melanoma, and acral lentiginous melanoma. Antigenic markers are important in the pathologic evaluation. The S-100 and HMB-45 markers can be used to confirm the diagnosis; HMB-45 is more specific than S-100. Most melanomas arise from a pre-existing nevus. Prognostic features include worse survival for patients with increased vertical height and level of invasion. Ulceration is also a poor prognostic sign. Nodular melanoma has the worst survival. A tumor that is 4 mm or less in thickness has a 5-year survival rate of 37%. For initial lesions, surgical excision is important and a 1-cm margin usually is removed. Elective lymph node dissection is controversial. Patients with intermediate-thickness melanomas (0.76 to 4 mm) have an increased risk of regional metastasis. In lesions thicker than this, the risk of distant occult disease is significant; therefore, lymph node dissection is not likely useful in this group. In nonrandomized studies an improved survival is suggested in the intermediate-thickness group with lymph node dissection. Therefore, it would be reasonable to have considered a lymph node dissection at the time of this patient's initial lesion. Two randomized trials, however, showed no definite survival benefit. Adjuvant therapy after resection is the subject of many clinical trials using vaccines and interferon but is not of proven benefit. (*DeVita et al*)

40.(A—False; B—True; C—False; D—True) *Discussion:* LCIS is characterized by tumor within the breast lobules. If the tumor is invasive (infiltrating lobular carcinoma) beyond the lobules, an "Indian filing" pathologic appearance is often present (see the figure *below*). LCIS is believed to be a marker of increased breast cancer risk. In fact, the risk of future cancer is increased equally in the affected and the contralateral breast. Therefore, it is not usually recommended that a mastectomy be performed because the risk of breast recurrence is just as high in the contralateral breast. Given the increased risk of breast cancer, however, further options have been considered.

The results of a clinical trial using tamoxifen in women at high risk for breast cancer includes patients with LCIS. The results of this study will not be known for many years, however, and therefore tamoxifen should not be used outside of a clinical trial. Other options that have been considered, although not routinely recommended, include bilateral prophylactic mastectomies. Infiltrating lobular carcinoma, in contrast, is treated like infiltrating ductal carcinoma. (*Cecil, Ch. 208; DeVita et al*)

41.(A—True; B—True; C—False; D—True) *Discussion:* Seminoma is the most common single germinal cell

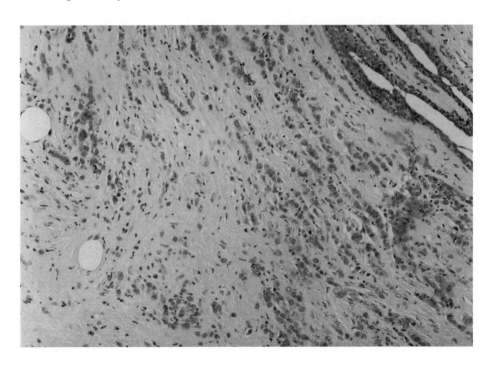

tumor, accounting for 40% of such tumors. Embryonal cell carcinoma, teratocarcinoma, and choriocarcinoma, or combined histologies, account for the rest. In about 85% of patients with nonseminomatous testicular cancer, the beta-hCG or AFP level is elevated. In contrast, in patients with seminoma, the AFP level is normal and the beta-hCG level may be elevated in about half. In fact, patients with the diagnosis of seminoma with elevated AFP level should be suspected of having nonseminomatous tumor. The half-life of AFP is 5 to 7 days and that of beta-hCG 24 to 36 hours. Beta-hCG may be elevated in other malignancies, pregnancy, and marijuana use. One cause of a false-positive hCG assay is an increased luteinizing hormone level. This can be distinguished by repeating the hCG assay after an injection of testosterone. (*Cecil, Ch. 158*)

42.(A—True; B—True; C—True; D—False) *Discussion:* About 79% of patients presenting with seminoma are stage I (disease confined to the testis). Patients with stage I disease have a greater than 90% long-term survival rate. Seminoma is very radiosensitive. For patients with stage I disease, it is standard to treat with prophylactic irradiation to the regional lymphatics. Patients with stage II seminoma with extensive disease (defined as greater than 5 cm) are at risk for failure with radiotherapy alone. It is therefore reasonable to treat these patients with chemotherapy initially, with a cure rate of approximately 90%. Alternatively, patients may be followed after irradiation of the infradiaphragmatic lymphatics, with follow-up and plans to treat with chemotherapy in the event of relapse. (*DeVita et al*)

43.(A—False; B—False; C—True; D—True) *Discussion:* Fever in a neutropenic patient is a medical emergency. The risk of infection increases with a neutrophil count of <1000 (the absolute neutrophil count is calculated as the percentage of neutrophils and bands times the total white blood cell count). Patients should be cultured immediately and started on broad-spectrum antibiotics. The coverage must include *Pseudomonas* and other gram-negative organisms. Additionally, if infection of a catheter is suspected or fever persists after initiation of antibiotics, coverage for gram-positive cocci should be added with drugs such as vancomycin. If fever persists after 5 to 7 days and the patient is still neutropenic, coverage for fungi should be added. The use of G-CSF is best after the next cycle of treatment in patients who have had fever and neutropenia. In this setting it has been shown to decrease the duration of hospitalization and the number of infections. It should not be given during the administration of chemotherapy because it could increase myelotoxicity. Its use at the time of neutropenia is not generally recommended. (*Cecil, Ch. 163*)

44.(A—False; B—True; C—True; D—False) *Discussion:* Back pain in patients with metastatic disease can be a symptom of spinal cord compression. Patients are treated in an emergent fashion because generally ambulation is maintained best in patients treated prior to paralysis. Evaluation usually consists of obtaining MRI. Treatment consists of radiation therapy. If compression occurs in an area of prior radiation or worsens through radiation, surgery is the next option. Most patients with cord compression have abnormal bone radiograms. (*Cecil, Ch. 163*)

45.(A—True; B—True; C—False; D—True) *Discussion:* In the United States, about 1 million people develop cancer each year. The leading causes of cancer among men (in order from most to least common) are prostate, lung, and colorectal carcinoma. The leading cancers seen in women are breast, colorectal, and lung carcinoma. For men and women, lung cancer is the leading cause of death. For women, the second most common cause of death is breast cancer and, for men, colorectal cancer. Rates of gastric and cervical cancer have declined, although proximal gastric cancers are increasing (gastric cardia). (*Cecil, Ch. 157; DeVita et al*)

46.(A—False; B—False; C—True; D—True);
47.(A—True; B—False; C—False; D—True) *Discussion:* Patients with metastatic carcinoma of unknown primary comprise 5 to 10% of cancer patients. Pathologic evaluation should be performed and should include immunostains, electron microscopy, and genetic analysis. The histologic categories include poorly differentiated neoplasms (in about 40%), well- and moderately differentiated adenocarcinoma (accounting for 40% of all carcinoma of unknown primary site), and squamous cell carcinoma (10 to 15%). For patients with well- or moderately differentiated adenocarcinoma, lung and pancreas primaries account for 40% at autopsy. Others include colon and biliary carcinoma. Above the diaphragm, lung cancer is the most common primary tumor found; below the diaphragm a metastasis is most likely pancreatic in origin. Prostate, breast, and ovarian cancer are rare as primaries in this group of patients. Radiographic evaluation could include mammography and CT of the chest, abdomen, and pelvis. However, CT scans usually detect untreatable malignancies. For patients with poorly differentiated cancers, multiple etiologies are possible. All patients should have beta-hCG, AFP, and PSA markers checked. Certainly, the possible presence of treatable tumors such as germ cell, breast, prostate, and lymphoma should be evaluated. Treatment of well- and moderately differentiated tumors usually consists of 5-FU combinations. Treatment for certain subtypes of tumors is more specific. For example, peritoneal carcinomatosis in women is treated as ovarian cancer, with surgery and a cisplatin chemotherapy regimen. In patients with poorly differentiated carcinoma, treatment with a cisplatin regimen can result is a good response in a subset. (*Cecil, Ch. 164; Greco et al*)

48.(All are True) *Discussion:* Multidrug resistance represents the ability of tumor cells to develop resistance to multiple chemotherapeutic agents of different structure and mechanism. One mechanism of multidrug resistance is the expression of the P glycoprotein pump. Another is the alteration of topoisomerase II and overexpression or alteration of genes that control programmed cell death (apoptosis). P glycoprotein is a pump coded by the *mdr-1* gene. It acts as a transporter protein and actively pumps out various chemotherapeutic agents. P glycoprotein is found in leukemia, lymphoma, breast cancer, and renal cell carcinoma. The expression appears to increase after the institution of chemotherapy. Agents that appear to be substrates include anthracyclines (such as Adriamycin), epipodophyllotoxins (such as etoposide), vinca alkaloids (such as vincristine), taxol, and mitomycin C. Studies are ongoing in an effort to alter this form of resistance. Agents such as dex-verapamil (an isomer of verapamil with less cardiac effects) or cyclosporin can inhibit P glycoprotein and may have a role in combination with various chemotherapeutic agents that are substrates. For example, an ongoing phase II clinical trial consists of the use of dex-verapamil and taxol chemotherapy in patients with metastatic breast cancer. Verapamil is a calcium channel blocker and is not likely to be clinically useful because it is cardiaotoxic in doses needed to achieve alteration of drug resistance. (*Cecil, Ch. 165*)

49.(A—True; B—True; C—False; D—True) *Discussion:* The syndrome of inappropriate antidiuretic hormone secretion (SIADH) can occur in patients with small cell lung cancer or brain metastases, in patients with pulmonary infection, or during treatment with cyclophosphamide and vincristine. The usual presentation is with hyponatremia, high urinary osmolality (higher than the plasma osmolality), and high urinary sodium concentrations. Tumor-associated SIADH should be treated by treating the underlying cancer. (*Cecil, Ch. 159; DeVita et al*)

50.(A—True; B—False; C—True; D—True) *Discussion:* Both methotrexate and 5-FU are antimetabolites. 5-FU is metabolized to FdUMP, which forms a covalent complex with thymidine synthetase. FdUMP competitively blocks the action of thymidine synthetase and prevents the formation of deoxythymidine triphosphate, a DNA precursor. Leucovorin (5-formylotetrahydrofolate) will increase the binding of the 5-FU metabolite and has been shown in clinical studies to enhance its effect. Methotrexate is an antifolate. It inhibits dihydrofolate reductase, which is important in the maintenance of intracellular folates for DNA synthesis. Following uptake of methotrexate by a folate transport system, methotrexate binds to dihydrofolate reductase. Polyglutamates of methotrexate are also formed that inhibit dihydrofolate reductase and thymidylate synthetase. Resistance to methotrexate can occur from reduced polyglutamation or elevated levels of dihydrofolate reductase. (*Cecil, Ch. 162*)

51.(A—False; B—True; C—True; D—False);
52.(A—False; B—False; C—True; D—True);
53.(A—True; B—True; C—True; D—False) *Discussion:* The unique pathologic finding in Hodgkin's disease is the Reed-Sternberg cell or a variant among normal lymphocytes, plasma cells, and fibrous stroma. These cells are important for the diagnosis, but cells simulating these cells have also been found in reactive lymphoid hyperplasia so they should not be considered pathognomonic. The histologic types of Hodgkin's disease include nodular sclerosing (70%), lymphocyte predominant (15%), mixed cellularity (10%) and lymphocyte depleted (5%). Mixed cellularity and lymphocyte-depleted disease are more commonly seen in advanced stages. Stage I represents involvement of a single lymph node region. Stage II represents involvement of two or more lymph node regions on the same side of the diaphragm. Stage III disease represents involvement on both sides of the diaphragm, and stage IV involvement of extranodal sites beyond the spleen. The classification a represents no symptoms and b represents fever, drenching sweats, or weight loss. Pruritis is associated with Hodgkin's disease but does not influence the staging. Staging laparotomy is

important for patients being considered for radiation therapy because some will be upstaged by the procedure and require chemotherapy. Patients with stage Ia and IIa disease can be treated with radiation therapy only. Patients with b symptoms consisting of fever or weight loss should be treated with chemotherapy, because there is a higher rate of recurrence with radiation alone. Patients with stage III or IV disease are generally treated with chemotherapy. Patients with large mediastinal masses, defined as greater than one third of the thoracic width, are treated with chemotherapy followed by mediastinal radiation. (*DeVita et al.*)

54.(A—True; B—True; C—True; D—False) *Discussion:* Brain metastasis occurs in about one fourth of all patients with cancer. The most common primary tumors include lung, breast, gastrointestinal, urinary, and melanoma in order from most to least common. However, the tumor type most likely to have cerebral spread is melanoma, with 65% of patients developing this during the course of the disease. Treatment consists of steroids, radiation, and, in patients with solitary metastases, surgery. (*Cecil, Ch. 163*)

55.(A—False; B—False; C—True; D—False) *Discussion:* Superior vena cava syndrome is the obstruction of blood flow through the superior vena cava. The first case ever described was a case of syphilitic aortic aneurysm in 1757. Now malignancy is the most common cause. Lung cancer represents 65% of malignant causes. Small cell lung cancer is the most common histologic subtype, found in 38% of patients who have lung cancer with the superior vena cava syndrome. The second most common subtype is squamous cell cancer. Lymphoma is the third most common. The most common symptom is dyspnea, in 63% of patients. A biopsy should be attempted. Treatment depends on the tumor type. With small cell lung cancer, both chemotherapy and radiation are often given. For lymphoma, chemotherapy alone is usually sufficient. Surgery is rarely indicated when malignany causes superior vena cava syndrome. (*Cecil, Ch. 163*)

56.(All are True); 57.(A—False; B—True; C—False; D—True) *Discussion:* Risk factors for esophageal carcinoma include tylosis (a condition involving hyperkeratosis of the palms and soles, inherited as an autosomal dominant disorder), achalasia, Barrett's esophagitis (60 to 86% of patients with adenocarcinoma have associated Barrett's esophagitis), caustic injury, alcohol, and smoking. The most common presenting symptoms include dysphagia and weight loss, seen in 90% of patients. The major histologic type is squamous cell carcinoma. The incidence is higher in blacks than in whites. However, the incidence of adenocarcinoma in whites is higher than in blacks. Recently, the incidence of adenocarcinomas of the esophagus and gastric cardia has increased. Treatment is surgery in patients with early disease. However, with surgery the 5-year survival is less than 10%. The most common reason for inoperability is invasion of the tracheobronchial tissue. Patients with unresectable disease survive longer with radiation and chemotherapy compared to radiation alone. (*DeVita et al, Herskovic et al*)

58.(A—False; B—True; C—True; D—False) *Discussion:* Clinical trials are an important part of medicine. Given our inability to cure most cancers, novel agents and approaches must be tested. Once an agent has shown promise in an animal model, trials in humans are considered. A phase I trial evaluates the toxicity of a new agent. The trial is usually constructed to continue dose escalation until a maximum tolerated dose is obtained. The starting dose is usually based on the maximal tolerated dose found in the animal model. A phase II trial usually evaluates the tumor response in a specific tumor type. In a phase II trial, therefore, measurable disease is important to assess response. A phase III trial evaluates, in a randomized fashion, the efficacy of an agent compared directly to the standard agent or agents. Usually, large numbers of patients are required. (*DeVita et al*)

59.(A—True; B—True; C—True; D—False) *Discussion:* Plasma cell neoplasms usually have high rates of synthesis and secretion of immunoglobulin. The serum protein electrophoresis or urinary electrophoresis is positive in 99% of patients. The beta$_2$-microglobulin level is an important prognostic factor. Patients with hyperviscocity are best treated by plasmapheresis. Increased viscosity is more likely to occur with immunoglobulin production. The bone scan is classically normal because the tumor activates the osteoclasts and not the osteoblasts. Alkaline phosphatase is typically normal because this is also produced by the osteoblasts. Treatment with chemotherapy is usually initiated when patients become symptomatic or advanced. (*DeVita et al*)

60.(A—True; B—False; C—True; D—True) *Discussion:* Topoisomerases are enzymes that alter the topologic structure of DNA by inducing DNA breaks and reunion. The epipodophyllotoxins, such as etoposide, act through targeting this enzyme. Drug resistance to these agents may be associated with abnormalities of topoisomerase II and decreased enzyme activity. Etoposide (VP-16) is a product of extracts of the root of the mayapple or mandrake. Cross-resistance can occur with other topoisomerase II inhibitors such as amsacrine and doxorubicin. This mechanism of resistance is distinct from P glycoprotein (the classic form of multidrug resistance). In fact, resistance can occur to both etoposide and doxorubicin through this mechanism, without the resistance to other agents that are substrates to P glycoprotein, such as vincristine. Agents that inhibit topoisomerase I are a separate class of agents that include the various camptothecin analogues (topotecan, CPT-11, and 9-aminocamptothecin). These agents have activity against a variety of tumor types and are in clinical trials currently. (*Cecil, Ch. 162*)

61.(A—True; B—False; C—True; D—True) *Discussion:* Proximal muscle weakness with reduced deep tendon reflexes, along with autonomic dysfunction, such as incontinence, and sparing of the ocular and bulbar muscles, is characteristic of the Eaton-Lambert syndrome. Myasthenia gravis, in contrast, has preserved sensation and deep tendon reflexes and commonly results in ocular or bulbar manifestations. The diagnosis is aided by the an electromyogram revealing an increased muscle response to each stimulation secondary to the accumulation of acetylcholine in the synaptic cleft. The Tensilon test has a poor response in Eaton-Lambert syndrome, unlike in myasthenia gravis. The Eaton-Lambert syndrome is most commonly seen in small cell carcinoma of the lung. Treatment mainly consists of initiation

of treatment of the primary cancer. Paraneoplastic syndromes do not affect the staging of a patient. (*Cecil, Ch. 158 and 160*)

62.(A—True; B—True; C—False; C—True) *Discussion:* Interferon is a cytokine that has antiviral and immunoregulatory properties. It has activity against hairy cell leukemia, other hematologic malignancies, and Kaposi's sarcoma and appears to enhance the effect of some chemotherapy agents such as 5-FU, possibly by increasing the 5-FU metabolite FdUMP, which inhibits thymidine synthetase. Interferon also has some effect in renal cell cancer and melanoma. Interferon-alpha is currently approved for use in hairy cell leukemia and Kaposi's sarcoma. The most frequent toxicities include a flu-like syndrome, with fever, muscle aches, and anorexia. (*DeVita et al*)

63.(A—True; B—True; C—True; D—False) *Discussion:* Malignant pericardial effusion occurs most commonly in lung, breast cancer, melanoma, lymphoma, and leukemia. The usual presentation is neck vein cancer, distention and pulsus paradoxus. Symptoms include dyspnea. An echocardiogram is the initial diagnostic study of choice. Local treatment includes pericardiocentesis, or the formation or a pericardial window. The cytologic examination will demonstrate malignant cells in 80 to 90% of patients. (*DeVita et al*)

64.(A—True; B—False; C—False; D—True) *Discussion:* Apoptosis is an energy-dependent process of programmed cell death. Many chemotherapeutic agents ultimately cause cell death via this route. Tumor cell resistance can occur by failure to undergo apoptosis. The wild-type *p53* tumor suppressor gene is often required for the induction of apoptosis. The *bcl-2* oncogene appears to block apoptosis; *bcl-2* may therefore act to prolong tumor cell life. Indeed, targeting these pathways may prove effective in improving current chemotherapeutic results. (*Cecil, Ch. 165*)

65.(C); 66.(F); 67.(A); 68.(D); 69.(E); 70.(B) *Discussion:* Duke's stage C colon carcinoma is defined pathologically as tumor involving the bowel wall and lymph nodes. Treatment with 5-FU and levamisole has been demonstrated to improve survival in this group. For patients with metastatic colon carcinoma, however, 5-FU and leucovorin has been most commonly used with some response. Patients with advanced ovarian cancer have been treated with various cisplatin-containing regimens after resection. Cisplatin and cytoxan has been standard. However, a recent study comparing taxol and cisplatin to this regimen has demonstrated an improved response to the former treatment. Patients with stage I and II breast cancer are often treated with adjuvant therapy. Recently, a meta-analysis was performed that combined the results of 133 clinical trials and 75,000 women. This analysis provides a foundation for our general conclusions about adjuvant treatment; additionally, it can guide our clinical decisions and future efforts at improving therapy. The overview demonstrated that combination chemotherapy improved disease-free survival and overall survival in all age groups, whether they had negative or positive lymph nodes. Specifically, premenopausal women had a 37% reduction in recurrence and postmenopausal women had a 22% reduction in recurrence. The benefit of tamoxifen also reduced the odds of recurrence and death in all age groups. Although these benefits occurred in women of any age, with tamoxifen or chemotherapy, the benefit appeared greater for chemotherapy in premenopausal and for tamoxifen in postmenopausal patients. The benefits were less for patients with estrogen receptor–negative tumors. Therefore, the premenopausal patient who has negative estrogen receptors should receive chemotherapy. The postmenopausal woman with estrogen-positive receptors should be treated with tamoxifen. Combined therapy using tamoxifen and chemotherapy is the subject of current clinical trials. Patients with metastatic breast cancer who have progressed after standard chemotherapy such as CMF or CAF could be treated with taxol. Taxol has been isolated from the Pacific yew tree and appears active in this group of patients. (*Cecil, Ch. 162; Early Breast Cancer Trialists Collaborative Group; DeVita et al*)

71.(B); 72.(A); 73.(E); 74.(C); 75.(D) *Discussion:* Paraneoplastic syndromes result from distant tumor effects. The possible mechanisms for these syndromes include the secretion of tumor products, production of proteins by normal cells in response to the tumor, and antibodies produced in response to malignancy. Some syndromes include the overproduction of hormones such as adrenocorticotropic hormone (ACTH). The clinical features of ectopic ACTH syndrome include hypokalemia, hyperglycemia, edema, muscle weakness, centripetal obesity, cutaneous striae, moon facies, buffalo hump, and hyperpigmentation. The most frequent tumors causing ectopic ACTH are small cell lung cancer or a carcinoid tumor. Other sites of tumors include thymus, thyroid, esophagus, stomach, pancreas, small intestine, appendix, salivary gland, ovary, testis, uterine cervix, and prostate. However, most of these other tumor sites that have demonstrated clinically apparent ACTH excess are of carcinoid or a small cell lung cancer–type tissue structure. Acanthosis nigricans is a skin lesion characterized by the presence of symmetrical brown areas of hyperpigmentation and exaggerated skin markings located in the axilla and neck. This is associated with gastric and other abdominal cancers. The lesions may be caused by the production by the tumor of transforming growth factor alpha. Although rare compared to acanthosis nigricans, the sign of Leser-Trelat (the sudden development of seborrheic keratoses) is also associated with gastrointestinal malignancies. Necrolytic migratory erythema consists of circinate and gyrate areas of blistering and erosive erythema on limbs. This is pathognomonic of a glucanonoma. Sweet's syndrome consists of fever, neutrophilia, and multiple painful cutaneous plaques with a neutrophilic dermal infiltrate. It is seen most often in hematologic malignancies. Tylosis is a hereditary disorder consisting of hyperkeratosis of the palms and soles. It is an autosomal dominant disorder and confers a 95% risk of esophageal carcinoma by the age of 65. (*Cecil, Ch. 158*)

76.(E); 77.(A); 78.(D); 79.(B); 80.(C); 81.(F) *Discussion:* Cytogenetic abnormalities are important in the understanding and diagnosis of cancer. Many oncogenes have been identified. The *BRCA-1* gene abnormality has been recently identified and confers a high risk of breast and ovarian cancer in women. It appears to be inherited in an autosomal dominant fashion. The *HER-2* oncogene is overexpressed or amplified in 20 to 30% of invasive breast cancers and is correlated with poor outcome. The 14;18 translocation is frequently detected in follicular lymphomas in which the

bcl-2 oncogene is present. *bcl-2* overexpression can block apoptosis (programmed cell death). The 15;17 translocation is seen in acute promyelocytic leukemia and causes the fusion of the retinoic acid receptor alpha with PML (a transcription factor). The Li-Fraumeni syndrome is caused by the inactivation of a tumor suppressor gene, *p53*. This consists of multiple cancers, including breast and colon. The translocation of 9;22 brings together the *abl* oncogene and *bcl-2* and is found in chronic myelogenous leukemia. (*Cecil, Ch. 156*)

82.(D); 83.(B); 84.(A); 85.(C); 86.(E) *Discussion:* Cyclophosphamide is an alkylating agent. It is transformed in the liver to an active metabolite and acrolein. Acrolein can cause hemorrhagic cystitis. Bladder toxicity is reduced by extensive hydration and the use of a uroprotectant agent called mesna. Vincristine is a plant alkaloid and acts by disrupting microtubules. Its major toxicity is a peripheral neuropathy, causing both sensorimotor and autonomic dysfunction (muscular weakness, paresthesias, constipation). Tamoxifen is an antiestrogen used in the treatment of breast carcinoma. It also has some estrogenic properties, including beneficial effects on bone density and lipids. Perhaps the most serious toxicity is endometrial carcinoma, which occurs in about 6:1000 patients who use tamoxifen. Other toxicities include phlebitis, weight gain, hot flashes, and retinal abnormalities. Idarubicin is an anthracycline antibiotic similar to doxorubicin and daunorubicin. Anthracyclines can cause cardiac toxicity, usually manifested by myocardial injury. Prior to treatment with anthracyclines, myocardial function should be assessed and the total dose kept to a limit, because the toxicity increases with increased total cumulative dose. Cytarabine is an antimetabolite acting as a pyrimidine antagonist. In high-dose therapy, chemical conjunctivitis is common but reduced with the use of steroid eye drops. Additionally, high-dose therapy can cause cerebellar toxicity. (*Cecil, Ch. 162*)

87.(E); 88.(B); 89.(F); 90.(B); 91.(D) Nonseminomatous testicular carcinoma stage A (Walter Reed stage I) is confined to the testis, stage B (Walter Reed stage II) has spread to the retroperitoneum, and stage C (Walter Reed stage III) indicates metastatic disease. The treatment for stage I nonseminomatous germ cell tumors is controversial. Because of the inaccuracy of clinical staging, retroperitoneal lymphadenectomy remains as the standard surgical therapy. The 2- to 5-year survival rate in patients after orchiectomy and retroperitoneal lymph node dissection is greater then 90%. Approximately 25% of patients who are clinically stage I are understaged. Because 75% of clinical stage I patients who undergo retroperitoneal lymph node dissection are found to have pathologic stage I disease, most undergo this procedure without therapeutic benefit. In some patients, a surveillance program is initiated instead of retroperitoneal lymph node dissection. However, this requires rigorous follow-up, including tumor marker evaluations each month for the first year and CT scans every 2 to 3 months for the first 2 years. In patients with pathologically negative retroperitoneal lymph nodes, only 10% will recur. In patients with pathologically staged stage II disease, 50% will have no recurrence without any postoperative treatment. The group that recurs can be treated with chemotherapy at that time, and so some advocate ether treatment with chemotherapy postoperatively or close surveillance. Treatment for disseminated (stage III) disease has included systemic chemotherapy with bleomycin, etoposide, and cisplatin (BEP). This regimen will cause a response in about 70% of patients, with about 60% long-term survivors. (*DeVita et al.*)

92.(C); 93.(B); 94.(A); 95.(D); 96.(E); 97.(F) *Discussion:* Benzene can cause aplastic anemia and leukemia. Leukemia usually develops within 5 years. Most cases have been a variant of acute myelogenous leukemia. Estrogens increase the risk of endometrial carcinoma. Combined use of estrogen and progesterone has been associated with a reduced risk of endometrial and ovarian cancer. Estrogen replacement therapy may also increase the risk of breast cancer. Etiologic factors for hepatocellular carcinoma include aflatoxin and, for hepatic angiosarcoma, vinyl chloride and Thorotrast. Arsenic can increase the risk of skin cancer. Other causes of skin cancer include the soot from a chimney in chimney sweeps causing scrotal squamous carcinoma. Etiologic factors for renal cell carcinoma include cigarette smoking, phenacetin analgesic abuse, and exposure to asbestos. Etiologic factors for bladder cancer include aniline dye, aryl amines, and cigarette smoking. Chronic bladder irritation has been correlated to squamous cell carcinoma of the bladder, such as chronic urinary tract infections and parasites (schistosomiasis). (*Cecil, Ch. 155; DeVita et al*)

98.(C); 99.(A); 100.(D); 101.(B) *Discussion:* Small cell cancer of the lung is staged and treated differently than non–small cell carcinoma. Staging for small cell cancer consists of determining the extent of disease. Patients with disease limited to a hemithorax can be treated with combined radiation and chemotherapy. Surgical resection is not usually performed. Bone marrow biopsies should be performed; they are positive in 20 to 30% of patients, representing extensive disease. Extensive disease is best treated with systemic chemotherapy only. Patients with small cell lung cancer treated with chemotherapy who attain a complete remission have a survival of about 18 months. Patients with non–small cell carcinoma can have hypercalcemia. This is rare, however, in small cell carcinoma. Biphosphonates, such as pamidronate, are useful for treatment. The hypercalcemia should be corrected before further treatment. Non–small cell lung carcinoma is best treated with surgical resection if the mediastinal lymph nodes are not involved. If the mediastinal lymph nodes are extensively involved and surgery is not possible, patients are often treated with a combined approach, using both chemotherapy and radiation. Randomized clinical trials have shown a benefit to the addition of chemotherapy to radiation in patients with localized unresectable non–small cell lung cancer. (*DeVita et al; Dillman et al*)

BIBLIOGRAPHY

Bennett JC, Plum F (eds): Cecil Textbook of Medicine. 20th ed. Philadelphia, WB Saunders Company, 1996.

Crawford ED, Eisenberger MA, McLeod DG, et al: A controlled trial of leuprolide with and without flutamide in prostatic carcinoma. N Engl J Med 321:419, 1989.

DeVita VT Jr, Hellman S, Rosenberg SA (eds): Cancer: Principles and Practice of Oncology. 4th ed. Philadelphia, JB Lippincott, 1993.

Dillman R, Seagren S, Proprert K, et al: A randomized trial of induction chemotherapy plus high-dose radiation versus radiation alone in stage III non-small cell lung cancer. N Engl J Med 323:940, 1990.

Early Breast Cancer Trialists Collaborative Group: Systemic treatment of early breast cancer by hormonal, cytotoxic, or immune therapy. Lancet 339:71, 1992.

Fisher B, Redmond C, Poisson R, et al: Eight-year results of a randomized clinical trial comparing total mastectomy and lumpectomy with or without irradiation in the treatment of breast cancer. N Engl J Med 320:822, 1989.

Fisher B, Costantino J, Redmond C, et al: Lumpectomy compared with lumpectomy and radiation therapy for the treatment of intraductal breast cancer. N Engl J Med 328:1581, 1993.

Gastrointestinal Tumor Study Group: Controlled trial of adjuvant chemotherapy following curative resection for gastric cancer. Cancer 49:1116, 1982.

Greco FA, Vaughn WK, Hainsworth JD: Advanced poorly differentiated carcinoma of unknown primary site: Recognition of a treatable syndrome. Ann Intern Med 104:547, 1986.

Herskovic A, Martz K, Al-Sarraf M, et al: Combined chemotherapy and radiotherapy compared with radiotherapy alone in patients with cancer of the esophagus. N Engl J Med 326:1563, 1992.

Kalser MH, Ellenberg SS: Pancreatic cancer: Adjuvant combined radiation and chemotherapy following curative resection. Arch Surg 120:899, 1985.

Miki Y, Swensen J, Shattuck-Eidens D, et al: A strong candidate for the breast and ovarian cancer susceptibility gene BRCA1. Science 266:66, 1994.

Moertel CG: Chemotherapy for colorectal cancer. N Engl J Med 330:1136, 1994.

Moertel CG, Fleming TR, MacDonald JS, et al: Levamisole and fluorouracil for adjuvant therapy of resected colon carcinoma. N Engl J Med 322:352, 1990.

Porter AT, McEwan AJB, Powe JE, et al: Results of a randomized phase-III trial to evaluate the efficacy of strontium-89 adjuvant to local field external beam irradiation in the management of endocrine resistant metastatic prostate cancer. Int J Radiat Oncol Biol Phys 25:805, 1993.

Silverstein MJ, Cohlan BF, Gierson ED, et al. Duct carcinoma in situ: 227 cases without microinvasion. Eur J Cancer 28:630, 1992.

Toribara NW, Sleisenger MH: Screening for colorectal cancer. N Engl J Med 332:861, 1995.

PART 6

HEMATOLOGY

John E. Humphries

DIRECTIONS: For questions 1 to 96, choose the ONE BEST answer to each question.

1. In a patient with complete sudden marrow shutdown, peripheral blood cytopenias appear in which order, from earliest to latest?

- A. Red cells—granulocytes—platelets
- B. Platelets—granulocytes—red cells
- C. Granulocytes—platelets—red cells
- D. Granulocytes—red cells—platelets

2. Distinguishing between anemia caused by recent retroperitoneal hemorrhage and that caused by recent intravascular hemolysis can be difficult. Which ONE of the following laboratory abnormalities is most useful in differentiating between these two diagnoses?

- A. Reticulocytosis
- B. Elevated lactate dehydrogenase (LDH)
- C. Unconjugated hyperbilirubinemia
- D. Polychromasia
- E. None of the above

3. In the patient with chronic, slowly developing anemia caused by occult blood loss with a hematocrit of 19%, compensatory mechanisms include all of the following EXCEPT

- A. Decreased 2,3-diphosphoglyceric in red cells
- B. Increased cardiac output
- C. Decreased peripheral vascular resistance
- D. Increased erythropoietin production

4. A 25-year-old woman is found to be anemic. Her family history is positive for gallstones in many family members at a young age. This combination suggests the diagnosis of

- A. Vitamin B_{12} deficiency
- B. Alpha-thalassemia trait
- C. Iron deficiency
- D. Hereditary spherocytosis
- E. Paroxysmal nocturnal hemoglobinuria

5. A patient being seen in the outpatient clinic for evaluation of fatigue is found to have a microcytic anemia. The best screening test to differentiate between iron deficiency anemia and anemia of chronic disease is

- A. Serum ferritin
- B. Reticulocyte count
- C. Serum iron
- D. Percent transferrin saturation
- E. Bone marrow iron stores

6. In a patient with a mild microcytic anemia, the finding of an elevated level of hemoglobin A_2 suggests the diagnosis of

- A. Alpha-thalassemia
- B. Sickle trait
- C. Beta-thalassemia
- D. Hereditary spherocytosis
- E. Hereditary persistence of fetal hemoglobin

7. In a patient with anemia, macrocytosis may be produced by all of the following EXCEPT

- A. Reticulocytosis
- B. Vitamin B_{12} deficiency
- C. Folate deficiency
- D. Myelodysplastic syndrome
- E. Sideroblastic anemia

8. In the patient suffering from chronic alcoholism, macrocytosis is often observed. Most often this macrocytosis is related to

- A. Reticulocytosis
- B. Alcohol use
- C. Folate deficiency
- D. Vitamin B_{12} deficiency
- E. Liver disease

9. Hemolytic anemia is characterized by all of the following laboratory abnormalities EXCEPT

- A. Increased LDH
- B. Increased reticulocytes
- C. Increased bilirubin
- D. Increased haptoglobin
- E. Increased urine hemosiderin

10. In a patient with aplastic anemia, to evaluate for the possibility of Fanconi's anemia as the cause, which of the following tests should be performed?

- A. Ham's test
- B. Cytogenetic evaluation
- C. Bone marrow biopsy and aspiration
- D. Hemoglobin electrophoresis

11. Common features of patients with symptomatic, idiopathic myelodysplastic syndrome include all of the following EXCEPT

- A. Age greater than 60 years
- B. Cytogenetic abnormalities on examination of bone marrow cells

C. Presentation with symptoms of anemia
D. Most eventually convert to acute leukemia

12. Acquired pure red cell aplasia has been associated with all of the following EXCEPT

A. Parvovirus
B. Dilantin
C. Thymoma
D. Systemic lupus erythematosus
E. Prior chemotherapy

13. Which of the following is NOT usually a contributor to anemia in alcoholic cirrhosis?

A. Vitamin B_{12} deficiency
B. Blood loss from gastritis and/or esophageal varices
C. Folate deficiency
D. Red cell membrane lipid abnormalities
E. Hypersplenism

14. Endocrine disorders are often associated with the development of anemia. Which of the following disorders is NOT associated with anemia?

A. Cushing's syndrome
B. Hypothyroidism
C. Hypopituitarism
D. Hyperthyroidism
E. Hypogonadism

15. Which of the following may enhance rather than diminish iron absorption in the gastrointestinal tract?

A. Tea
B. Cereals
C. Antacids
D. Vitamin C
E. Tetracycline

16. Iron deficiency anemia and anemia of chronic disease may have all of the following features in common EXCEPT

A. Microcytosis
B. Decreased red cell iron in the bone marrow
C. Decreased serum iron
D. Increased serum transferrin
E. Decreased transferrin saturation

17. A patient is seen for evaluation of mild anemia. Her dietary history reveals that she adheres to a strict vegan diet. With relation to her diet, this patient is at risk for developing deficiency of which of the following as a potential cause for her anemia?

A. Iron
B. Vitamin B_{12}
C. Pyridoxine
D. Folate
E. Copper

18. Which of the following conditions is NOT associated with anemia caused by folate deficiency?

A. Alcohol use
B. Tropical sprue
C. Partial gastrectomy
D. Dilantin therapy
E. Pregnancy

19. Which of the following laboratory abnormalities is NOT consistent with severe pernicious anemia?

A. Circulating nucleated red blood cells
B. Increased reticulocytes
C. Macro-ovalocytes
D. Hypersegmented neutrophils

20. Which of the following is NOT a feature of hereditary spherocytosis?

A. Ankle ulcers
B. Splenomegaly
C. Gallstones
D. Jaundice
E. Aseptic hip necrosis

21. Glucose-6-phosphate dehydrogenase deficiency is characterized by all of the following EXCEPT

A. Heinz body formation
B. Increased susceptibility of red cells to oxidative damage
C. Inability to maintain glutathione levels in red cells
D. Decreased intracellular ATP
E. X-linked inheritance

22. Features that differentiate immunoglobulin (Ig) G– and IgM-mediated autoimmune hemolytic anemia include all of the following EXCEPT

A. Temperature range of activity
B. Complement dependence
C. Splenic versus hepatic clearance
D. Clearance by macrophage Fc receptors
E. Clearance by macrophage complement receptors
F. Response to splenectomy

23. Of the following potential treatments for autoimmune hemolytic anemia, which is preferred for the treatment of IgM-mediated hemolytic anemia, in contrast to the lack of efficacy of this therapy for the treatment of IgG-mediated hemolytic anemia?

A. Plasmapheresis
B. Splenectomy
C. Cyclophosphamide
D. Corticosteroids

24. Which of the following is NOT usually associated with paroxysmal nocturnal hemoglobinuria?

A. Spherocytes on peripheral smear
B. Iron deficiency
C. Leukopenia
D. Thrombosis
E. Chronic hemolysis

25. In the evaluation of a patient for possible drug-induced hemolytic anemia, testing in the laboratory requires the addition of the possible involved drug to the test for all of the following drugs EXCEPT

A. Quinidine
B. Chlorpromazine
C. Aldomet

D. Penicillin
E. Cephalothin

26. Which of the following hemoglobins is NOT normally found in a 5-year-old?

A. α_2, β_3
B. α_2, γ_2
C. α_2, δ_2
D. α_2, ϵ_2

27. Which of the following statements regarding human hemoglobin is true?

A. Each hemoglobin molecule consists of four alpha chains and two beta chains.
B. For each alpha gene there are two alleles and for each beta gene there are two alleles.
C. When one alpha gene is defective, approximately 50% of the hemoglobin is affected.
D. Patients with a genetic defect in one beta gene may be symptomatic.

28. Iron overload caused by transfusion therapy for beta-thalassemia major frequently leads to all but which of the following clinically relevant conditions if chelation therapy is not used?

A. Growth retardation
B. Cirrhosis
C. Diabetes mellitus
D. Hypothyroidism
E. Congestive heart failure

29. Sudden worsening of anemia in patients with hemoglobin SS should NOT be related to

A. Parvovirus B19 infection
B. Splenic sequestration
C. Bone marrow infarct or necrosis
D. Folate deficiency
E. Iron deficiency

30. Transfusions or exchange transfusions for patients with sickle cell anemia are NOT indicated for the treatment or prevention of

A. Stroke
B. Priapism
C. Pregnancy
D. Acute splenic sequestration

31. Which of the following is a recognized complication of sickle cell trait?

A. Painful crises
B. Splenic dysfunction
C. Hematuria
D. Aplastic crisis
E. Epistaxis

32. Compared to patients with sickle cell disease (hemoglobin SS), patients with SB^+ thalassemia have a greater frequency of

A. Painful crises
B. Priapism
C. Aplastic crisis
D. Proliferative retinopathy

33. In patients receiving repeated transfusions, once a patient has had a febrile nonhemolytic transfusion reaction, the patient should receive which of the following products to decrease the chance of reaction?

A. Leukocyte-depleted red blood cells
B. Washed red blood cells
C. Frozen red blood cells
D. Irradiated red blood cells

34. Four hours after a transfusion of packed red blood cells to a previously healthy trauma victim with no prior history of transfusions, the patient develops hypotension. Which of the following is NOT a potential etiology in this patient?

A. Allergic reaction
B. Hemolytic transfusion reaction
C. IgE deficiency in the recipient
D. IgA deficiency in the recipient
E. Sepsis

35. Blood donated for use in transfusions in the United States is currently tested for all of the following EXCEPT

A. Human T-cell lymphotropic virus (HTLV)-I
B. Epstein-Barr virus
C. Hepatitis B
D. HTLV-II
E. Hepatitis C

36. Epinephrine leads to neutrophilia via

A. Increased bone marrow production of neutrophils
B. Increased release of neutrophils from the bone marrow
C. Release of neutrophils from the spleen
D. Decreased neutrophil adhesion
E. Prolonged neutrophil lifespan

37. The inability of the neutrophil to generate superoxide anion is the defect underlying which disorder?

A. Chédiak-Higashi syndrome
B. Chronic granulomatous disease
C. Myeloperoxidase deficiency
D. Bernard-Soulier syndrome

38. Lymphocytopenia is usually NOT observed in

A. Patients receiving corticosteroid therapy
B. Patients receiving alkylating agent chemotherapy
C. Protein-calorie malnutrition
D. Mononucleosis

39. Features that help to distinguish leukocytosis caused by infection from that caused by chronic myelogenous leukemia (CML) include all of the following EXCEPT

A. Leukocyte alkaline phosphatase (LAP)
B. Basophil count
C. Presence or absence of the Philadelphia chromosome
D. Splenomegaly
E. Lymphocyte count

40. Clinical and laboratory features that help to distinguish polycythemia vera from secondary erythrocytosis include all of the following EXCEPT

    A. Erythropoietin level
    B. Splenomegaly
    C. Red cell mass
    D. Basophil count

41. Which of the following is NOT a typical clinical feature of polycythemia vera?

    A. Splenomegaly
    B. More than 50% of patients develop thrombotic or hemorrhagic complications
    C. Peak incidence at approximately 60 years of age
    D. In more than 50% of patients it eventually transforms into leukemia
    E. Phlebotomy is the main form of initial therapy

42. At the time of diagnosis, most patients with essential thrombocythemia have

    A. Splenomegaly
    B. Thrombosis
    C. Hemorrhage
    D. Erythromelalgia
    E. No symptoms

43. The presence of which of the following clinical and laboratory features is NOT usually useful in distinguishing between reactive thrombocytosis and essential thrombocythemia?

    A. Splenomegaly
    B. Lymphadenopathy
    C. Decreased fibrinogen
    D. Elevated interleukin (IL)-6 level
    E. None of the above

44. Among the chronic myeloproliferative disorders, the best mean survival is observed in

    A. Essential thrombocythemia
    B. Polycythemia vera
    C. CML
    D. Agnogenic myeloid metaplasia
    E. Chronic lymphocytic leukemia (CLL)

45. In patients with CML, the *bcr-abl* translocation may be found in which bone marrow precursors?

    A. Erythroid
    B. Myeloid
    C. Megakaryocytic
    D. Lymphoid
    E. All of the above

46. Which of the following clinical laboratory abnormalities is NOT frequently found in patients with CML?

    A. Thrombocytosis
    B. Elevated LAP level
    C. Elevated vitamin B_{12} level
    D. Elevated LDH level
    E. Increased uric acid level

47. Which of the following is NOT a poor prognostic factor for patients with CML?

    A. Absence of the Philadelphia chromosome
    B. Thrombocytopenia

    C. Hepatomegaly
    D. Basophilia
    E. Decreased LAP level

48. Of the following potential therapies for patients with hairy cell leukemia, which has NOT been shown to be effective?

    A. Interferon-alpha
    B. 2-Deoxycoformycin
    C. 2-Chlorodeoxyadenosine
    D. Corticosteroids

49. Which of the following is NOT a disorder primarily involving B lymphocytes rather than T lymphocytes?

    A. Hairy cell leukemia
    B. Large granular lymphocyte leukemia
    C. Infectious mononucleosis
    D. CLL

50. Chemotherapy for patients with CLL is NOT usually indicated for the treatment of

    A. Autoimmune hemolytic anemia
    B. Fever and night sweats
    C. Massive lymphadenopathy
    D. Leukostasis
    E. Richter's transformation

51. Patients with Bloom syndrome, Fanconi's anemia, and Down's syndrome are all at increased risk of developing

    A. Pernicious anemia
    B. Non-Hodgkin's lymphoma
    C. Hemochromatosis
    D. Acute leukemia
    E. Multiple myeloma

52. Acute promyelocytic leukemia has been associated with which chromosomal abnormality?

    A. Inversion of chromosome 16
    B. 9;22 translocation
    C. 15;17 translocation
    D. Trisomy 8
    E. 8;14 translocation

53. Which of the following is NOT a good prognostic factor in acute myelogenous leukemia (AML)?

    A. 15;14 translocation
    B. 8;21 translocation
    C. Inversion of chromosome 16
    D. Monosomy 7

54. The development of acute adult T-cell leukemia is associated with

    A. Herpesvirus
    B. Epstein-Barr virus
    C. *bcl-1* Oncogene
    D. *ras* Oncogene
    E. HTLV-I

55. Diffuse, rather than localized, lymphadenopathy is typical of all of the following disorders EXCEPT

    A. Non-Hodgkin's lymphoma
    B. Acquired immunodeficiency syndrome (AIDS)
    C. Dilantin therapy

D. Hodgkin's disease
E. Angioimmunoblastic lymphoma

56. Detailed staging by physical exam and radiologic studies is most important for the treatment and prognosis in which of the following disorders?

A. Multiple myeloma
B. AML
C. Non-Hodgkin's lymphoma
D. Hodgkin's disease
E. Hairy cell leukemia

57. Terminal differentiation of eosinophils is promoted by

A. Granulocyte colony-stimulating factor (G-CSF)
B. Erythropoietin
C. Granulocyte-macrophage colony-stimulating factor (GM-CSF)
D. IL-5
E. IL-7

58. The finding of Charcot-Leyden crystals suggests the presence of what disease?

A. Non-Hodgkin's lymphoma
B. Plasma cell dyscrasia
C. Hypereosinophilic syndrome
D. Hemoglobin SC disease
E. Hemochromatosis

59. Which of the following is not necessary for the diagnosis of idiopathic hypereosinophilic syndrome?

A. Eosinophil count greater than 1.5×10^9/per liter for longer than 6 months
B. Negative evaluation for parasitic diseases
C. Negative evaluation for allergic disorders
D. Signs and symptoms of organ involvement by eosinophils
E. Increased numbers of eosinophils in biopsy or sputum specimen

60. Approximately what percentage of patients greater than 70 years of age have monoclonal gammopathies of unknown significance?

A. 1%
B. 3%
C. 5%
D. 10%
E. 20%

61. Which of the following is NOT a common finding in multiple myeloma patients at diagnosis?

A. Hypercalcemia
B. Serum M spike
C. Greater than 10% bone marrow plasma cells
D. Lytic bone lesions
E. Urine M spike

62. Recognized contributions to renal failure in patients with multiple myeloma include all of the following EXCEPT

A. Hypercalcemia
B. Light chain deposition
C. Infiltration of the kidney by myeloma cells
D. Amyloidosis
E. Hyperuricemia

63. Development of anorexia, confusion, and constipation in a patient with multiple myeloma usually indicates

A. Chemotherapy side effects, especially of vincristine
B. Polyneuropathy related to the M protein
C. Hyperviscosity
D. Hypercalcemia
E. Hyperuricemia

64. Without treatment, median survival for patients with multiple myeloma is

A. 6 months
B. 1 year
C. 2 years
D. 5 years
E. 10 years

65. Raynaud's phenomenon and cyanosis in a patient with an M protein is most likely related to

A. Hypercalcemia
B. Hyperviscosity
C. Cryoglobulinemia
D. Elevated IL-6 levels
E. Amyloidosis

66. The most frequent hemostatic defect detected on laboratory evaluation in patients with amyloidosis is

A. Decreased Factor X level
B. Acquired von Willebrand's disease
C. Thrombocytopenia
D. Prolonged prothrombin time
E. Prolonged thrombin time

67. In the diagnostic evaluation of amyloidosis, the test with the most favorable combination of diagnostic yield and safety is

A. Bone marrow biopsy
B. Sural nerve biopsy
C. Rectal biopsy
D. Abdominal fat biopsy
E. Liver biopsy

68. Most patients found to have an IgM M protein have

A. Waldenström's macroglobulinemia
B. CLL
C. Monoclonal gammopathy of unknown significance
D. Lymphoma
E. Multiple myeloma

69. The major source of IgM production in the normal healthy adult is

A. Thymus
B. Liver
C. Bone marrow
D. Spleen
E. Deep internal lymph nodes

70. The term for denatured hemoglobin in red cells removed from the red cells by pitting in the spleen is called

A. Howell-Jolly body
B. Heinz body
C. Russell body

D. Charcot-Leyden crystal

E. Auer rod

71. Splenomegaly is a common finding in all of the following disorders EXCEPT

A. CLL

B. Cirrhosis

C. Metastatic colon cancer

D. Infectious mononucleosis

E. Polycythemia vera

72. Therapeutic splenectomy may be clinically beneficial in all of the following disorders EXCEPT

A. CML

B. Hereditary spherocytosis

C. Immune thrombocytopenic purpura (ITP)

D. Gaucher's disease

E. Traumatic splenic rupture

73. Which of the following immune functions may be compromised following splenectomy?

A. IgM production

B. Properdin production

C. Cell-mediated immunity

D. Complement-mediated opsonization

E. All of the above

74. In the treatment of adult AML with allogeneic bone marrow transplantation, bone marrow purging and administration of methotrexate following transplant are methods primarily intended to

A. Increase the chance of engraftment of the donor marrow

B. Shorten the time to engraftment

C. Decrease the chance of developing graft-versus-host disease

D. Decrease the risk of recurrence of AML

E. Decrease the risk of hepatic veno-occlusive disease

75. Autologous bone marrow transplantation has led to long-term remission in some patients with all of the following disorders EXCEPT

A. CML

B. Non-Hodgkin's lymphoma

C. Acute lymphoblastic leukemia

D. Sickle cell anemia

E. Multiple myeloma

76. Spontaneous bleeding is unusual at a platelet count greater than (choose the lowest appropriate number):

A. 5×10^9 per liter

B. 10×10^9 per liter

C. 20×10^9 per liter

D. 50×10^9 per liter

E. 100×10^9 per liter

77. The most appropriate initial therapy for a 5-year-old with acute ITP and a platelet count of 30×10^9 per liter without apparent bleeding is

A. Corticosteroids

B. Intravenous immunoglobulin

C. Splenectomy

D. Observation

E. Platelet transfusion

78. In adults, the most rapid rise in the platelet count in the treatment of ITP is produced by

A. Intravenous immunoglobulin

B. Splenectomy

C. Corticosteroids

D. Danazol

79. Which of the following is NOT commonly found in both disseminated intravascular coagulation (DIC) and thrombotic thrombocytopenic purpura (TTP)?

A. Anemia

B. Hemolysis

C. Decreased fibrinogen

D. Peripheral smear schistocytes

E. Microvascular thrombosis

80. Therapeutic options shown to be effective for the prevention of uremic bleeding include all of the following EXCEPT

A. Dialysis

B. Estrogens

C. Desmopressin acetate (DDAVP)

D. Cryoprecipitate

E. Erythropoietin

F. Fresh frozen plasma

81. A 23-year-old woman with a history of epistaxis since childhood and a platelet count of 25×10^9 per liter, with large platelets seen on peripheral smear, is seen for evaluation. Platelet aggregation studies show normal response to all agonists except ristocetin. This patient most likely has

A. Glanzmann's thrombasthenia

B. ITP

C. von Willebrand's disease

D. Bernard-Soulier syndrome

E. Hermansky-Pudlak syndrome

82. Pulmonary arterovenous malformations and epistaxis are features of

A. Bernard-Soulier syndrome

B. Osler-Weber-Rendu syndrome

C. Kasabach-Merritt syndrome

D. Chédiak-Higashi syndrome

E. Hermansky-Pudlak syndrome

83. Which of the following is NOT a vitamin K–dependent protein?

A. Protein C

B. Factor II

C. Factor VII

D. Antithrombin III

E. Factor IX

84. Deficiency of which blood coagulation protein is associated with bleeding?

A. Factor XIII

B. Prekallikrein

C. Protein S

D. Factor XII

E. High-molecular-weight kininogen

85. In the presence of excess extrinsic pathway inhibitor (or tissue factor pathway inhibitor) activation, what factor sustains coagulation activation?

    A. Prothrombin (Factor II)
    B. Factor VIII
    C. Factor IX
    D. Factor X
    E. Factor XI

86. Activities of thrombin include all of the following EXCEPT

    A. Activation of platelets
    B. Cleavage of Factor V
    C. Activation of Factor XIII
    D. Activation of protein S
    E. Activation of protein C

87. A young man with hemophilia A gives his family history. Which individual could NOT also have the same inherited defect?

    A. Brother
    B. Maternal grandfather
    C. Maternal uncle
    D. Maternal great grandfather
    E. Son

88. For severe hemophilia A patients with significant bleeding, effective replacement therapy options include all of the following EXCEPT

    A. Cryoprecipitate
    B. Recombinant Factor VIII
    C. Fresh frozen plasma
    D. Chemically purified Factor VIII
    E. Monclonal Factor VIII

89. In patients with mild hemophilia A, measures shown to provide improved hemostasis for simple dental extractions without Factor VIII replacement include all of the following EXCEPT

    A. DDAVP
    B. Epsilon-aminocaproic acid
    C. Tranexamic acid
    D. Aprotinin

90. Approximately what percentage of patients with severe hemophilia A develop Factor VIII inhibitors?

    A. 2%
    B. 5%
    C. 15%
    D. 25%
    E. 50%

91. Features distinguishing severe von Willebrand's disease from severe hemophilia A include all of the following EXCEPT

    A. Bleeding time
    B. Activated partial thromboplastin time (aPTT)
    C. Pattern of inheritance
    D. von Willebrand factor level
    E. Platelet aggregation studies

92. Of the disorders listed below, the most common inherited bleeding disorder is

    A. Hemophilia A
    B. Platelet storage pool disorder
    C. Osler-Weber-Rendu syndrome
    D. Hemophilia B
    E. von Willebrand's disease

93. Causes of a bleeding disorder to be suspected in a patient with a normal bleeding time, prothrombin time, and aPTT include all of the following EXCEPT

    A. Alpha$_2$-antiplasmin deficiency
    B. Factor XIII deficiency
    C. Mild von Willebrand's disease
    D. Dysfibrinogenemia
    E. Prekallikrein deficiency

94. Abnormality of which of the following procoagulant factors is associated with a prothrombotic tendency?

    A. Factor VIII
    B. Factor XIII
    C. Factor VII
    D. Factor V
    E. Factor XI

95. Patients with lupus anticoagulants typically have a prothrombotic tendency; however, some patients have bleeding related to their lupus anticoagulants. Common causes of bleeding in such patients include all of the following EXCEPT

    A. Prothrombin deficiency
    B. Factor V deficiency
    C. Thrombocytopenia
    D. Platelet dysfunction

96. The cause of TTP is

    A. Vascular prostacyclin deficiency
    B. Production of extra-large von Willebrand factor multimers
    C. Anti–endothelial cell antibodies
    D. Bacterial-induced platelet activation
    E. Still unknown

DIRECTIONS: For questions 97 to 103, decide whether each statement is true or false. Any combination of answers, from all true to all false, may occur.

97. Which of the following statements is/are true about anemia?

A. Absence of increased reticulocytes in a patient with anemia excludes the diagnosis of acute hemolytic anemia.

B. Iron deficiency should be considered in the differential diagnosis of a normocytic anemia with a low reticulocyte count because the mean corpuscular volume often falls after the hematocrit.

C. A normal hematocrit and a normal MCV exclude the possibility that psychiatric problems may be related to vitamin B_{12} deficiency.

D. In a patient with vitamin B_{12} deficiency, the finding of a positive anti–intrinsic factor antibody assay confirms the diagnosis of pernicious anemia and obviates the need for further evaluation, such as a Schilling's test.

E. Currently, most patients with aplastic anemia under the age of 45 are initially treated with allogeneic bone marrow transplantation.

98. Which of the following statements is/are true with regard to the functions of the spleen?

A. In patients with severe hereditary spherocytosis, splenectomy essentially cures the hemolysis and ankle ulcers.

B. In autoimmune hemolytic anemia, IgG- and IgM-coated red cells are cleared predominantly by the spleen.

C. In patients with hairy cell leukemia, splenectomy is usually curative.

D. Splenectomy appears to be safe and effective for the treatment of refractory human immunodeficiency virus (HIV) related ITP.

99. Which of the following statements is/are true concerning the thalassemias?

A. Patients with beta-thalassemia major usually do not become anemic until after 6 months of life.

B. The most severe form of beta-thalassemia may be associated with hydrops fetalis.

C. Adults with hemoglobin SS who also have alpha-thalassemia (− alpha/ − alpha; two of four genes defective) typically have a higher hematocrit than sickle cell patients without alpha-thalassemia.

D. Despite advances in the understanding of the pathophysiology and treatment of complications of patients with sickle cell anemia, the mean life expectancy remains less than 50 years.

100. Which of the following statements is/are true about blood and blood products?

A. In order for a patient to have a severe ABO-based transfusion reaction to the transfusion of red cells (e.g., a patient with type B blood receiving blood from a patient with type A blood), prior exposure of the patient to type A blood through either pregnancy or prior transfusion is required.

B. Patients receiving whole blood transfusions require type-specific blood transfusion. For example, a patient with type O blood should receive only type O blood and a patient with type A blood should receive only type A blood. By contrast, patients receiving packed red cells require less specific matching. For example, a patient with type B blood may receive type O blood and a patient with type AB blood may receive either type A or type B blood.

C. The circulating neutrophil, despite having a nucleus, can no longer divide.

D. Eradication of an antibody to Factor VIII using prednisone and/or cyclophosphamide is more successful in patients with inherited hemophilia than in patients without hemophilia who acquire an autoantibody to Factor VIII later in life.

101. Which of the following statements is/are true regarding the various types of hematologic malignancies?

A. Cytogenetic remissions in CML may be induced by either bone marrow transplantation or interferon-alpha.

B. In low-grade small cell lymphoma, although peripheral lymph node and spleen involvement is often seen, bone marrow involvement is uncommon.

C. Aggressive chemotherapy often leads to cure in patients with high-grade lymphoma, in contrast to routine failure to achieve long-term remission in low-grade lymphoma.

D. Depending on stage, either radiation therapy alone or chemotherapy may be curative in Hodgkin's disease.

E. Regardless of etiology, when the platelet count exceeds 1000×10^9 per liter, the platelet count should be lowered by medication or by plateletpheresis.

102. Which of the following statements is/are true regarding the gammopathies?

A. A negative serum protein electrophoresis excludes a possible diagnosis of multiple myeloma.

B. Fewer than one third of patients with monoclonal gammopathy of unknown significance eventually develop multiple myeloma.

C. In familial Mediterranean fever, although colchicine is helpful in preventing painful episodes, it does not prevent progressive amyloidosis and renal failure.

103. Which of the following statements is/are true with regard to disorders of hemostasis?

A. Although growth factors for erythrocytes (erythropoietin) and neutrophils (G-CSF) have been discovered, the growth factor for megakaryocytes for the treatment of thrombocytopenia remains elusive.

B. Analogous to the direct Coombs test for the diagnosis of immune hemolytic anemia, antiplatelet antibody assays now provide accurate diagnostic results in the evaluation of patients for possible ITP.

C. Once treated successfully, the large majority of patients with TTP will suffer no relapses.

PART 6

HEMATOLOGY

ANSWERS

1.(C) *Discussion:* Granulocytes are rapidly turned over and have the shortest intravascular lifespan (6 to 12 hours). The next shortest lifespan is for platelets (7 to 10 days). The lifespan of the red cells is longest (approximately 120 days). Therefore, when bone marrow production suddenly ceases, the granulocytes disappear first, then platelets, and finally the red cells. (*Cecil, Ch. 127; Beutler et al, Ch. 24; Lee et al, Ch. 31*)

2.(E) *Discussion:* In response to blood loss and decreased oxygen-carrying capacity, renal erythropoietin secretion is increased, leading to increased red cell production by the bone marrow. These new young cells appear as reticulocytes and, on Wright's stain, demonstrate a bluish discoloration termed polychromasia. Hemoglobin released either from red cells destroyed within the vascular space or into large internal spaces, such as the retroperitoneum, is converted into unconjugated hemoglobin. Red cells destroyed in the intravascular space or degraded in extravascular spaces release LDH. Therefore, differentiating these two disorders can be very difficult, sometimes requiring search for a source of bleeding angiographically, or for possible causes of hemolysis and serial observations of the hematocrit, reticulocyte count, and bilirubin. Other bleeding, such as gastrointestinal bleeding, would not lead to hyperbilirubinemia or an elevated LDH. (*Cecil, Ch. 128; Lee et al, Ch. 32*)

3.(A) *Discussion:* In order to maintain oxygen delivery to tissues in the face of chronically decreased hemoglobin, blood flow to tissues is increased through a combination of increased cardiac output and decreased peripheral vascular resistance. The kidneys detect the decreased oxygen-carrying capacity and increase their synthesis of erythropoietin. The concentration of 2,3-diphosphoglyceric acid increases, thereby decreasing the oxygen affinity of hemoglobin and increasing release of oxygen to hypoxic tissues. (*Cecil, Ch. 129; Beutler et al, Ch. 40; Lee et al, Ch. 23*)

4.(D) *Discussion:* Hereditary spherocytosis is an autosomal dominant disorder of the red cell cytoskeletal proteins. Patients typically have chronic hemolysis with anemia, jaundice, and splenomegaly resulting from work hypertrophy. Up to 85% of adults develop pigment gallstones. Whereas alpha-thalassemia, with the loss of three of the four alpha genes (hemoglobin H), produces a clinically symptomatic chronic hemolytic anemia associated with jaundice and splenomegaly, loss of only one or two of the alpha hemoglobin genes (alpha-thalassemia trait) is usually asymptomatic and is not associated with anemia. Vitamin B_{12} deficiency, iron deficiency, and paroxysmal nocturnal hemoglobinuria are not inherited disorders. Both vitamin B_{12} deficiency and paroxysmal nocturnal hemoglobinuria have features of hemo-

lytic anemia. (*Cecil, Ch. 129; Beutler et al, Ch. 52; Lee et al, Ch. 33*)

5.(A) *Discussion:* In both of these disorders, the reticulocyte count, serum iron, and percent transferrin saturation are decreased; therefore, these tests do not discriminate between iron deficiency anemia and anemia of chronic disease. In a clinically stable patient such as the one described, the ferritin should provide an accurate representation of the body's iron stores at a much lesser cost than assessing bone marrow iron stores, in terms of both dollars and patient discomfort. In an acutely ill patient or a patient with a chronic inflammatory condition, such as rheumatoid arthritis, the ferritin level may be elevated through its behavior as an acute-phase reactant. This may diminish the diagnostic value of serum ferritin; in this situation, the bone marrow examination may be more appropriate. (*Cecil, Ch. 129; Beutler et al, Ch. 46; Lee et al, Ch. 25*)

6.(C) *Discussion:* Hemoglobin A refers to a tetramer of two alpha hemoglobin chains and two normal beta hemoglobin chains. Hemoglobin A_2 refers to two alpha hemoglobin chains and two delta hemoglobin chains. Hemoglobin A_2 normally accounts for up to 2.5% of adult hemoglobin, the remainder being hemoglobin A with a tiny amount of fetal hemoglobin (two alpha chains and two gamma chains). In patients with beta-thalassemia, the production of beta chains is decreased, so the proportion of hemoglobin made up by hemoglobin A_2 becomes increased. (*Cecil, Ch. 129; Beutler et al, Ch. 38; Lee et al, Ch. 39*)

7.(E) *Discussion:* Sideroblastic anemias may be inherited or acquired and are characterized by the finding of an increased number of red cell precursors in the bone marrow having an increased amount of perinuclear iron. Red cells in sideroblastic anemia are usually hypochromic and *microcytic*. Reticulocytes are large cells; therefore, if the number of reticulocytes is significantly increased, this may shift the MCV upward. In the megaloblastic anemias (vitamin B_{12} and folate deficiency), there is a loss of synchrony between development of cytoplasm and nucleus, leading to greater cytoplasm development and larger cells. Myelodysplastic syndromes are typically characterized by large, dysmorphic red cells. (*Cecil, Ch. 136 and 137; Beutler et al, Ch. 45 and 72*)

8.(B) *Discussion:* Up to 96% of patients abusing alcohol develop macrocytosis. This appears to be a direct effect of alcohol on the bone marrow and is not related to folate deficiency. Less frequently, alcoholics develop folate deficiency; clues to this diagnosis include macro-ovalocytes and hypersegmented neutrophils on peripheral smear examination. With acute blood loss from varices or gastritis, reticulocytosis may occur. Liver disease may also be associated with a mild macrocytosis. Vitamin B_{12} deficiency is not associated with alcohol abuse. (*Cecil, Ch. 129; Beutler et al, Ch. 47; Lee et al, Ch. 24*)

9.(D) *Discussion:* With destruction of red cells and release of hemoglobin and red cell enzymes, such as LDH, a variety of laboratory abnormalities may be detected. Serum LDH level increases. In response to destruction of red cells, anemia, and a decrease in oxygen-carrying capacity, red cell production increases, resulting in reticulocytosis. Hemoglobin released from destroyed red cells is bound by haptoglobin and cleared from the circulation by the liver, leading to a *decrease* in the serum haptoglobin level. Hemoglobin is converted to bilirubin, leading to an increased serum unconjugated bilirubin level. When the haptoglobin becomes depleted, hemoglobin may be excreted in the urine. Much of this hemoglobin is reabsorbed by proximal tubular cells. In these cells, the iron is incorporated into hemosiderin. The tubular cells containing hemosiderin are then sloughed into the urine. (*Cecil, Ch. 129; Lee et al, Ch. 32*)

10.(B) *Discussion:* Cytogenetic studies in patients with Fanconi's anemia have shown a variety of chromosomal abnormalities most likely resulting from an increased susceptibility to chromosomal breakage. The Ham's test is used for the diagnosis of paroxysmal nocturnal hemoglobinuria, which may also present as aplastic anemia. In this test, increased susceptibility of red cells to complement-mediated lysis is detected. The bone marrow biopsy and aspirate show no diagnostic features in Fanconi's anemia. The hemoglobin electrophoresis result would be normal in this disorder. (*Cecil, Ch. 130; Beutler et al, Ch. 127; Lee et al, Ch. 31*)

11.(D) *Discussion:* Idiopathic myelodysplastic syndromes are a group of clonal disorders of the bone marrow characterized by any combination of cytopenias presenting predominantly in patients greater than 60 years of age. Although patients may have pancytopenia at presentation, most commonly the presentation is one of a gradual onset of anemia. Cytogenetic abnormalities are found in up to 80% of patients. Only approximately 20% of patients convert to acute leukemia. (*Cecil, Ch. 130; Beutler et al, Ch. 26; Lee et al, Ch. 74*)

12.(E) *Discussion:* Whereas prior chemotherapy most often produces nonspecific damage to the bone marrow leading to involvement of all three cell lines (platelets, granulocytes, and red cells), other disorders may produce a red cell–specific damage. Parvovirus appears to infect bone marrow red cell precursors. In most patients a transient interruption in red cell production passes without symptoms; however, in patients with chronic hemolytic anemia, such as sickle cell disease, severe anemia may develop. Dilantin may produce a variety of cytopenias, including pure red cell aplasia. Up to 7% of patients with thymomas may have pure red cell aplasia, possibly related to T cell–mediated immunosuppression of red cell precursors. Systemic lupus erythematosus may be associated with pure red cell aplasia, in some cases as a result of IgGs directed against red cell precursors. (*Cecil, Ch. 130; Beutler et al, Ch. 41; Lee et al, Ch. 31*)

13.(A) *Discussion:* Chronic alcohol use leading to cirrhosis can be associated with the development of anemia of several causes. Patients with cirrhosis are at increased risk of gastrointestinal blood loss (e.g., from esophageal varices or gastritis). This can produce an acute anemia or lead to iron deficiency anemia. Alcohol's interference with folate metabolism, combined with decreased dietary folate, may lead to megaloblastic anemia resulting from folate deficiency. Alcohol may directly suppress bone marrow cell production. Cirrhosis with portal hypertension produces splenomegaly. This can lead to pooling of red cells, white cells, and platelets in the spleen. In addition, splenomegaly is associated with an increase in plasma volume leading to a decrease in the hematocrit, producing a "pseudoanemia" because there is no change in red cell mass. In patients with cirrhosis, red cells accumulate excess cholesterol. This produces membrane abnormalities that can be observed on peripheral smear examination as spur cells, and is accompanied by a shortened red cell survival. Chronic alcoholics are at increased risk for the development of sideroblastic anemia. In patients with alcoholic cirrhosis, vitamin B_{12} levels are usually normal or increased. (*Cecil, Ch. 131; Beutler et al, Ch. 45; Lee et al, Ch. 67*)

14.(A) *Discussion:* Hypothyroidism is frequently associated with anemia. Potential causes include a loss of a direct effect of thyroid hormone on promotion of erythropoiesis. In addition, patients with hypothyroidism may be at increased risk of developing iron deficiency as a result of gastric achlorhydria. Autoimmune thyroiditis is often associated with pernicious anemia. Ten to 25% of patients with hyperthyroidism are anemic; however, as yet there is no satisfactory explanation. Androgens promote erythropoiesis; the hematocrit in adult men is higher than that in women and, with castration or gonadal dysfunction in men, the hematocrit decreases to the level found in women. The anemia of hypopituitarism may be related to loss of downstream hormones such as thyroxine or androgens or directly caused by a decrease in growth hormone. Patients with Addison's disease often have a decrease in the red cell mass but, because there is also a decrease in the plasma volume, the hematocrit usually remains normal. Conversely, patients with Cushing's syndrome typically have a mild erythrocytosis rather than anemia. The etiology remains obscure. (*Cecil, Ch. 131; Beutler et al, Ch. 43; Lee et al, Ch. 30*)

15.(D) *Discussion:* Ingested iron must be in the reduced form (ferrous) in order to be absorbed. Ingestion of simple reducing agents, such as ascorbate or succinate, may enhance reduction of iron and thereby enhance iron absorption. Many other substances appear to complex with iron in the gastrointestinal tract and interfere with iron absorption. These include tetracycline, phytates in cereals, tannates in tea, and antacids. Antacids may also impair enzymatic release of iron from ingested food in the stomach. These may be important considerations in the evaluation of iron replacement therapy in patients with iron deficiency. (*Cecil, Ch. 132; Beutler et al, Ch. 34; Lee et al, Ch. 26*)

16.(D) *Discussion:* In both iron deficiency anemia and anemia of chronic disease, there is a failure to deliver iron to erythroid precursors. Therefore, red cell iron is absent in both disorders; however, bone marrow storage iron is increased in anemia of chronic disease but absent in iron deficiency anemia. Both disorders show hypochromic, microcytic anemia on peripheral smear examination consistent with failure to deliver adequate iron to developing red cells in the marrow. Serum iron and transferrin are decreased in both disorders; however, in iron deficiency anemia there is an increase in serum transferrin, or total iron-binding capacity, whereas in anemia of chronic disease transferrin is usually decreased. Serum ferritin may also help differentiate these disorders, being very low in iron deficiency anemia and elevated in anemia of chronic disease. (*Cecil, Ch. 132; Beutler et al, Ch. 46*)

17.(B) *Discussion:* Deficiency of all of these substances may, at least theoretically, produce anemia. The vegan diet excludes all animal products, including milk and eggs. This diet contains less than 10% of the normal amount of vitamin B_{12} and can lead to vitamin B_{12} deficiency and anemia. The vegan diet is rich in folate and contains adequate iron, pyridoxine, and copper. Pyridoxine deficiency has been described as a potential cause of anemia only rarely, but interference with pyridoxine by isoniazid therapy for tuberculosis may be associated with an anemia that is responsive to pyridoxine therapy. Copper deficiency may produce anemia, but copper is ubiquitous in the diet and even in the water supply, and dietary requirements are very small. Therefore, copper deficiency as a cause of anemia is rare but has been described in patients with kwashiorkor and on long-term hyperalimentation. (*Cecil, Ch. 133; Beutler et al, Ch. 47; Lee et al, Ch. 7 and 24*)

18.(C) *Discussion:* Folate is absorbed predominantly in the jejunum and requires very little if any gastric processing, in contrast to iron and vitamin B_{12}. Therefore, diseases of the small intestine rather than the stomach may be associated with folate deficiency. The diet of the alcoholic may be relatively low in folate, and alcohol may interfere with folate absorption and metabolism. Folate requirements are increased during pregnancy. Dilantin therapy is associated with evidence of folate deficiency; however, the exact mechanism(s) remain unclear. Possible causes include folate malabsorption and accelerated folate catabolism. (*Cecil, Ch. 133; Beutler et al, Ch. 45; Lee et al, Ch. 24*)

19.(B) *Discussion:* In megaloblastic anemia caused by vitamin B_{12} deficiency, there is a decreased ability of the marrow to make new red blood cells; therefore, there is a decrease in the reticulocyte count and thus in polychromasia on peripheral smear examination. Nonetheless, there also exist several features of a hemolytic anemia related to shortened lifespan of the deficient red cells, which leads to an elevated level of LDH and decreased serum haptoglobin. Because of loss of synchrony between development of the nucleus and of the cytoplasm, cells with excess cytoplasm and a high MCV are produced and are often oval in appearance. With severe megaloblastic anemia, nucleated red blood cells appear in the peripheral blood. Disordered nuclear development is also manifested by hypersegmentation of the neutrophils. (*Cecil, Ch. 133; Beutler et al, Ch. 45; Lee et al, Ch. 24*)

20.(E) *Discussion:* Hereditary spherocytosis is a chronic hemolytic disorder associated with increased bilirubin concentrations, producing jaundice and pigment gallstones. Work hypertrophy leads to splenomegaly. Patients with hereditary spherocytosis and other chronic hemolytic disorders, such as sickle cell disease, are at risk for developing ankle ulcers; the etiology is unclear but may be related to decreased red cell deformability. By contrast, with disorders such as sickle cell disease, hereditary spherocytosis is *not* associated with occlusion or obstruction of larger vessels and is therefore not associated with painful crises or avascular necrosis of the head of the femur. (*Cecil, Ch. 134; Beutler et al, Ch. 52 and 56; Lee et al, Ch. 33*)

21.(D) *Discussion:* Glucose-6-phosphate dehydrogenase (G6PD) is an enzyme in the pentose phosphate pathway for metabolism of glucose in red cells and is the primary source of red cell nicotinamide adenine dinucleotide phosphate (NADPH). NADPH is required for regeneration of intracellular glutathione, which plays a major role in protecting the red cell from oxidative injury. The gene for G6PD is located on the X chromosome. Individuals with G6PD deficiency are usually asymptomatic unless exposed to oxidative stresses, such as ingestion of antimalarials and sulfa drugs. This triggers oxidation of hemoglobin and hemolysis. Denatured hemoglobin precipitates in red cells and can be detected using a supravital stain, such as methyl violet. This precipitate is called a Heinz body. Defects in other red cell enzymes responsible for the generation of ATP may also produce hemolysis, thought to be due to decreased intracellular ATP. An example of this type of inherited disorder is pyruvate kinase deficiency. (*Cecil, Ch. 134; Beutler et al, Ch. 54*)

22.(E) *Discussion:* Most autoimmune hemolytic anemias caused by IgG have their greatest activity at body temperature (warm). Complement may or may not be activated. Red cells coated with IgG are cleared predominantly by splenic macrophage Fc receptors. If complement is activated, these red cells become coated with C3b and their clearance in the spleen is accelerated; these cells may be cleared by either splenic or hepatic macrophage complement receptors. In IgM-mediated hemolytic anemia, the IgM typically binds to red cells at temperatures below 30°C (cold), in the extremities. Complement is activated and, when the red cells return to the central circulation, the IgM falls off, leaving only complement on the red cells. These complement-coated red cells are then cleared by macrophage complement receptors in the liver or spleen, but predominantly in the liver. Because of greater splenic clearance in IgG-mediated hemolytic anemia, response to splenectomy is much greater than for IgM-mediated hemolytic anemia. (*Cecil, Ch. 135; Beutler et al, Ch. 64 and 65; Lee et al, Ch. 41*)

23.(A) *Discussion:* In IgG-mediated hemolytic anemia, response to splenectomy occurs in over 50% of patients, whereas response to splenectomy in IgM-mediated hemolytic anemia is seen in very few patients. Similarly, the majority of patients with IgG-mediated disease respond to prednisone therapy and very few with IgM-related anemia respond. Responses to cyclophosphamide may be observed in either disease. Because IgM, in contrast to IgG, is almost exclusively intravascular, plasmapheresis can be a very effective therapy for IgM-mediated hemolytic anemia. (*Cecil, Ch. 135; Lee et al, Ch. 41*)

24.(A) *Discussion:* Paroxysmal nocturnal hemoglobinuria is an acquired clonal marrow disorder associated with chronic hemolysis and pancytopenia. A defect in red cell membrane proteins leads to increased susceptibility to complement-mediated red cell lysis. Intermittent episodes of hemoglobinuria often lead to sufficient loss of iron to produce iron deficiency. A striking predisposition to thrombosis occurs in patients with paroxysmal nocturnal hemoglobinuria. Although the etiology remains unclear, possibilities include complement-mediated activation of platelets and a release of red cell stroma during hemolysis, leading to coagulation activation. Unlike other hemolytic anemias, such as autoimmune hemolytic anemia and hereditary spherocytosis, spherocytes are *not* usually observed on peripheral smear examination. (*Cecil, Ch. 135; Beutler et al, Ch. 25; Lee et al, Ch. 44*)

25.(C) *Discussion:* Drug-induced hemolytic anemias can be divided into three groups based on pathophysiologic mechanism. In the hapten-type mechanism, the drug combines with the red cell surface; this complex induces an immune response. The antibody recognizes this complex; therefore, preincubation of the drug with test red cells is required. Examples of this type include penicillins and cephalosporins. A second mechanism involves formation of an antibody to a specific drug, followed by deposition of this complex on the red cell. To test for this, the patient serum must be preincubated with drug prior to incubation with test red cells. Examples of this include quinidine and chlorpromazine. Finally, a drug may lead to the production of an autoantibody directed against red cells. This antibody does not require interaction with the drug to attach to the red cell, and therefore addition of the drug is *not* required for *in vitro* diagnostic testing. Aldomet produces hemolytic anemia by the latter method. (*Cecil, Ch. 135; Lee et al, Ch. 41*)

26.(D) *Discussion:* Normal adult hemoglobin is greater than 97% hemoglobin A, which consists of two alpha chains and two beta chains. Up to 2.5% of the hemoglobin may be hemoglobin A_2, which consists of two alpha chains and two delta chains. Approximately 0.5 to 1.5% hemoglobin F may be found throughout life; hemoglobin F is made up of two alpha chains and two gamma chains. The epsilon chains are found only during weeks 4 through 13 of gestation. (*Cecil, Ch. 136; Beutler et al, Ch. 8*)

27.(D) *Discussion:* The hemoglobin molecule is a tetramer, consisting of a dimer of alpha chains combined with a dimer of two other chains; in hemoglobin A this is two beta chains, in hemoglobin A_2 this is two delta chains. For the beta and delta chains, there are two alleles of a single gene (e.g., a patient has two copies of the beta gene). For the alpha chain, there are two genes with four alleles, making the number of possible combination of defects for the alpha genes more complex. Patients with alpha-thalassemia may be deficient in one, two, three, or all four genes. Defects often produce only a partial synthetic defect, such that in beta-thalassemia with one normal gene, the defective gene may produce some hemoglobin yet less than normal, and the patient may have a sufficient amount of hemoglobin. Patients missing only one of the four alpha genes are usually neither symptomatic nor anemic. (*Cecil, Ch. 136; Beutler et al, Ch. 55; Lee et al, Ch. 39*)

28.(B) *Discussion:* With frequent red cell transfusions, iron overload develops and iron is deposited in almost all organs, but particularly affects the endocrine glands. Iron deposition in the heart, if not reversed, leads to congestive heart failure, the major cause of death in patients with severe thalassemias. Iron deposition in endocrine glands produces deficiencies of growth hormone, insulin, and thyroxine. Despite significant deposition of iron in the liver, clinical cirrhosis is relatively uncommon, compared to that in adults with iron overload associated with inherited hemochromatosis. (*Cecil, Ch. 136; Lee et al, Ch. 39*)

29.(E) *Discussion:* In the patient with a chronic hemolytic disorder, a constant demand for increased erythropoiesis exists to compensate for premature red cell destruction. Influences on the bone marrow that might go unnoticed or produce a very mild clinical problem in the patient without ongoing hemolysis can produce dramatic, sudden, and life-threatening anemia in a patient with chronic hemolysis. Infection of bone marrow red cell precursors by parvovirus B19 is the most common cause of an aplastic crisis in children with sickle cell anemia. Other recognized causes include splenic sequestration and bone marrow infarction. Patients with chronic hemolysis have increased folate requirements and may develop a megaloblastic crisis. Iron deficiency is less common and produces a less acute aggravation of anemia. (*Cecil, Ch. 137; Lee et al, Ch. 38*)

30.(C) *Discussion:* Decreasing the percentage of sickled cells by transfusion or exchange transfusion has recognized benefit in the treatment and prevention of stroke, acute splenic sequestration, and refractory priapism. Transfusion therapy does not appear to be necessary during pregnancy. (*Cecil, Ch. 137; Beutler et al, Ch. 56; Lee et al, Ch. 38*)

31.(C) *Discussion:* Patients with sickle trait may have a very slightly shortened red cell lifespan but do not develop clinically relevant hemolysis. Patients do not have painful crises, do not develop splenic dysfunction, and are not at increased risk for aplastic crises. Several patients have been reported who developed splenic infarction while traveling in unpressurized aircraft at high altitudes. There may be a slight increase in the risk of thromboembolism. Intermittent hematuria is a recognized manifestation of sickle cell trait and may be related to renal papillary ischemia. Other hemorrhage, including epistaxis, is not a feature of sickle cell trait. (*Cecil, Ch. 137; Beutler et al, Ch. 56; Lee et al, Ch. 38*)

32.(D) *Discussion:* Whereas patients with sickle cell trait are asymptomatic, those who inherit both a sickle beta gene and a beta$^+$ thalassemia gene may be symptomatic, although usually much less so than patients with sickle cell anemia. In sickle cell trait, red cells contain both hemoglobin A and hemoglobin S, with hemoglobin A predominating. In SB$^+$ thalassemia, red cells contain more hemoglobin S than hemoglobin A, with the percentage of hemoglobin A ranging from 3 to 25. The presence of some hemoglobin A in the red cells decreases most sickle cell–related complications, including painful crises, priapism, and aplastic crises. However, these patients have a greater risk of proliferative retinopathy, perhaps related to the higher hematocrit found in SB$^+$ thalassemia patients compared to sickle cell patients. (*Cecil, Ch. 137*)

33.(A) *Discussion:* Febrile nonhemolytic transfusion reactions appear to be related to reaction to leukocyte antigens present on white cells in the red cell transfusion. Most of these reactions can be prevented by passing the red cells through a leukocyte filter. Frozen red cells have a much greater shelf life but are more expensive and are best used for treatment of patients with unusual blood types. Washed red blood cells are indicated for transfusions in patients with demonstrated hypersensitivity to plasma or IgA deficiency. Irradiated blood cells are given to immunocompromised recipients to kill lymphocytes and prevent graft-versus-host disease. (*Cecil, Ch. 138; Beutler et al, Ch. 151; Lee et al, Ch. 21*)

34.(C) *Discussion:* Hypotension following blood transfusion is a nonspecific sign. The differential diagnosis includes (1) allergic reaction to plasma proteins, (2) hemolytic transfusion reaction caused by ABO incompatibility or other mismatch, (3) anaphylactic reaction to IgA in an IgA-deficient recipient, and (4) sepsis caused by bacterial contamination of the blood product. IgE deficiency in the recipient is *not* a cause of transfusion reactions. (*Cecil, Ch. 138; Beutler et al, Ch. 151*)

35.(B) *Discussion:* Donated blood in the United States is tested for antibodies to HTLV-I, HTLV-II, hepatitis B, hepatitis C, and HIV. Serologic tests for syphilis and an alanine aminotransferase assay are also performed. A test for cytomegalovirus is not routinely performed but may be important prior to transfusing the immunocompromised recipient. Up to 90% of blood donors have antibodies to Epstein-Barr virus (EBV); likewise, most recipients are immune. Transmission of EBV and mononucleosis has been reported in immunocompromised recipients; however, blood for donation is not routinely tested for EBV. (*Cecil, Ch. 138; Beutler et al, Ch. 151; Lee et al, Ch. 21*)

36.(D) *Discussion:* Large numbers of neutrophils are found in different compartments, including the bone marrow, spleen, and tissues, as well as circulating and attached to the vascular endothelium. Neutrophilia is observed with stress even in patients after splenectomy, excluding the spleen as a source of increased neutrophils during stress. After injection of epinephrine, neutrophilia is observed within 20 minutes, excluding increased production and alteration in lifespan. Release of bone marrow neutrophils usually includes a large percentage of less mature neutrophils, including bands and metamyelocytes, as is seen with acute infections. Mature neutrophils adhere to the vascular endothelium; epinephrine appears to acutely decrease neutrophil adhesion, releasing large numbers of mature neutrophils into the circulation. (*Cecil, Ch. 139; Beutler et al, Ch. 82; Lee et al, Ch. 9*)

37.(B) *Discussion:* In order to kill catalase-positive microorganisms, the neutrophil must ingest them and then kill them by generating a respiratory burst, which includes superoxide anion formation. Patients with chronic granulomatous disease are unable to generate superoxide anion and are thus unable to handle infections by organisms such as *Staphylococcus aureus* and *Serratia marcescens,* and suffer recurrent lymphadenitis and other infections typically involving the skin, lung, and bones. Chédiak-Higashi syndrome is an autosomal dominant disorder associated with decreased neutrophil chemotaxis, disordered neutrophil granule function, and increased susceptibility to recurrent pyogenic infections. Myeloperoxidase deficiency is a clinically silent disorder associated with delayed neutrophil phagosome microbicidal activity resulting from the inability to generate hypochlorous acid. Bernard-Soulier syndrome is an inherited platelet function defect not associated with neutrophil dysfunction. (*Cecil, Ch. 139; Beutler et al, Ch. 83; Lee et al, Ch. 9*)

38.(D) *Discussion:* Lymphocytopenia may be an important clue to an underlying diagnosis, but the differential diagnosis includes a broad variety of disorders, such as inherited immune disorders, chronic and acute infections, responses to drug therapy, and a variety of systemic disorders. Corticosteroid therapy produces a shift of lymphocytes from the circulation. Alkylating agent chemotherapy destroys circulating lymphocytes and may also damage lymphocyte progenitors. Protein-calorie malnutrition is the most common cause of impaired lymphocyte production worldwide and may contribute to impaired immune response. Infection by EBV and cytomegalovirus may produce a mononucleosis syndrome that is associated with lymphocytosis rather than lymphocytopenia. (*Cecil, Ch. 140; Beutler et al, Ch. 101*)

39.(E) *Discussion:* Extreme leukocytosis ($>40 \times 10^9$ leukocytes per liter) may be caused by a leukemoid reaction to severe infection or lymphoid tumor, such as Hodgkin's disease. CML is a clonal disorder of a pluripotential stem cell of the bone marrow. Features that help to distinguish these two causes of granulocytosis include the LAP level, which is decreased in CML while it is normal or elevated in leukemoid reactions. The basophil count is usually elevated in CML and normal in reactive granulocytosis. The presence of the Philadelphia chromosome is diagnostic for CML. Lymphocytosis may occur in CML or in many of the disorders producing a leukemoid reaction, and therefore does not help to distinguish these disorders. Splenomegaly is present in greater than 90% of patients with CML at presentation but is only rarely found in leukemoid reactions. (*Cecil, Ch. 140; Beutler et al, Ch. 82 and 28; Lee et al, Ch. 75*)

40.(C) *Discussion:* Erythrocytosis may be absolute or relative, depending on whether the elevated hemoglobin concentration/increased hematocrit is accompanied by an elevated red cell mass. Absolute erythrocytosis may be primary, caused by polycythemia vera, or secondary to a variety of causes including cardiopulmonary disorders, exposure to high altitudes, and inappropriate erythropoietin secretion by tumors. The red cell mass elevation defines absolute erythrocytosis but does not help distinguish primary from secondary causes. In polycythemia vera, the erythropoietin level is very low, whereas in secondary polycythemia, the erythropoietin level is normal or elevated. Splenomegaly and basophilia are common in polycythemia vera and unusual in secondary states. (*Cecil, Ch. 141; Beutler et al, Ch. 29 and 40; Lee et al, Ch. 45*)

41.(D) *Discussion:* Splenomegaly is found in over three quarters of patients with polycythemia vera. The mean age at diagnosis is approximately 60 but has been reported from the teens to the 90s. Approximately 50% of patients have thrombotic complications, including stroke and Budd-Chiari syndrome. Hemorrhage is less common and usually minor, including easy bruising and mucosal bleeding. Initial therapy with phlebotomy usually results in prompt resolution of most symptoms, including headache, lethargy, and dizziness. Long-term therapy remains controversial. Transformation to AML occurs in fewer than 20% of patients. Thrombotic complications remain a major cause of death in patients with this disease. (*Cecil, Ch. 141; Beutler et al, Ch. 29; Lee et al, Ch. 45*)

42.(E) *Discussion:* Most patients with essential thrombocythemia are now detected by an abnormal routine complete blood count and are asymptomatic. Splenomegaly is detectable in only 30 to 40% of patients at diagnosis but, if present, may help distinguish essential thrombocythemia from reactive thrombocytosis. Hemorrhagic and thrombotic complications frequently complicate the course of this disorder but, with the inclusion of the platelet count on routine complete blood counts, are less frequent presenting features than previously. Erythromelalgia is an unusual burning or throbbing pain in the extremities, particularly the digits, which responds rapidly to aspirin treatment and may occur in a minority of patients during their course. (*Cecil, Ch. 141; Beutler et al, Ch. 31; Lee et al, Ch. 54*)

43.(B) *Discussion:* Reactive thrombocytosis occurs with a variety of clinical disorders but is most common in inflammatory disorders, in which IL-6 levels are elevated as part of the acute-phase response. IL-6 levels are normal in essential thrombocythemia. The fibrinogen level also increases as part of the acute-phase response. Although splenomegaly occurs in fewer than half of patients with essential thrombocythemia at diagnosis, it is unusual in patients with reactive thrombocytosis. Lymphadenopathy is uncommon in essential thrombocythemia but also in most cases of reactive thrombocytosis. (*Cecil, Ch. 141; Beutler et al, Ch. 31; Lee et al, Ch. 54*)

44.(A) *Discussion:* Most patients with essential thrombocythemia have a normal life expectancy. Median survival of patients with polycythemia vera is between 10 and 15 years. The median survival of patients with agnogenic myeloid metaplasia is approximately 5 years and that of patients with CML is between 2 and 5 years, depending on associated risk factors and stage of disease at diagnosis. CLL is not a myeloproliferative disorder. (*Cecil, Ch. 141; Beutler et al, Ch. 28 and 31; Lee et al, Ch. 54*)

45.(E) *Discussion:* The chromosomal rearrangement between chromosomes 9 and 22 resulting in the fusion of the *abl* oncogene on chromosome 9 and the breakpoint cluster region (*bcr*) on chromosome 22 appears to occur in a pluripotent stem cell and therefore is passed along to erythroid, myeloid, megakaryocytic, and lymphoid precursors. (*Cecil, Ch. 142; Beutler et al, Ch. 28*)

46.(B) *Discussion:* CML is a clonal disorder of a pluripotent marrow stem cell disorder. Patients have increased numbers of granulocytes, and up to 50% also have thrombocytosis. Granulocytes synthesize increased amounts of transcobalamin I and III, leading to an increase in the level of vitamin B_{12}. Elevations of uric acid and LDH are frequent findings in CML. LAP production in CML granulocytes is markedly *decreased* compared to that in normal granulo-

cytes. By contrast, LAP is usually increased in polycythemia vera. (*Cecil, Ch. 142; Beutler et al, Ch. 28; Lee et al, Ch. 75*)

47.(E) *Discussion:* Recognized important poor prognostic factors in CML include the absence of the Philadelphia chromosome and basophilia. Hepatomegaly and thrombocytopenia also appear to convey a poorer prognosis. In patients going into blast crisis, the LAP level often increases dramatically. The LAP level may also increase during acute infection and in some patients under good control in the chronic phase. Overall, therefore, a low LAP score cannot be interpreted as a poor prognostic factor. (*Cecil, Ch. 142; Beutler et al, Ch. 28; Lee et al, Ch. 75*)

48.(D) *Discussion:* Up to 90% of patients treated with interferon-alpha respond; however complete response occurs in fewer than 10% and most responders relapse within 2 years. 2-Chlorodeoxyadenosine and 2-deoxycoformycin are purine analogues to which nearly all patients with hairy cell leukemia respond, with durable complete remissions in up to 50%. Treatment with corticosteroids is *not* associated with clinical response and appears to increase the frequency of infectious complications. (*Cecil, Ch. 142; Beutler et al., Ch. 107; Lee et al., Ch. 82*)

49.(B) *Discussion:* Hairy cell leukemia and CLL are clonal disorders of lymphocyte origin. Essentially all hairy cell leukemias and approximately 95% of CLLs are of B cell origin. Infectious-mononucleosis is characterized by infection of B lymphocytes by EBV; T lymphocytes are not infected by this virus. Large granular lymphocyte leukemia is a clonal disorder of either T cell or natural killer cell, but not B cell, origin. (*Cecil, Ch. 142; Beutler et al., Ch. 108; Lee et al., Ch. 65, 78, and 82*)

50.(A) *Discussion:* CLL is a clonal disorder, predominantly of B cell origin, associated with increased numbers of mature-appearing lymphocytes in the peripheral blood, liver, spleen, bone marrow, and lymph nodes. Patients with newly diagnosed CLL may not require therapy for many years, and there are no proven cures. Indications to commence chemotherapy include anemia or thrombocytopenia related to bone marrow involvement or hypersplenism; massive symptomatic lymphadenopathy or splenomegaly; significant symptoms such as fever, night sweats, weight loss, and leukostasis; and conversion to an aggressive lymphoma (Richter transformation). Autoimmune disorders often associated with CLL, including autoimmune hemolytic anemia and ITP, are better treated with corticosteroids or other specific therapy rather than chemotherapy. (*Cecil, Ch. 142; Beutler et al., Ch. 106; Lee et al., Ch. 78*)

51.(D) *Discussion:* Patients with chromosomal abnormalities or chromosomal instability have an increased risk of developing AML. Recognized abnormalities include trisomy 21 (Down's syndrome), Fanconi's anemia (autosomal recessive disorder with increased susceptibility to chromosomal breakage), and Bloom syndrome (autosomal recessive disorder with spontaneous chromosome breakage). (*Cecil, Ch. 143; Beutler et al., Ch. 27; Lee et al., Ch. 73*)

52.(C) *Discussion:* Examination of chromosomes in patients with AML shows that specific morphologic subtypes of AML are associated with specific chromosomal abnormalities. In certain cases in which morphologic examination is equivocal, finding specific chromosomal defects helps to confirm the specific subtype of acute leukemia, which has importance regarding prognosis and selection of therapy. Chromosomal abnormalities are found in approximately 50% of cases. Inversion of a portion of chromosome 16 is found in the M4 subtype of AML, associated with increased eosinophils and a relatively good prognosis. The 9;22 translocation (Philadelphia chromosome) may be found in CML or acute lymphoblastic leukemia. The 15;17 translocation appears to be unique to acute promyelocytic leukemia, involves the retinoic acid receptor, and is associated with an increased incidence of coagulation disturbances. Trisomy 8, the most common chromosomal abnormality found in AML patients, is not associated with a particular AML subtype but may convey a poorer prognosis. The 8;14 translocation is found in Burkitt's lymphoma and involves the *c-myc* proto-oncogene. (*Cecil, Ch. 143; Beutler et al., Ch. 27; Lee et al., Ch. 73*)

53.(D) *Discussion:* Inversion of a portion of chromosome 16 and the 15;17 translocation are relatively good prognostic factors and are discussed in the answer to question 52. The 8;21 translocation is often seen in the M2 subtype of AML, is often associated with loss of the Y chromosome, and may convey a better prognosis. Loss of a chromosome 5 or 7 or gain of a chromosome 8 are frequent findings in many subtypes of AML and are associated with a poorer prognosis. (*Cecil, Ch. 143; Beutler et al., Ch. 27; Lee et al., Ch. 73*)

54.(E) *Discussion:* Chromosomal translocations associated with leukemias and lymphomas frequently lead to altered expression of oncogenes. Infections with certain viruses are associated with increased risk of development of virus-specific lymphoma or leukemia. Infection with the human retrovirus HTLV-I appears to play an important role in the development of acute T-cell leukemia, which is endemic in Southern Japan and the Caribbean. Infection with EBV, a herpesvirus, is associated with the development of endemic Burkitt's lymphoma. Another herpesvirus, herpesvirus 6, has been associated with lymphoproliferative disorders. Translocation of the *bcl-1* oncogene on chromosome 11 is associated with a variety of non-Hodgkin's lymphomas, and alterations in the *ras* oncogene have been detected in myelodysplastic syndromes and AML. (*Cecil, Ch. 143; Beutler et al., Ch. 27 and 111; Lee et al., Ch. 80*)

55.(D) *Discussion:* Diffuse lymphadenopathy is an important clue to disease but is very nonspecific. Certain disorders, however, typically present with diffuse lymphadenopathy, whereas others more often present with localized or regional lymphadenopathy. Lymphadenopathy associated with non-Hodgkin's lymphoma, warfarin treatment, AIDS and angio-immunoblastic lymphadenopathy is usually diffuse. In Hodgkin's disease, by contrast, lymph node involvement is often localized and the disease spreads contiguously. Careful staging is important in Hodgkin's disease because, if localized, the disease may be cured by local radiotherapy alone. This is in contrast to non-Hodgkin's lymphoma, which is very rarely restricted to one site at diagnosis. (*Cecil, Ch. 144; Beutler et al., Ch. 110; Lee et al., Ch. 79*)

56.(D) *Discussion:* At the time of diagnosis, multiple myeloma, AML, hairy cell leukemia, and to a large extent the non-Hodgkin's lymphomas are widespread. Therefore, these patients usually require systemic chemotherapy rather than localized treatment with radiation. By contrast, Hodgkin's lymphoma frequently presents with localized disease amenable to curative radiotherapy. (*Cecil, Ch. 145*)

57.(D) *Discussion:* Growth factors in general have a number of activities and do not affect just one cell type or act at just one stage of cellular development. G-CSF is produced by monocytes and endothelial cells and stimulates granulocyte and macrophage progenitors. Erythropoietin is produced primarily by the renal tubular interstitial cells and acts on erythroid precursors. GM-CSF is produced by T cells, endothelial cells, and fibroblasts and stimulates production of granulocytes, macrophages, and eosinophils, and to some extent acts on erythroid precursors. IL-5 is produced by T cells and stimulates B cell proliferation and supports proliferation, maturation, and function of eosinophils. IL-7 is produced by leukocytes and activates B cells. (*Cecil, Ch. 148; Beutler et al., Ch. 22; Lee et al., Ch. 3*)

58.(C) *Discussion:* Charcot-Leyden crystals are formed from the eosinophil protein lysophospholipase, and may be found in sputum, feces, and tissues in patients with the hypereosinophilic syndrome but are also seen in other eosinophilic inflammatory disorders. (*Cecil, Ch. 148; Beutler et al., Ch. 73*)

59.(E) *Discussion:* Eosinophilia is a relatively frequently encountered laboratory abnormality. Most often it is transient and related to an allergic or infectious disorder. In order to make the diagnosis of the idiopathic hypereosinophilic syndrome, it is necessary to demonstrate persistence of eosinophilia for greater than 6 months, show no evidence of causative parasitic (e.g., trichinosis, schistosomiasis, echinococcus) or allergic (e.g., asthma, drug reaction, urticaria) disorders, and have evidence of organ dysfunction related to the eosinophilia (e.g., endomyocardial fibrosis, skin rash, splenomegaly). It is *not* necessary to document infiltration of tissues by eosinophils. (*Cecil, Ch. 148; Beutler et al., Ch. 84; Lee et al., Ch. 60*)

60.(B) *Discussion:* Approximately 3% of patients over 70 years of age have a detectable level of M protein, and this may approach 20% in patients in their 90s. Because only a minority of these patients progress to myeloma, because no curative treatment for myeloma exists, and because of the patient population, simple observation and follow-up without treatment is the preferred approach. (*Cecil, Ch. 149; Beutler et al., Ch. 113; Lee et al., Ch. 83*)

61.(A) *Discussion:* The presence of >10% bone marrow plasma cells is necessary for the diagnosis of multiple myeloma. At diagnosis, 80% of patients with myeloma have a serum M spike and 75% have a urine M spike. Lytic skeletal lesions are present in the majority of patients at diagnosis, although some may present with diffuse osteoporosis rather than discrete skeletal lesions. Hypercalcemia is present in only approximately 25% of patients at diagnosis, although its presence may be a clue to the diagnosis of multiple myeloma. (*Cecil, Ch. 149; Beutler et al., Ch. 113; Lee et al., Ch. 83*)

62.(C) *Discussion:* Renal failure is a common complication in patients with multiple myeloma. Most commonly this is caused by hypercalcemia or precipitation of light chains in the kidney. Hyperuricemia may also contribute to renal failure, and occasionally amyloid deposition in the kidney may precipitate renal failure. Myeloma cells are not usually found in the kidneys. Renal failure is better prevented than treated once it has developed. (*Cecil, Ch. 149; Lee et al., Ch. 84*)

63.(D) *Discussion:* Hypercalcemia is a frequent complication in patients with multiple myeloma. It may cause dehydration, renal failure, and encephalopathy. The primary cause of hypercalcemia appears to be increased osteoclast bone resorption. Hyperviscosity occurs in fewer than 10% of patients with multiple myeloma and may also present with confusion. However, anorexia and constipation are not typical features of hyperviscosity. (*Cecil, Ch. 149; Beutler et al., Ch. 115; Lee et al., Ch. 84*)

64.(A) *Discussion:* Without treatment, the median survival of patients with multiple myeloma is approximately 6 months. The most common causes of death are infection and renal failure. With therapy, median survival increases to about 3 years. Allogeneic bone marrow transplantation from a human leukocyte antigen (HLA)-matched related donor may produce a 40% long-term remission rate in young patients. (*Cecil, Ch. 149; Beutler et al., Ch. 114; Lee et al., Ch. 84*)

65.(C) *Discussion:* Some M proteins have the property of precipitating at temperatures reached in the peripheral circulation found in the extremities. These are usually either IgM or IgG and are found in 5 to 10% of patients with multiple myeloma and up to 20% of patients with Waldenström's macroglobulinemia. Approximately 40% of patients with cryoglobulinemia will have Raynaud's phenomenon (distal cyanosis and necrosis of the digits). Hyperviscosity usually produces more central symptoms such as fatigue, dizziness, blurred vision, and headache. (*Cecil, Ch. 149; Beutler et al., Ch. 115; Lee et al., Ch. 85 and 88*)

66.(E) *Discussion:* Hematologic abnormalities, including thrombocytopenia, are relatively uncommon in patients with amyloidosis. Thrombocytosis may be observed in up to 10% of these patients. Hemostatic defects are common. Most commonly, patients bruise easily as a result of infiltration of the amyloid protein into blood vessels, producing fragility. Factor X may bind to the amyloid protein, leading to a detectable deficiency and prolonging the prothrombin time; however, this is a relatively rare finding. The thrombin time is prolonged in up to 40% of patients, most often as a result of interference with fibrin polymerization by an M protein. (*Cecil, Ch. 149; Beutler et al., Ch. 117; Lee et al., Ch. 87*)

67.(D) *Discussion:* The diagnosis of amyloidosis is dependent on demonstration of amyloid on a tissue biopsy. Given the frequent association with hemostatic defects in this disorder, hemorrhagic complications are an important concern in selecting tissue for biopsy. Biopsy of abdominal fat yields a diagnosis in approximately 80% of patients and is associated with few complications. Rectal biopsy has a similar yield but carries a higher risk of hemorrhage. Liver, bone marrow,

and sural nerve biopsies are all more invasive procedures. (*Cecil, Ch. 149; Beutler et al., Ch. 117; Lee et al., Ch. 87*)

68.(C) *Discussion:* As with IgG, most patients with an IgM M spike have a monoclonal gammopathy of unknown significance at diagnosis. Only 17% have Waldenström's macroglobulinemia. Lymphoma and CLL each account for about 5%. IgM myelomas are rare. (*Cecil, Ch. 149; Beutler et al., Ch. 114; Lee et al., Ch. 85*)

69.(D) *Discussion:* The spleen serves several important functions in the body's immune system. Humoral immune response involves the activation of B cells in the spleen in response to infection. Plasmablasts secrete immunoglobulin, beginning with IgM; the spleen is the major source of IgM in the body. The spleen also plays a role in cellular immune response to infection. The spleen contains many phagocytic cells, which remove foreign antigens and microorganisms from the circulation. Removal of the spleen compromises these functions and predisposes the patient to overwhelming infection, most commonly caused by pneumococcus and meningococcus. (*Cecil, Ch. 150; Beutler et al., Ch. 5; Lee et al., Ch. 12*)

70.(B) *Discussion:* Howell-Jolly bodies are nuclear remnants left in red cells after they depart from the bone marrow. These bodies are removed from circulating red cells by the spleen. The Heinz body represents denatured hemoglobin formed in a variety of disorders such as G6PD deficiency after exposure to oxidative stresses. Heinz bodies are removed from circulating red cells by pitting in the spleen. Russell bodies are collections of immunoglobulin within plasma cells observed in multiple myeloma. Charcot-Leyden crystals are precipitates of the eosinophil protein lysophospholipase, found in eosinophilic disorders. Auer rods are long, fused primary granules containing peroxidase and lysosomal enzymes found in blasts in patients with AML. (*Cecil, Ch. 148 and 150; Lee et al., Ch. 84*)

71.(C) *Discussion:* The spleen is frequently involved in hematologic neoplasms, such as lymphomas and leukemias. Bone marrow fibrosis leads to extramedullary hematopoiesis in disorders such as agnogenic myeloid metaplasia and polycythemia vera. Infectious mononucleosis is usually associated with splenomegaly related to T cell proliferation. Cirrhosis with portal hypertension produces congestion and enlargement of the spleen. Work hypertrophy by phagocytic cells in disorders such as autoimmune hemolytic anemia and hereditary spherocytosis also produces splenomegaly. Metastasis of solid tumor to the spleen as a cause of splenomegaly is extraordinarily rare. (*Cecil, Ch. 150; Lee et al., Ch. 67*)

72.(A) *Discussion:* Splenectomy decreases hemolysis and prevents other complications in patients with hereditary spherocytosis. In patients with ITP, splenectomy produces a response in up to 80%. Splenectomy in patients with Gaucher's disease improves symptoms and corrects cytopenias. Splenectomy following traumatic rupture may be necessary to prevent exsanguination. Splenectomy appears to be of no clinical benefit in CML despite often massive splenomegaly. (*Cecil, Ch. 150; Beutler et al., Ch. 69; Lee et al., Ch. 67*)

73.(E) *Discussion:* Because the spleen plays a role in humoral and cellular immunity, splenectomy has an impact on cell-mediated immunity; antibody production, especially of IgM; and properdin production and complement-mediated opsonization. The spleen is the major site of IgM production; however, following splenectomy, this function appears to be adequately resumed elsewhere in the lymphatic system. The spleen is also the major site of properdin production, necessary for complement-mediated opsonization. The ability of the spleen to filter and capture microorganisms is not well compensated following splenectomy. Therefore, a major deficit following splenectomy is susceptibility to overwhelming infection by encapsulated bacteria, such as pneumococcus and meningococcus. (*Cecil, Ch. 150; Beutler et al., Ch. 5; Lee et al., Ch. 13*)

74.(C) *Discussion:* Engraftment of immunocompetent donor T cells appears to be responsible for the development of graft-versus-host disease following allogeneic bone marrow transplantation. Methods to decrease the numbers or activity of T cells in the donated marrow, such as purging the marrow, are aimed at decreasing the frequency of this complication. Methotrexate is administered following transplant as an immunosuppressant to decrease the activity of these donor T cells for the same purpose. Cyclosporine and corticosteroids are additional agents used to prevent graft-versus-host disease. (*Cecil, Ch. 151; Beutler et al., Ch. 18*)

75.(D) *Discussion:* Autologous bone marrow transplantation showed promise initially in malignant disorders in which the bone marrow was not involved. This allowed escalation of the dosing of chemotherapy with rescue reinfusion of preserved autologous marrow. However, techniques that allow removal of malignant cells from the bone marrow *ex vivo* have permitted the extension of the use of autologous transplantation to hematologic malignancies involving the marrow. These include non-Hodgkin's lymphoma, CML, acute lymphoblastic leukemia, and multiple myeloma. In all of these disorders, patients have received autologous transplants, with long-term remission in some patients. Autologous transplantation in sickle cell anemia would fail to correct the genetic defect, whereas allogeneic transplantation has been curative. (*Cecil, Ch. 151; Beutler et al., Ch. 18*)

76.(C) *Discussion:* Significant spontaneous bleeding is rare with a platelet count above 20×10^9 per liter. With surgery, the platelet count should exceed 50×10^9 per liter to avoid excessive blood loss. In patients undergoing induction chemotherapy, it has been routine to infuse platelets whenever the patient's platelet count falls below 20×10^9 per liter; however, in the absence of active bleeding or fever, a lower threshold such as 5 to 10×10^9 per liter might be safe and practical. (*Cecil, Ch. 152; Beutler et al., Ch. 126*)

77.(D) *Discussion:* Up to 90% of children with acute ITP will have complete long-term remissions by 6 months with no treatment. Therefore, simple observation of asymptomatic children with ITP, particularly with platelet counts greater than 20×10^9 per liter, is a reasonable approach. For more severe ITP or in the presence of bleeding, therapeutic intervention with corticosteroids or intravenous immunoglobulin is appropriate. Only for refractory severe ITP should splenectomy be considered. Transfusion of platelets

is of very little benefit because the infused platelets are rapidly cleared from the circulation, and they carry the risk of transmission of infectious agents. (*Cecil, Ch. 152; Beutler et al., Ch. 129; Lee et al., Ch. 50*)

78.(B) *Discussion:* Up to 80% of adults with ITP will show a rise in the platelet count with corticosteroid therapy, with responses usually requiring 3 to 7 days to appear. Treatment with intravenous immunoglobulin shows a similar degree of success but the rise in the platelet count appears earlier, within 2 to 3 days. In those patients with ITP who are going to respond to splenectomy, the platelet count elevation is often observed within 24 hours. Danazol therapy usually requires 4 to 6 weeks before a response is observed and is therefore more useful as a steroid-sparing agent. (*Cecil, Ch. 152; Beutler et al., Ch. 129; Lee et al., Ch. 50*)

79.(C) *Discussion:* DIC and TTP are both microangiopathic hemolytic anemias. Therefore, in both disorders patients are anemic and have evidence of hemolysis (increased LDH, decreased haptoglobin). Peripheral smear schistocytes resulting from the passage of red cells through microvascular thrombi are present in both disorders. In TTP these microvascular thrombi are composed primarily of platelets, whereas in DIC fibrin predominates. Abnormalities of coagulation, such as consumption of fibrinogen, are almost universal in patients with acute DIC but are very unusual in patients with TTP. (*Cecil, Ch. 152; Beutler et al., Ch. 128; Lee et al., Ch. 51*)

80.(F) *Discussion:* Patients with uremia have a hemostatic defect mostly resulting from platelet dysfunction caused by exposure of platelets to the uremic environment. Another important contributor to increased bleeding diathesis is severe anemia (<26% hematocrit). Agents shown, at least anecdotally, to shorten the prolonged bleeding time and/or lead to cessation of bleeding in uremic patients include conjugated estrogens, DDAVP and cryoprecipitate. The mechanism whereby hemostasis is promoted by these agents in uremic patients is poorly understood. Improvement in the uremic environment by dialysis produces a temporary enhancement of platelet function. Maintenance of a hematocrit of greater than approximately 26%, either by administration of erythropoietin or red cell transfusions, appears to improve *in vivo* platelet function in flowing blood by forcing the platelet from the center of the blood vessel toward the vascular endothelium of the blood vessel, where its function is required. (*Cecil, Ch. 152; Beutler et al., Ch. 133; Lee et al., Ch. 55*)

81.(D) *Discussion:* Glanzmann's thrombasthenia is an autosomal recessive platelet function disorder caused by defective or absent platelet glycoprotein IIb/IIIa complex, the receptor for fibrinogen. Hermansky-Pudlak syndrome is an autosomal recessive inherited platelet storage pool disorder associated with albinism. Platelet number and size are normal in both of these disorders. Patients with von Willebrand's disease may present with lifelong epistaxis but usually have a normal platelet count. One exception is subtype IIb of von Willebrand's disease, in which mild thrombocytopenia (rarely less than 50×10^9 per liter) may occur. ITP is an acquired disorder that may be associated with epistaxis and large platelets on peripheral smear; however, lifelong symptoms would not be expected. Not surprisingly, many patients with Bernard-Soulier syndrome, an autosomal recessive platelet function disorder caused by defective or deficient platelet glycoprotein Ib receptor for von Willebrand factor, often undergo splenectomy as treatment for "refractory ITP" before the true diagnosis is recognized. Platelet number in patients with Bernard-Soulier is usually less than 100×10^9 per liter; however, because platelet size is significantly increased, the absolute platelet mass in the body may be normal. (*Cecil, Ch. 152; Beutler et al., Ch. 132; Lee et al., Ch. 55*)

82.(B) *Discussion:* Osler-Weber-Rendu syndrome (hereditary hemorrhagic telangiectasia) is an autosomal dominant disorder caused by disordered formation of capillaries, venules, and arterioles. These abnormal vessels are fragile and prone to rupture, causing mucosal hemorrhage, most commonly epistaxis. Progressive malformation in the microvasculature may lead to arteriovenous malformations, most often found in the gastrointestinal tract, leading to chronic gastrointestinal blood loss and iron deficiency anemia, and in the lung, producing hemoptysis. Telangiectases are most commonly found on the lips, face, tongue, palms, and fingers. Bernard-Soulier syndrome, Chédiak-Higashi syndrome, and Hermansky-Pudlak syndrome are inherited diseases with platelet function defects; patients may present with epistaxis but do not have arteriovenous malformations. Kasabach-Merritt syndrome (giant cavernous hemangiomas) is a congenital disorder associated with internal or superficial hemangiomas and is typically associated with the development of a chronic DIC-like picture. (*Cecil, Ch. 152; Beutler et al., Ch. 134; Lee et al., Ch. 53 and 57*)

83.(D) *Discussion:* The liver is the primary synthetic source of most coagulation factors and natural anticoagulants. Several of these proteins require post-translational modification in the liver in a vitamin K–dependent process. The vitamin K–dependent procoagulant factors include Factors II, VII, IX, and X. The vitamin K–dependent natural anticoagulants include protein C and protein S. Deficiency of another vitamin K–dependent factor, protein Z, has recently been reported in association with a mild familial bleeding diathesis. (*Cecil, Ch. 153; Beutler et al., Ch. 139; Lee et al., Ch. 57*)

84.(A) *Discussion:* Deficiency of Factor XIII is associated with a bleeding disorder characterized by delayed bleeding and poor wound healing. Factor XIII is a transglutaminase activated by thrombin that plays important roles in cross-linking fibrin to form a stable clot and in cross-linking alpha$_2$-antiplasmin into the fibrin clot to protect it from degradation by plasmin. Protein S acts as a natural anticoagulant, serving as a cofactor for activated protein C; deficiency of protein S is associated with a prothrombotic tendency. Deficiencies of the high-contact pathway factors (Factor XII, prekallikrein, and high-molecular-weight kininogen) often produce dramatic prolongations of the aPTT but are *not* associated with a bleeding diathesis. (*Cecil, Ch. 153; Beutler et al., Ch. 137; Lee et al., Ch. 56*)

85.(C) *Discussion:* Prior diagrams of the coagulation cascades showing convergence of the intrinsic and extrinsic pathways into the common pathway without interaction above the common pathway have been replaced with a new pathway with Factor VII at the center. This was precipitated by the discovery and understanding of the extrinsic pathway inhibitor (EPI), also known as tissue factor pathway inhibitor. The current model shows the release or exposure of tissue factor leading to Factor VII activation as the primary *in vivo* initiator of coagulation. Activated Factor VII activates both Factor X and Factor IX; however, EPI rapidly complexes with Factor Xa and this complex then acts as a Factor VIIa inhibitor and effectively shuts down the tissue factor:Factor VIIa complex. Activated Factor IX continues to activate Factor X, leading to the conversion of prothrombin to thrombin and thus to the formation of fibrin from fibrinogen. (*Cecil, Ch. 153; Beutler et al., Ch. 123*)

86.(D) *Discussion:* Thrombin is generated from prothrombin by the action of activated Factor X in the presence of activated Factor V, calcium, and phospholipid. Thrombin is a very potent enzyme with many important hemostatic effects. Thrombin activates platelets, converts fibrinogen to fibrin, activates the major cofactors of coagulation (Factors V and VIII), and activates Factor XIII, which crosslinks the fibrin clot. Thrombin also has an anticoagulant function; when bound to thrombomodulin, an endothelial cell surface protein, thrombin activates protein C, one of the natural anticoagulants. Protein S is not activated by thrombin but instead, after being acted on by thrombin, may lose its anticoagulant activity. (*Cecil, Ch. 153; Beutler et al., Ch. 123; Lee et al., Ch. 19*)

87.(E) *Discussion:* The gene for Factor VIII is located on the X chromosome. Therefore, men with a defective gene will have lower Factor VIII levels than women with one defective gene and one normal gene. In addition, lyonization may occasionally produce women with significantly decreased Factor VIII levels, and rare women may be homozygous for defective Factor VIII genes. Because of this X linkage, a man with hemophilia will inherit the defective X chromosome *only* from his mother, who received her abnormal X from either her father (maternal grandfather) *or* her mother. On average, a woman carrier will pass the abnormal X chromosome to half of her sons. The mother's brother (maternal uncle) may have received the defective X chromosome from his mother (maternal grandmother). The patient's mother may have received the defective X chromosome from her mother (maternal grandmother), who may have inherited it from her father (maternal great grandfather). A certain percentage of patients have hemophilia caused by new mutations, so that the family history will be negative. A man with hemophilia A will pass the defect to all of his daughters and none of his sons. (*Cecil, Ch. 153; Lee et al., Ch. 56*)

88.(C) *Discussion:* Where once patients with hemophilia A required the infusion of large amounts of plasma, now concentrates of Factor VIII protein, chemically or immunologically purified or made by recombinant genetic technology, are available to permit normalization of Factor VIII levels even in patients with severe hemophilia (<1% Factor VIII). This progress over the past 20 years has, of course, not been without significant adverse effects, dominated by the widespread transmission of infectious agents in concentrates of Factor VIII produced from pools of plasma from thousands of donors. Transfusion-related HIV and hepatitis C are major causes of morbidity and mortality in adults with severe hemophilia A. Cryoprecipitate is produced from plasma and is enriched for Factor VIII. Although not virally inactivated, it comes from a much smaller donor pool than the purified factor concentrates. This product may under certain circumstances be appropriate for replacement therapy in hemophilia A patients; however, current viral inactivation methods used in the production of Factor VIII products derived from human plasma and the availability of recombinant Factor VIII appear to make cryoprecipitate a less safe product. Fresh frozen plasma contains only 1 unit of Factor VIII per milliliter and is not virally inactivated; therefore, this product is both relatively ineffective and less safe than other factor replacement options. (*Cecil, Ch. 153; Beutler et al., Ch. 135*)

89.(D) *Discussion:* The administration of blood products, including factor concentrates, to patients with hemophilia over the past 20 years has been associated with a high frequency of transmission of viruses, including HIV and hepatitis B and C. Although current methods of viral inactivation of factor concentrates and the availability of recombinant Factor VIII have greatly diminished viral transmission, it remains wise to avoid blood product administration when it is possible to do so safely. For patients with mild hemophilia A (5 to 30% Factor VIII) undergoing a minor procedure such as a dental extraction, it is often possible to provide adequate hemostasis without administration of Factor VIII. Agents with utility in this setting include (1) DDAVP, which stimulates an increase in the Factor VIII level in many patients with mild hemophilia A, and (2) antifibrinolytic agents (epsilon-aminocaproic acid and tranexamic acid), which help prevent premature clot lysis. Whether aprotinin, an agent with inhibitory activity against plasmin and kallikrein, is beneficial in prevention of bleeding in this setting is unknown. (*Cecil, Ch. 153; Beutler et al., Ch. 135*)

90.(C) *Discussion:* Approximately 15% of patients with severe hemophilia A will develop clinically significant Factor VIII antibodies during their lifetimes. These inhibitors usually develop during childhood, occur following repeated Factor VIII infusions, and if of high titer may render infusion of human Factor VIII concentrates totally ineffective. Methods for obtaining hemostasis in these patients include administration of prothrombin complex concentrate (Factors II, VII, IX, and X), chemically activated prothrombin complex concentrate, porcine Factor VIII, or recombinant activated Factor VII. (*Cecil, Ch. 153; Beutler et al., Ch. 135*)

91.(B) *Discussion:* Both severe hemophilia A and severe von Willebrand's disease may be characterized by decreased Factor VIII level and aPTT prolongation. Important differences include (1) the pattern of inheritance (hemophilia A is X linked and von Willebrand's disease is autosomal); (2) the bleeding time is usually normal in hemophilia A and usually prolonged in severe von Willebrand's disease; (3) the von Willebrand factor level is normal in hemophilia A; and (4) platelet aggregation studies usually show abnormal response to ristocetin in von Willebrand's disease but are normal in hemophilia A. (*Cecil, Ch. 153; Beutler et al., Ch. 135 and 138*)

92.(E) *Discussion:* von Willebrand's disease is by far the most common inherited bleeding disorder, with some estimates of frequency as high as 1% of the population being affected. Hemophilia A occurs in 0.5 to 1 per 10,000 but is the most common coagulation factor deficiency (not including von Willebrand's disease), and may account for up to three quarters of all inherited factor deficiencies. Hemophilia B occurs in roughly 1 in 50,000. Osler-Weber-Rendu syndrome (hereditary hemorrhagic telangiectasia) has a similar frequency. The platelet storage pool disorders (e.g., Hermansky-Pudlak syndrome and Chédiak-Higashi syndrome) are very rare autosomal recessive disorders. (*Cecil, Ch. 153; Beutler et al., Ch. 138; Lee et al., Ch. 56*)

93.(E) *Discussion:* In the patient with a strong history of bleeding consistent with a coagulation or platelet defect, a normal platelet count, bleeding time, prothrombin time, and aPTT should not be the end of the evaluation. A variety of clinically significant hemostatic defects may be overlooked in this setting. In particular, Factor XIII and elements of the fibrinolytic system (alpha$_2$-antiplasmin or plasminogen activator inhibitor-1 deficiency) are not assessed by the above four screening tests. Mild von Willebrand's disease is notoriously difficult to diagnose, and patients often have both a normal aPTT and normal bleeding time. Inherited abnormal fibrinogens may predispose to bleeding yet not affect the results of screening tests. In order to exclude these diagnoses, testing in a special coagulation laboratory is usually necessary. Prekallikrein deficiency is not associated with a bleeding diathesis. (*Cecil, Ch. 153; Lee et al., Ch. 48*)

94.(D) *Discussion:* Despite thorough investigation of families with frequent thromboemboli, the majority fail to have one of the recognized inherited hypercoagulable states, such as deficiency of antithrombin III, protein C, or protein S. Recently, several investigators discovered a mutation in coagulation Factor V that renders it resistant to inactivation by activated protein C. Preliminary epidemiologic studies suggest that this defect may account for up to 30% of inherited hypercoagulable states, whereas deficiencies of antithrombin III, protein C, and protein S may each account for approximately 5%. (*Cecil, Ch. 153; Beutler et al., Ch. 144*)

95.(B) *Discussion:* The clinical relevance of the finding of a lupus anticoagulant continues to be defined. However, clinical epidemiologic evidence suggests a true association of the presence of a lupus anticoagulant with an increased risk of thrombosis, particularly if the lupus anticoagulant persists beyond 3 months and if the patient also has a connective tissue disorder, such as systemic lupus erythematosus. Nonetheless, it has also become apparent that some patients with lupus anticoagulants may have mild to moderate bleeding tendencies. Recognized causes of bleeding in this setting include associated prothrombin deficiency, thrombocytopenia, and platelet dysfunction. Up to 15% of patients with lupus anticoagulants may have a significant antibody-mediated depression in the prothrombin level. (*Cecil, Ch. 153; Beutler et al., Ch. 140*)

96.(E) *Discussion:* Although a dramatic reversal in the clinical outcome of patients with TTP was observed with the introduction of plasma exchange therapy, very little progress has been made in determining the pathogenesis of this unusual disorder. Some evidence exists supporting each of several different theories, including an acquired deficiency in vascular endothelial cell prostacyclin, abnormalities in the processing of extra-large von Willebrand factor multimers secreted by vascular endothelial cells, development of anti–endothelial cell antibodies, and platelet activation by bacteria; however, these remain theories and the exact etiology remains obscure. (*Cecil, Ch. 153*)

97.(A—False;   B—True;   C—False;   D—True; E—False) *Discussion:* In response to an acute decrease in red blood cells, the time from detection of decreased oxygen-carrying capacity by the kidneys, to increased synthesis and release of erythropoietin, to bone marrow response with accelerated red cell production, to the release of an increased number of reticulocytes into the circulation may be 5 to 10 days. Therefore, for up to 5 days following acute hemolysis, one should not expect to see an elevated reticulocyte count, and a normal reticulocyte count should not be interpreted as evidence against hemolysis or for a bone marrow production problem (A).

In the development of iron deficiency, with depletion of bone marrow iron stores, the following sequence of laboratory abnormalities occurs with increasing severity of iron deficiency: (1) decreased ferritin and transferrin saturation, (2) decreased hemoglobin, and (3) decreased MCV. With mild, early iron deficiency anemia, the MCV may be normal. Review of a peripheral smear at this point may demonstrate anisocytosis and a population of hypochromic, microcytic cells, although the *mean* corpuscular volume remains normal. Therefore, iron deficiency should be included in the differential diagnosis of a normocytic anemia (B).

Up to 44% of patients with neuropsychiatric problems caused by vitamin B_{12} deficiency may *not* be anemic, and up to one third may have a normal MCV. Therefore, a normal complete blood count with normal red cell indices should not be used as a reason not to pursue the possibility of vitamin B_{12} deficiency as a cause of neuropsychiatric problems (C), which can be quite diverse, including not only impaired vibration and position sense but also memory loss, weakness, hallucinations, urinary incontinence, and depression.

The development of vitamin B_{12} deficiency as a result of pernicious anemia is related to interference with vitamin B_{12} absorption in the gastrointestinal tract. Intrinsic factor, produced by gastric parietal cells, binds to ingested vitamin B_{12} and is essential for subsequent effective absorption of vitamin B_{12} in the small intestine. Detection of antibodies to intrinsic factor is highly specific for the diagnosis of pernicious anemia but may be found in only approximately one half of patients with this disorder. If such antibodies are found, the diagnosis is made and there is no need for the more cumbersome Schilling's test (D).

The major options for the treatment of patients with aplastic anemia include immunosuppression with antithymocyte globulin and/or cyclosporine or allogeneic bone marrow transplantation. Which of these produces the best outcome continues to be studied but often depends on the individual patient and includes important variables such as patient age, prior transfusion history, and, most importantly, the availability of an appropriate match. At this time, related-donor match transplants are reasonably successful and may be the preferred treatment in patients with a related HLA-matched donor; outcome with unrelated donors is much poorer. Because only approximately one third of patients will have HLA-matched sibling donors, the majority of patients are currently treated initially with immunosuppression (E). (*Cecil, Ch. 129, 130, and 133; Beutler et al., Ch. 18 and 45; Lee et al., Ch. 24, 26, 31, and 32*)

98.(A—True; B—False; C—False; D—True) *Discussion:* Hereditary spherocytosis is an autosomal disorder, usually dominant, of the red cell cytoskeleton associated with chronic hemolysis. The abnormal red cells are destroyed prematurely by the spleen. Following splenectomy, the anemia resolves, although red cell survival remains shortened (A). Ankle ulcers also disappear after splenectomy. If splenectomy fails to correct the anemia, one should either question the diagnosis or search for an accessory spleen. Because splenectomy increases the risk of infection, it should probably be delayed until after the age of 5 to 10 years and be performed only in patients with severe hemolysis, symptomatic anemia, or gallstones.

In the presence of IgG autoantibodies attached to circulating red cells, splenic macrophage Fc receptors remove the red cells from the circulation. Splenic macrophages do *not* have receptors for IgM. In IgM-mediated hemolytic anemia, complement is activated and C3b is deposited on the red cells, leading to predominantly hepatic rather than splenic clearance. Therefore, based on this, one would anticipate clinical improvement following splenectomy in patients with IgG-mediated hemolytic anemia but not IgM-mediated hemolytic anemia (B). Clinically, this is borne out, although improvement may be seen in some patients with IgM-mediated disease, perhaps because the spleen is a major source of IgM production in the adult.

Hairy cell leukemia is a clonal disorder of B lymphocytes associated with a characteristic lymphocyte morphology on peripheral smear and palpable splenomegaly in up to 80% of patients. Splenectomy was often performed in the past for diagnostic and therapeutic purposes, producing significant improvement in symptoms and cytopenias in most patients. However, because the disease is not restricted to the spleen, splenectomy is not curative, and patients usually develop progressive cytopenias as a result of bone marrow involvement (C).

Splenectomy in HIV-related ITP produces responses in up to 80% of patients, which may be lasting in almost 50 to 70%. Splenectomy is also followed by an increase in the absolute CD4 count; however, the clinical significance of this is unclear. There is no evidence that splenectomy in this population produces increased morbidity or mortality (D). (*Cecil, Ch. 134, 135, 142, and 150; Beutler et al., Ch. 52, 103, and 107; Lee et al., Ch. 33, 41, and 66*)

99.(A—True; B—False; C—True; D—True) *Discussion:* In newborns, the predominant hemoglobin is hemoglobin F, made up of two alpha chains and two gamma chains. By 6 months of age, gamma chain production has decreased greatly and has been replaced by beta chain synthesis. Hemoglobin F is replaced therefore, defects hemoglobin A, consisting of two alpha chains and two beta chains. Because of this delay in beta chain appearance, defects in beta chain synthesis do not become clinically apparent until after 6 months of age (A). Defects in all four alpha chains lead to stillbirth at 34 to 40 weeks' gestation (B). The alpha chains are required for the majority of fetal hemoglobins and are important throughout fetal development.

Although patients without sickle cell anemia who have alpha-thalassemia may develop a mild anemia, the coinheritance of alpha-thalassemia with sickle cell anemia is associated with a higher hematocrit (C). This is related to the concentration of hemoglobin in the red cells; sickling is dependent on the hemoglobin concentration within the red cell. With alpha-thalassemia there is less hemoglobin; this produces less sickling and less hemolysis, and thereby a higher hematocrit.

The current life expectancy for males with sickle cell disease is 42 years and that for women is 48 years (D). This has increased over the years as a result of improvements in general medical care rather than greater understanding of the pathophysiology of this disease. Bone marrow transplantation remains experimental, and the potential role of gene therapy in this disorder remains to be clarified. (*Cecil, Ch. 136 and 137; Beutler et al., Ch. 8, 55, and 56; Lee et al., Ch. 38*)

100.(A—False; B—True; C—True; D—False) *Discussion:* Unlike other alloantibodies and autoantibodies, antibodies to the ABO antigens occur *without* prior exposure. Therefore, a patient with type A blood has antibodies to type B blood despite the absence of prior exposure and will have a severe hemolytic transfusion reaction if type B blood is transfused (A). A patient with type O blood has antibodies to both types A and B but their red cells possess neither A nor B antigens. Patients with type AB blood do not have antibodies to type A or B but their red cells have both A and B antigens. Therefore, a patient with type O blood can only receive type O red blood cell transfusions, whereas patients with type A, B, or AB blood can receive type O blood (B).

The development of the mature granulocyte begins with the myeloblast. Progressive differentiation proceeds through the promyelocyte and myelocyte stages. The myelocyte is the last stage in which division occurs. Following the myelocyte stage, the nucleus begins to deform, becoming a metamyelocyte followed by the band. The mature, segmented neutrophil found in the peripheral blood is incapable of division but may continue to synthesize proteins (C).

Because patients with inherited severe hemophilia A lack normal Factor VIII, up to 15% of patients develop isoantibodies to Factor VIII after repeated treatments with it. Immunosuppression with corticosteroids and cyclophosphamide is not usually effective in eradicating the inhibitor; however, induction of immune tolerance with frequent infusions of Factor VIII may be associated with long-term disappearance of the antibody in many patients. Patients with acquired hemophilia A caused by the appearance of an autoantibody directed against Factor VIII frequently respond to treatment with corticosteroids alone or with the addition of cyclophosphamide, particularly if the initial antibody titer is not high (D). (*Cecil, Ch. 138, 139, and 153; Beutler et al., Ch. 73, 135, and 140; Lee et al., Ch. 21*)

101.(A—True; B—False; C—True; D—True; E—False) *Discussion:* Allogeneic bone marrow trans-

plantation in patients with CML may produce long-term survival in 40 to 70%, associated with eradication of the Philadelphia chromosome. In patients in the chronic phase of CML, treatment with interferon-alpha produces hematologic remission in up to 75%, approximately one third show a decreased number of Philadelphia chromosome–positive cells, and in a small number of patients the Philadelphia chromosome disappears altogether. However, testing with polymerase chain reaction shows persistence of the *bcr-abl* gene. Therefore, this cannot be considered curative but rather a prolongation of the chronic phase (A).

At diagnosis, lymphoma cells in low-grade small cell lymphoma are widespread, involving the spleen, liver, lymph nodes, and bone marrow (B). Another low-grade lymphoma, the mucosa-associated lymphoid tissue lymphoma, may be localized to the gastrointestinal tract at diagnosis and not involve the marrow until late in the course. Intermediate-grade lymphomas more commonly affect extranodal sites than the low-grade lymphomas, but at presentation the marrow is less frequently involved. Marrow involvement sought morphologically may overlook minor involvement detectable by molecular genetic studies. Because of this, autologous bone marrow transplantation for patients with non-Hodgkin's lymphoma, even those without apparent marrow involvement, should probably include a method for purging the autologous marrow of lymphoma cells.

In the subtyping of non-Hodgkin's lymphoma, the diagnosis of low-grade rather than high-grade lymphoma represents a situation of good news and bad news, the good news being the rather indolent course and the bad news being the near-certain inability to cure the disease. By contrast, the more aggressive lymphomas, if responsive, can be cured by chemotherapy (C).

Early-stage Hodgkin's disease (stage I or II) may be approached with radiation therapy alone with curative intent, resulting in long-term disease-free survival in 85 to 90% of patients. More advanced stages require combination chemotherapy but, even in the most advanced stages, up to 75% of patients are curable. Patients initially treated with radiation therapy who relapse are still curable; there is a 70 to 90% complete remission rate with combination chemotherapy (D).

Essential thrombocythemia, one of the myeloproliferative disorders, is a clonal disorder involving predominantly the megakaryocyte lineage. This disorder may be asymptomatic or may be associated with either hemorrhagic or thrombotic complications. Reactive thrombocytosis involves elevation of the platelet count, usually transiently, in association with a variety of clinical disorders. In patients with reactive thrombocytosis, platelet function is normal and therefore is not associated with hemorrhagic risk. In patients with a history of thromboembolic disease or significant atherosclerotic disease, some practitioners administer antiplatelet agents; however, lowering of the platelet count by medication or pheresis is rarely needed. Among patients with essential thrombocythemia, there is general agreement that lowering of the platelet count is indicated in those with thrombotic or hemorrhagic complications; however, controversy remains regarding whether to treat asymptomatic patients (E). (*Cecil,*

Ch. 141, 142, 145, and 152; Beutler et al., Ch. 18, 28, 31, and 110; Lee et al., Ch. 54, 75, and 79)

102.(A—False; B—True; C—False) *Discussion:* Minimal criteria for the diagnosis of multiple myeloma include the demonstration of greater than 10% plasma cells in the bone marrow and at least one of the following: (1) serum M protein, (2) urine M protein, or (3) lytic bone lesions. Only 80% of patients with myeloma have a serum M spike, and only 75% have a urine M spike. Up to 10% of patients may have a nonsecreting myeloma or express an IgD M spike not readily detected by routine laboratory methods. Therefore, demonstration of an M spike is *not* required for the diagnosis of multiple myeloma (A).

Only 20 to 25% of patients with a monoclonal gammopathy of unknown significance progress to overt multiple myeloma even when followed for up to three decades (B). Others may show an increase in the quantity of M protein without lytic lesions or bone marrow plasmacytosis. Because this is a disorder of elderly patients, approximately 50% of patients die of other unrelated causes.

Familial Mediterranean fever is an inherited disorder associated with recurrent attacks of fever, pain, and inflammation, including pericarditis, arthritis, and pleuritis. This disorder is often associated with amyloidosis and progressive renal failure. Clinical trials show that long-term treatment with colchicine prevents most acute attacks and can prevent the development of amyloidosis and renal failure (C). Colchicine is not beneficial for an acute attack once it has begun.

(Cecil, Ch. 139 and 149; Beutler et al., Ch. 113 and 114; Lee et al., Ch. 83 and 84)

103.(A—False; B—False; C—True) *Discussion:* The identification of hematopoietic growth factors has been a very labor-intensive endeavor. Erythropoietin was identified first, followed by a host of other colony-stimulating factors and interleukins, including G-CSF. These are now in routine clinical use. The cytokine for megakaryocyte proliferation and platelet production has taken the longest to identify despite intense efforts. Recently, a potential thrombopoietin was cloned and is currently undergoing laboratory evaluation (A).

Platelets normally contain a large amount of IgG in their alpha granules and also may have IgG bound to their surfaces. In immune thrombocytopenia, patients develop autoantibodies directed predominantly against platelet membrane glycoprotein IIb, IIIa, or Ib/IX. Despite much effort toward the development of a clinically useful diagnostic test for ITP based on the detection of antiplatelet antibodies, no currently available test appears to have sufficient sensitivity and specificity to be useful (B).

TTP was once a disorder associated with rapid fatality—90% mortality within 3 months of diagnosis. With the introduction of plasmapheresis as primary therapy, more than 80% of patients enter remission. In addition, fewer than 25% of patients relapse and 10% of patients suffer a chronic relapsing course (C). *(Cecil, Ch. 152; Beutler et al., 118, 128, and 152; Lee et al., Ch. 17 and 51)*

BIBLIOGRAPHY

Bennett JC, Plum F (eds): Cecil Textbook of Medicine. 20th ed. Philadelphia, WB Saunders Company, 1996.

Beutler E, Lichtman MA, Coller BS, Kipps TJ (eds): Williams Hematology. 5th ed. New York, McGraw-Hill, 1995.

Lee GR, Bithell TC, Foerster J, Athens JW, Lukens JN (eds): Wintrobe's Clinical Hematology. 9th Ed. Philadelphia, Lea & Febiger, 1993.

PART 7

GASTROINTESTINAL DISEASE

Peter F. Ells and Joseph M. Polito, III

DIRECTIONS: For questions 1 to 28, choose the ONE BEST answer to each question.

1. A prolonged prothrombin time (PT) is a bad prognostic sign in the setting of acute hepatitis. All of the following statements support its utility EXCEPT

   A. Hepatic synthesis of clotting factors is necessary to maintain a normal PT.
   B. Some of the clotting factors the liver synthesizes have short half-lives (<1 day).
   C. It requires severe liver injury to suppress synthesis to levels associated with a prolongation of the PT.
   D. Parenteral vitamin K administration will normalize the elevated PT seen in fulminant hepatic failure.

2. All of the following statements concerning alpha$_1$-antitrypsin (A1AT) deficiency are true EXCEPT

   A. Liver disease is associated with the Z allele and particularly the homozygotes for Z (PiZZ).
   B. Approximately 10% of PiZZ individuals develop neonatal liver disease.
   C. Adults with PiZZ who did not suffer from overt neonatal disease have a 10% chance of developing cirrhosis.
   D. Identification of PiZZ homozygotes is important because replacement of A1AT is now possible and will prevent liver disease.
   E. Liver biopsy in individuals with a Z allele will show periodic acid–Schiff–positive, diastase-resistant globular deposits of the abnormal A1AT. Because this occurs in both homozygotes and heterozygotes, the presence of such globules on biopsy cannot be used to positively confirm etiology.

3. A 28-year-old white man presents because his father was diagnosed as having hereditary hemochromatosis. His father is a 54-year-old whose liver biopsy showed increased hepatic iron with a hepatic iron index of 5.5. His son feels well and has a normal physical examination. He takes no medications and has no significant medical history. His serum transaminases and liver biochemistries are normal. What is the most appropriate approach to decide whether the son has hemochromatosis?

   A. Do human leukocyte antigen (HLA) typing on father and son and look for identical alleles
   B. Measure iron, transferrin saturation, and ferritin level
   C. Obtain a computed tomography (CT) scan of the liver

   D. Obtain a magnetic resonance imaging (MRI) study of the liver
   E. Screening of any type is inappropriate because only homozygotes are affected and siblings are more commonly affected than the proband children

4. All of the following statements about chronic pancreatitis are true EXCEPT

   A. Alcohol is a common etiologic factor.
   B. Exocrine insufficiency with steatorrhea occurs early when lipase output has been reduced by less than 10%.
   C. Pancreatic calcification is an important diagnostic finding in chronic pancreatitis.
   D. Diabetes can occur as a result of islet cell damage.
   E. The pain associated with chronic pancreatitis is easily differentiated from the pain of acute pancreatitis.

5. Peptic ulcer disease has long been considered to be a chronic illness. Recent scientific discoveries have suggested a way to change the natural history of ulcer disease. To do this, one would

   A. Quit a stressful job
   B. Take chronic histamine-2 (H$_2$) blocker therapy
   C. Take intermittent H$_2$ blocker therapy
   D. Treat and eradicate *Helicobacter pylori*
   E. Avoid hot (spicy) foods

6. Patients with ileitis or ileal resection may develop diarrhea. Which statement *most* accurately reflects the pathophysiology underlying the symptoms?

   A. Bile acids may be deconjugated in an inflamed distal ileum, leading to maldigestion of fats and steatorrhea.
   B. Steatorrhea develops in patients whose distal ileum is inflamed because of malabsorption of fats by the ileal mucosa even in the presence of adequate bile acid levels.
   C. When bile acid absorption in the ileum is reduced as a result of regional ileitis, the elevated levels of bile acids in the colon will trigger steatorrhea.
   D. In cases of ileal resection, following which bile acids cannot be deconjugated in the ileum, the appearance of the conjugated bile acids in the stools accounts for a characteristic foamy appearance and light, buoyant density.

E. In relatively mild to moderate ileitis, the failure to recover bile salts by the receptor-mediated route may trigger a watery diarrhea, but steatorrhea is likely to develop only in more severe ileitis or after extensive resection.

7. The presence of fecal leukocytes in a sample of stool or rectal mucus is consistent with all of the following causes of diarrhea EXCEPT

A. *Campylobacter jejuni*
B. *Shigella sonnei*
C. *Giardia lamblia*
D. Ulcerative colitis
E. *Entamoeba histolytica*

8. All of the following are indications for cholecystectomy in a patient with gallstones EXCEPT

A. Vague abdominal discomfort, bloating, and flatulence
B. Biliary colic
C. Acute cholecystitis
D. Calcification of the gallbladder (porcelain gallbladder)
E. Acute pancreatitis without other obvious causes

9. In the evaluation of a jaundiced patient with a cholestatic biochemical pattern, various imaging studies may be useful. The choice of appropriate study depends on the urgency of the situation, the likelihood of extrahepatic obstruction, and local expertise and availability. All of the following studies are a useful part of our diagnostic armamentarium EXCEPT

A. Sonography
B. Hepatobiliary scintigraphy (HIDA, DISIDA, or PIPIDA scans)
C. CT
D. Endoscopic retrograde cholangiopancreatography (ERCP)
E. Percutaneous transhepatic cholangiography (PTC)

10. All of the following are risk factors for development of ulcer disease EXCEPT

A. Daily use of nonsteroidal anti-inflammatory drugs (NSAIDs)
B. Gastric infection with *H. pylori*
C. Severe emotional stress
D. Cigarette smoking
E. Gastrin-secreting tumors

11. All of the following are true statements regarding Crohn's disease EXCEPT

A. An increased prevalence is seen among Ashkenazi Jews.
B. Incidence has been rising steadily over the past 20 years.
C. Cigarette smoking is a risk factor for disease.
D. An autosomal recessive pattern of inheritance is seen.

12. The single feature that best distinguishes Crohn's disease from ulcerative colitis is

A. Presence of ileal disease
B. Rectal bleeding
C. Continuous colonic involvement on endoscopy

D. Noncaseating granulomas
E. Crypt abscesses

13. A 40-year-old white man presents with a 4-year history of dysphagia, weight loss, and nocturnal aspiration. An upper gastrointestinal (GI) series reveals a moderately dilated esophagus with a smooth, tapered distal "beak." All of the following are true statements regarding management of this disorder EXCEPT

A. Further evaluation with upper endoscopy is not indicated.
B. Long-term pharmacologic therapy is unlikely to be effective.
C. Pneumatic dilation is appropriate initial therapy.
D. Esophageal manometry is likely to reveal incomplete relaxation of the lower esophageal sphincter with swallowing and absent peristalsis.

14. Upper endoscopy is indicated in all of the following situations EXCEPT

A. A 62-year-old man with a nonhealing gastric ulcer on upper GI series after 6 weeks of acid suppressive therapy
B. A 26-year-old human immunodeficiency virus–positive woman with odynophagia
C. A 32-year-old man with newly diagnosed familial adenomatous polyposis
D. A 65-year-old woman with absent bowel sounds, rigid abdomen, rebound tenderness, and a history of peptic ulcer disease

15. Bilateral salivary gland enlargement and decrease in salivary secretion can occur with all of the following EXCEPT

A. Sjögren's syndrome
B. Sarcoidosis
C. Bacterial sialoadenitis
D. Mumps

16. All the following are true regarding arteriovenous malformations of the gastrointestinal tract EXCEPT

A. Can be diagnosed and treated during colonoscopy
B. Can be diagnosed with angiography
C. May require hemicolectomy for treatment
D. Are more common in the left colon than in the right colon

17. A 65-year-old white man with a history of dilated cardiomyopathy presents with a sudden onset of severe abdominal pain associated with passing of maroon-colored stool. Abdominal exam is nonspecific and reveals only very mild tenderness to deep palpation. Laboratory studies reveal an elevated white blood cell (WBC) count and abdominal radiographs of the abdomen reveal small bowel ileus with submucosal edema (thumbprinting). Which of the following is the next appropriate therapeutic/diagnostic procedure?

A. Colonoscopy
B. Upper endoscopy
C. Mesenteric angiography
D. Upper GI small bowel series
E. Indium scan

18. A 38-year-old white woman with an 18-year history of heavy alcohol use presents with nausea, vomiting, and epigastric pain radiating to the back worsened by eating.

Plain films of the abdomen revealed diffuse calcifications of the pancreas. Which of the following is indicated to confirm the diagnosis of pancreatitis?

    A. An abdominal CT scan
    B. ERCP
    C. Secretin tests with duodenal aspiration
    D. Stool trypsin concentration
    E. No further testing necessary

19. All of the following are potential complications of pancreatitis EXCEPT

    A. Ascites
    B. Pancreatic abscess
    C. Pancreatic pseudocyst
    D. Hypercalcemia
    E. Acute renal failure

20. Each of the following is considered a risk factor for gastric adenocarcinoma EXCEPT

    A. Peptic ulcer disease
    B. Adenomatous polyps of the stomach
    C. Dietary nitrosamines
    D. Common variable immunodeficiency
    E. Previous gastric surgery for peptic ulcer disease

21. A 69-year-old white woman presents with cramping lower abdominal pain of acute onset, accompanied by rectal bleeding, vomiting, and fever. Barium enema reveals a localized area of ''sawtooth'' irregularity in the colon. At colonoscopy, such lesions are most likely to be present at which one of the following?

    A. Splenic flexure
    B. Midtransverse colon
    C. Cecum
    D. Mid-descending colon
    E. Ascending colon

22. Which of the following common causes of bacterial food poisoning results in symptoms from the ingestion of food contaminated with preformed toxins?

    A. *Staphylococcus aureus*
    B. *Salmonella enteritidis*
    C. *Clostridium botulinum*
    D. *Listeria monocytogenes*
    E. A and C

23. All of the following influence the risk of cancer in adenomatous polyps EXCEPT

    A. Polyp location
    B. Polyp size
    C. Degree of dysplasia
    D. Histologic type (villous verse tubular)

24. All of the following polyposis syndromes have an autosomal dominant pattern of inheritance EXCEPT

    A. Familial adenomatous polyposis
    B. Hereditary nonpolyposis colorectal cancer syndrome (Lynch syndrome)
    C. Gardner's syndrome
    D. Juvenile polyposis
    E. All of the above

25. All of the following statements regarding anal fissures are true EXCEPT

    A. They present with painful defecation.
    B. They are most commonly located in the anterior midline.

    C. They may be a manifestation of Crohn's disease.
    D. They may be associated with a sentinel skin tag at the anal verge.

26. A 42-year-old white man comes to the emergency room with a history of passing black, tarry stools that day. He has no other medical problems and takes no medications. His blood pressure is 110/70 mm Hg, with a resting pulse of 92 beats per minute. Blood is drawn and sent for study. The next step should be

    A. Do an emergent upper endoscopy
    B. Transfuse with 2 units of packed red blood cells
    C. Determine his blood pressure and pulse in the sitting and standing positions
    D. Await the result of his hemoglobin and hematocrit before other action
    E. Order an emergency bleeding scan

27. A 60-year-old white man presents with left lower quadrant (LLQ) pain, loose stools, and fever. He has no significant past medical history. Physical exam reveals normal vital signs except for a temperature of 38.7°C and LLQ tenderness to palpation. There is guarding in the LLQ, but no definite mass can be palpated. Laboratory evaluation is normal except for a 15,000 WBC count. Plain abdomen and upright radiographs are normal. All of the following would be reasonable parts of an initial plan EXCEPT

    A. Empiric therapy with broad-spectrum antibiotics
    B. Surgical consultation
    C. Flexible sigmoidoscopy
    D. Barium enema
    E. CT scan

28. A 50-year-old white man is admitted because of jaundice and pruritus. Evaluation reveals biliary obstruction caused by a pancreatic mass. The mass is proven to be an adenocarcinoma by fine-needle aspiration. Because of multiple filling defects in the liver on CT scan, a palliative approach is taken and a stent placed endoscopically to relieve obstruction. One week after stent placement, he returns for follow-up. He feels well; his pruritus is gone, and his urine color is normal, but he continues to be jaundiced. Laboratory studies show

	Just Prior to Stent Placement	7 Days Later
Bilirubin	12.0 mg/dl	6.0 mg/dl
Alanine transaminase (ALT)	102	50
Asparatate transaminase (AST)	79	39
Serum alkaline phosphate	720 u/L	492 u/L
Urine bilirubin	Positive	Negative

Which is the most appropriate action?

    A. Obtain a sonogram to assess duct size
    B. Replacement of the stent, because it is probably clogged
    C. Establishment of drainage by a percutaneous transhepatic route
    D. Consideration of surgery to create a choledochoenterostomy
    E. Continued observation without therapeutic intervention at this time

DIRECTIONS: For questions 29 to 46, determine whether EACH choice is true or false. Any combination of answers, from all true to all false, may occur.

29. A 23-year-old male graduate student presents because of a recent discovery of an elevated bilirubin level. He feels well and has a normal physical examination. His chemistry profile is normal except for an elevated bilirubin level. Laboratory studies show a total bilirubin level of 2.6 mg per deciliter and a direct bilirubin level of 0.3 mg per deciliter. Which of the following statements is/are true?

A. The most common cause of these abnormalities is Gilbert's syndrome.
B. Chronic hemolysis could give a similar picture, so appropriate testing for hemolysis is indicated.
C. His urine will test positive for bilirubin.
D. The biochemical findings are also consistent with type I Crigler-Najjar syndrome.

30. A 20-year-old white woman presents to the emergency room with jaundice and malaise of 2 weeks' duration. She had noted dark urine for several days and was recently noted by a friend to have icteric sclera. Her boyfriend had some form of hepatitis several months before. The patient is on no medications and has no significant medical history. Her physical examination is normal except for scleral and cutaneous icterus; she is alert and oriented. Initial laboratory studies reveal the following results:

ALT	1206
AST	983
Alkaline phosphatase (normal <120 u/L)	183 u/L
Bilirubin	8.6 mg/dl
PT	12.2 sec
Hematocrit	39%
WBC count	8900/μL

Hepatitis serologies are pending. Which of the following statements is/are true?

A. Admission is required because of the danger of fulminant hepatic failure in this setting.
B. An imaging study (sonogram or CT) is indicated to rule out dilated intrahepatic ducts.
C. This is most likely acute viral hepatitis, and the patient can be safely discharged with outpatient follow-up pending serologic results.
D. Although not necessary, a liver biopsy would provide useful etiologic and prognostic information.

31. Which of the following statements is/are true about laboratory tests used to assess liver disease?

A. An elevation of ALT is generally more sensitive and more specific for liver injury than is an elevation of AST.
B. Acute biliary obstruction, as may occur during passage of a gallstone, can cause transient elevations of serum transaminase levels of 1000 IU or more.
C. Serum alkaline phosphatase activity increases can be attributed to a hepatobiliary origin if there is an elevation in serum levels of 5′-nucleotidase,

leucine aminopeptidase, or gamma-glutamyltranspeptidase (GGTP).
D. Although it is prudent to pursue the cause of an elevated alkaline phosphatase level, as many as one third of patients with isolated elevation of hepatobiliary alkaline phosphatase activity have no demonstrable liver or biliary disease.
E. GGTP is a sensitive and specific test for hepatobiliary disease.

32. A 45-year-old white woman with a long history of primary biliary cirrhosis (PBC) is admitted because of fever and abdominal pain. Previous evaluation includes several liver biopsies that documented the progression from stage I (florid duct lesion) to stage IV (cirrhosis with cholestasis). Her bilirubin level was 12 mg per deciliter on last determination. Physical examination reveals a thin, jaundiced, chronically ill–appearing woman; her temperature is 38.1°C pulse is 100 beats per minute, and blood pressure is 110/60 mm Hg. There is gross abdominal distention with bulging flanks and shifting dullness. There is trace pedal edema. Laboratory studies show

Bilirubin	13.6 mg/dl
Alkaline phosphatase	1256 u/L
Hemoglobin	12.2 g/dl
WBC count	14,500/μl
Platelet	98,000/μl
PT	16.2 sec
Serum albumin	2.8 g/dl

A sample of ascitic fluid shows

Albumin	0.9 g/dl
WBCs	650/μl
Polymorphonuclear leukocytes	90%
Mononuclear cells	10%
Gram's stain	No organisms seen

Which of the following statements is/are true?

A. A diagnostic paracentesis should be delayed until the PT is normalized either by parenteral vitamin K replacement or infusion of fresh frozen plasma.
B. The ascites is likely secondary to portal hypertension.
C. The cell count suggests spontaneous bacterial peritonitis and is an indication for empiric broad-spectrum antibiotics.
D. Paracentesis should only be done under sonographic guidance.
E. Once the infection is controlled, the patient should be evaluated for transplantation.

33. Which of the following statements is/are true concerning the eradication of *H. pylori*?

A. Most individuals with *H. pylori* who present with nonulcer dyspepsia have symptomatic cures when *H. pylori* is eradicated.

B. Infection cure predicts a markedly reduced rate of ulcer recurrence.
C. All patients with evidence of *H. pylori* infection should be treated to decrease their risk of developing gastric cancer.
D. Successful treatment can be documented by repeating serology in 4 to 6 weeks.
E. Appropriate antimicrobial therapy leads to eradication in greater than 80% of cases.

34. Which of the following is/are considered to be extraintestinal manifestations of inflammatory bowel disease?

A. Ankylosing spondylitis
B. Sclerosing cholangitis
C. Uveitis
D. Erythema nodosum
E. Large joint arthritis

35. Which of the following statements concerning ulcerative colitis is/are true?

A. Toxic megacolon may complicate severe ulcerative colitis.
B. Corticosteroids are useful as maintenance therapy after acute exacerbation of disease.
C. Proctocolectomy represents a cure.
D. The duration of disease and extent of colonic involvement influences long-term colon cancer risk.
E. Ulcerative colitis typically extends from the rectum in a continuous manner.

36. Which of the following statements regarding medical therapy of inflammatory bowel disease is/are true?

A. Topical mesalamine (enema) therapy is effective in treating distal proctocolitis.
B. Metronidazole is useful in inducing remission of active ulcerative colitis.
C. Elemental diets have therapeutic benefit in active Crohn's disease.
D. Corticosteroids should be discontinued in pregnant women with inflammatory bowel disease.
E. Therapy with sulfasalazine may be limited by allergy to the sulfa moiety.

37. Which of the following is/are risk factors for squamous cell cancer of the esophagus?

A. Tobacco
B. Lye ingestion
C. Achalasia
D. Alcohol
E. Squamous papilloma

38. Which of the following statements concerning Zenker's diverticula is/are true?

A. They are most commonly seen in the midesophagus.
B. They are classically seen in patients with scleroderma.
C. They may present with recurrent aspiration.
D. The patient is at increased risk of perforation during upper endoscopy.
E. They should never be treated surgically.

39. Which of the following is/are indications for colonoscopy?

A. A 28-year-old woman with a 3-year history of left-sided ulcerative colitis confirmed on flexible sigmoidoscopy last year, and asymptomatic on conservative medical therapy
B. A 45-year-old woman with guaiac-positive stools
C. A 60-year-old man with a single 1-cm sessile polyp in the descending colon found on screening sigmoidoscopy
D. A 70-year-old asymptomatic man 1 year after right hemicolectomy for colon cancer

40. Which of the following statements regarding flexible fiberoptic sigmoidoscopy is/are true?

A. It will detect at least 60% of colon cancers and polyps when used for screening.
B. It is an appropriate method for removing an isolated pedunculated sigmoid polyp.
C. It is indicated as a routine preoperative examination in patients undergoing elective abdominal surgery for noncolonic disease.
D. It is the method of choice for screening asymptomatic individuals at risk for colorectal carcinoma.

41. Which of the following is/are in the differential diagnosis of acute right lower quadrant pain?

A. Ectopic pregnancy
B. Ruptured ovarian cyst
C. *Yersinia* ileal colitis
D. Diverticulitis

42. Which of the following is/are true statements concerning radiation enterocolitis?

A. Injury usually develops when total dosage exceeds 5000 rads.
B. Stricture formation is a late complication.
C. Surgical resection should routinely be recommended.
D. Arteritis and mucosal ischemia may result from significant exposure levels.

43. A 63-year-old man with a history of diverticulosis presents with gradual onset of constant LLQ pain and fever. Fullness and tenderness is noted in the LLQ on exam. Laboratory studies reveal a marked leukocytosis with a left shift. Early appropriate diagnostic/therapeutic options include

A. Abdominal CT scan
B. Colonoscopy
C. Broad-spectrum intravenous antibiotics
D. Abdominal radiography

44. Which of the following statements is/are true about the relationship of *H. pylori* and superficial gastritis of the antrum?

A. Gastritis has been induced by self-administration of *H. pylori*.
B. *H. pylori* causes a similar syndrome in many animals.
C. *H. pylori* is present in virtually all patients with superficial gastritis.
D. The gastritis resolves once the infection is cured.
E. The epidemiologic patterns for the occurrence of *H. pylori* and superficial gastritis are identical.

45. Which of the following statements is/are true about the epidemiology of pancreatic cancer?

    A. Carcinoma of the pancreas is more common in men than women.

    B. Coffee consumption is a very strong risk factor in the development of pancreatic cancer.

    C. The incidence of pancreatic cancer has increased recently.

    D. The vast majority of pancreatic cancers are derived from the cells of the pancreatic duct.

    E. With new diagnostic tests, the 5-year survival rate of pancreatic cancer now approaches 50%.

46. A 24-year-old female graduate student is evaluated for abdominal pain. The pain is crampy and involves the lower abdomen. It is usually followed by passage of loose stools with pain relief. Her symptoms occur almost weekly. They seem to be worsened by anxiety or emotional stress. She is occasionally constipated. She tolerates milk and dairy products without difficulty. Her symptoms have been unchanged since college yet she has never seen a physician for these problems. Family history reveals that her 55-year-old uncle was recently diagnosed as having colon cancer. The patient is concerned she may have a serious illness. Her symptoms have not interfered with her usual activities. Physical exam is normal. Stool obtained on rectal is hemoccult-negative. A complete blood count sedimentation rate, and serum electrolyte analysis are normal. Stool tests for ova and parasites are negative. Which of the following is/are appropriated next steps?

    A. Flexible sigmoidoscopy

    B. Colonoscopy

    C. Treatment with a mild sedative/hypnotic

    D. Psychiatric consultation

    E. Gastroenterology consultation

DIRECTIONS: Questions 47 to 81 are matching questions. For each numbered item, choose the most likely associated lettered item from those provided. Each numbered item has ONLY ONE answer. Within each set of questions, each answer may be used once, more than once, or not at all.

QUESTIONS 47–53

Match each of the following statements with the type of hepatitis described.

  A. Hepatitis A
  B. Hepatitis B
  C. Hepatitis C
  D. Hepatitis D
  E. Hepatitis E

47. Although 50% of adults who develop acute disease will normalize their transaminase levels within 6 months, most of this group have evidence of continued viral replication despite the normal transaminase levels.

48. This virus is most readily transmitted by sexual contact.

49. This is an incomplete virus that requires the presence of another hepatitis virus to infect or replicate.

50. Prompt administration of immune serum globulin to appropriate contacts is effective in preventing infection.

51. Whereas 90 to 95% of adults who develop acute disease will clear the virus, 5 to 10% will develop chronic disease.

52. Acute disease is associated with a case fatality rate as high as 20% for pregnant women.

53. This virus is the most common cause of point-source epidemics in the United States; it never causes chronic disease.

QUESTIONS 54–59

For each of the following risk factors for gallstone formation, select the mechanism for this increased risk.

  A. Increased biliary secretion of cholesterol
  B. Bile salt deficiency
  C. Poor gallbladder emptying
  D. Chronic biliary infection and stasis
  E. Increased biliary secretion of unconjugated bilirubin

54. Obesity

55. Chronic hemolysis

56. Parenteral alimentation

57. Bile duct strictures

58. Female sex or estrogen use

59. Ileal inflammation or ileal resection

QUESTIONS 60–63

Match the following stool fluid electrolyte results with the most likely mechanism.

  A. Osmotic diarrhea caused by a nonmetabolizable substance (e.g., magnesium citrate)
  B. Osmotic diarrhea caused by a metabolizable substance (e.g., lactose malabsorption)
  C. Secretory diarrhea (e.g., cholera)
  D. Dilution of stool by added water

	Na^+ (mEq/L)	K^+ (mEq/L)	Stool Osmolarity (mOsm/kg H_2O)
60.	5	5	22
61.	90	35	280
62.	40	20	280
63.	40	20	500

QUESTIONS 64–68

Match the following effects with the associated compounds.

  A. Sulfasalasine
  B. Azathioprine
  C. Glucocorticosteroids
  D. Metronidazole
  E. Olsalasine (Dipentum)

64. Competitively inhibits intestinal folate absorption

65. Reversible sperm abnormalities

66. Peripheral neuropathy

67. Allergic pancreatitis

68. Secretory diarrhea

QUESTIONS 69–72

For each of the following patients, select the next most appropriate therapeutic or diagnostic step.

  A. Omeprazole 20 mg daily and esophageal dilation
  B. Surgical antireflux procedure
  C. Ambulatory 24-hour esophageal pH study
  D. Therapeutic trial of antireflux measures (elevation of head of bed, smoking cessation, avoidance of food or fluid prior to bedtime) and antacids after meals and at bedtime
  E. Acid infusion test (Bernstein)

69. A 32-year-old woman with daily heartburn after meals and when supine. No other symptoms are present.

70. A 50-year-old man with a long history of frequent heartburn treated intermittently with antacids. He now presents with solid food dysphagia; upper GI series and endoscopy reveal a short distal esophageal stricture without evidence of malignancy on biopsy.

71. A 45-year-old man with distal esophageal stricture requiring monthly dilation while on omeprazole therapy.

72. A 34-year-old man with an 18-month history of persistent reflux symptoms and evidence of esophagitis on endoscopy despite maximum medical therapy.

QUESTIONS 73–77

For each of the following clinical syndromes, select the most likely abnormality listed. (*Note:* use each answer only once.)

A. Transient cystic duct obstruction
B. Cystic duct obstruction
C. Common bile duct obstruction
D. Common bile duct obstruction with infection
E. Cholecystolithiasis

73. Acute cholecystitis

74. Obstructive jaundice

75. Cholangitis

76. No symptoms

77. Biliary pain or colic

QUESTIONS 78–81

For each condition, select the characteristic most closely associated with it.

A. Desmoid tumors and mandibular osteomas
B. Melanotic spots on the lips, buccal mucosa, and skin
C. Medulloblastoma
D. Fingernail dystrophy, alopecia, and cutaneous hyperpigmentation

78. Gardner's syndrome

79. Cronkhite-Canada syndrome

80. Peutz-Jeghers syndrome

81. Turcot's syndrome

GASTROINTESTINAL DISEASE

ANSWERS

1.(D) *Discussion:* Although there may be vitamin K depletion in cholestasis as a result of other factors, the prolongation of PT seen in severe acute hepatitis is secondary to insufficient hepatic synthesis of rapidly turning-over clotting factors. Severe disease is necessary to cause such a degree of insufficiency, and many patients with significant prolongation will proceed to acute liver failure with encephalopathy. (*Cecil, Ch. 117*)

2.(D) *Discussion:* Liver disease in A1AT deficiency is related to retention of the abnormal protein in the hepatocytes. This contrasts with the risk of pulmonary disease, which seems to be related to the enzyme activity. Those with the null mutation produce no A1AT have and a high rate of pulmonary disease but do not get liver disease. (*Cecil, Ch. 121*)

3.(B) *Discussion:* Liver disease only occurs in patients homozygous for the disorder. Because the son can get only one allele from his father, the only way he can be homozygous is if he gets a hemochromatosis gene from his mother. Because the gene frequency is 5 to 8%, this is certainly likely enough to recommend screening. The abnormal iron accumulation begins at birth and is cumulative. Normal iron studies at a young age do not necessarily rule out the disorder, and repeated measurements over time may be necessary. This is especially true of women, who accumulate iron at lower rates because of menstrual losses. HLA typing is useful in assessing the risk of disease in siblings; if the sibling shares both haplotypes with the proband, they probably also share the same hemochromatosis genes, because these are very closely linked. However, this screening method is not useful across generations. Although patients with full-blown hemochromatosis may have suggestive abnormalities on CT or MRI, these studies are neither sensitive nor specific. When abnormal screening iron studies are found, a liver biopsy with quantification of total hepatic iron is necessary to confirm the diagnosis. (*Cecil, Ch. 121; Edwards and Kushner*)

4.(B) *Discussion:* At least 70 to 80% of patients with chronic pancreatitis are chronic alcohol abusers. Malabsorption is a late finding and occurs when pancreatic secretion of enzymes is decreased by 90% or more. Approximately 30% of patients with chronic pancreatitis will have diffuse or focal pancreatitis calcification; although not sensitive for the disease, it is quite specific. Diabetes will occur in about 70% of patients as a result of progressive loss of islets; half will require insulin. Chronic pancreatitis presents with initial episodes that are indistinguishable from acute pancreatitis in approximately 40% of patients. Another 40% will have an insidious onset of pain, with the remainder presenting with complications. (*Cecil, Ch. 107; Sleisenger & Fordtran, Ch. 81*)

5.(D) *Discussion:* There is no good evidence to link emotional stress or spicy foods with peptic ulcer disease. Chronic H_2-receptor antagonists can decrease ulcer recurrence as long as they are taken regularly; once stopped, relapse is common. Neither chronic nor intermittent H_2-receptor antagonist use changes the natural history. Eradication of *H. pylori* dramatically decreases the relapse rate. (*Cecil, Ch. 99; NIH Consensus Statement*)

6.(E) *Discussion:* Bile salts are necessary for normal fat absorption. Deconjugated bile salts can be absorbed passively in the small intestine. The absorption of conjugated bile salts occurs by a receptor-mediated route in the ileum. Ileal loss or damage can lead to malabsorption of bile salts. If the length of diseased or resected ileum is great enough (usually <100 cm), the liver is not able to compensate by increased bile salt synthesis and malabsorption occurs. With smaller resection or less extensive disease, the liver can compensate and prevent malabsorption. However, unabsorbed bile salts have a secretory effect on the colonic mucosa. Cholestyramine is effective therapy. (*Cecil, Ch. 102*)

7.(C) *Discussion:* The presence of large numbers of WBCs in stool is diagnostic of inflammation and should suggest infection with *Shigella, E. histolytica, Salmonella, Campylobacter,* invasive *Escherichia coli,* or *Neisseria gonorrhoeae.* Those organisms that cause diarrhea by a noninvasive mechanism are not associated with pus in the stool. Pus is usually abundant in active ulcerative colitis. (*Cecil, Ch. 102*)

8.(A) *Discussion:* In general, asymptomatic gallstones are not an indication for surgery. Studies have shown no difference in the frequency of symptoms such as vague abdominal pain, bloating, and flatulence between patients with and without gallstones. One attack of biliary colic usually portends future colic in most patients. Although the risk of gallbladder cancer, which is uncommon but seems to occur only in those with gallstones, is not great enough to warrant cholecystectomy in all patients with gallstones, the risk is great enough in the setting of a calcified gallbladder to recommend surgery. Pancreatitis caused by gallstones seems to be related to passage of a stone through the papilla of Vater. When the pancreatitis has resolved, a cholecystectomy is indicated to prevent future attacks. If the pancreatitis is progressive or slow to resolve, it may be necessary to rule out persistent obstruction. (*Cecil, Ch. 126; Johnston and Kaplan; Ransohoff and Gracie*)

9.(B) *Discussion:* A patient with obvious viral hepatitis does not benefit from any imaging study. In general, sonography is the preferred modality because it is inexpensive and noninvasive. It may be difficult in the presence of bowel gas or obesity. It is also somewhat dependent on the skill of the examiner. CT may be preferred if there is a high suspicion of malignancy because it will give additional information. Neither modality can identify all patients with extrahepatic obstruction. If the likelihood of extrahepatic obstruction is considered strong on solely clinical grounds, direct cholangiography may be the appropriate first choice. The choice between ERCP and PTC depends to some extent on local expertise as well as level of obstruction expected and other factors. (*Cecil, Ch. 113 and 126*)

10.(C) *Discussion:* Daily NSAID use significantly increases the risk of ulcer disease (risk ratio, 10- to 20-fold). Gastric infection with *H. pylori* increases risk about five- to sevenfold. Cigarette smoking doubles the risk. It is difficult to be precise about the relative risk of ulcer in Zollinger-Ellison syndrome because discovery of an ulcer is usually the reason to measure gastrin. At least 90% of those with Zollinger-Ellison syndrome have gastric or duodenal ulcer. (*Cecil, Ch. 99.2 and 99.6*)

11.(D) *Discussion:* Approximately 20% of patients with Crohn's disease have similarly affected relatives. However, no clear genetic pattern of inheritance has been defined. (*Cecil, Ch. 104*)

12.(D) *Discussion:* "Backwash ileitis" can occur in ulcerative colitis. Rectal bleeding and continuous involvement of the colon may be seen in both Crohn's disease and ulcerative colitis. The presence of crypt abscesses does not distinguish ulcerative colitis from Crohn's disease; however, noncaseating granulomas, when present, are pathognomonic of Crohn's disease. (*Cecil, Ch. 104*)

13.(A) *Discussion:* Infiltrating carcinoma of the gastroesophageal junction (pseudoachalasia) may present with radiographic findings similar to those of achalasia; therefore, endoscopy with retroflex examination of the gastric cardia is indicated. Achalasia is best treated with mechanical disruption of the lower esophageal sphincter. Long-term pharmacologic therapy is generally not helpful. Characteristic manometric findings in achalasia include incomplete relaxation of the lower esophageal sphincter with swallowing and absent peristalsis. (*Cecil, Ch. 97*)

14.(D) *Discussion:* Esophagogastroduodenoscopy should be performed on all patients with nonhealing gastric ulcers to rule out malignancy. Upper endoscopy is useful in the diagnosis of infectious esophagitis, which often presents as odynophagia in immunocompromised individuals. Patients with familial adenomatous polyposis should be screened every 1 to 3 years with upper endoscopy to rule out concurrent gastroduodenal adenomas. Suspected or known perforation is a contraindication to upper endoscopy. (*Cecil, Ch. 94 and 97; Rustgi*)

15.(C) *Discussion:* Bilateral salivary gland enlargement with decreased salivary secretion is commonly caused by infection with the mumps virus in children. Sjögren's syndrome is characterized by decreased salivary secretion and the gradual development of bilateral firm and nontender salivary glands in approximately one third of patients. Other causes of bilateral salivary gland enlargement include chronic granulomous diseases such as sarcoidosis and lep-rosy. Bacterial sialoadenitis most commonly presents as a unilateral enlargement of a major salivary gland, which is tender to palpation and may have a purulent exudate expressible from the duct. (*Cecil, Ch. 96*)

16.(D) *Discussion:* Arteriovenous malformations of the gastrointestinal tract may occur as solitary lesions or they may be multiple. Arteriovenous malformations can be successfully diagnosed with angiography or colonoscopy and can be treated during colonoscopy with laser therapy or heater probe. They are most frequently located in the cecum, and occasionally a right hemicolectomy may be required for definitive treatment. (*Cecil, Ch. 105*)

17.(C) *Discussion:* Acute onset of severe abdominal pain out of proportion to physical findings associated with gastrointestinal bleeding in an elderly patient with heart disease should suggest the diagnosis of acute mesenteric ischemia. Early use of mesenteric angiography is critical for diagnosis and therapy. Failure to diagnose this disorder before intestinal infarction occurs is associated with a mortality rate of 70 to 90%. The intra-arterial use of papavarin during mesenteric angiography may be helpful in both occlusive and nonocclusive mesenteric ischemia. (*Cecil, Ch. 105*)

18.(E) *Discussion:* Diagnosis of chronic pancreatitis requires positive documentation of two of the following: symptoms, abnormal test for pancreatic functions, and radiologic studies. The presence of pancreatic calcification in a patient with epigastric pain radiating to the back worsened by eating is sufficient for the diagnosis of chronic pancreatitis. (*Cecil, Ch. 107*)

19.(D) *Discussion:* Local complications of pancreatitis may include pseudocyst formation, pancreatic abscess, hemorrhage, and pancreatic ascites. Acute renal failure may be caused by circulatory shock and an elevation in renal vascular resistance. Hypocalcemia occurs in up to 30% of patients from a combination of hypoalbuminemia and calcium precipitation in areas of fat necrosis. (*Cecil, Ch. 107*)

20.(A) *Discussion:* Dietary nitrosamines are powerful carcinogens in animal studies and are thought to be important as a cause of gastric cancer. Adenomatous polyps are rare; however, they occasionally give rise to carcinoma. Subtotal gastric resection for benign peptic ulcer disease may result in a chronic atrophic gastritis, which is a long-term risk factor for gastric cancer. Immunologic deficiencies may predispose to gastric cancer. Peptic ulcer disease is not a risk factor for gastric cancer, although gastric adenocarcinoma may present as a gastric ulcer. (*Cecil, Ch. 100*)

21.(D) *Discussion:* The splenic flexure is one of the "watershed" areas of the colon between two adjacent arterial supplies where ischemia is more likely to develop. (*Cecil, Ch. 105*)

22.(E) *Discussion:* Staphylococcal food poisoning and food-borne botulism is caused by ingestion of food containing bacterial-produced toxins. *Salmonella enteritidis* and *Listeria monocytogenes* produce symptoms from ingestion of bacteria and proliferation in the intestine. (*Cecil, Ch. 109*)

23.(A) *Discussion:* Size, histologic type, and epithelial dysplasia are all important factors in the transformation of adenomatous polyps to carcinomas. Colonic location of polyps does not appear to influence the risk of cancer. (*Cecil, Ch. 106*)

24.(E) *Discussion:* Familial adenomatous polyposis, Gardner's syndrome, Peutz-Jeghers syndrome, and juvenile polyposis are all believed to be inherited in an autosomal dominant pattern. (*Cecil, Ch. 106*)

25.(B) *Discussion:* Anal fissures are located in the posterior midline in over 90% of cases as a result of straining at stool or passing a hard stool. The presence of an anal fissure off the midline should alert one to the possibility of Crohn's disease, sexually transmitted disease, or anal cancer. (*Cecil, Ch. 110*)

26.(C) *Discussion:* In upper gastrointestinal tract bleeding, immediate resuscitation is the first goal, with specific diagnosis postponed until it is safe. In acute bleeding, the hemoglobin may not reflect the degree of volume loss. The presence of shock indicates an acute blood volume loss of at least 15 to 20%. Postural decreases in blood pressure indicate an acute loss of 10 to 15%. The decision whether to transfuse immediately is made after assessing the degree of volume loss, presence of anemia, and whether bleeding continues or has stopped. Although not foolproof, passage of a nasogastric tube with aspiration of gastric contents can provide information as to the site (upper versus lower) and severity of the bleeding. (*Cecil, Ch. 95*)

27.(C) *Discussion:* Endoscopy is contraindicated in the presence of diverticulitis because of the possibility of perforation. If studies raise the possibility of colon cancer or inflammatory bowel disease, endoscopy may be appropriate later. Because of the theoretical risk of perforation, an abdominal CT scan has become the imaging test of choice. Barium enema can be complementary because CT is not 100% sensitive or specific. (*Cecil, Ch. 112*)

28.(E) *Discussion:* Chronic obstruction (or hepatitis) can lead to a substantial amount of bilirubin becoming bound to albumin. This tightly bound bilirubin is cleared slowly, with a half-life similar to that of albumin—17 days. Because it is tightly bound to albumin, bilirubin is not filtered at the glomerulus and does not appear in the urine. Because such protein-bound bilirubin can account for varying amounts of the total bilirubin (8 to 90%), a slow resolution of hyperbilirubinemia alone does not imply stent failure. In this patient, because the bilirubinuria has cleared and all other parameters of cholestasis are improving, no further intervention is necessary. (*Cecil, Ch. 115; Zakim and Boyer, Ch. 11*)

29.(A—True; B—True; C—False; D—False) *Discussion:* Gilbert's syndrome is very common (occurs in up to 7% of the population). Thus it is the most common cause of isolated elevation of unconjugated bilirubin. Chronic hemolysis can also present with hyperbilirubinemia resulting from increased production of bilirubin. Because unconjugated bilirubin is very poorly soluble in water, it circulates tightly bound to albumin, is not filtered by the glomeruli, and does not appear in the urine. Type I Crigler-Najjar syndrome is an almost uniformly lethal, nearly complete inability to conjugate bilirubin. It presents in neonates with very high levels of bilirubin. (*Cecil, Ch. 115; Berk and Noyer*)

30.(A—False; B—False; C—True; D—False) *Discussion:* With a normal PT, fulminant hepatic failure is unlikely to develop. As long as the patient can maintain hydration, discharge is appropriate and safe. The presentation is very suggestive of acute viral hepatitis. Because the chance of biliary obstruction is very low, an imaging study is not necessary. If hepatitis serologies are negative (hepatitis C antibody can take weeks to develop, so negative serology does not rule out hepatitis C) and the patient is not improving, an imaging study might be appropriate at a later date. Although the histologic pattern is slightly different among viral etiologies, it is not enough to allow confident etiologic diagnosis by histology. Serologic studies are more definitive, safer, and less costly. In addition, the biopsy does *not* provide any useful prognostic data in acute viral hepatitis. Liver biopsy is rarely indicated in acute hepatitis. (*Cecil, Ch. 117*)

31.(A—True; B—True; C—True; D—True; E—False) *Discussion:* AST is commonly elevated in diseases of skeletal or cardiac muscle, whereas ALT is not. Most patients with hepatic necrosis will have higher levels of ALT than AST. A notable exception is alcoholic liver disease, in which AST routinely exceeds ALT. This seems to reflect a change in the intracellular concentration of these enzymes because acute necrosis of some other etiology in an alcoholic (e.g., acetaminophen toxicity) results in very high levels of serum transaminase but with the same relative ratio (i.e., AST ≫ ALT). Whereas the biochemical pattern seen in chronic obstruction is dominated by elevation of the alkaline phosphatase level with mild elevation of transaminases, acute obstruction can cause transient increases to greater than 1000 IU. Because bone disease is associated with elevation in the alkaline phosphatase measurement, other enzymes are useful to confirm a hepatobiliary source. Although measurement of the hepatic isoenzyme is possible, it is usually more practical to rely on measurement of these other enzymes. Although an elevated alkaline phosphatase level may be the only clue to bile duct pathology or infiltrative disease (such as primary or metastatic cancer, lymphoma, leukemia or sarcoidosis), it does not always imply liver or biliary disease. The GGTP level usually parallels that of the alkaline phosphatase. However, it can be increased by the ingestion of ethanol or other inducers of the microsomal enzymes (e.g., phenobarbital) in the absence of liver disease. It is also increased after myocardial infarction, in neuromuscular diseases, in pancreatic disease, and in diabetes. (*Cecil, Ch. 113 and 116*)

32.(A—False; B—True; C—True; D—False; E—True) *Discussion:* When there is a large amount of ascites, diagnostic sampling is usually safe without sonography. Use of a small-bore needle to sample enough fluid for diagnostic purposes is safe even with an elevated PT. Delay in order to correct the PT is not indicated if there is a suspicion of PBC. The serum-ascites albumin gradient is 1.9, which makes the ascites likely secondary to portal hypertension. An ascites polymorphine nuclear leukocyte count of >250 per cubic millimeter is enough for a presumptive diagnosis of PBC. Therapy should cover gram-negative and gram-positive bacteria. A third-generation cephalosporin is a good empiric choice. It is important to assess response by resampling of ascites. Because PBC is recurrent and has a

2-year survival of less than 50%, referral for transplantation is indicated. Because a bilirubin level of >10 mg per deciliter in PBC also portends a poor prognosis, this referral should be urgent. (*Cecil, Ch. 115 and 126*)

33.(A—False; B—True; C—False; D—False; E—True) *Discussion:* Most patients with *H. pylori* superficial gastritis are asymptomatic. Nonulcer dyspepsia seems to be related to abnormalities of visceral sensation. Although treatment to eradicate *H. pylori* is a reasonable option in those who do not respond to other management, infection cure does not eliminate symptoms in most patients. In those with duodenal ulcer in whom *H. pylori* is eradicated, the recurrence rate was 2% at 12 months as opposed to 85% in those in whom *H. pylori* persisted. There is epidemiologic evidence to associate *H. pylori* infection with gastric adenocarcinoma of the body and antrum. However, gastric cancer occurs in individuals with no evidence of *H. pylori* infection. In the United States, fewer than 1% of *H. pylori*–infected individuals develop gastric cancer. The effect of treatment of *H. pylori* infection on gastric cancer risk has not been studied adequately. As of February, 1994, the NIH Consensus Statement recommends treatment of those patients with gastric or duodenal ulcer. Antibody levels decrease slowly following successful eradication. A dramatic fall 6 to 12 months following treatment indicates successful eradication. Breath testing is the best noninvasive test at documenting successful eradication; however, it is not routinely indicated. The issue of which antimicrobial regimen is best is still unclear. The best results have occurred with triple therapy—bismuth subsalicylate, tetracycline, and metronidazole for 2 weeks. Antimicrobial therapy is usually combined with antisecretory therapy; acid-pump inhibitors seem superior to H_2-receptor antagonists. The concern about patient compliance with a four-drug regimen requiring four doses per day has led to multiple trials of various two-drug regimens. The most popular have used twice-a-day omeprazole with high doses of amoxicillin or clarithromycin. Not all studies have documented success rates greater than 80% with these regimens. It is to be expected that current research will soon clarify this important point. (*Cecil, Ch. 98, 99, and 100; NIH Consensus Statement; Walsh and Peterson*)

34.(All are True) *Discussion:* All are disorders associated with inflammatory bowel disease. Large joint arthritis and erythema nodosum generally coincide with active bowel disease and will respond to treatment of intestinal inflammation. Uveitis and ankylosing spondylitis are associated with the HLA-B27 haplotype, and may run a course independent of the activity of bowel disease. Sclerosing cholangitis is more frequently associated with ulcerative colitis than Crohn's disease, and its progression is not affected by treatment of intestinal inflammation, including colectomy. (*Cecil, Ch. 104; Shrumpf et al*)

35.(A—True; B—False; C—True; D—True; E—True) *Discussion:* Corticosteroids are effective in controlling active disease and inducing remission; however, they have not been shown to prevent relapse in ulcerative colitis or Crohn's disease and have significant long-term side effects. Ulcerative colitis but not Crohn's disease is cured by proctocolectomy; pancolitis represents a greater risk for colon cancer than left-sided disease. Cancer risk increases with increasing duration of disease as well. (*Cecil, Ch. 104; Podolsky*)

36.(A—True; B—False; C—True; D—False; E—True) *Discussion:* Mesalamine and corticosteroid enemas are effective in treating active proctocolitis. Metronidazole may successfully induce remission of active Crohn's disease, especially with parenteral involvement, but is not helpful in ulcerative colitis. Active Crohn's disease responds favorably to elemental diets as well as to parenteral nutrition. Pregnant women with active inflammatory bowel disease may be safely treated with corticosteroids and/or sulfasalazine. Sulfasalazine is cleaved by colonic bacteria to its active moiety, 5-aminosalicylic acid, and a sulfa moiety, which may cause allergic reactions in patients with sulfa sensitivity. (*Cecil, Ch. 104*)

37.(A—True; B—True; C—True; D—True; E—False) *Discussion:* Squamous papilloma of the esophagus are papillary structures lined by normal squamous epithelium and do not have malignant potential. (*Cecil, Ch. 97; Sleisenger and Fordtran*)

38.(A—False; B—False; C—True; D—True; E—False) *Discussion:* Zenker's diverticula occur above the upper esophageal sphincter at the level of the pharynx and may present with recurrent aspiration of undigested food particles hours after eating. Scleroderma is generally associated with multiple wide-mouth diverticula throughout the length of the esophagus. When large enough to be clinically problematic, Zenker's diverticula are effectively treated with a diverticulectomy and cricopharyngeal section. (*Cecil, Ch. 97*)

39.(A—False; B—True; C—True; D—True) *Discussion:* Endoscopic screening for dysplasia should begin after 7 years of extensive colitis. Left-sided disease may have a lower risk for carcinoma, and later initiation of surveillance colonoscopy (after 12 to 15 years of disease) may be reasonable. Guaiac-positive stools, screening for synchronous polyps in patients in whom a polyp has been found on sigmoidoscopy, and 1-year follow-up after colorectal cancer resection are all appropriate indications for colonoscopy. (*Cecil, Ch. 94 and 104; Levin et al*)

40.(A—True; B—False; C—False; D—True) *Discussion:* Flexible fiberoptic sigmoidoscopy is indicated for screening asymptomatic patients at risk for colorectal neoplasm, in the evaluation of suspected distal colonic disease in patients having no indication for colonoscopy, and to complete the examination of the colon in patients having barium enema. Sixty per cent of colorectal cancers and polyps occur in the distal 60 cm of the colon reached by flexible fiberoptic sigmoidoscopy. Polypectomy should not be performed during sigmoidoscopy because inadequate preparation of the colon presents a risk of explosion during electrocautery; thus one should proceed with colonoscopy to rule out synchronous polyps or cancer. (*Cecil, Ch. 106*)

41.(All are True) *Discussion:* Pelvic or gynecologic disorders should be considered with all female patients with acute right lower quadrant pain. Ruptured ovarian cysts generally occur at midcycle and are not accompanied by fever.

Yersinia infection generally involves the ileum and may present as right lower quadrant pain. Diverticula are generally left sided but may present with right lower quadrant pain in the setting of cecal diverticulitis. (*Cecil, Ch. 112*)

42.(A—True; B—True; C—False; D—True) *Discussion:* At higher doses of radiation (>5000 rads), submucosal damage and arteritis may result in late complications, including stricture formation and bleeding from diffuse vascular ectasias. Such patients are at an increased risk of operative resection because of damage to adjacent bowel segments leading to problems with reanastomosis of the bowel. As a result, patients should be referred to surgery only when more conservative measures have failed. (*Cecil, Ch. 112*)

43.(A—True; B—False; C—True; D—True) *Discussion:* Diverticulitis typically presents as fever and constant LLQ pain in older patients. Abdominal CT is the test of choice and may reveal thickened colonic wall or abscess formation. Abdominal radiographs are helpful in excluding perforation and other potential etiologies such as ischemic colitis. Colonoscopy is contraindicated in the setting of acute diverticulitis because of the risk of perforation. Intravenous antibiotic therapy is appropriate for moderate to severe disease, while mild disease may be managed with oral antibiotics on an outpatient basis. (*Cecil, Ch. 112*)

44.(A—True; B—False; C—True; D—True; E—True) *Discussion:* Both self-administration of and accidental infection with *H. pylori* have caused gastritis. No reservoir other than human gastric mucosa has been identified. (*Cecil, Ch. 98; Marshall et al*)

45.(A—True; B—False; C—True; D—True; E—False) *Discussion:* The male/female sex ratio is 2:1 in most studies of pancreatic cancer. Whereas early epidemiologic studies showed an association, multiple recent studies have shown no association between pancreatic cancer and coffee consumption. The incidence of pancreatic cancer has increased recently, the reasons for this increase are not clear. Ninety per cent are adenocarcinomas of ductal origin and 5% are of islet cell origin. The 5-year survival is under 2%. Although new diagnostic tests are available, they have not yet been proven to be breakthroughs in the early diagnosis of pancreatic cancer. (*Cecil, Ch. 108; Warshaw and Fernandez–Del Castillo*)

46.(A—True; B—False; C—False; D—False; E—False) *Discussion:* This patient has irritable bowel syndrome (IBS). Her symptoms are mild and have not interfered with her daily routine. She has not sought medical attention for years and is now prompted to seek evaluation because of fear of colon cancer. It is possible to make a tentative positive diagnosis of IBS and do limited diagnostic testing tailored to individual patients. A flexible sigmoidoscopy is usually indicated, whereas a colonoscopy is not. Once her fear of colon cancer has been addressed by the results of the flexible sigmoidoscopy and by reassurance that her symptoms do not suggest a serious problem, she may return to her previous well-compensated state. Pharmacologic therapy should be reserved for a limited trial in patients with intractable symptoms. It is best tailored to the specific symptom, constipation or diarrhea. Mild IBS is best treated by a primary care physician who will develop a therapeutic relationship with the patient. Consultants should be reserved for confirmation in difficult cases or for intractable cases. (*Cecil, Ch. 101; Drossman and Thompson; Camilleri and Prather*)

47.(C); 48.(B); 48.(D); 50.(A); 51.(B); 52.(E); 53.(A) *Discussion:* Observation of patients with post-transfusion non-A, non-B hepatitis show that 50 to 60% have elevated transaminase levels for over 12 months. It is clear that the vast majority of such cases are due to hepatitis C. Now that we have tests to measure hepatitis C virus (hepatitis C RNA by polymerase chain reaction or branched-chain DNA assay), it is clear that at least half of those patients with persistently normal transaminases have hepatitis C virus RNA and are "chronic carriers." Hepatitis A and E are fecal-orally transmitted, with hepatitis A having a 2- to 7-day period of viremia with the potential for needle stick or blood-borne transmission. Hepatitis C can be passed by sexual contact but at a much lower rate than hepatitis B. Hepatitis D is always passed with hepatitis B and only can establish infection when hepatitis B infection occurs. If immune serum globulin is given to individuals exposed to hepatitis A, it can prevent or modify infection. It should be given as soon as possible, preferably within 2 to 3 days, but can be effective as long as 2 weeks after exposure. In some instances, no clinical illness develops but patients develop long-term immunity, suggesting a primary immunization or modified infection. Anywhere from 2 to 10% of otherwise healthy adults infected with hepatitis B become chronically infected; hepatitis B surface antigen persists for longer than 6 months. Among Americans and Europeans, the spontaneous clearance rate of these chronic carriers is 1 to 2% per year. The rate of initial clearance is lower in younger individuals, with greater than 90% of those infected neonatally becoming chronic carriers. Hepatitis E is associated with a case fatality rate of approximately 1 to 2%. In pregnant females this rate is as high as 20% and is highest for those infected in the third trimester. The reason for this is unknown. Hepatitis A accounts for essentially all water-borne, point-source, or institutional epidemics in the United States and Europe. In India, Central Asia, Pakistan, China, Southeast Asia, North Africa, the former Soviet Union, and Mexico, hepatitis E has caused large epidemics of water-borne hepatitis. Although cases have been reported among travelers returning to the United States from endemic areas, there are as yet no endogenous cases of hepatitis E. (*Cecil, Ch. 117; Tong et al*)

54.(A); 55.(E); 56.(C); 57.(D); 58.(A); 59.(B) *Discussion:* Multiple factors interplay to predispose to cholesterol and pigment gallstones. Obesity and estrogen are associated with increased levels of biliary cholesterol secretion. Crohn's disease is associated with an increased risk of cholesterol gallstones because of bile salt deficiency caused by increased fecal loss. Although these mechanisms lead to supersaturation of bile with cholesterol, this is not sufficient for formation of cholesterol gallstones. One of the best understood risks are conditions associated with defective gallbladder emptying. This occurs in parenteral alimentation, very-low-fat weight reduction diets, and pregnancy, wherein progesterone impairs emptying (as well as lower esophageal sphincter function) and estrogen increases biliary cholesterol. Hemolytic conditions cause increased biliary secretion of unconjugated bilirubin and result in the precipitation of calcium bilirubinate. These are black pigment stones and are typically radiopaque. Brown pigment stones contain calcium bilirubinate as well as calcium soaps of fatty acids and usually form in bile ducts as a result of infection and stasis, which leads to deconjugation of bilirubin in the biliary system. (*Cecil, Ch. 115 and 126*)

60.(D); 61.(C); 62.(A); 63.(B) *Discussion:* Because the gastrointestinal tract does not have a diluting mechanism, the osmolarity of fecal fluid is never less than the osmolarity of plasma. A very low stool osmolarity in a patient with "diarrhea" suggest an addition of water to simulate diarrhea (question 60). In question 61 there is no osmotic gap and this, in association with excess stool volumes >1 liter, suggests a secretory diarrhea. In question 62, there is a significant osmotic gap with normal measured stool osmolarity, but stool osmolarity is higher than plasma. This can be a result of bacterial metabolism of larger carbohydrates into smaller molecules, with resultant higher osmotic activity. In question 63, stool osmolarity was equal to plasma at the time of elimination. This metabolism occur in the collection container before measurement of stool osmolarity. (*Cecil, Ch. 102 and 103; Eherer and Fordtran*)

64.(A); 65.(A); 66.(D); 67.(B); 68.(E) *Discussion:* Long-term sulfasalazine therapy may result in folate deficiency as a result of competitive inhibition of intestinal folate absorption. Supplementation with folic acid (1 mg daily) is indicated in such patients. The sulfapyridine moiety of sulfasalazine is thought to be responsible for the reversible oligospermia and abnormal sperm morphology seen in men taking this medication. Peripheral neuropathy is frequently seen in patients on metronidazole for prolonged periods or at higher doses (>1 gram daily). Allergic pancreatitis is seen in up to 15% of patients on azathioprine. A toxic pancreatitis is rarely seen with sulfasalazine therapy. Olsalazine use may be limited by worsening diarrhea in 6% of patients as a result of increased intestinal secretion. (*Cecil, Ch. 104; Das*)

69.(D); 70.(A); 71.(B); 72.(B) *Discussion:* Gastroesophageal reflux is a common disorder that frequently presents with epigastric substernal discomfort after meals or when supine. When no other symptoms or systemic signs of illness are present, conservative antireflux measures, as well as antacids or standard-dose H_2 blockers, are indicated. Benign peptic strictures may be treated with dilation with good symptomatic relief. Concurrent use of H_2 blockers or omeprazole may reduce the need for repeat dilations. Strictures requiring frequent repeat dilations (every few weeks), as well as patients with intractable symptoms despite at least 6 months of maximum medical therapy, are candidates for antireflux surgery. (*Cecil, Ch. 97; Sontag*)

73.(B); 74.(C); 75.(D); 76.(E); 77.(A) *Discussion:* Obstruction caused by a stone is the primary cause of all manifestations of gallstone disease. The mere presence of stones in the gallbladder does not cause symptoms, and between 60 and 80 per cent of patients with gallstones are asymptomatic. When there is transient cystic duct obstruction, biliary pain results. If the obstruction is persistent, chemical inflammation occurs and acute cholecystitis results. Early in the course of acute cholecystitis, the bile is sterile, so bacterial infection does not play a primary role. When a stone obstructs the common bile duct, jaundice will result; as with acute cholecystitis, the bile is initially sterile. When bacterial infection occurs, cholangitis results. Since the infected bile may be under high pressure, purulent cholangitis, with severe sepsis, may complicate cholangitis (*Cecil, Ch. 126*)

78.(A); 79.(D); 80.(B); 81.(C) *Discussion:* Gardner's syndrome differs from familial adenomatous polyposis by the presence of benign extraintestinal growths, including osteomas and desmoid tumors, in Gardner's syndrome. Peutz-Jeghers syndrome is characterized by melanotic spots on the lips, buccal mucosa, and skin as well as multiple hamartomatous polyps throughout the gastrointestinal tract. Turcot's syndrome is defined as the presence of hereditary adenomatous polyposis and tumors of the central nervous system. Cronkhite-Canada syndrome is characterized by diffuse gastrointestinal polyposis associated with alopecia, dystrophy of the fingernails, and cutaneous hyperpigmentation. (*Cecil, Ch. 106*)

BIBLIOGRAPHY

Bennett JC, Plum F (eds): Cecil Textbook of Medicine. 20th ed. Philadelphia, WB Saunders Company, 1996.

Berk PD, Noyer C: Bilirubin metabolism and hereditary hyperbilirubinemias 6: Familial unconjugated hyperbilirubinemias. Semin Liver Dis 14:356, 1994.

Camilleri M, Prather CM: The irritable bowel syndrome: Mechanisms and a practical approach to management. Ann Intern Med 116:1001, 1992.

Das KM: Sulfasalazine therapy in inflammatory bowel disease. Gastroenterol Clin North Am 18:35, 1989.

Drossman DA, Thompson WG: The irritable bowel syndrome: Review and a graduated multicomponent treatment approach. Ann Intern Med 116:1009, 1992.

Edwards CQ, Kushner JP: Screening for hemochromatosis. N Engl J Med 328:1616, 1993.

Eherer AJ, Fordtran JS: Fecal osmotic gap and pH in experimental diarrhea of various causes. Gastroenterology 103:545, 1992.

Helicobacter pylori in peptic ulcer disease. NIH Consens Statement FEB 7–9:12(1) 1–22, 1994.

Johnston DE, Kaplan MM: Pathogenesis and treatment of gallstones. N Engl J Med 328:412, 1993.

Levin B, Lennard-Jones J, Riddell RH, et al: Surveillance of patients with chronic ulcerative colitis. Bull WHO 69:121–126, 1991.

Marshall BJ, Armstrong JA, McGechie DB, et al: Attempt to fulfill Koch's postulate for *Campylobacter pylori*. Med J Aust 142:436, 1985.

Podolsky D: Inflammatory bowel disease. N Engl J Med 325:928–937, 1008–1016, 1991.

Ransohoff DF, Gracie WA: Treatment of gallstones. Ann Intern Med 119:608, 1993.

Rustgi A: Hereditary gastrointestinal polyposis and non-polyposis syndromes. N Engl J Med 331:1694–1702, 1994.

Shrumpf E, Fausa O, Elgjock, et al: Hepatobiliary complications of inflammatory bowel disease. Semin Liver Dis 8:201, 1988.

Sleisenger MH, Fordtran JS (eds): Gastrointestinal Disease: Pathophysiology, Diagnosis, Management. 4th ed. Philadelphia, WB Saunders Company, 1988.

Sontag SJ: The medical management of reflux esophagitis: Role of antacids and acid inhibition. Gastroenterol Clin North Am 19:683, 1990.

Tong MJ, El-Farra NS, Reikes AR, et al: Clinical outcomes after transfusion-associated hepatitis C. N Engl J Med 232:1463, 1995.

Walsh JH, Peterson WL: Treatment of *Helicobacter pylori* infection in the management of peptic ulcer disease. N Engl J Med 333:984, 1995.

Warshaw AL, Fernandez-Del Castillo C: Pancreatic carcinoma. N Engl J Med 326:455, 1992.

Zakim D, Boyer TD (eds): Hepatology. 2nd ed. Philadelphia, WB Saunders Company, 1990.

PART 8

INFECTIOUS DISEASES

Peter G. Pappas

DIRECTIONS: For questions 1 to 67, choose the ONE BEST answer to each question.

QUESTIONS 1–3

A 33-year-old human immunodeficiency virus (HIV)–positive male patient presents with headache, confusion, low-grade fever, and sinus fullness for 1 week. There is no history of an opportunistic infection, but a recent CD4 count is 55 cells per cubic millimeter. His medications include trimethoprim-sulfamethoxazole (TMP/SMX) once daily and zidovudine (AZT) 600 mg daily. On examination, there is moderate bilateral papilledema. The patient is mildly confused, but there are no other focal neurologic findings. A computed tomography (CT) scan with contrast is negative. A lumbar puncture reveals an opening pressure of 320 mm H_2O and the fluid is noted to be slightly turbid. Cerebrospinal fluid (CSF) protein and glucose levels are normal, and there are 10 white blood cells (WBCs) per cubic millimeter. Other studies are pending.

1. What is the most likely diagnosis?

   A. Pneumococcal meningitis
   B. Toxoplasma encephalitis
   C. Drug-induced encephalopathy
   D. Cryptococcal meningitis
   E. Progressive multifocal leukoencephalopathy (PML)

2. All of the following would be useful diagnostic tests in this patient EXCEPT

   A. CSF cryptococcal antigen titer
   B. Serum cryptococcal antigen titer
   C. CSF India ink preparation
   D. *Toxoplasma gondii* serum titers
   E. CSF Venereal Disease Research Laboratory (VDRL) test

3. Which of the following is the most appropriate initial and long-term therapy for this patient?

   A. Fluconazole, 200 mg daily for initial and chronic therapy
   B. Amphotericin B, 0.7 mg per kilogram intravenously (IV) for 14 days, followed by fluconazole 200 mg daily chronically
   C. Amphotericin B, 0.3 mg per kilogram IV, plus 5-flucytosine, 150 mg per kilogram daily for 6 weeks, then stop therapy
   D. Amphotericin B, 0.7 mg per kilogram IV for 14 days, followed by amphotericin B, 1 mg per kilogram IV weekly thereafter

QUESTIONS 4–6

A 45-year-old man sustained a gunshot wound to the abdomen leading to a hemicolectomy, partial jejunal resection, and splenectomy. He is placed on ampicillin, gentamicin, and clindamycin preoperatively. He becomes afebrile on postoperative day 2, but develops fever again on day 6 to 39.2°C without an apparent source. The patient is clinically stable. Peripheral WBC count is 19,500 per microliter with a left shift. A subclavian vein central venous catheter has been present since surgery. A chest roentgenogram is negative. Blood, urine, and abdominal wound drainage cultures are obtained.

4. What is the best approach to anti-infective therapy at this time?

   A. Add vancomycin to current regimen
   B. Add fluconazole to current regimen
   C. Add ceftazidine to current regimen
   D. Stop current regimen, begin aztreonam and vancomycin
   E. Stop all antibiotics

The patient remains clinically stable but persistently febrile. There are no new clinical findings and peripheral leukocytosis persists. Two of four blood cultures drawn 48 hours earlier are positive for budding yeasts.

5. What is the most appropriate intervention?

   A. Replace central venous catheter over a guidewire, do not add antifungal therapy
   B. Replace central venous catheter at a new site, begin antifungal therapy
   C. Do not manipulate central venous catheter, begin antifungal therapy
   D. Begin antifungal therapy, schedule patient for abdominal CT scan
   E. The blood cultures represent contamination; no intervention is necessary

6. *Torulopsis glabrata* is isolated from two blood cultures. Which of the following is the best therapy in this clinical situation in a patient with normal renal function?

   A. Fluconazole, 400 mg daily
   B. Amphotericin B, 0.6 mg per kilogram daily
   C. Amphotericin B, 0.6 mg per kilogram daily, plus flucytosine, 150 mg per kilogram daily
   D. Amphotericin B, 0.6 mg per kilogram daily, plus fluconazole, 400 mg daily

QUESTIONS 7-9

Five months following exposure to a household case of active pulmonary tuberculosis, a 28-year-old HIV-positive man presents with fever, chills, rash, weight loss, and nonproductive cough for 2 weeks. A CD4 count 3 months ago was 380 cells per cubic millimeter. A chest roentgenogram reveals basilar interstitial infiltrates without cavities, adenopathy, or pleural effusion. A purified protein derivative test with controls reveal cutaneous anergy.

7. Which of the following is the most likely explanation for this illness?

A. *Pneumocystis carinii*
B. Cytomegalovirus
C. *Toxoplasma gondii*
D. *Streptococcus pneumoniae*
E. *Mycobacterium tuberculosis*

The patient is placed empirically on parenteral cefotaxime, erythromycin, and TMP/SMX. Five days later, fever and nonproductive cough continue, pulmonary infiltrates have progressed, and the patient is clinically worse.

8. What is the most appropriate intervention?

A. Begin empiric intravenous ganciclovir
B. Add intravenous pentamidine, stop TMP/SMX
C. Begin empiric amphotericin B
D. Begin empiric antituberculosis regimen, schedule bronchoscopy
E. Schedule open lung biopsy, continue current regimen

9. A bronchoalveolar lavage specimen reveals numerous acid-fast bacilli. What is the appropriate therapeutic intervention?

A. Begin clarithromycin, ethambutol, and amikacin
B. Begin isoniazid and rifampin
C. Begin four-drug antituberculous therapy
D. Suspecting multidrug-resistant *M. tuberculosis*, begin six-drug therapy
E. Await culture results, then start specific therapy

10. Risk factors for disseminated (extrapulmonary) tuberculosis include all of the following EXCEPT

A. Age less than 2 years
B. HIV infection
C. Solid organ transplantation
D. Hypogammaglobulinemia
E. Advanced age

11. All of the following statements regarding the epidemiology of tuberculosis are true EXCEPT

A. Tuberculosis is the major infectious cause of morbidity and mortality in the world.
B. The majority of cases in the United States occur among racial minorities.
C. There has been a small but steady decline in cases of tuberculosis in the United States from 1984 to the present.
D. Immigration has been significantly associated with newly diagnosed cases in the United States.
E. Among household contacts of patients with active

pulmonary tuberculosis, fewer than 50% become infected.

12. A 33-year-old HIV-positive man with a history of IV drug use presents with fever and diffuse bilateral pneumonia and hypoxia (Po$_2$ 55 torr). He is taking no medications. His last CD4 count was 89 cells per cubic millimeter. What is the LEAST likely cause of pneumonia in this patient?

A. *Mycobacterium tuberculosis*
B. *Mycobacterium avium-intracellulare*
C. *Pneumocystis carinii*
D. Cytomegalovirus
E. *Histoplasma capsulatum*

13. Which of the following is the LEAST likely cause of a solitary intracerebral lesion in a patient with advanced HIV disease (CD4 count ≤ 200 cells per cubic millimeter)?

A. *Toxoplasma gondii*
B. *Mycobacterium tuberculosis*
C. *Cryptococcus neoformans*
D. *Aspergillus fumigatus*
E. B-cell lymphoma

14. Which of the following is not a direct consequence of HIV infection on the nervous system?

A. Peripheral neuropathy
B. Vacuolar myelopathy
C. Aseptic meningitis
D. PML

15. Which of the following is the most common cause of cholangiopathy in a patient with acquired immunodeficiency syndrome (AIDS)?

A. Cytomegalovirus
B. Kaposi's sarcoma
C. Lymphoma
D. *Cryptococcus neoformans*

16. A 47-year-old HIV-positive man presents with acute ocular discomfort and rapidly progressive visual loss in the right eye. Funduscopic exam reveals widespread pale, peripheral and central necrotic retinal lesions. There is associated mild conjunctivitis and keratitis. What is the likely cause of this patient's ocular findings?

A. Cytomegalovirus
B. *Toxoplasma gondii*
C. *Histoplasma capsulatum*
D. Herpes simplex virus
E. *Staphylococcus aureus*

17. Common causes of pancytopenia in patients with HIV infection include each of the following EXCEPT

A. Kaposi's sarcoma
B. *Histoplasma capsulatum*
C. Parvovirus B19
D. *Mycobacterium avium-intracelluare*

18. Which of the following is the most common adverse effect associated with AZT?

A. Peripheral neuropathy
B. Megaloblastic anemia
C. Pancreatitis
D. Hepatitis

19. All of the following statements about HIV infection are true EXCEPT

- A. In many high-risk populations, the incidence of HIV infection has increased.
- B. AIDS has disproportionately affected certain racial and ethnic groups.
- C. Most pediatric cases result from perinatal transmission.
- D. HIV infection is predominantly a disease of white gay males.
- E. Women represent an increasing proportion of HIV-infected individuals in most countries

20. Which is the most efficient method of HIV transmission?

- A. Vertical transmission from a mother with AIDS to a neonate
- B. Heterosexual vaginal intercourse
- C. Hollow needle stick from HIV-positive patient
- D. Deep kissing with an HIV-positive individual
- E. Receptive anal intercourse with an HIV-positive partner

21. Immunologic abnormalities among patients with advanced HIV disease include each of the following EXCEPT

- A. Absolute decrease in CD4 lymphocytes
- B. Decrease in qualitative function of CD4 and CD8 lymphocytes
- C. Quantitative and qualitative B lymphocyte abnormalities
- D. Natural killer cell qualitative deficiency
- E. Macrophage and monocyte depletion through viral cytopathic effort

22. Important host immune responses that limit spread of HIV include all of the following EXCEPT

- A. Neutralizing antibodies produced by B lymphocytes
- B. Antibody-dependent cellular cytotoxicity
- C. Natural kill cells
- D. Cytotoxic T lymphocytes
- E. Monocytes/macrophages

23. Which of the following is NOT a common cause of genital ulcer disease in the developing world?

- A. *Treponema pallidum*
- B. *Neisseria gonorrhoeae*
- C. Herpes simplex virus
- D. *Calymmatobacterium granulomatis*
- E. *Haemophilus ducreyi*

24. Which of the following is most closely associated with the risk of acquiring a sexually transmitted disease?

- A. The number and type of different sexual partners
- B. Receptive anal intercourse
- C. A recent history of gonorrhea
- D. Intravenous drug use
- E. Male sex

25. What percentage of women with mucopurulent cervicitis are infected with *Chlamydia trachomatis*?

- A. Less than 10%
- B. 10–30%

C. 30–50%
D. 50–80%
E. 80–100%

26. Which of the following is NOT a cause of nongonococcal urethritis in males?

- A. *Chlamydia trachomatis*
- B. Herpes simplex virus
- C. *Ureaplasma urealyticum*
- D. *Trichomonas vaginalis*
- E. *Haemopilus ducreyi*

QUESTIONS 27 AND 28

A 20-year-old sexually active female college student presents with vaginal irritation, scant discharge, and odor for 1 week. There is no dysuria. She denies any history of sexually transmitted disease.

27. Which of the following is the most likely cause of her current complaints?

- A. Primary genital herpes
- B. *Trichomonas* vaginitis
- C. *Candida* vaginitis
- D. Gonococcal cervicitis
- E. Bacterial vaginosis

A vaginal exam reveals a thin, grayish discharge with an unpleasant odor, no genital lesions, and minimal cervical friability. Analysis of vaginal secretions reveals the following: pH 6.5, scant leukocytes, 3^+ clue cells, and positive "whiff" test with addition of potassium hydroxide. No trichomonads or yeasts are seen microscopically.

28. What is the likely causative organism(s)?

- A. *Chlamydia trachomatis*
- B. Herpes simplex virus
- C. *Neisseria gonorrhoeae*
- D. Mixed infection with *Gardnerella vaginalis, Mobiluncus* sp., and other genital anaerobes.
- E. *Ureaplasma urealyticum*

QUESTIONS 29 AND 30

A 69-year-old man with mild dementia is noted to have a serum VDRL titer of 1:16 and a positive fluorescent treponemal antibodies (FTA) test. The remainder of his evaluation is negative, including a spinal fluid analysis that reveals normal protein and glucose, fewer that five leukocytes, and a negative CSF VDRL test. There is no history of prior treatment for syphilis. What is the most appropriate therapy?

- A. Aqueous penicillin G, 20 million units IV for 14 days
- B. Procaine penicillin, 600,000 units intramuscularly daily for 14 days
- C. Benzathine penicillin, 2.4 million units intramuscularly weekly for three doses
- D. Ceftriaxone, 2 grams IV daily for 10 days
- E. No therapy is necessary

30. If the patient was allergic to beta-lactamase antimicrobials, what would be the best alternative therapy?

A. TMP/SMX (800 mg/160 mg) bid for 30 days
B. Ciprofloxacin, 500 mg bid for 30 days
C. Erythromycin, 500 mg qid for 14 days
D. Doxycycline, 100 mg bid for 30 days
E. Azithromycin, 2-gram single dose

31. Each of the following syndromes has been etiologically linked to *Chlamydia trachomatis* infection EXCEPT

A. Reiters' syndrome
B. Nonbacterial prostatitis
C. Follicular conjunctivitis and corneal pannus with visual loss
D. Endometritis
E. Neonatal pneumonitis

32. *Coxiella burnetii* may cause each of the following EXCEPT

A. Acute lobar pneumonia
B. Chronic cavitary pneumonia
C. Chronic granulomatous hepatitis
D. Culture-negative endocarditis

33. Which of the following is NOT characteristic of Rocky Mountain spotted fever (RMSF)?

A. Severe headache
B. Thrombocytopenia
C. Mucous membrane lesions
D. Pulmonary infiltrate
E. High mortality in untreated patients

34. Which of the following is NOT a late complication of Lyme borreliosis?

A. Pauciarticular arthritis
B. Bell's palsy
C. Erythema chronicum migrans
D. Acrodermatitis chronica atrophicans
E. Complete heart block

35. Which of the following statements about the laboratory features of Lyme borreliosis is true?

A. The organism is readily cultured from blood and spinal fluid.
B. Special stains of skin biopsies are readily available and quite useful.
C. Because of cross-reactive antigens, many patients will have positive VDRL test results.
D. Serologic assays are essential in the diagnosis of Lyme borreliosis.
E. The diagnosis of Lyme borreliosis is clinical and epidemiologic; standardized laboratory tests are unavailable and of limited value.

36. Which of the following is NOT characteristic of infection with *Ehrlichia chaffeensis?*

A. Leukocytosis
B. Thrombocytopenia
C. Headache
D. Erythematous rash
E. CSF pleocytosis

37. Which of the following situations merits aggressive reduction of fever?

A. A 21-year-old otherwise healthy woman with acute pyelonephritis and temperature of 39.8°C
B. A healthy 2-year-old boy with acute onset fever to 39.2°C with no apparent source
C. A 74-year-old chronically ill woman with pneumonia and temperature of 39.4°C
D. An 18-year-old man with acute myelogenous leukemia, neutropenia, and fever to 39.2°C
E. A 56-year-old man with recent myocardial infarction and fever to 38.8°C

38. Which of the following plasma proteins do not increase during the acute-phase response?

A. Alpha$_1$-antitrypsin
B. Fibrinogen
C. Factor VIII
D. Plasminogen
E. Albumin

39. Which of the following is the most common type of nosocomial infection?

A. Urinary tract infection
B. Pneumonia
C. Wound infection
D. Intravenous catheter–related bacteremia
E. Antibiotic-associated diarrhea

40. Among the following types of nosocomial infections, which of the following has the most significant impact on mortality and excess hospital stay?

A. Urinary tract infection
B. Pneumonia
C. Surgical wound infection
D. Bacteremia
E. Antibiotic-associated diarrhea

41. Which of the following methods might have the most significant impact in decreasing nosocomial infections?

A. Effective hand washing
B. Judicious use of antibacterial prophylaxis
C. Frequent central venous catheter changes
D. Barrier precautions for all patients
E. Universal precautions for all patients

QUESTIONS 42–44

An otherwise healthy 33-year-old man plans to join the Peace Corps and will be assigned to Thailand for 2 years. He is leaving in approximately 6 months and has come to your clinic requesting pretravel advice and recommendations regarding vaccination. On questioning, he states that all of his vaccinations are ''up to date,'' but cannot provide any specifics as to when he received these vaccinations. Which of the following is not a recommended vaccination in this patient?

A. Hepatitis A
B. Hepatitis B
C. Yellow fever
D. Tetanus
E. Oral polio vaccine

43. Which would be the most appropriate antimalarial prophylaxis provided he remains in the urban areas of Thailand?

A. Doxycycline, 100 mg daily
B. Chloroquine, 300 mg weekly
C. Fansidar weekly
D. Mefloquine, 250 mg weekly
E. No malaria prophylaxis is necessary provided he remains in urban areas of Thailand

44. Other suggestions for this patient would include each of the following EXCEPT

A. Avoid undercooked seafood, raw vegetables, and unbottled drinks
B. Avoid sexual intercourse, especially without the use of a condom
C. Consider preexposure rabies vaccination
D. Begin norfloxacin, 400 mg daily, on entering the country to prevent to traveler's diarrhea
E. If travel to rural areas occurs, use mosquito netting and diethyltoluamide (DEET)

45. Which of the following describes the mechanism of penicillin resistance among isolates of *Streptococcus pneumoniae?*

A. Beta-lactamase
B. Alteration of penicillin-binding proteins
C. Altered permeability
D. Altered internuclear binding sites

46. Which of the following antimicrobial agents has the best penetration to CSF in the absence of inflammation?

A. Penicillin G
B. Ceftriaxone
C. Gentamicin
D. Chloramphenicol

47. Which of the following antimicrobial agents is NOT a common cause of drug-induced fever?

A. Sulfonamide
B. Penicillin
C. Cephalosporines
D. Vancomycin
E. Aminoglycosides

48. The most important virulence factor of *Streptococcus pneumoniae* is

A. Elaboration of beta-lactamase
B. Hemolysin
C. Polysaccharide capsule
D. Resistance to lysosomal enzymes
E. Production of hyaluronidase

49. For which of the following individuals is pneumococcal vaccine currently NOT recommended?

A. A 35-year-old man with alcohol-induced cirrhosis
B. An 18-month-old boy, otherwise healthy
C. A 50-year-old woman with diet-controlled diabetes mellitus
D. A 19-year-old woman with sickle cell disease
E. A 74-year-old man with ischemic heart disease

QUESTIONS 50 AND 51

A 54-year-old woman with a history of chronic mastoiditis is admitted with acute meningitis. CSF reveals gram-positive cocci in pairs and chains and *Streptococcus pneumoniae* is isolated by culture. The patient is initially placed on high-dose intravenous penicillin G but fails to respond clinically and, on the third day following admission, these susceptibility data are available:

Drug	MIC (μg/ml)
Penicillin G	≥ 4
Cefotaxime	≥ 8
Imipenem	≥ 4

50. Which of the following is the most appropriate therapy at this time?

A. Continue high-dose penicillin G (20,000,000 units per day) but add rifampin, 600 mg daily
B. Begin ceftriaxone, 2 grams every 12 hours
C. Intravenous erythromycin, 1 gram every 6 hours
D. Vancomycin, 15 mg per kilogram every 12 hours
E. Chloramphenicol, 1 gram IV every 6 hours

An appropriate therapeutic change is made, and the patient improves clinically; however, on day 7, the patient is noted to have decreasing mental status progressing to obtundation. Exam reveals an afebrile patient barely arousable to verbal stimuli. A neurologic exam is remarkable for cranial nerve palsy and altered mental status. Funduscopic exam reveals bilateral papilledema.

51. What is the likely explanation for the patient's current clinical status?

A. Antibacterial therapy is inadequate and she has progressive meningitis
B. Increased intracranial pressure with focal neurologic findings
C. The patient has had a cerebrovascular accident
D. Findings are likely due to metabolic abnormality such as hyperglycemia

52. Which of the following organisms is LEAST likely to cause infective endocarditis in a native aortic valve?

A. *Staphylococcus aureus*
B. *Enterococcus. faecalis*
C. Group A streptococcus
D. *Haemophilus parainfluenzae*
E. *Escherichia coli*

53. Which of the following is not necessarily an indication for surgical intervention in infective endocarditis?

A. Congestive heart failure
B. Multiple systemic emboli
C. Persistently positive blood cultures despite adequate antimicrobial therapy
D. Myocardial abscess
E. Fungal endocarditis

54. Which of the following cardiac lesions is LEAST likely to predispose to endocarditis?

A. Prosthetic valve
B. Previous history of native valve endocarditis

C. Coarctation of the aorta
D. Atrial septal defect
E. Mitral valve prolapse with a regurgitant murmur

QUESTIONS 55 AND 56

A previously healthy 48-year-old woman is admitted to the hospital with undifferentiated fever. Her examination on admission is entirely unremarkable except for a temperature of 39.7°C. Her laboratory tests are unrevealing except for mild leukocytosis. On the second hospital day, three of three blood cultures are positive for *Staphylococcus aureus* susceptible to oxacillin. She is placed on oxacillin, 2 grams every 6 hours, and responds clinically within the next 48 hours. A repeat cardiac exam is unremarkable and a transthoracic echocardiogram reveals no valvular vegetations.

55. What is the likelihood that this patient has infective endocarditis?

A. Less than 10%
B. 10–20%
C. 30–40%
D. Greater than 50%

56. What is the most appropriate therapy for this patient given the current data?

A. Continue oxacillin for 2 weeks
B. Continue oxacillin for 4 to 6 weeks
C. Discontinue oxacillin, begin vancomycin for 2 weeks
D. Discontinue oxacillin, begin vancomycin for 4 to 6 weeks
E. Continue oxacillin and add gentamicin, 3 mg per kilogram daily, and rifampin, 600 mg daily, for 2 weeks

57. *Staphylococcus xylosus* is isolated from three blood cultures from a patient who underwent mitral valve replacement with a homograft 6 months ago for myxomatous degeneration. The patient has been minimally febrile over the last 2 to 3 weeks but has no other symptoms. Which of the following statements is correct?

A. *Staphylococcus xylosus* is a contaminant and should be disregarded. Repeat blood cultures.
B. Obtain additional blood cultures and begin vancomycin and gentamicin.
C. Obtain additional blood cultures and transthoracic echocardiogram; do not start antimicrobials unless echocardiogram reveals valvular vegetations.
D. Contact the cardiac surgeon immediately because this patient will ultimately require prosthetic valve replacement.

58. Which of the following is the most likely cause of acute bacterial meningitis (ABM) in a 62-year-old alcoholic man with no other significant health history?

A. *Streptococcus pneumoniae*
B. *Neisseria meningitidis*
C. *Haemophilus influenzae*
D. *Staphylococcus aureus*
E. *Listeria monocytogenes*

QUESTIONS 59–61

A 40-year-old man living in the United States for the past 15 years has recently returned from a month-long visit to his native country, India. He presents with fever, abdominal pain, constipation, and headache. The patient states that he took malaria prophylaxis but no other medications or pretravel vaccinations. He appears to be very reliable. Based solely on this information, what is the LEAST likely cause of his illness?

A. *Plasmodium vivax* malaria
B. Typhoid fever
C. Brucellosis
D. Acute hepatitis A
E. Ameobic liver abscess

The physical exam is remarkable for an ill-appearing man with temperature of 40°C. The abdomen is slightly distended and tender and the liver is nonpalpable, but the spleen is moderately enlarged and nontender. There is no rash, and no other physical findings.

60. Which test is LEAST likely to be helpful in this setting?

A. Upright abdominal roentgenogram
B. Blood cultures
C. Abdominal ultrasound
D. Hepatitis A, B, and C serology and liver function tests
E. Peripheral blood smear

61. The patient is hospitalized and started on intravenous fluids. On day 3 of hospitalization, blood cultures are positive for an aerobic gram-negative rod identified as probable *Salmonella* sp. What is the most appropriate initial therapy in this patient?

A. Ampicillin, 2 grams IV every 6 hours
B. Chloramphenicol, 1 gram IV every 6 hours
C. Ciprofloxacin, 400 mg IV every 12 hours
D. TMP/SMX, 160/800 mg orally every 12 hours
E. Both A and B

62. Which of the following is the most common cause of diarrhea in travelers?

A. *Salmonella enteritidis*
B. *Shigella flexneri*
C. *Campylobacter jejuni*
D. *Giardia lamblia*
E. Enterotoxigenic *Escherichia coli*

63. Which of the following enteric pathogens is most likely to be associated with bacteremia and metastatic infection?

A. *Campylobacter fetus*
B. *Vibrio cholerae*
C. *Shigella sonnei*
D. *Salmonella typhi*
E. *Salmonella choleraesuis*

64. Among the following antimicrobials, which does NOT have excellent *in vitro* activity versus significant anaerobic bacterial pathogens?

A. Chloramphenicol
B. Metronidazole
C. Clindamycin

D. Imipenem
E. All have excellent anaerobic activity

65. A 26-year-old male student complains of abdominal cramps, belching, excess flatus, and watery diarrhea for 6 weeks following a 1-month tour of Russia. He describes no fever but has lost 12 pounds. Which of the following viruses likely explains his symptoms?

A. *Cryptosporidium parvum*
B. *Giardia lamblia*
C. Enterotoxigenic *E. coli*
D. *Salmonella enteritidis*
E. *Shigella sonnei*

66. Which of the following viruses possess the enzyme reverse transcriptase?

A. Rabies virus
B. Herpes simplex virus types I and II
C. Parvovirus B19
D. Human T-cell lymphotrophic virus type I (HTLV-I)
E. Marburg and Ebola viruses

67. Which of the following respiratory viruses is LEAST likely to cause bronchitis?

A. Influenza A
B. Influenza B
C. Respiratory syncytial virus
D. Rhinovirus
E. Coronavirus

DIRECTIONS: For questions 68 to 115, decide whether EACH statement is true or false. Any combination of answers, from all true to all false, may occur.

68. Poor prognostic indicators among patients with cryptococcal meningitis include which of the following?

A. Obtundation
B. High CSF cryptococcal antigen titer
C. Underlying immune deficiency
D. Headache
E. CSF white blood cell count >20 cells per cubic millimeter

69. Which of the following statements about infection with *Blastomyces dermatitidis* is/are true?

A. Most acute infections are asymptomatic.
B. Bone is the most common extrapulmonary site of involvement.
C. Serology is the most rapid and reliable diagnostic method.
D. Itraconazole, 200 to 400 mg daily for 6 months, is the therapy of choice for uncomplicated infections.
E. Widespread dissemination and fatal infections are frequently seen in immunocompromised patients.

70. Clinical and epidemiologic features of coccidioidomycosis include which of the following?

A. Person-to-person respiratory transmission is commonly seen.
B. Presumptive diagnosis is made by detection of specific serum antibodies.
C. Solitary pulmonary nodules and thin-walled cavities are characteristic.
D. Extrapulmonary dissemination is seen commonly in immunocompromised patients.
E. Coccidioidal meningitis may go into spontaneously remission.

71. Which of the following statements about histoplasmosis is/are true?

A. Immunocompetent patients with acute pulmonary disease usually require antifungal therapy.
B. Relapsing pulmonary and disseminated disease is common after discontinuation of therapy.
C. A diagnosis is usually based on serologic assays.
D. Oral ulcerations are associated with disseminated disease.
E. Most patients with AIDS present with localized disease.

72. Which of the following statements about Hansen's disease (leprosy) is/are true?

A. It is highly contagious to household contacts.
B. *Mycobacterium leprae* is easily cultivated in laboratory media.
C. Lepromatous leprosy may result from a selective T lymphocyte unresponsiveness to *M. leprae* antigen.
D. Palpable peripheral nerves are usually found in patients with lepromatous leprosy.
E. Large numbers of organisms are characteristic in lesions of polar tuberculoid leprosy.

73. Which of the following is/are relative indications for corticosteroid therapy?

A. Tuberculous pericarditis
B. Tuberculous meningitis
C. Disseminated histoplasmosis
D. Disseminated blastomycosis
E. Miliary tuberculosis

74. Which of the following is/are acceptable regimens for uncomplicated pulmonary tuberculosis caused by susceptible organisms?

A. Isoniazid (INH) plus rifampin (RIF) for 9 months
B. INH, RIF, and pyrazinamide (PAZ) for 2 months, then INH and RIF for 4 months
C. INH, RIF, PZA, and ethambutol (EMB) for 2 months, then INH and RIF for 4 months
D. INH and EMB for 18 months

75. Which of the following individuals should receive INH prophylaxis for 6 to 12 months?

A. A 35-year-old HIV-positive black man with 6-mm reactive tuberculin skin test
B. A 17-year-old Vietnamese woman with negative chest roentgenogram and 12-mm reactive tuberculin skin test
C. A 28-year-old diabetic woman with negative chest roentgenogram and 8-mm reactive tuberculin skin test
D. A 74-year-old man who lives in a nursing home who is asymptomatic and whose chest roentgenogram reveals biapical fibronodular scarring; a tuberculin skin test is reactive to 7 mm.
E. A 55-year-old woman who is otherwise healthy with a positive tuberculin skin test to 16 mm; her test was nonreactive 2 years ago and a recent chest roentgenogram is normal

76. For which of the following infections in HIV-infected patients is primary prophylaxis generally recommended?

A. *Pneumocystis carinii*
B. *Toxoplasma gondii*
C. *Histoplasma capsulatum*
D. *Cryptococcus neoformans*
E. *Mycobacterium avium-intracellulare*

77. Common causes of chronic diarrhea in patients with advanced (CD4 count $\leq$ 200 cells/mm^3) HIV disease include which of the following?

A. *Cryptosporidium parvum*
B. *Microsporidia* sp.
C. HIV enteropathy
D. Cytomegalovirus
E. *Clostridium difficile*

78. Which of the following neoplasms are more common in HIV-infected than non–HIV-infected patients?

A. Hodgkins' disease
B. B-cell lymphoma

C. Cervical carcinoma
D. Anal carcinoma
E. Gastric adenocarcinoma

79. Which of the following statements about HIV-associated nephropathy (HIVAN) is/are true?

A. About 90% of patients with HIVAN are black.
B. About 80% are intravenous drug users.
C. Heavy proteinuria usually precedes end-stage renal disease.
D. The renal lesion is usually focal and segmental glomerulosclerosis.
E. HIVAN occurs almost exclusively in patients with advanced HIV disease.

80. Which of the following rheumatologic syndromes is/are associated with HIV infection?

A. Sicca syndrome
B. Systemic lupus erythematosus
C. Hypersensitivity vasculitis
D. Reiters' disease
E. Polymyositis

81. In which of the following patients is/are antiretroviral therapy generally considered desirable?

A. Symptomatic, CD4 count < 200 cells per cubic millimeter
B. Asymptomatic, CD4 count < 200 cells per cubic millimeter
C. Symptomatic, CD4 count 200 to 500 cells per cubic millimeter
D. Asymptomatic, CD4 count 200 to 500 cells per cubic millimeter
E. Asymptomatic, CD4 count > 500 cell per cubic millimeter

82. Potential causes of CD4 depletion in HIV-infected patients include which of the following?

A. Direct viral cytopathic effect
B. Syncytia formation
C. Autoimmune destruction
D. Apoptosis
E. Impaired regeneration from the peripheral T-cell compartment

83. Which of the following statements about the biology of HIV-1 and HIV-2 is/are true?

A. Both are single-standard RNA viruses.
B. The viruses have approximately 80% genetic homology.
C. Both viruses demonstrate marked genetic variability.
D. Both viruses are closely related to simian immunodeficiency viruses isolated from African green monkeys and sooty mangabeys.
E. Both viruses lead to immunodeficiency at similar rates.

84. The differential diagnosis of pelvic inflammatory disease (PID) includes which of the following?

A. Appendicitis
B. Hemorrhagic ovarian cyst

C. Ectopic pregnancy
D. Ovarian torsion
E. Endometriosis

85. Which of the following organisms has/have been commonly linked to acute and chronic salpingitis?

A. *Neisseria gonorrhoeae*
B. *Chlamydia trachomatis*
C. *Bacteroides* sp.
D. Aerobic gram-negative rods
E. *Staphylococcus aureus*

86. Which of the following is/are complications associated with salpingitis?

A. Infertility
B. Ectopic pregnancy
C. Ovarian cysts
D. Chronic pelvic pain
E. Abnormal uterine bleeding

87. Which of the following is/are characteristic of disseminated gonococcal infection?

A. Mostly occurs in females
B. Diffuse pustular rash, usually with >100 lesions
C. Organisms usually seen in Gram's stain of joint fluid
D. Most patients are culture negative
E. May cause rapidly progressive infective endocarditis

88. Together with doxycycline, which of the following is/are acceptable single-dose therapies for gonococcal pharyngitis?

A. Ceftriaxone, 125 mg intramuscularly
B. Ofloxacin, 400 mg orally
C. Ciprofloxacin, 500 mg orally
D. Cefixime, 400 mg orally
E. Amoxicillin/clavulanate, 500 mg orally

89. A 30-year-old man presents with a solitary, painful genital ulcer and right inguinal adenopathy. A presumptive diagnosis of chancroid is made. What is acceptable therapy in this situation?

A. Ceftriaxone, 250 mg intramuscularly
B. Azithromycin, 1.0 gram orally (single dose)
C. Tetracycline, 500 mg orally four times daily for 7 days
D. Amoxicillin, 500 mg orally three times daily for 5 days
E. Erythromycin, 500 mg four times daily for 7 days

90. Which of the following statements about current syphilis epidemiology is/are true?

A. Direct contact, usually sexual, is responsible for most transmission.
B. The disease is most common in poor, rural settings.
C. The disease is only slightly more common in blacks than in whites.

D. The current epidemic has been linked to sex in exchange for drugs.

E. HIV transmission is probably enhanced with primary syphilis.

91. The laboratory diagnosis of secondary syphilis is supported by which of the following?

A. Positive culture for *Treponema pallidum*

B. Positive darkfield image of an oral mucosal lesion, with motile spirochetes

C. Positive VDRL test and microhemagglutinin–*Treponema pallidum* (MHA-TP) test

D. Positive VDRL test and negative FTA test

92. Which of the following statements is/are true regarding illness caused by *Chlamydia* species?

A. *C. pneumoniae* frequently causes disease outside of the respiratory system.

B. Pneumonia caused by *C. pneumoniae* is generally milder than that caused by *C. psittaci*.

C. *C. psittaci* is transmitted person to person by aerosol.

D. *C. pneumoniae* and *C. psittaci* infections are most easily diagnosed by cell culture.

E. Tetracycline is the drug of choice for *C. pneumoniae* and *C. psittaci*.

93. Which of the following statements is/are true about human ehrlichiosis?

A. Most cases are tick borne.

B. There are at least two *Ehrlichia* species that cause human disease.

C. The disease is as least as severe as RMSF.

D. The disease is particularly common in the western United States.

E. Tetracycline or doxycycline is the drug of choice.

94. Which of the following proteins have pyrogenic activity?

A. Tumor necrosis factor alpha

B. Interleukin-1 alpha

C. Interleukin-6

D. Interferon alpha

E. Interferon gamma

95. The combination of ticarcillin and clavulanic acid provides enhanced antibacterial activity against which of the following organisms?

A. Penicillin-resistant, oxacillin-susceptible *Staphylococcus aureus*

B. Beta-lactamase–producing *Bacteroides fragilis*

C. Oxacillin-resistant *S. aureus*

D. *Pseudomonas aeruginosa*

E. Penicillin-resistant pneumococcus

96. Under which of the following circumstances is combination antimicrobial therapy warranted?

A. Uncomplicated viridans streptococcal endocarditis

B. Enterococcal endocarditis

C. Fever in the neutropenic patient

D. *S. aureus* bacteremia caused by contaminated central venous catheter

E. *E. coli* bacteremia complicating pyelonephritis

97. Clinical and laboratory findings commonly associated with *Mycoplasma pneumoniae* infections include which of the following?

A. Bullous myringitis

B. Bilateral interstitial infiltrates on chest radiograph

C. Encephalitis

D. Erythema multiforme

E. Hemolytic anemia

98. Which of the following is/are features of aerobic gram-negative bacillary pneumonia?

A. Most cases are community-acquired

B. Clinical course may be indolent or fulminant

C. Extensive lung necrosis is common

D. Mortality rates are usually <20%

E. Sputum culture is a poor indicator of the etiology of pneumonia

99. Which of the following is/are risk factors for legionnaires disease?

A. Cigarette smoking

B. Age over 50 years

C. Glucocorticosteroid use

D. Cytotoxic chemotherapy

E. Neutropenia

100. Specific therapy for legionnaires disease may include which of the following?

A. Erythromycin, 500 to 1000 mg every 6 hours

B. Clarithromycin, 500 mg twice daily

C. Ciprofloxacin, 500 mg twice daily

D. Ceftriaxone, 2 grams daily

E. Doxycycline, 100 mg twice daily, plus rifampin, 600 mg daily

101. For which of the following procedures is antimicrobial prophylaxis warranted in a patient with a bicuspid aortic valve?

A. Tooth extraction

B. Cystoscopy

C. Bronchoscopy with flexible scope for bronchoalveolar lavage

D. Incision and drainage of a superficial abscess

E. Esophageal dilation

102. Which of the following is/are risk factors for invasive disease caused by *Staphylococcus aureus?*

A. Nasal carriage with *S. aureus*

B. Chronic hemodialysis

C. IV drug abuse

D. Non–insulin-requiring diabetes mellitus

E. Chronic eczematous dermatitis

103. Which of the following statements about the use of glucocorticosteroids as adjunctive therapy in acute bacterial meningitis (ABM) is/are true?

A. Steroids are indicated in all patients with severe ABM.

B. The main benefit of steroids in patients with ABM is to decrease mortality.

C. Children with *Haemophilus influenzae* meningitis who receive adjunctive steroids have fewer neurologic deficits following recovery.

D. It is important to begin steroids prior to or simultaneous with antibacterial agents.

E. There are clear benefits to patients with ABM caused by organisms other than *H. influenzae* who receive adjunctive glucocorticosteroids.

104. Which of the following statements regarding infection with *Bordetella pertussis* is/are correct?

A. Nonimmune household contacts contract disease less than 50% of the time.

B. Vaccination and/or natural infection confer life-long immunity.

C. Marked peripheral lymphocytosis is characteristic of acute infection.

D. A protracted convalescent stage sometimes lasting 3 months is common.

E. Treatment with erythromycin in the paroxysmal stage clearly ameliorates symptoms and shortens the duration of the disease.

105. Which of the following statements is/are true regarding human infection with *Francisella tularensis?*

A. Ticks are a major vector.

B. Pneumonia may result from skinning or eviscerating an infected rabbit.

C. It may mimic disease caused by *Sporothrix schenckii.*

D. Diagnosis is usually based on isolates from blood cultures.

E. Ceftriaxone is the drug of choice for systemic disease.

106. Which of the following is/are characteristic of nocardiosis?

A. Underlying host usually has impaired humoral immunity

B. Multi-loculated brain abscesses

C. Isolation from sputum may occur in absence of radiographic or clinical disease

D. Multiple organ involvement is common, especially in immunocompromised hosts

E. Sulfur granules are often seen in clinical specimens from involved sites

107. Which of the following agents is/are effective therapies for herpes simplex virus infections?

A. Acyclovir

B. Vidarabine

C. Trifluorothymidine

D. Ribavirin

E. Ganciclovir

108. Which of the following should receive influenza vaccine routinely?

A. Persons age 65 years or older

B. Physicians, nurses, and other health care workers

C. Nursing home residents

D. Solid organ transplant recipients

E. Anyone wishing to reduce the risk of influenza

109. Which of the following should receive measles vaccine?

A. A 43-year-old otherwise healthy man traveling to central Africa

B. A 17-year-old pregnant girl

C. A healthy 12-month-old boy

D. A 35-year-old man with AIDS

E. A 20-year-old male college student without a history of vaccination

110. Which of the following has/have been associated with infection with Epstein-Barr virus (EBV)?

A. Nasopharyngeal carcinoma

B. Hodgkin's disease

C. Post-transplantation lymphoproliferative disorder

D. Central nervous system B-cell lymphoma

E. Burkitt's lymphoma

111. Which of the following disorders has/have been strongly associated with HTLV-I infection?

A. Topical spastic paraparesis

B. AIDS

C. Adult T-cell lymphoma

D. PML

E. Dementia

112. Which of the following hemorrhagic fever viruses are commonly transmitted in the nosocomial setting?

A. Yellow fever virus

B. Lassa fever virus

C. Dengue virus

D. Crimean-Congo hemorrhagic fever virus

E. Ebola virus

113. Which of the following are complications of fulminant falciparum malaria?

A. Acute renal failure

B. Pulmonary edema

C. Seizures

D. Severe anemia

E. Abdominal pain and diarrhea

114. Which of the following *Plasmodium* sp. has/have a chronic intrahepatic stage?

A. *Plasmodium malariae*

B. *Plasmodium ovale*

C. *Plasmodium vivax*

D. *Plasmodium falciparum*

115. A traveler returning from West Africa has fever, severe headache, and anemia. A diagnosis of falciparum malaria is made. Which of the following is/are appropriate therapies?

A. Chloroquine

B. Mefloquine

C. Quinine

D. Halofantrine

E. Pyrimethamine plus sulfadoxine

DIRECTIONS: Questions 116 to 196 are matching questions. For each numbered item, choose the most likely associated lettered item from those provided. Each numbered item has ONLY ONE answer. Within each set of questions, each answer may be used once, more than once, or not at all.

QUESTIONS 116–121

For each fungal organism, select the appropriate microscopic morphology.

A. Large spherule (75 μm) containing endospores
B. Budding yeasts with pseudohyphae
C. Multiple budding "pilot wheel" yeasts
D. Small (2- to 6-μm) cigar-shaped budding yeasts
E. Broad-based budding yeasts with doubly refractile cell walls
F. Small (4- to 6-μm) budding yeasts with large polysaccharide capsule

116. *Paracoccidiodes brasiliensis*

117. *Blastomyces dermatitidis*

118. *Candida albicans*

119. *Coccidioides immitis*

120. Cryptococcal meningitis

121. *Sporothrix schenckii*

QUESTIONS 122–127

Match the following descriptions with the appropriate organisms.

A. *Bacillus anthracis*
B. *Sporothrix schenckii*
C. *Mycobacterium chelonae*
D. *Blastomyces dermatitidis*
E. *Leishmania tropica*
F. *Nocardia asteroides*

122. A 33-year-old male gardener with nodular lymphangitis involving the right dorsal hand and forearm

123. A 51-year-old female renal transplant recipient with painful erythematous nodules involving the left lower extremity

124. A 57-year-old female diabetic with a right lower lobe pulmonary infiltrate and multiple ring-enhancing lesions on brain CT

125. A 41-year-old male textile worker with a 2 × 2-cm painless black eschar over the left wrist

126. A 76-year-old male retired farmer with a right perihilar mass on chest roentgenogram and five large violaceous plaques on the face and hands

127. A 25-year-old male Persian Gulf War veteran with a 3 × 4-cm painful ulceration with heaped up borders over the left shoulder

QUESTIONS 128–132

Match the following descriptions with the most appropriate antifungal compounds.

A. Fluconazole
B. Itraconazole
C. Amphotericin B
D. Flucytosine
E. Ketoconazole

128. Empiric therapy in persistently febrile neutropenic patients receiving broad-spectrum antibacterials

129. Significant gastrointestinal, hepatic, and bone marrow toxicity

130. Markedly decreased absorption in achlorhydria

131. Oral therapy for mild to moderate invasive aspergillosis

132. Oral drug of choice for coccidioidal meningitis

QUESTIONS 133–136

Match the following characteristic clinical and/or laboratory features with the appropriate spirochetes.

A. *Treponema carateum*
B. *Borrelia recurrentis*
C. *Leptospira interrogans*
D. *Borrelia burgdorferi*

133. Positive darkfield image for motile spirochetes from a papular skin lesion

134. Organisms may be cultured from urine in recently febrile patients

135. Multiple vascular erythematous lesions with central clearing ranging from 3 to 20 cm in diameter

136. Spirochetes on peripheral blood smear, high mortality

QUESTIONS 137–142

Match the clinical or epidemiologic features with the appropriate rickettsial organism.

A. *Rickettsia conorii*
B. *Rickettsia akari*
C. *Rickettsia rickettsii*
D. *Rickettsia typhi*
E. *Rickettsia prowazekii*
F. *Coxiella burnetii*
G. *Ehrlichia equi*

137. Humans infected through body louse feces, recurrent symptoms years after primary illness

138. Tache noir

139. Rash is uncharacteristic

140. Rodent reservoir, truncal rash, moderate illness

141. Mouse reservoir, papulovesicular rash, self-limited illness

142. Severe headache, history of tick exposure, petechial rash, multisystem involvement

QUESTIONS 143–147

Match the mechanism of action with the appropriate class of antimicrobial agent.

A. Vancomycin
B. Aminoglycosides
C. Macrolides (erythromycin, clarithromycin)
D. Trimethoprim
E. Quinolones

143. Binds to the 30-S ribosomal unit

144. Binds to the 50-S ribosomal unit

145. Binds to the peptidoglycan precursors

146. Binds DNA gyrase

147. Inhibits dihydrofolate reductase

QUESTIONS 148–151

Match the following disease processes with the most appropriate beta-hemolytic streptococcus.

A. Group A streptococcus (*S. pyogenes*)
B. Group B streptococcus (*S. agalactiae*)
C. Group C streptococcus
D. Group F streptococcus

148. Periappendiceal abscess

149. Necrotizing fasciitis

150. Recurrent cellulitis in a saphenous vein harvest site

151. Diabetic foot infection with cellulitis and chronic osteomyelitis

QUESTIONS 152–155

Select the appropriate *Clostridium* sp. for each of the descriptions.

A. *Clostridium tetani*
B. *Clostridium botulinum*
C. Both
D. Neither

152. Ingestion of preformed toxin causes disease

153. Organism produces toxin once it is inside the host

154. A major clinical manifestation is profuse, watery diarrhea

155. Specific antitoxin is given for suspected cases

QUESTIONS 156–160

Match the following clinical descriptions with the associated viruses.

A. Adenovirus type 7
B. Mumps
C. Measles
D. Rubella
E. Parvovirus B19

156. Significantly decreased cell-mediated immunity during acute infection and recovery phase

157. Pharyngoconjunctival fever in a first grader

158. Monoarticular arthritis in a 23-year-old pregnant woman

159. Unilateral orchitis and aseptic meningitis in an adolescent boy

160. Congenitally infected infants may shed virus in urine and saliva for up to 1 year following birth

QUESTIONS 161–164

Match each clinical description with the appropriate arthropod-borne virus.

A. Western equine encephalitis
B. Eastern equine encephalitis
C. St. Louis encephalitis
D. California encephalitis

161. Likelihood of apparent disease greatest in early childhood; overall mortality 3 to 5%, mostly in children less than 5 years old

162. Likelihood of apparent disease increases with age; fatality rare in patients less than 20 years, approximately 30% in patients 65 or older

163. Epizootics in horses and exotic birds precede human epidemics; case fatality rate is 50 to 70%

164. Disease of younger, rural individuals living in proximity to deciduous hardwood forests; case fatality rate <1%

QUESTIONS 165–168

Match the following clinical descriptions with the correct trypanosome.

A. *Trypanosoma brucei brucei*
B. *Trypanosoma brucei rhodesiense*
C. *Trypanosoma brucei gambiense*
D. *Trypanosoma cruzi*

165. Megaesophagus with achalasia, recurrent aspiration pneumonia

166. Winterbottom's sign followed by chronic encephalopathy

167. High fever, rapid neurologic deterioration, evidence of disseminated intravascular coagulation

168. A nonhuman pathogen that causes wasting illness in cattle and wild animals

QUESTIONS 169–172

Match the following clinical descriptions with the appropriate human parasite.

A. *Schistosoma haematobium*
B. *Paragonimus westermanii*
C. *Clonorchis sinensis*
D. *Fasciolopsis buski*

169. Causes "endemic hemoptysis" and lung nodules in Southeast Asian population

170. Small bowel infestation may result in intestinal obstruction and protein-losing enteropathy

171. Associated with hematuria, dysuria, and hydronephrosis

172. Chronic human infection is associated with gallstones and cholangiocarcinoma

QUESTIONS 173–176

Match the following clinical associations with the appropriate nematode.

   A. *Strongyloides stercoralis*
   B. *Necator americanus*
   C. *Ascaris lumbricoides*
   D. *Trichinella spiralis*

173. Chronic iron deficiency anemia

174. Intestinal obstruction, abdominal pain in toddler

175. Fever, myalgias, and periorbital edema

176. Fever, hypotension, and gram-negative bacillary bacteremia

QUESTIONS 177–181

Match the following descriptions with the appropriate nontuberculous mycobacterium (NTM).

   A. *Mycobacterium avium-intracellulare*
   B. *Mycobacterium kansasii*
   C. *Mycobacterium marinum*
   D. *Mycobacterium abscessus*
   E. *Mycobacterium gordonae*

177. Most common cause of NTM lymphadenitis

178. Rapidly growing NTM; may cause cutaneous, pulmonary, or disseminated disease

179. Cutaneous ulcer in a fisherman

180. Pulmonary infection resembles *M. tuberculosis* but therapy is INH, RIF, and EMB for 18 months

181. Rarely a human pathogen; usually indicative of environmental contamination

QUESTIONS 182–185

Match the following disease processes with the associated *Bartonella* species.

   A. *Bartonella bacilliformis*
   B. *Bartonella henselae*
   C. *Bartonella quintana*
   D. *Bartonella elizabethae*

182. Painful lymphadenopathy in the right axilla 6 weeks following a cat scratch on the right index finger

183. Multiple painless erythematous, papular skin lesions located diffusely over the face, arms, and trunk in a patient with advanced HIV disease

184. Culture-negative aortic valve endocarditis in a homeless alcoholic man

185. Transmitted by the sandfly; leads to high fever and hemolytic anemia in the acute phase, verruga peruana in the chronic phase

QUESTIONS 186–189

Match the following genital ulcer syndromes with the most likely organism.

   A. *Treponema pallidum*
   B. *Hemophilus ducreyi*
   C. *Calymmatobacterium granulomatis*
   D. *Herpes simplex virus*

186. Multiple, elevated beefy granulomatous inguinal lesions

187. Multiple, painful, shallow ulcers

188. Solitary, painful ulcer with shaggy borders and undermining

189. Solitary, painless ulcer with surrounding induration

QUESTIONS 190–196

Match the following infectious complications with the most appropriate defect in host immunity.

   A. Neutropenia
   B. Decreased cell-mediated immunity
   C. Immunoglobulin A deficiency
   D. Complement deficiency
   E. Asplenia

190. *Legionella pneumophila* in a renal transplant patient

191. Severe babesiosis

192. Chronic giardiasis

193. Recurrent meningococcal disease

194. Hepatosplenic candidiasis

195. Overwhelming pneumococcal bacteremia

196. *Pseudomonas aeruginosa* bacteremia

INFECTIOUS DISEASES

ANSWERS

1.(D) *Discussion:* The patient likely has cryptococcal meningitis based on the findings of papilledema, a negative CT scan, and a consistent spinal fluid analysis. Sinus fullness is a common complaint among these patients. There is often little inflammation evident in the spinal fluid of patients with AIDS and cryptococcal meningitis, and the turbidity is likely due to abundant yeasts in the CSF. *Cryptococcus neoformans* is the most common fungal pathogen of the central nervous system and may cause disease in up to 10% of patients with AIDS in the United States. The clinical and laboratory presentation would be unusual for pneumococcal meningitis. PML usually presents with altered mental status and an abnormal CT scan. Toxoplasma encephalitis is unusual in a patient receiving prophylactic TMP/SMX and is usually associated with an abnormal CT scan. (*Cecil, Ch. 352 and 364*)

2.(E) *Discussion:* In a patient with suspected cryptococcal meningitis, both serum and CSF cryptococcal antigen are appropriate tests; CSF titers are positive in at least 95% of HIV-positive patients with cryptococcal meningitis, and serum titers are also positive in the majority of patients. An India ink test is a rapid test that is very likely to be positive in this patient, although it is generally less sensitive than cryptococcal antigen and fungal culture. *Toxoplasm gondii* serum antibody titers may be useful in patients who have negative assays, because only about 3 to 5% of patients with central nervous system toxoplasmosis have negative serum antibody titers. A VDRL test is not likely to be useful in this patient with papilledema, increased intracranial pressure, and turbid CSF with few leukocytes. Although central nervous system syphilis is increasingly common in this population, these clinical and CSF findings would be unusual. (*Cecil, Ch. 352*)

3.(B) *Discussion:* Cryptococcal meningitis in a patient with AIDS requires chronic, lifelong suppression because relapse off therapy is almost inevitable. Comparative trials suggest that fluconazole is effective induction therapy when compared to amphotericin B with or without 5-flucytosine, but a more rapid clinical and microbiologic response plus a better early outcome have led to the use of amphotericin B as induction therapy for most patients with cryptococcal meningitis. The addition of 5-flucytosine appears to provide only marginal benefit to amphotericin B when the latter is dosed at 0.7 mg per kilogram daily. Chronic suppressive therapy with fluconazole, 200 mg daily, is superior to amphotericin B administered weekly, with fewer relapses reported in chronic fluconazole suppression. (*Cecil, Ch. 352; Saag et al*)

4.(A) *Discussion:* Given this patient's history, there is likely an infections cause of fever and leukocytosis. The most likely possibilities include the development of a wound infection, an intra-abdominal abscess, or a central venous catheter–related infection. Stopping antibiotics is unreasonable at this juncture, and there is little evidence that changing to a different regimen or adding a broad-spectrum cephalosporin is useful. Furthermore, the empiric use of fluconazole in this setting is of no proven value. However, the addition of vancomycin to cover multidrug-resistant *Staphylococcus aureus* and *S. epidermidis* and multidrug-resistant enterococcus seems reasonable while awaiting further culture and laboratory data. (*Cecil, Ch. 270*)

5.(B) *Discussion:* The patient presumptively has candidemia, perhaps central venous catheter related. Positive blood cultures for *Candida* sp. are always considered significant and require some form of antifungal therapy, either systemic amphotericin B or fluconazole. Therapy is usually given for 1 to 2 weeks beyond resolution of clinical findings associated with candidemia. In presumed intravenous catheter–related candidemia, removal of the catheter is important. If a central venous catheter is essential, then replacement at a different site is important. Guidewire replacement is associated with a higher rate of persistent candidemia. (*Cecil, Ch. 354*)

6.(B) *Discussion: Torulopsis glabrata* is relatively resistant to fluconazole; therefore, in patients with systemic infections caused by this organism, amphotericin B is probably the antifungal agent of choice. Combination therapy with flucytosine is warranted for patients with disease unresponsive to amphotericin B alone. Combination therapy with amphotericin B and fluconazole is unproven for systemic fungal infections. (*Cecil, Ch. 354; Rex et al*)

7.(E) *Discussion:* The patient is moderately immunocompromised based on his depressed CD4 lymphocyte count, but is not in a range (<200 cells per cubic millimeter that is typical for patients with "classical" opportunistic infections in AIDS. Thus, *Pneumocystis carinii,* cytomegalovirus, and *Toxoplasma gondii* are unlikely pathogens. Furthermore, his illness is rather subacute for pneumococcal pneumonia. His recent exposure to a household contact with pulmonary tuberculosis, the subacute nature of his illness, and the radiographic findings are quite consistent with pulmonary tuberculosis in an HIV-infected patient. (*Cecil, Ch. 311 and 365*)

8.(D) *Discussion:* For the reasons given above, empiric antituberculous therapy is appropriate and probably should have been started at presentation. Empiric antifungal therapy is not warranted at this time, nor is empiric therapy for cytomegalovirus. It the patient is unable to produce sputum, then bronchoscopy is warranted. An open lung biopsy should be reserved for situations in which bronchoscopy has been unhelpful and the patients' clinical status dictates this aggressive approach. (*Cecil, Ch. 311*)

9.(C) *Discussion:* Given the likelihood of pulmonary tuberculosis, most authorities would recommend initial therapy with a four-drug regimen including INH, RIF, PAZ, and EMB or streptomycin. If a multidrug-resistant organism is requested based on clinical or epidemiologic data, then a six-drug initial regimen might be appropriate. (*Cecil, Ch. 311; Iseman*)

10.(D) *Discussion:* Extrapulmonary tuberculosis is more common in patients with underlying cell-mediated immune abnormalities. For instance, over 50% of patients with advanced HIV disease and tuberculosis have extrapulmonary involvement. Hypogammaglobulinemia is the only condition listed that is not associated with cell-mediated immune dysfunction. (*Cecil, Ch. 311*)

11.(C) *Discussion:* Following decades of declining rates of tuberculosis in the United States, a sudden increase in cases occurred in the mid-1980s corresponding to the AIDS epidemic. Coupled with less stringent public health practices that led to poorer compliance with medications, these two factors have led to major increases in tuberculosis incidence in certain major cities and in the nation as a whole. Tuberculosis rates worldwide have risen, and tuberculosis is now the leading cause of infectious morbidity and mortality. (*Cecil, Ch. 311*)

12.(B) *Discussion: Mycobacterium avium-intracellulare* is commonly isolated from patients with advanced HIV disease and is probably responsible for much of the wasting, fever, diarrhea, and pancytopenia seen in these patients. However, it is an uncommon cause of pulmonary disease in patients with AIDS, whereas the other pathogens listed commonly present as interstitial pneumonia. (*Cecil, Ch. 312 and 365*)

13.(D) *Discussion:* Solitary intracerebral lesions in patients with advanced HIV disease are most commonly caused by central nervous system lymphoma, cryptococcoma, and tuberculoma. *Toxoplasma gondii* will occasionally cause solitary lesions but is usually associated with multiple lesions. Aspergillosis is a rare cause of central nervous system mass lesions in this population. (*Cecil, Ch. 364*)

14.(D) *Discussion:* Peripheral neuropathy, vacuolar myelopathy, and aseptic meningitis are all direct consequences of nervous system involvement with HIV, a neurotropic virus. JC virus, a papovavirus, is the cause of PML in immunocompromised patients. (*Cecil, Ch. 364*)

15.(A) *Discussion:* Although a number of opportunistic pathogens may cause biliary disease among patients with AIDS, cytomegalovirus and *Cryptosporidium* are the two most common etiologies. Lymphoma and Kaposi's sarcoma can also cause obstructive cholangiopathy, but these are less common causes of biliary disease. (*Cecil, Ch. 366*)

16.(D) *Discussion:* The clinical description is most consistent with acute retinal necrosis, a syndrome most often caused by herpes simplex virus or varicella-zoster virus. Cytomegalovirus, *Toxoplasma gondii*, and *Histoplasma capsulatum* may also cause retinal destruction, but the process is usually much more indolent and less likely associated with conjunctivitis and keratitis. (*Cecil, Ch. 368*)

17.(A) *Discussion:* Pancytopenia in HIV-infected patients may result from disseminated infection with *Histoplasma capsulatum* and *Mycobacterium avium-intracellulare,* and these organisms are usually easily identified on examination of the bone marrow in these patients. Parvovirus B19, a cause of aplastic crisis in patients with chronic hemolytic anemias, can cause pancytopenia in immunocompromised patients. Kaposi's sarcoma rarely involves the bone marrow and is not usually associated with pancytopenia. (*Cecil, Ch. 369*)

18.(B) *Discussion:* Reversible megaloblastic anemia is commonly seen with the use of AZT. Pancreatitis and peripheral neuropathy are seen much more frequently with dideoxycytidine (ddC) and dideoxyinosine (ddI), respectively. (*Cecil, Ch. 391*)

19.(D) *Discussion:* Women, racial and ethnic minorities, and many high-risk groups such as IV drug users and heterosexually promiscuous persons represent the bulk of newly acquired HIV infections. The perception that AIDS remains a disease largely confined to gay white males is outdated. (*Cecil, Ch. 362*)

20.(A) *Discussion:* The efficiency of HIV transmission form an infected mother to a neonate ranges between 10 and 50%. Although considered high-risk activities, heterosexual intercourse, receptive and intercourse, and needle exposure are all less efficient (probably less than 1% per exposure) means of transmission. Kissing, including deep kissing, has not been associated with HIV transmission. (*Cecil, Ch. 362 and 367*)

21.(E) *Discussion:* HIV infection is associated with a host of immunologic abnormalities in addition to depletion of CD4 lymphocytes. The function of natural killer cells, CD4 and CD8 cells, and B lymphocytes may all be abnormal in HIV infection. Monocytes and macrophages, although infected with HIV and probably responsible for dissemination to other systems, such as the central nervous system, are not easily destroyed through viral cytopathic effect. (*Cecil, Ch. 360*)

22.(E) *Discussion:* The host response to HIV infection is not limited to cell-mediated immune responses. Neutralizing antibodies, antibody-dependent cellular cytotoxicity, and natural killer cells are involved in the host immune response. Monocytes and macrophages probably facilitate the spread of HIV in the host. (*Cecil, Ch. 360*)

23.(B) *Discussion:* Genital ulcer disease is perhaps the most common clinical presentation among patients seen in sexually transmitted diseases clinics in the developing world. In this setting, chancroid, herpes genitalis, syphilis, and donovanosis are seen with varying degrees of frequency. *Neisseria gonorrhoeae* infections, although common, are not a cause of genital ulcer disease. (*Cecil, Ch. 314, 316, 317, 318, and 339; Holmes et al, Ch. 59*)

24.(A) *Discussion:* A number of behaviors are conducive to acquisition and dissemination of sexually transmitted disease. However, none of these is as important as the number and type of different sexual partners. (*Cecil, Ch. 314*)

25.(C) *Discussion:* Numerous studies indicate that *Chlamydia trachomatis* is an important pathogen in women with mucopurulent cervicitis. It is for this reason that treatment with doxycycline or another antichlamydial agent is warranted in all cases of cervicitis, in addition to appropriate therapy for *Neisseria gonorrhoeae*. (*Cecil, Ch. 315 and 323, Holmes et al, Ch. 46*)

26.(E) *Discussion:* Nongonococcal urethritis in men may be caused by *Chlamydia trachomatis,* herpes simplex virus, *Ureaplasma urealyticum,* and *Trichomona vaginalis.* Up to 40% of cases have no proven etiology. *Haemophilus ducreyi* is a cause of genital ulcer disease and lymphadenopathy but does not cause nongonococcal urethritis. (*Cecil, Ch. 323; Holmes et al, Ch. 52*)

27.(E) *Discussion:* The patient's history is most consistent with vaginitis, and the description of foul odor and vaginal irritation sounds characteristic of bacterial vaginosis. Primary genital herpes presents as painful genital lesions and oftentimes as a systemic illness. (*Cecil, Ch. 314; Holmes et al, Ch. 47*)

28.(D) *Discussion:* Bacterial vaginosis is a mixed, "synergistic" vaginal infection caused by an overgrowth of certain vaginal flora. The inciting event is often inapparent, but the disorder is much more common in sexually active women than in virgins, suggesting its sexually transmitted nature. (*Holmes et al, Ch. 47*)

29.(C) *Discussion:* This patient appears to have latent syphilis, and standard therapy involves the administration of benzathine penicillin, 2.4 million units intramuscularly in three doses given 1 week apart. Although there is a very small chance that the patient is suffering from neurosyphilis, the normal CSF formula and negative CSF VDRL test argue against this, and most authorities would not treat for neurosyphilis. Because the patient has both positive serum VDRL and FTA tests, these results cannot be considered as biologic false-positive results, and, given no history of therapy, effective therapy for latent syphilis should be given. (*Cecil, Ch. 318*)

30.(D) *Discussion:* Among patients with prior histories of beta-lactam antibiotic intolerance, doxycycline or erythromycin given for 30 days is the best alternative. There are more data to support the use of doxycycline in this setting, although neither of these drugs is an effective therapy for neurosyphilis. (*Cecil, Ch. 318*)

31.(B) *Discussion: Chlamydia trachomatis* causes a number of illnesses in neonates, children, and adults, including neonatal afebrile pneumonia, endometritis, salpingitis, and the leading cause of blindness worldwide, trachoma. Reiters' syndrome has also been associated with chlamydial infections, particularly nongonococcal urethritis. Despite its prevalence as a genital pathogen, *Chlamydia trachomatis* has not been associated with nonbacterial prostatitis. (*Cecil, Ch. 323; Holmes et al, Ch. 16*)

32.(B) *Discussion:* Q fever, caused by the rickettsia-like organism *Coxiella burnetti,* is an airborne agent that causes acute pneumonia. Two chronic forms of the disease occur, granulomatous hepatitis and chronic infective endocarditis. Chronic cavitary pneumonia is not a clinical feature of Q fever. (*Cecil, Ch. 324*)

33.(C) *Discussion:* The characteristic rash of RMSF is petechial, beginning on the extremities and progressing centrally. Mucous membrane involvement is distinctly uncommon. Headache is common to all rickettsial diseases. Thrombocytopenia and pulmonary involvement are also common. Untreated RMSF has a mortality rate of approximately 25%. (*Cecil, Ch. 324*)

34.(C) *Discussion:* Lyme disease has multiple clinical manifestations, including early and late features. Among the late clinical features of the disease are carditis; pauciarticular arthritis; neurologic symptoms including Bells' palsy, asthenia, mental status changes, and peripheral neuropathy; and distal extremity changes occurring late in untreated disease (acrodermatitis chronica atrophicans). Erythema chronicum migrans is a pathognomonic clinical features of early Lyme disease. (*Cecil, Ch. 321*)

35.(E) *Discussion:* Lyme disease is a clinical and epidemiologic diagnosis, often supported by serologic tests or other laboratory data. Serologic assays are generally unreliable and not very reproducible between laboratories. Cultures of blood, CSF, and skin may be positive but require special techniques and are generally unavailable. Infection with *Borrelia burgdorferi* usually does not lead to a positive VDRL test. (*Cecil, Ch. 321*)

36.(A) *Discussion:* Human ehrlichiosis is caused by two organisms, *Ehrlichia chaffeensis* and *E. equi.* Both organisms infect leukocytes and are often found within the cytoplasm of circulating granulocytes (*E. equi*) and monocytes (*E. chaffeensis*). Leukopenia is a characteristic finding in patients with acute infection. Thrombocytopenia, headache, rash, and aseptic meningitis are common features of ehrlichiosis. (*Cecil, Ch. 324; Fishbein et al*)

37.(E) *Discussion:* Pyrexia (fever) is a response to various physical, chemical, and infectious agents and is generally not considered to be harmful. On the contrary, evidence suggests that fever may have a beneficial effect in the host defense against invading pathogens. It is usually unnecessary to control fever with antipyretics during acute infectious illnesses. However, it would be quite appropriate to control pyrexia in a patient recovering from a myocardial infarction to limit oxygen demand and myocardial damage. (*Cecil, Ch. 264*)

38.(E) *Discussion:* Albumin is not an acute-phase reactant as are fibrinogen, Factor VIII, plasminogen, and alpha$_1$-antitrypsin. Produced in the liver, albumin tends to fall in concentration during acute and chronic infections, particularly if nutrition is compromised. (*Cecil, Ch. 265*)

39.(A) *Discussion:* Although nosocomial pneumonia and surgical wound infections account for the greatest morbidity associated with nosocomial infections, nosocomial urinary tract infections are by far the most common. (*Cecil, Ch. 267*)

40.(B) *Discussion:* Nosocomial pneumonia is most commonly caused by aerobic gram-negative rods and is associated with significant excess hospital stay. Mortality often exceeds 30% for some of the more virulent pathogens such as *Pseudomonas aeruginosa* and *Enterobacter* sp. (*Cecil, Ch. 267 and 273*)

41.(A) *Discussion:* Although all of the methods listed might have an effect on nosocomial transmission of pathogens, handwashing is an effective and often overlooked technique. Most nosocomial infections occur as a result of a breakdown in this technique. (*Cecil, Ch. 267*)

42.(C) *Discussion:* Yellow fever is not endemic to Asia; therefore, pretravel vaccination is unnecessary. However, hepatitis A and B are hyperendemic to this and other developing countries; thus vaccination is recommended. Oral polio vaccine is given as a "booster" to previously vaccinated adults traveling to developing countries because polio remains endemic in many parts of the world. Revaccination for tetanus is recommended for all adults every 10 years. (*Cecil, Ch. 268 and 345*)

43.(D) *Discussion:* Chloroquine and Fansidar-resistant falciparum malaria exists in parts of Thailand, particularly rural areas. There are also mefloquine-resistant strains, but these are less common. Daily doxycycline is given to short-term travelers, but this seems impractical for a 2-year stay. Furthermore, residence in an urban area will significantly decrease the likelihood of malaria. (*Cecil, Ch. 268 and 374*)

44.(D) *Discussion:* Traveler's diarrhea occurs in as many as 50% of travelers to foreign countries; however, prophylaxis is generally unwarranted except for unusual circumstances. Therapy with norfloxacin is usually started at the onset of symptoms and continued for 3 to 5 days. Sexual intercourse is discouraged among travelers, particularly where the risk of HIV and hepatitis B exposure is significant. Rabies vaccination is also encouraged among travelers to developing countries where rabies among domestic animals remains common. (*Cecil, Ch. 268, 298, 314, and 374*)

45.(B) *Discussion:* The mechanism of penicillin resistance among pneumococcal isolates is alteration of penicillin-binding proteins. These isolates do not produce beta-lactamase. (*Cecil, Ch. 273; Applebaum*)

46.(D) *Discussion:* Penicillin G, ceftriaxone, and gentamicin achieve poor concentrations in the CSF in the absence of inflammation, whereas chloramphenicol is actually concentrated in the CSF, exceeding 50% of serum levels. (*Cecil, Ch. 270; Mandell et al, Ch. 15, 16, and 24*)

47.(E) *Discussion:* Drug-induced fever may be caused by virtually any antimicrobial agent, but aminoglycosides are clearly the least likely agents to cause this adverse effect. (*Cecil, Ch. 264*)

48.(C) *Discussion:* Unlike group A streptococcus, the pneumococcus is a relatively inert organism that is not particularly rich in destructive enzymes. The main virulence factor of the pneumococcus is the polysaccharide capsule, which inhibits phagocytosis. (*Cecil, Ch. 271; Mandell et al, Ch. 178*)

49.(B) *Discussion:* Pneumococcal vaccine is recommended for a variety of patient groups who are determined to be at high risk for pneumococcal disease. This includes diabetics; patients with chronic renal, hepatic, pulmonary and/or cardiac disease; patients with chronic hemolytic anemia; and all patients age 65 year or older. To date, young otherwise healthy children are not routinely given pneumococcal vaccine. (*Cecil, Ch. 271*)

50.(D) *Discussion:* The patient has meningitis caused by multidrug-resistant pneumococcus, and the therapy of choice is vancomycin. Chloramphenicol-resistant isolates are uncommon in the United States, but clinical results with susceptible strains indicate that treatment with chloramphenicol is associated with a worse outcome, perhaps because of its activity as a bacteriostatic agent. (*Cecil, Ch. 280; Applebaum*)

51.(B) *Discussion:* The patient has little evidence of recurrent meningitis given the absence of fever or meningismus. The insidious onset of her demise, as well as the papilledema and cranial nerve palsy, are consistent with increased intracranial pressure, which may be associated with bacterial meningitis even after effective therapy. (*Cecil, Ch. 280*)

52.(E) *Discussion:* Among the listed organisms, all are well-recognized valvular pathogens except for *Escherichia coli*. This organism and other enteric gram-negative rods are very uncommon pathogens on native valves but may cause prosthetic valve endocarditis, particularly in the early postoperative period. (*Cecil, Ch. 278*)

53.(B) *Discussion:* Systemic emboli associated with infective endocarditis generally occur before or shortly after effective therapy is initiated, becoming rare following several days of effective antimicrobial therapy. Congestive heart failure, myocardial abscess, and persistently positive blood cultures in spite of appropriate therapy are well-recognized indications for immediate valve replacement. Fungal endocarditis rarely responds to medical therapy alone and should be managed with antifungal therapy and surgical excision of the involved valve. (*Cecil, Ch. 278*)

54.(D) *Discussion:* Among the cardiac conditions listed, a congenital atrial septal defect is the only lesion that is unlikely to be associated with infective endocarditis and, in the absence of other cardiac abnormalities, does not require antibiotic prophylaxis prior to an invasive procedure. (*Cecil, Ch. 278*)

55.(C) *Discussion:* Several studies have indicated a difference in the likelihood of infective endocarditis among patients with *Staphylococcus aureus* bacteremia associated with a removable focus (e.g., central venous catheter) versus those with community-acquired *S. aureus* bacteremia without apparent source. In the former group the risk of infective endocarditis is less than 10%, whereas in the latter group the risk is 30 to 40%. (*Cecil, Ch. 278 and 279; Nolan and Beaty*)

56.(B) *Discussion:* Given the possibility that this patient has infective endocarditis, a 4- to 6-week course of oxacillin is appropriate. Neither the clinical exam nor a negative transthoracic echocardiogram reliably excludes the possibility of staphylococcal infective endocarditis. (*Cecil, Ch. 278 and 279*)

57.(B) *Discussion:* Bacteremia caused by coagulase-negative staphylococci is often considered to be insignificant and to represent contamination. However, in patients with intravascular prosthetic devices, these organisms can represent true pathogens. This patient likely has late prosthetic valve endocarditis due to *Staphylococcus xylosus*. The most appropriate management at this point would involve obtaining additional blood cultures and starting vancomycin and gentamicin until more data are available. (*Cecil, Ch. 278 and 279*)

58.(A) *Discussion: Streptococcus pneumoniae* is the most common cause of ABM in adults. Frequent underlying illnesses include alcoholism, diabetes mellitus, and chronic glucocorticosteroid use. (*Cecil, Ch. 280*)

59.(A) *Discussion:* If one assumes that the patient is reliable, the malaria caused by *Plasmodium vivax* is unlikely. Falciparum malaria, however, remains possible. Acute fever in the traveler should always lead to suspicion of malaria, typhoid, acute viral hepatitis, brucellosis, viral hemorrhagic fever, and complications of amebiasis. (*Cecil, Ch. 268; Mandell et al, Ch. 302*)

60.(A) *Discussion:* It is appropriate to obtain blood cultures, a peripheral blood smear to look for malaria forms, an abdominal ultrasound to look for intrahepatic abscess, and hepatitis serologies. An upright "plain film" of the abdomen is not likely to be helpful in this situation. (*Cecil, Ch. 268; Mandell et al, Ch. 302*)

61.(E) *Discussion:* The patient's history and positive blood cultures suggest that his illness is due to *Salmonella typhi*. Although all of the drugs listed have varying degrees of activity against this organism, chloramphenicol is the drug that has been associated with the best outcome and is the most commonly used drug worldwide for typhoid. Ampicillin is also active against most strains of *S. typhi*. (*Cecil, Ch. 292*)

62.(E) *Discussion:* Each of the organisms listed is a well-known cause of traveler's diarrhea. However, the greatest number of cases are caused by enterotoxogenic *Escherichia coli*. (*Cecil, Ch. 298*)

63.(E) *Discussion:* Among the organisms listed, only *Salmonella choleraesuis* is commonly associated with both bacteremia and metastatic infection, usually involving the aorta and other large arteries. *Salmonella* sp. are overall the most common gram-negative agents causing mycotic aneurysms. *Vibrio cholerae* is rarely bacteremic. (*Cecil, Ch. 293*)

64.(E) *Discussion:* Imipenem/cilastatin is the broadest antibacterial agent, and this includes a very broad anaerobic spectrum. Clindamycin, metronidazole, and chloramphenicol have excellent activity against anaerobic pathogens. (*Cecil, Ch. 270; Mandell et al, Ch. 17, 21, and 23*)

65.(B) *Discussion:* The patient describes chronic diarrhea, weight loss, excessive flatus, and belching but no fever or other signs of systemic illness. These features are classic for chronic intestinal giardiasis. Diarrhea caused by *Escherichia coli*, *Salmonella* sp., or *Shigella* sp. is usually acute, self-limited, and associated with fever. Cryptosporidiosis is usually associated with watery diarrhea, vomiting, and low-grade fever and may be difficult to distinguish from giardiasis. (*Cecil, Ch. 298 and 380*)

66.(D) *Discussion:* The retroviruses are unique in their ability to generate DNA from viral RNA through the action of the enzyme reverse transcriptase. This allows for the incorporation of proviral DNA into the host genome, making the virus a "permanent" part of the infected host cell. The only human retroviruses include HTLV-I, HTLV-II, HIV-1, and HIV-2. Each of these viruses possess reverse transcriptase. (*Cecil, Ch. 361*)

67.(D) *Discussion:* Rhinovirus, the respiratory virus often associated with the common cold, may lead to sinusitis and pharyngitis but rarely bronchitis. Influenza viruses A and B and respiratory syncytial virus classically lead to bronchitis and bronchiolitis, respectively, following a brief upper respiratory illness. Coronovirus has been associated with upper and lower respiratory involvement. (*Cecil, Ch. 329*)

68.(A—True; B—True; C—True; D—False; E—False) *Discussion:* There are several clearly defined risk factors for a poor outcome in cryptococcal meningitis. Among these factors are underlying immune dysfunction (especially HIV infection), absence of headache, altered mental status, high CSF and/or serum cryptococcal antigen titers, and a CSF WBC count of ≤20 cells per cubic millimeter. Thus, in this disease, the absence of inflammation as evidenced by a low CSF leukocyte count and absent headache portends a poor outcome. (*Cecil, Ch. 352*)

69.(A—True; B—False; C—False; D—True; E—True) *Discussion: Blastomyces dermatitidis* is a dimorphic fungus that is usually acquired through inhalation of infectious spores. Most acute infections are asymptomatic or cause a mild, self-limited, "atypical" pneumonia. Following the lungs, the skin is the most common site of involvement, although the skeletal system and male genitourinary system are also common extrapulmonary sites. The presumptive diagnosis of blastomycosis is based on the typical appearance of broad-based budding yeasts on histopathologic specimens. Diagnosis is confirmed by culture. Serology is not a reliable method of diagnosis at this time. Itraconazole has become the oral azole of choice for uncomplicated blastomycosis, replacing ketoconazole in this role. Severe, frequently fatal infections most often occur in immunocompromised patients and result from widespread disseminated and multiple visceral organ involvement. (*Cecil, Ch. 350; Pappas et al*)

70.(A—False; B—True; C—True; D—True; E—False) *Discussion:* Coccidioidomycosis is a deep fungal infection caused by the fungus *Coccidioides immitis*. Most infections occur through inhalation of infectious spores, but person-to-person transmission is rare. The typical chest roentgenographic findings include solitary infiltrates, nodules, and thin-walled cavities. Extrapulmonary dissemination is common among immunocompromised patients, especially those with AIDS. Coccidioidal meningitis is among the most serious extrapulmonary complications of this disease, and it is virtually always fatal if untreated. The diagnosis of coccidioidomycosis is based on isolation of the organism from clinical specimens, but a presumptive diagnosis can be made based on serologic assays. The most commonly utilized of these tests is the complement fixation assay. (*Cecil, Ch. 349*)

71.(A—False; B—True; C—False; D—True; E—False) *Discussion:* Acute infections with *Histoplasma capsulatum* are usually asymptomatic or mildly asymptomatic; even among those patients with acute pneumonitis, antifungal therapy is probably unnecessary. Relapsing disease is common following therapy for patients with chronic pulmonary and disseminated disease. Mucocutaneous findings associated with disseminated disease include rash, cutaneous nodules, ulcers, and oropharyngeal ulceration. Over 90% of patients with AIDS and histoplasmosis present with disseminated disease. (*Cecil, Ch. 348; Sarosi and Johnson*)

72.(A—False; B—False; C—True; D—True; E—False) *Discussion:* In contrast to public perception regarding leprosy, the disease is not highly contagious, afflicting fewer than 5% of household contacts. *Mycobacterium leprae* is not easily cultivated on artificial media in part because of its very slow growth rate. More severe disease (as seen with lymphomatous leprosy) may be in part caused by selective T-cell unresponsiveness to important *M. leprae* antigens. Because *M. leprae* is a neutrotopic organism, palpable nerves are found in all stages of the disease but are particularly common in later stages. Polar tuberculoid leprosy is among the milder forms of the disease and is associated with very few organisms on biopsy specimens. (*Cecil, Ch. 313*)

73.(A—True; B—True; C—False; D—False; E—False) *Discussion:* Few comparative studies have examined the empiric use of glucocorticosteroids in disseminated fungal and mycobacterial disease; however, most experts argue that steroids may be effective in preventing complications associated with meningeal and pericardial tuberculosis. There is less evidence to support empiric steroids for miliary tuberculosis, and no data to support their use in disseminated histoplasmosis or blastomycosis in the absence of adrenal insufficiency. (*Cecil, Ch. 311*)

74.(All are True) *Discussion:* Treatment for uncomplicated pulmonary tuberculosis has evolved significantly over the last four decades. The current regimen involves the use of three or four drugs for 2 months followed by dual therapy with INH and RIF for 4 months. Acceptable alternatives include INH and RIF for 9 months or INH and EMB for 18 to 24 months. (*Cecil, Ch. 311*)

75.(A—True; B—True; C—False; D—True; E—True) *Discussion:* The criteria for initializing INH prophylaxis have been recently adapted to apply to a very heterogenous group of patients. For patients who do not fall into "high-risk" groups, a positive skin test is defined as ≥15 mm induration. For severely immunocompromised patients, a positive test is ≥5 mm. For patients at "moderate risk" and those from high incidence areas, a positive skin test is ≥10 mm. (*Cecil, Ch. 311*)

76.(A—True; B—False; C—False; D—False; E—True) *Discussion:* Among the many opportunistic infections complicating advanced HIV disease, only two of the entities listed have been shown in clinical trials to warrant primary prophylaxis. Virtually all authorities agree regarding primary prophylaxis for *Pneumocystis caranii* pneumonia in patients with CD4 lymphocytes ≤200 cells per cubic millimeter. Debate exists over the use of rifabutin for prophylaxis of *Mycobacterium avium-intracellulare* infections, although published data support prophylaxis. Studies are in progress to determine the utility of primary prophylaxis for histoplasmosis, cryptococcosis, and toxoplasmosis in high-risk patients. (*Cecil, Ch. 372*)

77.(A—True; B—True; C—True; D—True; E—False) *Discussion:* Chronic diarrhea is common among HIV-infected patients and is often attributed to cryptosporidium, microsporidium, cytomegalo-virus, and HIV enteropathy. These entities are usually chronic, and are only marginally amenable to therapy. *Clostridium difficile* causes acute colitis in these patients and is treatable with oral vancomycin, metronidazole, bacitracin, or cholestyramine. (*Cecil, Ch. 366*)

78.(A—True; B—True; C—True; D—True; E—False) *Discussion:* Neoplasms are common among patients with AIDS, particularly those that have been linked to a viral etiology. This is particularly true of Hodgkin's disease and B-cell lymphoma, both of which have been linked to chronic EBV, and cervical and oral carcinoma, which have been linked to certain strains of human papillomaviruses. Presently, there is no good evidence to link gastric adenocarcinoma and HIV infection. (*Cecil, Ch. 369*)

79.(A—True; B—False; C—True; D—True; E—False) *Discussion:* HIVAN is most commonly seen in blacks, but only about 50% of patients with HIVAN have a history of IV drug use. The disease may occur at any time during the course of HIV disease, including patients with otherwise asymptomatic disease. Heavy proteinuria usually precedes end-stage renal disease caused by HIVAN. (*Cecil, Ch. 370*)

80.(All are True) *Discussion:* HIV is associated with a number of rheumatologic syndromes, although the etiology of these disorders are not completely understood. Clearly, there is an "autoimmune" component to HIV disease that may contribute not only to the development of rheumatologic syndromes but also to disease-progressive immunosuppression as measured by declining numbers of CD4 lymphocytes. (*Cecil, Ch. 370*)

81.(A—True; B—True; C—True; D—True; E—False) *Discussion:* Antiretroviral therapy is generally considered to be a useful adjunct to overall care in patients with symptomatic HIV disease regardless of CD4 counts. Asymptomatic patients who have CD4 counts ≤500 cells per cubic milliliter are usually offered therapy, whereas those whose CD4 lymphocyte counts exceed 500 cells per cubic millimeter are normally not offered therapy. (*Cecil, Ch. 371*)

82.(All are True) *Discussion:* It is important to realize that direct viral cytopathic effects cannot account for CD4 cell depletion alone. Even among patients with advanced disease, only about 1% of circulating CD4 cells are infected with HIV. Therefore, other mechanisms must be operative. (*Cecil, Ch. 360*)

83.(A—True; B—False; C—True; D—False; E—False) *Discussion:* Both HIV-1 and HIV-2 are single-stranded RNA retroviruses, but they possess only about 50% genetic homology. Both viruses demonstrate remarkable genetic diversity, accounting for the large degree of strain variation seen with HIV-1 and HIV-2. Both viruses probably descended from simian viruses, but only HIV-2 is related to African green monkey and sooty mangabey strains. HIV-1 probably descended from chimpanzee strains of simian immunodeficiency virus. HIV-1 generally has greater affinity for the CD4 molecule than HIV-2, possibly accounting for the more rapid immune destruction and disease progression seen among patients infected with HIV-1. (*Cecil, Ch. 361*)

84.(All are True) *Discussion:* PID is most often a clinical diagnosis, but it is easily confused with other important entities. For this reason, many authorities quip that PID really stands for ''pretty inaccurate diagnosis.'' A clinical diagnosis of PID is accurate only about 65 to 70% of the time based on laparoscopic studies. (*Cecil, Ch. 314; Holmes et al, Ch. 49 and 50*)

85.(A—True; B—True; C—True; D—True; E—False) *Discussion:* Traditionally, *Neisseria gonorrhoeae* and *Chlamydia trachomatis* are linked to acute and chronic salpingitis, respectively. In addition, aerobic gram-negative rods and anaerobes have been isolated from the fallopian tubes of a substantial proportion of women with chronic salpingitis. *Staphylococcus aureus* is rarely, if ever associated with salpingitis. (*Holmes et al, Ch. 49 and 50*)

86.(A—True; B—True; C—False; D—True; E—False) *Discussion:* The major complications associated with salpingitis include infertility and ectopic pregnancy. Indeed, approximately 20% of women experiencing an episode of salpingitis will become infertile. Chronic pelvic pain is commonly associated with chronic salpingitis, and may persist even following effective antimicrobial therapy. (*Cecil, Ch. 315 and 323; Holmes et al, Ch. 49 and 50*)

87.(A—True; B—False; C—False; D—True; E—True) *Discussion:* Disseminated gonococcal infection occurs predominantly in women; the majority have asymptomatic genital infections. The classic presentation is the development of characteristic pustular, necrotic lesions occurring on the extremities. These are usually fewer than 20 in number. Patients may experience tenosynovitis as well. Following this phase, many patients will develop monoarticular or pauciarticular arthritis that is usually culture and Gram's stain negative. The diagnosis is usually based on clinical findings. Rarely, an aggressive and rapidly destructive form of endocarditis may occur with fulminant disseminated gonococcal infection. (*Cecil, Ch. 315*)

88.(A—True; B—True; C—True; D—True; E—False) *Discussion:* There are several single-dose therapies for uncomplicated gonococcal urethritis, cervicitis, pharyngitis, and proctitis, all of which result in cure rates exceeding 95%. Amoxicillin, with or without clavulanate, is no longer recommended for therapy of any form of gono-

coccal infection because of the prevalence of beta-lactamase and chromosomally-mediated resistant strains. (*Cecil, Ch. 315*)

89.(A—True; B—True; C—False; D—False; E—True) *Discussion:* Ceftriaxone and azithromycin, given as single doses, are both effective therapies for chancroid. Erythromycin is also effective therapy but must be given in multiple doses for 1 week, thereby making compliance an important factor. Neither tetracycline nor amoxicillin is considered effective therapy for chancroid. (*Cecil, Ch. 317*)

90.(A—True; B—False; C—False; D—True; E—True) *Discussion:* Syphilis is a disease primarily transmitted through sexual contact, with few cases associated with nonsexual exposure. These are marked socioeconomic and racial factors that characterize the current epidemic. Most cases occur in poor, inner city environments, with blacks outnumbering whites about 25:1. Exchange of sex for drugs is a common epidemiologic feature. HIV transmission is very likely enhanced by the presence of an active primary genital lesion. (*Cecil, Ch. 318*)

91.(A—False; B—False; C—True; D—False) *Discussion: Treponema pallidum* is not culturable on artificial media; therefore, isolation of the organism is limited to very few research centers using animal models. The diagnosis of syphilis therefore rests on serologic assays and visualization of the organism from clinical specimens. Cutaneous and genital lesions that are positive by darkfield microscopic examination for motile spirochetes are sufficient for a diagnosis of primary syphilis. Specimens from oral mucosal lesions are not useful because of the presence of spirochetes that normally reside in the mouth. In primary syphilis serology may be negative, but in secondary syphilis both the screening nontreponemal assays (VDRL, rapid plasma reagin) and the confirmatory treponemal assays (FTA, MHA-TP) are virtually always positive. (*Cecil, Ch. 318*)

92.(A—False; B—True; C—False; D—False; E—True) *Discussion: Chlamydia pneumoniae* and *C. psittaci* both cause respiratory illness, although disease caused by the former is much milder than psittacosis. *C. psittaci* may also cause extrapulmonary disease, most notably infective endocarditis. Whereas *C. pneumoniae* is probably transmitted person to person, there is little evidence to suggest this for *C. psittaci*. Diagnosis of both infections is generally through serology because cell culture methodology is cumbersome and potentially dangerous. Tetracycline is the recommended drug of choice for both agents. (*Cecil, Ch. 323*)

93.(A—True; B—True; C—False; D—False; E—True) *Discussion:* Human ehrlichiosis has recently been described in the United States, and is due to *Ehrlichia chaffeensis* (human monocytic ehrlichiosis) and *E. equi* (human granulocytic ehrlichiosis). The disease resembles RMSF but is generally milder. Most cases appear to be tick borne and occur in the eastern and midwestern United States. The drug of choice for both forms of the disease is tetracycline (doxycycline). (*Cecil, Ch. 324; Fishbein et al*)

94.(All are True) *Discussion:* Each of the cytokines listed has pyrogenic activity. All are produced by macrophages and/or lymphocytes and are induced by a number of factors, most notably lipopolysaccharides (endotoxin) and other microbial products. (*Cecil, Ch. 264*)

95.(A—True; B—True; C—False; D—False; E—False) *Discussion:* The addition of a clavulanate to ticarcillin enhances the spectrum of ticarcillin to include beta-lactamase–producing gram-positive and anaerobic bacteria. Because many aerobic gram-negative bacilli produce several types of beta-lactamase, this combination is not necessarily more effective against these organisms. The addition of clavulanate to a penicillin does not improve activity against oxacillin-resistant *Staphylococcus aureus* and penicillin-resistant pneumococcus, neither of which produces beta-lactamase as a mechanism for resistance, but rather have altered penicillin-binding proteins. (*Cecil, Ch. 270; Mandell, Ch. 15*)

96.(A—True; B—True; C—True; D—False; E—False) *Discussion:* Combination antimicrobial therapy has proven efficacy in relatively few situations. In uncomplicated viridans streptococcal endocarditis, 2 weeks of gentamicin and penicillin is equivalent to 4 weeks of penicillin alone. Enterococcal endocarditis is virtually always treated with two agents, either penicillin or vancomycin plus an aminoglycoside. Fever in the neutropenic patient is empirically treated with two and often three compounds, although monotherapy with a broad-spectrum beta-lactam agent is sometimes used. Uncomplicated *Staphylococcus aureus* and *Escherichia coli* bacteremia do not usually warrant combination therapy. (*Cecil, Ch. 270*)

97.(All are True) *Discussion:* Mycoplasma pneumoniae has myriad systemic manifestations in addition to the well-described atypical pneumonia syndrome. Deaths caused by acute infection, although rare, usually result from encephalitis. (*Cecil, Ch. 272*)

98.(A—False; B—True; C—True; D—False; E—True) *Discussion:* Aerobic gram-negative bacillary pneumonia is largely a nosocomial complication with mortality rates that often exceed 30%. The clinical cause may be acute or indolent, and extensive tissue destruction with cavity formation is common. The etiologic diagnosis of pneumonia is often difficult, and sputum cultures correlate poorly with blood, pleural fluid, and tissue cultures. A good-quality sputum Gram's stain is probably at least as important as a sputum culture. (*Cecil, Ch. 273*)

99.(A—True; B—True; C—True; D—False; E—False) *Discussion:* Cigarette smoking, glucocorticosteroid use, and age over 50 years are well-described risk factors for legionellosis. Cytotoxic chemotherapy and neutropenia are not risk factors. (*Cecil, Ch. 275*)

100.(A—True; B—True; C—True; D—False; E—True) *Discussion: Legionella* infections respond to a number of antibacterial agents but are not effectively treated by currently available beta-lactams, except perhaps imipenem. Erythromycin, tetracycline, quinolones, and newer macrolides have excellent *in vitro* and *in vivo* activity. Rifampin is sometimes added in more refractory cases. (*Cecil, Ch. 275*)

101.(A—True; B—True; C—False; D—True; E—True) *Discussion:* Although antimicrobial prophylaxis is commonly practiced to prevent infective endocarditis in patients with pre-existing valvular lesions, its efficacy has been widely questioned. Nonetheless, procedures that are likely to be associated with transient bacteremia are conditions that warrant prophylaxis. Among the procedures listed, only bronchoscopy with bronchoalveolar lavage is not likely to be associated with bacteremia. (*Cecil, Ch. 278; Dajani et al*)

102.(A—True; B—True; C—True; D—False; E—True) *Discussion:* Invasive *Staphylococcus aureus* infection is usually preceded by skin colonization with the organism. Conditions that predispose to colonization include those that lead to breaks in the integrity of the skin. Examples of these conditions include chronic hemodialysis, IV drug abuse, insulin-requiring diabetes, and chronic dermatitis. (*Cecil, Ch. 279*)

103.(A—False; B—False; C—True; D—True; E—False) *Discussion:* The use of glucocorticosteroids in ABM has been studied only in children, particularly those with *Haemophilus influenzae* meningitis. The benefits derived from steroids appear to be in the prevention of neurodeficits, with a small impact on mortality. Assuming that the effect of steroids is mediated through limitation of inflammation, it is important to begin steroids prior to or simultaneous with the administration of antibiotics to minimize the effect of tumor necrosis factor. It is difficult to extrapolate the results of previous studies to adults with ABM and children with non–*H. influenzae* ABM. (*Cecil, Ch. 280 and 282; Odio et al*)

104.(A—False; B—False; C—True; D—True; E—False) *Discussion:* Pertussis is one of the more contagious respiratory infections, infecting 80% or more of nonimmune household contacts. Neither infection nor vaccination confers lifelong immunity, so that reinfection in previously vaccinated adults is not uncommon. Acute infection is often associated with marked lymphocytosis. Treatment with erythromycin is effective only in the early stages of infection, and the convalescent stage may last for several months. (*Cecil, Ch. 284*)

105.(A—True; B—True; C—True; D—False; E—False) *Discussion:* Tularemia may result from ingestion, inhalation, direct inoculation, or tick transmission of the etiologic agent, *Francisella tularensis*. Pneumonia may result from aerosol exposure or bacteremic spread. A sporotrichroid form may result from direct inoculation or tick exposure. The organism is fastidious and hazardous to deal with. Although streptomycin remains the drug of choice, tetracycline is a reasonable alternative in milder disease, although the relapse rate with tetracycline therapy is higher. (*Cecil, Ch. 301*)

106.(A—False; B—True; C—True; D—True; E—False) *Discussion:* Nocardiosis occurs most commonly in patients with impaired cellular immunity, with which multiple organ involvement is common. Central nervous system involvement is usually characterized by focal intracerebral lesions that are multi-inoculated. Sulfur granules are typical of actinomycosis, not *Nocardia,* infections. Isolation of *Nocardia* sp. from the sputum of immunocompetent individuals with chronic lung disease but without clinical or radiographic evidence of invasive disease constitutes colonization and need not be treated. (*Cecil, Ch. 307*)

107.(A—True; B—True; C—True; D—False; E—True) *Discussion:* Herpes simplex virus is susceptible to a number of antiviral agents, including acyclovir, ganciclovir, vidarabine, and trifluorothymidine, all of which are nucleoside analogues. Ribavirin is active against respiratory syncytial virus and certain hemorrhagic fever viruses. (*Cecil, Ch. 39*)

108.(All are True) *Discussion:* Influenza vaccine is safe, effective, and indicated in older individuals, nursing home residents, immunocompromised patients, all health care providers, and virtually anyone wishing to reduce the risk of influenza and its complications. (*Cecil, Ch. 332; Nichol et al*)

109.(A—False; B—False; C—True; D—False; E—True) *Discussion:* Although measles is uncommon in most developed countries, it continues to be highly endemic in many developing countries; thus healthy travelers to these areas should consider revaccination if born after 1957 (when vaccination became available). The vaccination consists of a live attenuated vaccine that is not given to pregnant women or immunocompromised patients. (*Cecil, Ch. 334*)

110.(All are True) *Discussion:* EBV has been linked to a number of neoplastic processes, including nasopharyngeal carcinoma, post-transplantation lymphoproliferative disorder, central nervous system B-cell lymphoma, and Burkitt's lymphoma. Hodgkin's disease is less strongly linked, but recent evidence suggests a relationship to EBV. (*Cecil, Ch. 341*)

111.(A—True; B—False; C—True; D—False; E—False) *Discussion:* HTLV-I infection is related to tropical spastic paraparesis (HTLV-I–associated myelopathy) and adult T-cell lymphoma. Rare associations with an AIDS-like illness and polymyositis are reported. (*Cecil, Ch. 342*)

112.(A—False; B—True; C—False; D—True; E—True) *Discussion:* Infections due to Lassa fever virus, Ebola virus, and Crimean-Congo hemorrhagic fever virus generally require strict isolation because of their propensity for nosocomial transmission. The majority of outbreaks involving these two viruses have involved significant numbers of health care workers, including the recent Ebola outbreaks. The remaining hemorrhagic fever viruses are not commonly transmitted person to person. (*Cecil, Ch. 345*)

113.(All are True) *Discussion:* Fulminant falciparum malaria is a severe disease that may cause multiorgan failure. Acute renal failure, pulmonary edema, and seizures are common manifestations of severe falciparum malaria and are associated with a mortality of at least 25%. (*Cecil, Ch. 374*)

114.(A—False; B—True; C—True; D—False) *Discussion:* Among the four human malaria parasites, only *Plasmodium vivax* and *P. ovale* have chronic intrahepatic stages which require treatment with primaquine to prevent relapse. (*Cecil, Ch. 374*)

115.(A—False; B—True; C—True; D—True; E—True) *Discussion:* Chloroquine-resistant *Plasmodium falciparum* is now widespread in endemic areas except for the Middle East and parts of Central America. Thus, a traveler returning from West Africa with falciparum malaria must be assumed to have chloroquine-resistant infection. Effective alternatives include mefloquine, quinine, and quinidine. Halofantine is less effective than mefloquine but acceptable. Pyrimethamine-sulfadoxine (Fansidar) continues to be a useful alternative, although resistant strains have emerged in certain areas. (*Cecil, Ch. 374*)

116.(C); 117.(E); 118.(B); 119.(A); 120.(F); 121.(D) *Discussion:* The microscopic morphologies described are characteristic of each of the matching organisms. Because cultures of many fungal organisms may require several weeks for adequate growth, a presumptive diagnosis of fungal infection is often made on the basis of microscopic morphology from histopathologic specimens. This is an essential component for the diagnosis of invasive fungal infection because serologic assays, except for some cases of cryptococcosis and coccidioidomycosis, are generally unreliable. (*Cecil, Ch. 347*)

122.(B); 123.(C); 124.(F); 125.(A); 126.(D); 127.(E) *Discussion:* Each of the organisms listed may cause the cutaneous ulcer syndrome. Because these disorders are similar in their clinical appearance and because culture confirmation is often delayed or unavailable, a biopsy with special studies for acid-fast bacilli, fungi, and other likely organisms is appropriate. Finally, a detailed history is important to determine exposure risks. (*Cecil, Ch. 301, 302, 307, 312, 350, and 377*)

128.(C); 129.(D); 130.(E); 131.(B); 132.(A) *Discussion:* Although orally available antifungal compounds have been a major advance in therapy, amphotericin B remains the drug of choice for febrile neutropenic patients. Fluconazole is active against most *Candida* sp., *Cryptococcus neoformans,* and the endemic fungi, including *Coccidiodes immitis.* Itraconazole is active against the endemic dimorphic fungi and is the only oral antifungal agent for invasive aspergillosis. The oral absorption of ketoconazole, and to a lesser extent itraconazole, is limited in the absence of gastric acidity. Flucytosine remains a drug to be used in combination with amphotericin B and monitored carefully for its many toxicities. (*Cecil, Ch. 347; Mandell et al, Ch. 31*)

133.(A); 134.(C); 135.(D); 136.(B) *Discussion:* Pinta, caused by the non-syphilitic treponeme *Treponema carateum,* is diagnosed by finding motile spirochetes from suspicious skin lesions. Serologic tests cross-react with syphilis serology. Leptospirosis may be diagnosed by serology or recovery of the organism from urine. Urine excretion of the organism may persist for weeks following clinical recovery. Lyme disease is a clinical diagnosis based on characteristic findings, including erythema chronicum migrans. Epidemic relapsing fever has an acute mortality in untreated patients of approximately 40%. The diagnosis is made by identification of spirochetes on peripheral blood smear during febrile episodes. (*Cecil, Ch. 319, 320, and 322*)

137.(E); 138.(A); 139.(F); 140.(D); 141.(B); 142.(C) *Discussion:* Brill-Zinsser disease is the reactivation form of latent *Rickettsia prowazekii* infection, characterized by mild typhus-like symptoms, often occurring years after initial infection. Tache noire is the characteristic eschar associated with Mediterranean spotted fever (Boutonneuse fever, North African tick typhus), which is caused by *R. conorii*. Rash is not characteristic of Q fever, caused by *Coxiella burnetti*. Murine typhus is a more benign illness than RMSF and is transmitted to humans via the rat flea. The rash of typhus begins in the trunk and face, spreading to the extremities. *R. akari* causes rickettsial pox, a benign illness characterized by a papulovesicular rash on the trunk and abdomen. RMSF, caused by *R. rickettsii*, is the most severe of the rickettsial illnesses and is associated with a 25% mortality in untreated cases. (*Cecil, Ch. 324*)

143.(B); 144.(C); 145.(A); 146.(E); 147.(D) *Discussion:* The non–beta-lactam antibacterial agents act through a number of mechanisms, including impaired synthesis of cell wall components (vancomycin), inhibition of protein synthesis through binding to ribosomes (aminoglycosides, macrolides), inhibition of DNA gyrase (quinolones), and inhibition of dihydrofolate reductase (trimethoprim). (*Cecil, Ch. 270; Mandell et al, Ch. 20, 24, 26, and 27*)

148.(D); 149.(A); 150.(C); 151.(B) *Discussion:* The beta-hemolytic streptococci are characterized clinically by marked propensity for tissue invasion and can be associated with severe systemic toxicity. *Streptococcus pyogenes* can be associated with necrotizing fasciitis and marked tissue necrosis. *S. agalactiae* is a common cause of diabetic foot infection and osteomyelitis. Cellulitis in the saphenous vein harvest site is usually attributed to group C streptococcus. Group F streptococcus and a related organism, *S. milleri*, are pus-forming organisms often found in soft tissue and intra-abdominal abscesses. Each of these organisms is susceptible to penicillin. (*Cecil, Ch. 276*)

152.(B); 153.(C); 154.(D); 155.(C) *Discussion:* Most cases of adult botulism are the result of ingestion of pre-formed toxin from *Clostridium botulinum*. Infant and wound botulism occur when the organism produces toxin following ingestion or contamination of a wound with viable *C. botulinum* spores. Tetanus is the result of toxin (tetanospasmin) produced by *C. tetani* and is usually associated with wound contamination with viable spores. Antitoxin is administered for both disorders as adjunctive therapy to supportive care. Profuse watery diarrhea is not a regular component of either tetanus or botulism. (*Cecil, Ch. 288 and 289*)

156.(C); 157.(A); 158.(E); 159.(B); 160.(D) *Discussion:* During and immediately following a bout of measles, many patients will develop cutaneous anergy. There are many reports of worsening of underlying infections such as tuberculosis following measles. Adenovirus type 7 is the most virulent of the adenoviruses and may cause pharyngoconjunctival fever or severe systemic disease. Parvovirus B19 may cause unexplained fever, anemia, and monoarticular arthritis in young pregnant women, who seem to be particularly prone to the development of this infection. Mumps is a leading cause of orchitis and aseptic meningitis in young, nonvaccinated adults. Infants and children with congenital rubella may shed virus in urine and saliva for months or years following birth. (*Cecil, Ch. 333, 334, 335, and 338*)

161.(A); 162.(C); 163.(B); 164.(D) *Discussion:* Arthropod-borne encephalitis viruses occur in summer and early fall. Mortality is unusual in patients with western equine encephalitis and California encephalitis. Mortality is common in eastern equine encephalitis (70%) and increases with age among patients with St. Louis encephalitis (up to 30%). Apparent disease is inversely related to age in western equine encephalitis. (*Cecil, Ch. 346*)

165.(D); 166.(C); 167.(B); 168.(A) *Discussion:* African trypanosomiasis is divided into two forms: Rhodesian and Gambian sleeping sickness. *Trypanosoma rhodesiense* causes a much more acute encephalopathy. Surinam is the drug of choice for humans. *T. brucei brucei* is a nonhuman pathogen that causes a chronic wasting illness in African livestock. All three agents are transmitted by the bite of the tsetse fly. American trypanosomiasis (Chagas' disease) is caused by *T. cruzii* and transmitted by the reduvid bug. Chronic manifestation include dilated cardiomyopathy and megaesophagus. (*Cecil, Ch. 375 and 376*)

169.(B); 170.(D); 171.(A); 172.(C) *Discussion:* *Schistosoma hematobium* is associated with hematuria and inflammation in and around the bladder and ureters. The inflammation is a result of egg deposition in the involved tissues. The lung fluke, *Paragonimus westermanii*, causes "endemic hemoptysis" and chronic pulmonary lesions in infected persons of Southeast Asia. *Clonorchis sinensis*, the Chinese liver fluke, resides in the smaller intrahepatic bile ducts and gallbladder. *Fasciolopsis buski*, the intestinal fluke, may cause intestinal obstruction and/or small bowel ulceration leading to diarrhea and protein-losing enteropathy. (*Cecil, Ch. 385 and 386*)

173.(B); 174.(C); 175.(D); 176.(A) *Discussion:* Chronic colonic infection with *Necator americanus* can lead to intestinal blood loss and iron deficiency anemia. *Ascaris* infections, because of the large size of the nematode (up to 12 inches), may cause abdominal pain and intestinal obstruction, expecially in younger children. Acute infection with *Trichinella spiralis* is associated with systemic symptoms and signs, including fever, myalgias, muscle tenderness, and periorbital edema. Hyperinfection with *Strongyloides stercoralis* is seen in immunocompromised patients and is often associated with gram-negative bacteremia, meningitis, shock, and multiorgan failure. (*Cecil, Ch. 387*)

177.(A); 178.(D); 179.(C); 180.(B); 181.(E) *Discussion:* NTM are an uncreasingly important group of pathogens, particularly among immunocompromised individuals. Each of these organisms can cause disseminated disease or may be localized to one organ system. *Mycobacterium avium-intracellulare* is the most common cause of NTM lymphadenitis. *M. marinum* exists in aquatic environments and may cause nodular lymphangitis. *M. kansasii* causes pulmonary disease similar to tuberculosis but requires prolonged three-drug therapy. *M. abscessus* is a rapidly growing NTM causing localized or disseminated disease in immunocompromised hosts. *M. gordonae* is usually an environmental contaminant, although occasionally it has been implicated in certain wound infections. (*Cecil, Ch. 312*)

182.(B); 183.(B); 184.(C); 185.(A) *Discussion:* *Bartonella henselae* causes the majority of cases of cat scratch disease, although some cases may be related to infection with a related organism, *Afipia felis*. Bacillary angiomatosis in AIDS patients is also caused by *B. henselae*, although *B. quintana* may be responsible for a small proportion of cases. A newly described entity of "culture-negative" endocarditis in homeless alcoholic men is largely due to *B. quintana*, although cases caused by *B. henselae* and *B. elizabethae* have been described. Classic bartonellosis, restricted to the Peruvian Andes, is caused by *B. bacilliformis*. (*Cecil, Ch. 309, 310, and 367*)

186.(C); 187.(D); 188.(B); 189.(A) *Discussion:* Genital ulcer disease is an intriguing syndrome with a number of etiologies, both infectious and noninfectious. Fully 20% of genital ulcers have no proven etiology. Clinical features are important in the diagnosis of genital ulcer disease because cultures are usually delayed or unavailable. Syphilitic chancres are usually solitary, indurated, and painless. Herpetic ulcers are usually shallow, multiple, nonindurated, and painful. Chancroid lesions are painful, deep, and generally noninindurated. Lesions of donovanosis are heaped-up, confluent, ulcerative lesions and are often painless. Considerable overlap in clinical features may occur; for instance, syphilis may present as multiple, painful indurated lesions. Nonetheless, the classic presentations are useful for clinical decision making. (*Cecil, Ch. 314, 316, 317, 318, and 339*)

190.(B); 191.(E); 192.(C); 193.(D); 194.(A); 195.(E); 196.(A) *Discussion:* Host immune abnormalities may include defects in cell-mediated immunity, humoral immunity, complement activity, qualitative or quantitative neutrophil dysfunction, and splenic abnormalities. Patients with asplenia (functional or surgical) are at risk for overwhelming sepsis resulting from encapsulated organisms such as pneumococcus, meningococcus, and *Haemophilia influenzae*. Asplenic patients may also develop severe manifestations of babesiosis. Neutropenic patients are at risk for overwhelming sepsis resulting from a number of bacteria and fungi, most notably aerobic gram-negative rods, *Staphylococcus* sp., and *Candida* sp. Patients with immunoglobulin A deficiency may develop chronic and recurrent sinopulmonary infections but are also at risk for chronic intestinal infections caused by *Giardia lamblia*. Cell-mediated immune dysfunction is seen in solid-organ transplant recipients, who are at risk for invasive protozoan, fungal, mycobacterial, and certain bacterial infections, including legionellosis. The classic presentation of patients with terminal complement deficiency is recurrent systemic infections with *Neisseria* sp. (*Cecil, Ch. 266; Buckley*)

BIBLIOGRAPHY

Applebaum PC: Antimicrobial resistance in *Streptococcus pneumoniae:* An overview. Clin Infect Dis 15:77, 1992.

Bennett JC, Plum F (eds): Cecil Textbook of Medicine. 20th ed. Philadelphia, WB Saunders Company, 1996.

Buckley HR: Immunodeficiency diseases. JAMA 268:2797–2806, 1992.

Dajani AS, Bisno AL, Chung KI, et al: Prevention of bacterial endocarditis: Recommendations by the American Heart Association. JAMA 264:2919, 1990.

Fishbein DB, Dawson JE, Robinson LE: Human ehrlichiosis in the United States, 1985 to 1990. Ann Intern Med 120:736–743, 1994.

Holmes KK, Mardh PA, Sparling PF, et al: Sexually Transmitted Diseases. 2nd ed. New York, McGraw-Hill, 1990.

Iseman MD: Treatment of multidrug-resistant tuberculosis. N Engl J Med 329:784, 1993.

Mandell GL, Bennett JE, Dolin R: Principles and Practice of Infectious Diseases. 4th ed. New York, Churchill Livingston, 1995.

Nichol KL, Lind A, Margolis KL, et al: The effectiveness of vaccination against influenza in healthy, working adults. N Engl J Med 333:889–893, 1995.

Nolan CM, Beaty HN: *Staphylococcus aureus* bacteremia: Current clinical patterns. Am J Med 60: 495–500, 1976.

Odio CM, Faingezicht I, Paris M, et al: The beneficial effects of early dexamethasone administration in infants and children with bacterial meningitis. N Engl J Med 324:1525–1531, 1991.

Pappas PG, Threlkeld MG, Bedsole GD, et al: Blastomycosis in immunocompromised patients. Medicine 72:311–325, 1993.

Rex JH, Bennett JE, Sugar AM, et al: A randomized trial comparing fluconazole with amphotericin B for the treatment of candidemia in patients without neutropenia. N Engl J Med 331:1325–1330, 1994.

Saag MS, Powderly WG, Cloud GA, et al: Comparison of amphotericin B with fluconazole in the treatment of acute AIDS-associated cryptococcal meningitis. N Engl J Med 326:83–89, 1992.

Sarosi GA, Johnson PC: Disseminated histoplasmosis in HIV-infected patients. Clin Infect Dis 14:560, 1992.

PART 9

RHEUMATOLOGY AND CLINICAL IMMUNOLOGY

Louis W. Heck, Jr.

DIRECTIONS: For questions 1 to 26, choose the ONE BEST answer to each question.

1. A 43-year-old woman presents with a 3-year history of progressive rheumatoid arthritis that has been partially responsive to various nonsteroidal anti-inflammatory medications and to low-dose oral corticosteroids. After the examination, you decide to treat her active arthritis with methotrexate, the most widely used and effective agent currently used to treat rheumatoid arthritis. Some of the facts about methotrexate therapy to tell her include

- A. Therapeutic effects are delayed so that clinical improvement is not generally seen for 3 to 6 weeks after initiation of treatment.
- B. Adverse effects may include oral ulcers, nausea, vomiting, pneumonitis, bone marrow suppression, and cirrhosis.
- C. Complete blood count, platelet count, alkaline phosphatase level, and serum glutamic-oxaloacetic transaminase (SGOT) level should be obtained every 4 to 6 weeks to monitor therapy.
- D. Birth control measures must be in use before methotrexate is started.
- E. All of the above

2. A 54-year-old woman complains of severe right shoulder pain localized mainly to the mid-humerus but also diffusely around the anterolateral shoulder. The onset was sudden and not precipitated by trauma. Physical examination reveals limited abduction with point tenderness over the subacromial bursa and the greater tuberosity of the humerus. A radiograph reveals a linear calcific density in the supraspinatus tendon. All of the following statements are true EXCEPT

- A. Treatment consists of cortisone injection into the subacromial bursa, nonsteroidal anti-inflammatory medications, and physical therapy.
- B. The calcific density is most likely calcium urate.
- C. This is a common clinical problem.
- D. The diagnosis could not be made by an arthrocentesis.
- E. Local tendon injury may be the major cause.

3. A 74-year-old woman complains of worsening left knee pain with weight bearing and ambulation. Examination of the knee reveals a small effusion without warmth, bony enlargement, and crepitus with flexion and extension of the knee. A diagnostic arthrocentesis is performed. Each of the following characteristics of the synovial fluid would be expected EXCEPT

- A. Pale yellow color
- B. Good viscosity
- C. Routine culture negative
- D. White blood cell count 800 per cu mm
- E. Glucose 22 mg per deciliter

4. A 42-year-old woman with seropositive rheumatoid arthritis has become disabled by pain and tightness behind the right knee. Physical examination reveals cystic swelling over the popliteal fossa and semimembranous tendon. Which of the following is the most appropriate next step?

- A. Arthrogram of the right knee
- B. Synovial biopsy of right knee
- C. Ultrasound study of right knee popliteal fossa
- D. Venogram of right lower extremity
- E. None of the above

5. All of the following conditions involve the distal interphalangeal (DIP) joint EXCEPT

- A. Multicentric reticulohistiocytosis
- B. Erosive osteoarthritis
- C. Psoriasis with nail changes
- D. Juvenile chronic arthritis
- E. Rheumatoid arthritis

6. Rheumatoid factor may be present in each of these conditions EXCEPT

- A. Adult Still's disease
- B. Subacute bacterial endocarditis
- C. Vasculitis syndromes
- D. Sarcoidosis
- E. Sjögren's syndrome

7. An 82-year-old woman was hospitalized for treatment of congestive heart failure. She developed a warm, painful right knee on the third hospital day. The most appropriate procedure would be

- A. Blood cultures followed by intravenous antibiotics
- B. Arthrocentesis for diagnostic/therapeutic purposes
- C. Intravenous colchicine

D. Allopurinol
E. Ultrasound study of right knee, including popliteal fossa

8. A 46-year-old man on hemodialysis for 12 years complains of insidious onset of painful nocturnal dysesthesias involving the thumb and three fingers, relieved by shaking the hand. Physical examination of the hand reveals thenar wasting and numbness over the fingers. Each of the following statements is true EXCEPT

A. Deposits of beta$_2$-microglobulin (AH) amyloid compressing the median nerve could produce these findings.
B. An entrapment neuropathy could explain these findings.
C. Paresthesias involving the radial side of the thumb, second, third, and fourth fingers suggest compression of the medial nerve.
D. Carpal tunnel syndrome could explain the above findings.
E. Deposits of amyloid of the primary type (AL) would be typical.

9. Ophthalmologic manifestations of rheumatoid arthritis may include all of the following EXCEPT

A. Secondary Sjögren's syndrome with sicca complex
B. Scleritis
C. Episcleritis
D. Corneal melts
E. Ischemic optic atrophy

10. All of the following are characteristic patterns of joint involvement in rheumatoid arthritis EXCEPT

A. Polyarticular involvement
B. Oligoarticular involvement
C. Symmetrical involvement
D. Involvement of the proximal interphalangeal (PIP), metacarpophalangeal (MCP) wrist, and metatarsophalangeal (MTP) joints
E. Frequent cervical spine involvement

11. A 32-year-old woman presents with left inguinal and groin pain of 1 week's duration that is worse with weight bearing and ambulation. Physical examination reveals full range of motion of the left hip. She walks with a limp. She had previously been treated with MOPP therapy for Hodgkin's disease. An anteroposterior film of the pelvis demonstrates no osseous abnormality. Which of the following tests would be most useful in making the diagnosis?

A. Serum rheumatoid factor
B. Erythrocyte sedimentation rate
C. Magnetic resonance imaging of left hip
D. Arthrogram of left hip
E. Blood alcohol level

12. Extra-articular manifestations of rheumatoid arthritis that may be associated with severe morbidity or mortality include

A. Rheumatoid vasculitis
B. Pericarditis
C. Cachexia
D. Rheumatoid nodule within the aortic valve
E. All of the above

13. Each of the following metabolic diseases may be associated with calcium pyrophosphate crystal deposition disease EXCEPT

A. Hypothyroidism
B. Hemochromatosis
C. Primary hyperoxaluria
D. Hyperparathyroidism
E. Gout

14. All of the following statements are true of nonsteroidal anti-inflammatory drugs in general EXCEPT

A. They have no major effect on the underlying disease process.
B. They tend to cause gastric irritation and to exacerbate peptic ulcers.
C. They may suppress vasodilatory functions of renal prostaglandins.
D. They may increase the pain threshold.
E. Most are readily absorbed after oral administration.

15. All of the following are consistent with the radiographic manifestation of pyrophosphate arthropathy EXCEPT

A. Cystic changes in bones of the wrist with triangular cartilage calcification
B. Periarticular calcification of the first MTP joint
C. Severe degenerative changes and subarticular cysts in knee
D. Linear subperiosteal resorption most marked in the radial border of the middle phalanx
E. Linear calcification of the hyaline cartilage of the knee

16. Each of the following is a potential side effect of weekly low-dose (5 to 15 mg) methotrexate used to treat rheumatoid arthritis EXCEPT

A. Leukopenia
B. Alopecia
C. Nephropathy
D. Stomatitis
E. Thrombocytopenia

17. A 32-year-old homosexual man presents for evaluation and treatment of left ankle pain of 2 weeks duration. Besides tenderness, swelling, and marked limitation of tibial-talar motion, he has swelling and tenderness over the Achilles' tendon insertion on the calcaneus; painful swelling over the left second and third MTP, PIP, and DIP joints; a clear mucoid penile discharge; hyperkeratosis of the soles and palms; and multiple erythematous plaque lesions with scaling over the trunk, arms, and legs. Each of the following would be appropriate diagnostic or treatment possibilities EXCEPT

A. Nonsteroidal anti-inflammatory drugs for 2 weeks to reduce joint pain and swelling
B. Request for patient consent for human immunodeficiency virus (HIV) screening
C. Gram's stain and culture of the urethral exudate for gonococcus
D. Strong consideration of adding methotrexate as a disease-modifying agent if there is no improvement within a 2- to 3-week period
E. Arthrocentesis for diagnostic and therapeutic purposes

18. Each of the following statements about immunoglobulin (Ig) structure and function are true EXCEPT

A. Among the various classes, the basic structure of all immunoglobulin molecules is similar

B. Both of the heavy and light chains of an IgG molecule have a variable region

C. Both of the heavy and light chains of an IgM molecule have a constant region

D. Complement fixation appears to depend on a structural determinant in the IgG V_2 region

E. The hypervariable regions are in intimate contact with the structural elements of the antigen

19. Each of the following antibodies have been found in patients with HIV infections EXCEPT

A. Antinuclear antibodies (ANAs)

B. Anticardiolipin antibodies

C. Cryoglobulins

D. Antilymphocyte antibodies

E. Anti–G protein antibodies

20. A 22-year-old black woman with systemic lupus erythematosus (SLE) develops worsening arthralgia and is given ibuprofen 800 mg three times per day. Two days later, she presents to the emergency room with headache, stiff neck, and fever. Cultures of the cerebrospinal fluid are negative for bacteria and fungi. The most appropriate next step would be to

A. Institute corticosteroids

B. Give intravenous cyclophosphamide

C. Discontinue the ibuprofen

D. Initiate Plaquenil therapy

E. Give intravenous corticosteroids and cyclophosphamide

21. A 32-year-old white woman presents with a 6-week history of fatigue, lymphadenopathy, and low-grade fever. At age 17, she required splenectomy for thrombocytopenia. In her early 20s, she had three miscarriages, one of which was followed by a deep venous thrombosis. Which laboratory tests would be most helpful in establishing a diagnosis?

A. ANA, anti–Sjögren's syndrome (anti-SSA and anti-SSB) antibodies

B. Rheumatoid factor, ANA, antiscleroderma (anti–SCL-70) antibodies

C. Antineutrophilic antibodies, antihistone antibodies

D. ANA, anticardiolipin antibodies, and anti-DNA antibodies

E. ANA, rheumatoid factor, and Lyme antibodies

22. A 65-year-old white man is admitted to the hospital for cholecystitis and undergoes cholecystectomy. Postoperatively, he develops a persistent low-grade fever, intermittent severe crampy abdominal pain, and purpuric lower extremity skin lesions. On the tenth hospital day, he develops a right footdrop and diplopia. The most appropriate next step in his diagnostic evaluation is to

A. Obtain a kidney biopsy

B. Obtain open lung biopsy

C. Obtain celiac and mesenteric angiography

D. Obtain a right temporal artery biopsy

E. Obtain a computed tomographic scan of the brain

23. A 50-year-old white man is transferred to your hospital with a presumptive diagnosis of tuberculosis. His chest radiograph shows nodular cavitary lesions in both lung fields. His urinalysis shows 50 red blood cells per high-power field and 3+ proteinuria. He is scheduled for bronchoscopy with transbronchial lung biopsy in the morning. That evening he has a sudden deterioration consisting of massive hemoptysis and progressive renal failure. The most appropriate therapeutic intervention at this point would be supportive management and

A. Intravenous corticosteroids

B. Antituberculous medications

C. Intravenous cyclophosphamide, 4 mg per kilogram

D. Oral cyclophosphamide, 2 mg per kilogram

E. Intravenous corticosteroids and intravenous cyclophosphamide, 4 mg per kilogram

24. Each of the following is characteristic of polymyalgia rheumatica EXCEPT

A. Mild joint inflammation

B. Stiffness of the shoulder and hip girdles

C. Weakness of the shoulder and hip girdles

D. Elevated erythrocyte sedimentation rate

E. Normochromic normocytic anemia

25. A 74-year-old man is noted to have purplish-discolored right third and fourth toes 4 days after coronary angiography and a creatinine level of 2.4 mg per deciliter (creatinine level was normal on admission). He has a history of adult-onset diabetes mellitus, hypertension, and 50 pack-years of smoking. Cholesterol crystal atheromatous embolization is suspected. Which of the following may be present?

A. Livedo reticularis

B. Elevated erythrocyte sedimentation rate and/or leukocytosis and/or eosinophilia

C. Prominent gastrocnemius pain or claudication

D. The source(s) of the cholesterol emboli are usually the abdominal aorta or iliofemoral arteries rather than from the more distal arteries

E. All of the above

26. An 83-year-old woman presented to the emergency room on stretcher with severe right hip and thigh pain after falling in the shower. Radiographs revealed generalized osteopenia and a displaced right femoral neck fracture. Each of the following statements about osteoporosis is true EXCEPT

A. Decreased bone mass is the major risk factor for sustaining a fracture as a result of minor trauma.

B. Lifestyle factors such as calcium intake, cigarette smoking, and ethanol use may modify bone mass.

C. The severity of bone loss is best assessed using plain bone radiographs.

D. There are no symptoms or physical findings in early osteoporosis.

E. The number of osteoporotic fractures in the United States is expected to increase dramatically in the next 40 years.

DIRECTIONS: For questions 27 to 48, decide whether EACH choice is true or false. Any combination of answers, from all true to all false, may occur.

27. Which of the following statements concerning cholesterol (atheromatous) emboli syndrome is/are true?

A. Precipitating factors can always be identified if diligently sought.
B. Dermal manifestations may include petechiae, hemorrhage, purplish-discolored toes, and digital gangrene.
C. Transient basophilia is commonly seen.
D. Cholesterol emboli most commonly arise from atheromatous plaque in the distal lower extremity arteries.
E. The administration of anticoagulants may be associated with episodes of embolization.

28. Glucocorticoid-induced osteoporosis is currently the most common cause of drug-related osteoporosis in the United States. Which of the following recommendations concerning management of glucocorticoid-induced osteoporosis is/are true?

A. Bone densitometry techniques may detect bone mineral depletion before fractures in patients on chronic glucocorticoid therapy.
B. Encourage the daily ingestion of 1500 mg of elemental calcium and 400 IU per day of vitamin D.
C. Decrease or stop all glucocorticoids when osteoporosis is detected.
D. Encourage weight-bearing activity and exercises.
E. Replace gonadal hormones in all postmenopausal women if there are no contraindications.

29. Which of the following statements concerning neutrophil/neutrophil-mediated tissue injury is/are true?

A. Proteinases released extracellularly may degrade matrix molecules.
B. Tissue-bound IgG/immune complexes are the major *in vivo* signal for degranulation.
C. The major lipid mediators released extracellularly are leukotriene A_4 and lipoxin B.
D. The major surface protein mediating adhesion is IIb/IIIa.
E. CD11b/CD18 functions as a receptor for iC3b (CR3) and thereby mediates phagocytosis or opsonized particles.

30. Which of the following statements concerning the antiphospholipid antibody syndrome is/are true?

A. It could not be associated with the sudden onset of left paresis in a previously healthy 28-year-old woman.
B. It could explain recurrent spontaneous abortion in a 24-year-old woman with an ANA 1:40 titer, speckled pattern.
C. Lupus anticoagulant and anticardiolipin antibody are always identical immunoglobulin molecules.
D. It could not explain ischemic necrosis of the forefoot in a previously healthy 24-year-old man.

E. Tests for anticardiolipin antibodies have a low degree of variability and excellent reproducibility and should be done in all hospital laboratories.

31. Which of the following statements concerning rheumatoid factor is/are true?

A. It is present in the blood of approximately 80% of patients with rheumatoid arthritis.
B. It is clearly implicated as causing rheumatoid arthritis.
C. In most cases it can be demonstrated to be an IgG antibody to autologous IgM.
D. Its production is restricted to the human leukocyte antigen (HLA) DR4 haplotype.
E. None of the above

32. Which of the following statements concerning B cells is/are true?

A. They can directly secrete antibodies.
B. Activation, proliferation, and differentiation require a variety of cytokines.
C. The binding region of the membrane immunoglobulin of each cell line is unique in its specificity.
D. They contain immunoglobulin genes located on chromosomes 2, 14, and 22.
E. Their major receptor is the T3 complex.

33. Which of the following statements concerning hemochromatosis is/are true?

A. Pyrophosphate arthropathy may affect the second and third MCP joints in approximately 50% of patients.
B. The diagnosis is made by an elevated serum ferritin level.
C. The diagnosis is made by liver biopsy showing increased iron within parenchymal cells.
D. Initiating weekly phlebotomies until tissue iron stores are depleted is the usual treatment.
E. Hepatic cirrhosis, cardiomyopathy, diabetes mellitus, and skin pigmentation may result from increased iron in tissues.

34. Which of the following statements concerning lumbosacral spine films is/are true?

A. Focal or generalized reduction in bone density may be observed in myeloma.
B. Progression of vertebral body osteomyelitis may lead to involvement of two adjacent vertebrae and the intervening disc space.
C. Localized rarefaction of the vertebral end-plate is the earliest radiographic change in vertebral osteomyelitis.
D. Metastatic neoplasms to the vertebral bodies characteristically invade the intervening disc space.
E. Alternate bands of osteosclerosis and resorption may be seen in renal osteodystrophy.

35. Which of the following statements concerning ankylosing spondylitis is/are true?

    A. Monoarthritis or oligoarthritis may precede the onset of back pain.

    B. The earliest recognizable radiographic change in the sacroiliac joints is fusion.

    C. Back pain and morning stiffness may diminish with activity and may recur after periods of inactivity.

    D. Lateral lumbosacral flexion may be assessed with the Schober's test.

    E. Aortic insufficiency may be an extra-articular manifestation.

36. Which of the following statements concerning osteoporosis is/are true?

    A. Bone mineral and matrix formation rates are always greater than resorption rates.

    B. Bone density in postmenopausal women is the most important determinant for hip and vertebral fractures.

    C. Dual-energy x-ray absorptiometry is the most accurate method for assessing bone density.

    D. Single- and dual-photon analysis is the most common technique to assess bone density.

    E. Prevention of symptomatic osteoporosis should be a top public health goal in the United States.

37. Which of the following statements about gonococcal arthritis is/are true?

    A. It is a rare problem in healthy, sexually active teenagers and young adults.

    B. The diagnosis is easy to make in most cases because of positive synovial fluid Gram's stain and culture.

    C. Causative organisms are gram-positive diplococci.

    D. The arthritis pattern is oligoarticular associated with tenosynovitis and skin lesions.

    E. Response to treatment of antibiotics/drainage is slow but definite.

38. Which of the following concerning matrix structure and functions is/are true?

    A. The collagens are the second most abundant class of proteins in the human body.

    B. Proteoglycans are the major noncollagenous structural proteins of articular cartilage.

    C. The major components of basement membranes are collagen type IV, laminin, entactin, and heparin sulfate proteoglycans.

    D. Genetic mutation associated with defects in type I collagen includes Ehlers-Danlos syndrome and osteogenesis imperfecta.

    E. Basement membrane alterations are frequently found in diabetes mellitus.

39. Which of the following statements concerning complement is/are true?

    A. CR1 may function to clear circulating immune complexes and enhance phagocytosis.

    B. A low CH_{50} (total hemolytic complement) may suggest C2 deficiency.

    C. A deficiency of C5, C6, C7, and C8 may be associated with recurrent disseminated staphylococcal infections.

    D. The two complement activation pathways (classic and alternative) may lead to the generation of the membrane attack complex.

    E. SLE-like syndromes and discoid lupus may be associated with C2 and C4 deficiency.

40. Which of the following statements concerning cytokines is/are true?

    A. Interleukin-1-alpha and -beta can produce fever, bone and cartilage resorption, and prostaglandin release.

    B. Tumor necrosis factor alpha can produce fever and macrophage activation and can stimulate bone resorption.

    C. Interleukin-2 is produced by T cells and may stimulate proliferation of T cells and natural killer cells.

    D. Interleukin-2 has antitumor activity.

    E. Interleukin-6 induces antibody secretion.

41. Which of the following statements concerning HLA is/are true?

    A. Over 100 diseases of diverse manifestations are associated with HLA.

    B. The majority of individuals with a given disease associated with HLA haplotype are afflicted with the disease.

    C. HLA-A molecules are found on virtually all cells.

    D. Certain regions within the DR4 and DR1 class II molecules with the same amino acid sequence may confer predisposition to rheumatoid arthritis.

    E. HLA-DR4 occurs in 95% of seropositive individuals with rheumatoid arthritis.

42. Which of the following statements concerning rheumatic manifestations of HIV infection is/are true?

    A. Fever, myalgias, and arthralgias are a distinctly uncommon manifestation of acute HIV seroconversion.

    B. A polymyositis-like illness characterized by myalgias, proximal muscle weakness, and wasting has been described as the initial manifestation of HIV infection.

    C. An oligoarticular arthritis associated with urethritis, conjunctivitis, painless oral ulcerations, and keratoderma blennorrhagicum are the hallmark of Reiter's syndrome in both HIV-infected and noninfected individuals.

    D. To date, xerophthalmia and xerostomia with abnormal salivary gland biopsies have not been described in HIV-infected individuals.

    E. All reported cases of HIV-related periarteritis nodosa have also been hepatitis B surface antigen positive, suggesting that true vasculitis does not occur with HIV infection.

43. Which of the following statements concerning polyarteritis nodosa is/are true?

    A. Characteristic pathologic findings in an involved vessel are leukocytoclastic vasculitis with nuclear debris.

B. The lesions tend to involve arteries of medium or small caliber, especially at bifurcations.

C. Eosinophilia with lung involvement is common.

D. Hypocomplementemia is characteristic.

E. Subcutaneous nodules are commonly found in this disease.

44. Which of the following statements regarding the vasculitis syndromes is/are true?

A. Wegener's granulomatosis is characterized by infiltration of various organs and vessels with cellular infiltrates consisting of atypical lymphoid and plasmacytoid cells.

B. Hypersensitivity vasculitis is often confined to the skin and often manifested by palpable purpura.

C. Temporal arteritis usually involves small intracranial arterioles and venules.

D. Takayasu's arteritis may involve the subclavian arteries.

E. Henoch-Schönlein purpura is usually progressive, leading to death or renal failure without appropriate therapeutic intervention.

45. Which of the following statements concerning SLE is/are true?

A. Although renal glomerular disease is common, renal tubular and interstitial inflammation is rare.

B. Anti-SSA antibodies (anti-Ro) have been associated with the development of congenital heart block in babies of mothers with SLE.

C. Vasculitic lesions of the skin usually portend central nervous system vasculitis.

D. Pleural fluid from patients with active SLE is usually exudative, with a low glucose level.

E. The chance that a black woman will develop SLE in her lifetime is approximately 1:250.

46. Which of the following statements is/are true?

A. Idiopathic midline destructive disease is usually treated with a combination of prednisone, cyclophosphamide, and radiation.

B. Elevation of the creatine phosphokinase level and a myopathic pattern in the electromyogram is useful in diagnosing polymyalgia rheumatica.

C. SLE patients with alopecia can be advised that hair will regrow, unless the scalp is involved with discoid lesions.

D. Renal transplantation is contraindicated in patients with end-stage renal failure caused by SLE.

E. A lupus anticoagulant has been identified that prolongs the partial thromboplastin time (PTT) by reacting with phospholipids used in the PTT assay and that is associated with thrombosis rather than bleeding.

47. Which of the following statements is/are true?

A. A neutrophilic leukocytosis and positive rheumatoid factor are often seen in patients with Wegener's granulomatosis.

B. Anticytoplasmic antibodies are highly specific for Wegener's granulomatosis.

C. Idiopathic midline destructive disease is a systemic vasculitis.

D. Lymphomatoid granulomatosis is a systemic vasculitis similar to polyarteritis nodosa.

E. All patients with Wegener's granulomatosis have lung involvement.

48. Which of the following statements concerning Lyme disease is/are true?

A. Erythema chronicum migrans occurs after an incubation period of 2 months in greater than 95% of affected patients.

B. Most affected patients develop arthritis, with monoarticular or oligoarticular arthritis in large joints.

C. Lyme antibody is frequently present early (2 to 4 weeks) in the disease.

D. The decision to treat patients with antibiotics in an endemic area should be based on serologic results.

E. The presence of Lyme antibodies may be of most use in the patient with either an atypical manifestation or unexplained recurrent attacks of monoarticular or oligoarthritis over several years.

DIRECTIONS: Questions 49 to 108 are matching questions. For each numbered item, choose the most likely associated lettered item from those provided. Each numbered item has ONLY ONE answer. Within each set of questions, each answer may be used once, more than once, or not at all.

QUESTIONS 49–52

Match the following histopathologic findings with the most likely associated rheumatic disease.

A. Calcific masses staining purple with hematoxylin
B. Dark pigmented hyaline cartilage fragments
C. Villi infiltrated by lymphocytes with synovial lining cell hyperplasia
D. Congophilia
E. Sheets of histiocytes and multinucleated giant cells

49. Ochronosis

50. Pigmented villonodular synovitis

51. Calcium pyrophosphate deposition disease

52. Rheumatoid arthritis

QUESTIONS 53–56

Match the following characteristic ocular manifestations with the rheumatic disease with which they are most likely to be associated.

A. Corneal melt
B. Ischemic optic atrophy
C. Anterior uveitis
D. Retinal vascular disease

53. Temporal arteritis

54. SLE

55. Rheumatoid arthritis

56. Ankylosing spondylitis

QUESTIONS 57–60

Match the following clinical syndromes with the radiographic description with which they are most likely associated.

A. Thyroiditis with thyroid acropachy
B. Synovial osteochondromatosis
C. Scleroderma
D. Gout
E. Acromegaly

57. Hand radiograph showing destruction of the tufts of the terminal phalanges

58. Shoulder radiograph demonstrating marked osteoarthritis with osteophyte formation

59. Punched-out erosion with overhanging bone

60. Lateral knee radiograph demonstrating multiple calcified loose bodies in a popliteal cyst

QUESTIONS 61–64

Match the following sets of clinical problems with the complication in dialysis patients with which they are most likely to be associated.

A. Bone pain, pathologic fractures, proximal muscle weakness, dementia
B. Carpal tunnel syndrome, subchondral cysts
C. Osteolysis of phalangeal tufts, pathologic fractures
D. Pruritus, periarthritis, acute joint pain
E. Hypertrophic skin changes, periosteal proliferation

61. Secondary hyperparathyroidism

62. Beta$_2$-microglobulin amyloid arthropathy

63. High serum calcium $\times$ phosphorus product

64. Aluminum-related osteomalacia

QUESTIONS 65–68

Match the following cutaneous manifestations with the most likely associated rheumatic disease.

A. Ringlike erythema that has elevated margins, expands peripherally, and leaves fading centers
B. Thrombocytopenic purpura
C. Periorbital swelling with erythema along the lid margins
D. Nonthrombocytopenic palpable purpura
E. Hemorrhagic vesicopustules

65. Rheumatic fever

66. Henoch-Schönlein syndrome

67. Disseminated gonococcal arthritis

68. Dermatomyositis

QUESTIONS 69–72

Match the following joint pattern findings with the disease with which they are most likely to be associated.

A. Inflammatory oligoarthritis in a 21-year-old man
B. Symmetric polyarthritis in a 32-year-old woman
C. Inflammatory monoarthritis of the first toe interphalangeal joint in a 58-year-old man
D. Monoarticular arthritis in a 6-year-old girl
E. Squaring of the base of the thumb in a 66-year-old woman

69. Gout

70. Reiter's syndrome

71. Rheumatoid arthritis

72. Pauciarticular juvenile chronic arthritis

QUESTIONS 73–76

Match the following characteristic findings with the disease with which they are most likely associated.

A. Digital clubbing, periostitis, and painful swelling of bones and joints

B. Asymptomatic pleural effusions
C. Upper lobe fibrosis
D. Transient arthritis affecting knees, ankles, and wrists
E. Swollen, tender DIP joints

73. Ankylosing spondylitis

74. Bronchogenic carcinoma

75. Sarcoidosis

76. Rheumatoid arthritis

QUESTIONS 77–80

Match the following clinical findings with the most likely associated rheumatic disease.

A. Thenar atrophy, decreased ability to oppose thumb to little finger
B. Fixed facial expression, rigidity of the left arm
C. Acute onset of sagging of the right eyebrow and drooping of the mouth on the right
D. Disturbances of micturition or impotence
E. Sudden, painless loss of vision in the left eye

77. Temporal arteritis

78. Ankylosing spondylitis

79. Lyme arthritis

80. Beta$_2$-microglobulin hemodialysis arthropathy

QUESTIONS 81–84

Match the following characteristic findings with the most likely associated endocrine disease.

A. Transient Raynaud's phenomenon
B. Vertebral body fractures
C. Finger digit sclerosis with PIP flexion contractures
D. Synovial fluid speckled with dark particles resembling brown pepper
E. Muscle weakness with elevated creatinine kinase level

81. Hyperparathyroidism

82. Hypothyroidism

83. Acromegaly

84. Diabetes mellitus

QUESTIONS 85–88

Match the following characteristic findings with the rheumatic syndromes associated with HIV infection with which they are most likely to be associated.

A. Presents as peripheral sensory or sensorimotor neuropathy
B. Sicca symptoms
C. Present in one third of HIV-infected patients
D. Oligoarticular arthritis associated with conjunctivitis, urethritis, painless oral ulcers, and circinate balanitis
E. Presence of nemaline rods

85. Myopathy

86. Arthralgias

87. Reiter's syndrome

88. Vasculitis

QUESTIONS 89–92

Match the following clinical syndromes with the manifestation which they are most likely to be associated.

A. Rheumatoid arthritis
B. SLE
C. Dermatomyositis
D. Hypersensitivity vasculitis
E. Periarteritis nodosa

89. Palpable purpura

90. Subcutaneous nodules

91. Gottron's papules

92. Hypopigmented skin lesion with central atrophy and telangiectasia

QUESTIONS 93–96

Match the following clinical syndromes with the most likely associated finding.

A. Wegener's granulomatosis
B. Sjögrens syndrome
C. SLE
D. Eosinophilic fascitis
E. Polyarteritis nodosa

93. C2 deficiency

94. Antibodies against a 29-kD cytoplasmic antigen of neutrophils

95. Renal tubular acidosis

96. Brawny, tender induration of the skin with retraction of subcutaneous tissue

QUESTIONS 97–100

Match the following clinical syndromes with the most likely associated finding.

A. Polyarteritis nodosa
B. SLE
C. Temporal arteritis
D. Behçets syndrome
E. Scleroderma

97. Cytoid bodies

98. Mononeuritis multiplex

99. Jaw claudication

100. Meningoencephalitis

QUESTIONS 101–104

Match the following laboratory findings with the condition with which they are most likely to be associated.

A. Anticardiolipin antibodies
B. Anti-SSA antibodies

   C.   Antihistone antibodies
   D.   Anti-Smith antibodies
   E.   Anti–SCL-70 antibodies

101. Recurrent abortions

102. Congenital heart block

103. Drug-induced lupus

104. SLE

QUESTIONS 105–108

Match the following clinical syndromes with the most likely associated symptoms.

   A.   Eosinophilia-myalgia syndrome
   B.   Eosinophilic fascitis syndrome
   C.   Fibromyalgia
   D.   Churg-Strauss syndrome
   E.   Toxic oil syndrome

105. Pulmonary and systemic vasculitis, eosinophilia, often occurring in patients with history of allergy or asthma

106. Intense and incapacitating generalized myalgia, fatigue, eosinophilia, and history of ingestion of L-tryptophan

107. Swelling and stiffness of the extremities, eosinophilia, occurring in patients following extreme physical exertion

108. Widespread pain in combination with tenderness at specific tender point sites

RHEUMATOLOGY AND CLINICAL IMMUNOLOGY

ANSWERS

1.(E) *Discussion:* All of the answers are correct. Methotrexate is currently the best drug used to treat rheumatoid arthritis, with initial improvement seen in 3 to 6 weeks and peak efficacy in 4 to 6 months. Adverse effects such as nausea, abdominal pain, and diarrhea are frequently seen, but serious toxicity is rare. Methotrexate is taken orally (7.5 to 15 mg per week), and tolerance may be increased by spacing the oral doses over 1 to 2 days, giving a single intramuscular injection each week, and daily folic acid (1 mg per day) supplementation. Laboratory tests such as complete blood count, platelet count, alkaline phosphatase, and SGOT are done every 4 to 6 weeks. The most toxic drug-related side effects are pancytopenia, neutropenia, thrombocytopenia, pneumonitis, and cirrhosis; all are reasons to stop the medications. Transient or sustained (1.5 to 2 times normal values) elevations in alkaline phosphatase and SGOT are commonly seen and in the majority of patients and generally do not portend the development of hepatic fibrosis. Methotrexate is known to be teratogenic and should not be given to women with child-bearing potential unless they are using an adequate method of birth control. Although the action of methotrexate to affect sperm, leading to defined fetal abnormalities, is unknown, men should discontinue methotrexate 3 to 4 months before attempting conception. (*Cecil, Ch. 237; Weinblatt*)

2.(B) *Discussion:* The clinical features and radiographic pattern are characteristic for calcific tendonitis, an extremely common rheumatic syndrome characterized by deposits of hydroxyapatite crystals within injured rotator cuff muscles near the humeral attachment region. It most commonly involves the supraspinatus tendon, but the infraspinatus and subscapularis tendon may also be involved. Conservative treatment is indicated and is successful in the vast majority of cases. (*Cecil, Ch. 252 and 255*)

3.(E) *Discussion:* Clinically, the patient has osteoarthritis of the left knee. Synovial fluid in patients with osteoarthritis is typically ''noninflammatory,'' meaning that the leukocyte count is less than 2000 per cubic millimeter. A low level of glucose in the synovial fluid would not be found in this patient but is suggestive of septic arthritis. (*Cecil, Ch. 236 and 254*)

4.(C) *Discussion:* The physical examination is suggestive of a distended Baker's cyst, but physical examination alone is not diagnostic, particularly if there has been a dissection or rupture. Ultrasound has been found to be very useful in making a diagnosis of popliteal cyst with or without dissection. An arthrogram could also demonstrate a popliteal cyst but is less desirable because it is an invasive procedure. A venogram of the right lower extremity could be performed

if a deep venous thrombosis was suspected clinically, but would not be indicated in this case. (*Cecil, Ch. 237; Primer*)

5.(E) *Discussion:* Although hand involvement is very common in rheumatoid arthritis and occurs in approximately 95% of patients, DIP joint involvement is distinctly unusual. The most commonly involved joints in the rheumatoid hand are the PIPs, MCPs, and wrist joints in a symmetrical manner. (*Resnick and Niwayama*)

6.(A) *Discussion:* Patients with adult Still's disease are ''seronegative'' and lack serum rheumatoid factor. Rheumatoid factors are antibodies specific for the region of the Fc portion of human IgG. Although present in 75 to 80% of rheumatoid arthritis cases, primarily those with HLA-DR4 haplotype, they are by no means specific for this disorder and are found in normal subjects as well as patients with a variety of other inflammatory illnesses. (*Cecil, Ch. 236 and 237*)

7.(B) *Discussion:* Clinically, the patient has a monoarthritis most likely caused by a crystal-associated arthritis such as pseudogout or gout. She could also have septic arthritis, although this would be less likely. Gout and pseudogout can be rapidly and definitively diagnosed by proper examination of joint fluid, and infection can also be ruled out in this manner. (*Cecil, Ch. 233 and 252*)

8.(E) *Discussion:* Clinically, the patient has carpal tunnel syndrome, an entrapment neuropathy in which the median nerve is compressed within the carpal tunnel area. A new type of amyloid protein identified as beta$_2$-microglobulin has been demonstrated in bone and carpal tunnel tissue of patients undergoing long-term (usually greater than 10 years) hemodialysis. It is hoped that modifications of the dialysis membranes may result in improved beta$_2$-microglobulin clearance with diminished tissue deposition. (*Cecil, Ch. 248*)

9.(E) *Discussion:* Ischemic optic atrophy is not routinely seen in patients with rheumatoid arthritis but may be a major ophthalmic manifestation of giant cell arteritis, Wegener's granulomatosis, and, less commonly, SLE. (*Cecil, Ch. 237 and 246*)

10.(B) *Discussion:* Clinically, rheumatoid arthritis is a symmetric polyarthritis especially involving the PIP, MCP, wrist, and MTP joints. Many of these joints will develop definite articular deformities over time. Cervical spine involvement is common. Rarely is an oligoarticular pattern observed except in the early course of this illness. (*Cecil, Ch. 237*)

11.(C) *Discussion:* Osteonecrosis is one of the most common causes of hip pain and incapacity in patients with a variety of diseases who have been treated with corticosteroids. A major problem in diagnosing osteonecrosis relates to the lag between the onset of symptoms (pain and limp) and defined radiographic changes. Magnetic resonance imaging has been shown to be extremely valuable in evaluating high-risk patients who are symptomatic but radiographically normal. (*Resnick and Niwayama*)

12.(E) *Discussion:* All of the answers are correct. Rheumatoid arthritis may be associated with a number of systemic features that may be associated with severe morbidity or mortality. (*Cecil, Ch. 237*)

13.(C) *Discussion:* There is an association of calcium pyrophosphate crystal deposition disease with several metabolic diseases, including primary hyperparathyroidism, hemochromatosis, hypothyroidism, gout, familial hypocalciuric hypercalcemia, hypomagnesemia, and hypophosphatasia, but not with primary hyperoxaluria, which is associated with the tissue deposition of calcium oxalate crystals. The development of premature symptomatic osteoarthritis associated with the features of chondrocalcinosis should initiate a search for underlying associated disorders. In general, treatment of the primary disorder, such as hyperparathyroidism, hemochromatosis, or hypothyroidism, does not lead to resorption of calcium pyrophosphate deposition. Phlebotomy treatment of hemochromatosis may actually exacerbate the arthritis. (*Cecil, Ch. 189, 252, and 256;* Primer)

14.(D) *Discussion:* Most nonsteroidal anti-inflammatory drugs are aspirin-like in that they reduce but do not completely eliminate the signs and symptoms of inflammation. A major effect on the underlying disease process has not been demonstrated. They have a broad range of pharmacologic activities, the most well described of which is the inhibition of cyclo-oxygenase, the enzyme that catalyzes the conversion of arachadonic acid to prostaglandins, prostacycline, and thromboxanes. Although nonsteroidal anti-inflammatory agents are well tolerated, they can be associated with a spectrum of adverse reactions. The most notable of these are the gastrointestinal effects, such as the tendency to produce gastritis and antral prepyloric ulcers. (*Cecil, Ch. 235 and 237*)

15.(D) *Discussion:* Linear subperiosteal resorption is seen in primary or secondary hyperparathyroidism. The other manifestations are common radiographic manifestations of calcium pyrophosphate deposition disease. (*Resnick and Niwayama*)

16.(C) *Discussion:* Nephropathy is not an adverse manifestation of oral methotrexate. Methotrexate is usually administered orally ranging from 1 to 3 doses per week separated by 8 to 12 hours. Typically, this protocol results in a reduction in the immunosuppressive and toxic reactions of the drug. Although the mechanism of action may be primarily through inhibition of synovial cell proliferation, its toxicity is primarily associated with effects on rapidly dividing cells such as bone marrow and intestinal epithelium. (*Cecil, Ch. 237; Weinblatt*)

17.(D) *Discussion:* The data presented indicate that the patient has typical Reiter's syndrome, which may or may not be associated with HIV infection. Efforts should be made to screen for HIV, rule out gonorrhea, and refrain from using immunosuppressant drugs such as methotrexate because these may be contraindicated in a patient who is HIV positive. (*Cecil, Ch. 238 and 370*)

18.(D) *Discussion:* There are five classes of immunoglobulin molecules in humans (IgG, IgA, IgM, IgG, and IgE), which have the same basic four-chain structure, including two heavy (H) and two light (L) chains, but which differ in their chemical and physical properties. Complement activation by the classical pathway appears to be associated with the constant region of IgG, with IgG_1 and IgG_3 subclasses being the most effective. (*Cecil, Ch. 221*)

19.(E) *Discussion:* A variety of antibodies have been found in patients with HIV infections, but to date no anti–G protein antibodies have been reported. Antinuclear, antilymphocyte, antineutrophil, antiplatelet, antiphospholipid, rheumatoid factor, and cryoglobulins have all been demonstrated to occur in patients with HIV infections. The relationship of these antibodies to the rheumatologic diseases associated with the HIV infection is unclear. (*Cecil, Ch. 370*)

20.(C) *Discussion:* Nonsteroidal anti-inflammatory drugs are commonly used to treat the arthralgias and arthritis in patients with SLE. However, the use of ibuprofen in patients with SLE has been associated with the development of a drug-induced aseptic meningitis. Aseptic meningitis secondary to sulindac and tolmetin has also been described. (*Cecil, Ch. 240*)

21.(D) *Discussion:* The picture of recurrent miscarriages and deep venous thromboses is suggestive of an anticardiolipin antibody syndrome associated with SLE. Thus it would be important to determine whether anticardiolipin antibodies are present as well as to substantiate a diagnosis of SLE. (*Cecil, Ch. 240*)

22.(C) *Discussion:* This patient has multiorgan manifestations suggesting a systemic necrotizing vasculitis with prominent mesenteric artery involvement. Celiac and mesenteric angiography would be the procedure of choice. Biopsy of other accessible involved tissues, such as the skin and sural nerve, would also be appropriate. (*Cecil, Ch. 244*)

23.(E) *Discussion:* The involvement of the lower respiratory tract as well as renal involvement suggests Wegener's granulomatosis. Treatment of Wegener's granulomatosis with cyclophosphamide has resulted in marked improvement in outcome of this condition. Because of the severity and sudden deterioration, intravenous corticosteroids and intravenous cyclophosphamide would be indicated. (*Cecil, Ch. 245*)

24.(C) *Discussion:* Polymyalgia rheumatica is a common clinical syndrome in patients older than 55 years old and is characterized by stiffness and soreness in the shoulder and hip girdle areas. It is sometimes associated with mild joint swelling. Laboratory findings include normocytic/normochromic anemia and elevated sedimentation rate. Weakness of the proximal upper and lower extremity muscles is distinctly unusual and suggests a proximal myopathy such as polymyositis. (*Cecil, Ch. 246*)

25.(E) *Discussion:* All of the answers are correct. Cholesterol crystal (atheromatous) embolization is a common occurrence in patients with advanced atherosclerotic disease but is frequently either not recognized or misdiagnosed as "vasculitis." The exact incidence is currently unknown but it is associated with significant morbidity and mortality. With a rise in the number of geriatric patients with atherosclerosis, the recognition of this disorder is critical to prevent unnecessary diagnostic studies and treatment with high-dose corticosteroids/cytotoxic agents, which are of no benefit. The source of most cholesterol emboli is the abdominal aorta or iliofemoral arteries, but cardiac and thoracic aorta sources have been described. Episodes of embolization may occur spontaneously or may be temporally associated with surgery or invasive arterial studies (days) or response to anticoagulant or thrombocytic therapy (weeks). The clinical manifestations may mimic periarteritis nodosa, with fever, accelerated hypertension, and progressive renal failure; abdominal pain with bleeding or bowel infarction; multiple dermal manifestations such as livedo reticularis, purplish-discolored toes, and digital gangrene; intense thigh and gastronemius tenderness; and laboratory findings of elevated erythrocyte sedimentation rate, creatinine, and creatine phosphokinase and leukocytosis, eosinophilia, anemia, and proteinuria. (*Fine et al*)

26.(C) *Discussion:* Osteoporosis is characterized by a reduction in bone mass 2.5 standard deviations below the normal premenopausal mean value. Instead of a single disease, it is heterogeneous and influenced by hereditary, lifestyle, and hormonal factors. It is most treacherous in that the first manifestations may be fractures of the hip and spine, with enormous human and economic costs. Bone mass is inversely related to the risk of hip and spine fractures. Routine bone radiographs do not adequately quantify bone mineral density. (*Cecil, Ch. 217*)

27.(A—False; B—True; C—False; D—False; E—True) *Discussion:* See answer to question 25.

28.(All are True) *Discussion:* There is no question that glucocorticoid therapy has been beneficial to many patients with a variety of acute and chronic inflammatory disease. However, a common complication of chronic glucocorticoid treatment is severe bone mineral loss and subsequent fracture. Glucocorticoids influenced many aspects of calcium and bone metabolism. For example, they may inhibit osteoblast-mediated matrix synthesis; decrease intestinal absorption or calcium and phosphorus; diminish the circulating levels of estrogen, testosterone, follicle-stimulating hormone, and luteinizing hormone; and increase parathyroid hormone secretion, leading indirectly to osteoclast-mediated bone resorption. Some recommendations for management include using the lowest possible dose of glucocorticoids (completely stopping this treatment is not possible in most patients), encouraging ingestion of 1500 mg of elemental calcium (calcium carbonate and calcium citrate contain 40% and 11% elemental calcium, respectively), estrogen replacement (if no contraindication) in postmenopausal women, regular weight-bearing exercise therapy, and measurement of bone mineral density. (*Cecil, Ch. 217, Lane et al*)

29.(A—True; B—True; C—False; D—False; E—True) *Discussion:* Neutrophils contain within their granules potent proteinases such as elastase and collagenase that can cleave a number of matrix proteins. The major stimulus for the extracellular release of these proteases is by tissue-bound IgG immune complexes binding to the neutrophil Fc receptor. In addition to the release of proteinases, neutrophils may release reactive oxygen species and lipid-derived inflammatory substances such as platelet activating factor, leukotriene B_4, and lipoxin A. CR3 (CDE11/CD18) may demonstrate increased expression with neutrophil activation and binds to iC3b. IIb/IIIa is a major protein complex of platelets, not neutrophils. (*Cecil, Ch. 235*)

30.(A—False; B—True; C—False; D—False; E—False) *Discussion:* The presence of antiphospholipid antibodies has been associated with arterial and venous thrombosis, premature stroke syndromes, mesenteric artery insufficiency, and recurrent or multiple spontaneous abortions in patients with lupus or lupus-like illnesses. The lupus anticoagulant (associated with a prolonged PTT) and the anticardiolipin antibody have been shown to be different antibodies but may be present together in approximately 70% of patients. As stressed in the text, measurement of anticardiolipin antibody levels is difficult and should only be done in reference laboratories with multiple controls. (*Cecil, Ch. 236 and 240*)

31.(A—True; B—False; C—False; D—False; E—False) *Discussion:* Rheumatoid factor is typically an IgM antibody recognizing Fc determinants of the autologous IgG molecule and is present in the serum of approximately 75 to 80% of patients with rheumatoid arthritis. It is not specific for rheumatoid arthritis and is found in the serum of patients with a variety of inflammatory disorders, such as sarcoidosis and leprosy. It does not cause the disease and is not restricted to the HLA-DR4 haplotype. (*Cecil, Ch. 236 and 237*)

32.(A—False; B—True; C—True; D—True; E—False) *Discussion:* B cells arise from progenitor cells in the bone marrow. Their activation, proliferation, and differentiation into antibody-secreting plasma cells requires a variety of cytokines. Within their surface membranes, B cells have receptors, allowing them to recognize foreign antigenic determinants. These receptors are membrane immunoglobulins of unique specificity. The T3 complex is part of the T-cell receptor complex. (*Cecil, Ch. 221*)

33.(A—True; B—False; C—True; D—True; E—True) *Discussion:* Hemochromatosis is transmitted as an autosomal recessive disease associated with increased absorption of iron from the gastrointestinal tract, with increased tissue deposition of iron within the liver, heart, pancreas, and skin. Although the serum ferritin level is usually elevated, this is by no means diagnostic and occurs with a variety of disorders. The diagnosis is made by liver biopsy, which demonstrates increased parenchymal iron by staining as well as by quantitative liver iron measurement. Chondrocalcinosis is a common radiographic manifestation associated with hemochromatosis, primarily involves the second or third MCP joints, and occurs in about 50% of patients. Treatment consists of weekly phlebotomies to decrease the iron content of tissues, but this may aggravate the arthritis. (*Cecil, Ch. 189 and 256*)

34.(A—True; B—True; C—True; D—False; E—True) *Discussion:* Plain radiographs of the lumbosacral spine are indicated primarily in older patients complaining of back pain. These may show patterns of permeative bone destruction such as in myeloma or osteomyelitis. Osteomyelitis of the vertebral body is characterized by localized rarefaction of the vertebral end-plate progressing to destruction of the vertebral body and then to involvement of two adjacent vertebrae and the intervening disc space. Typically, metastatic neoplasms may involve the vertebral body but characteristically spare the intervening disc space. Myeloma may present with either focal, punched-out lesions or generalized reduction in bone density. Patients with renal osteodystrophy may show alternate bands of osteosclerosis and resorption, the so-called rugger jersey sign. (*Resnick and Niwayama*)

35.(A—True; B—False; C—True; D—False; E—True) *Discussion:* Symptoms of ankylosing spondylitis typically occur in the postpubescent male and consist of back and buttock pain and morning stiffness that diminishes with activity and recurs after periods of rest. Approximately 25% of patients may have an associated peripheral arthritis that is transient or, in a few cases, prolonged. Patients have reduced anterior lumbosacral flexion as measured by the Schober's test. The radiographic changes in the adolescent boy are delayed and may not be manifest until the patients are in their early 20s, but consist of sacroiliac irregularities with areas of sclerosis and/or erosions (widening). Fusion is typically a late radiographic manifestation. Patients may have extra-articular manifestations that include iritis, apical lung fibrosis, conduction disturbances, and aortic insufficiency. (*Cecil, Ch. 238; Resnick and Niwayama*)

36.(A—False; B—True; C—True; D—True; E—True) *Discussion:* Complications of postmenopausal osteoporosis, particularly severe morbidity from hip and vertebral fractures, represent a major health problem within the United States. Typically, bone mineral appears normal but is reduced in amount, suggesting that there is a disorder in which the formation of mineralized bone does not equal the resorption rate. Quantitative assessment of bone density is possible with dual-energy x-ray absorptiometry. This is a relatively new technique that should replace the more commonly used single- and dual-photon analysis in the future. (*Cecil, Ch. 217*)

37.(A—False; B—False; C—False; D—True; E—False) *Discussion:* The gonococcus is a gram-negative diplococcus that, when disseminated, may cause arthritis. Disseminated gonococcemia is an extremely common problem in healthy, sexually active teenagers and young adults. Physical presentation is that of an oligoarticular/monoarticular arthritis associated with tenosynovitis and skin lesions that vary from small pustules to vesicopustules with central necrotic centers. Diagnosis is frequently presumptive because it is a fastidious organism that is difficult to culture, requiring increased amounts of carbon dioxide and specialized media (Thayer-Martin). Response to treatment with antibiotics is dramatic. (*Cecil, Ch. 239*)

38.(A—False; B—True; C—True; D—True; E—True) *Discussion:* Collagens are the most abundant protein in the human body and constitute approximately 30% of the total protein. They serve diverse functions. Defects of type I collagen, the most abundant collagen type, have been associated with genetic syndromes including Ehlers-Danlos syndrome and osteogenesis imperfecta. In the formation of specialized collagens, collagen interacts with other components to make functional basement membranes. Type II collagen is the major fibrillar component of hyaline articular cartilage, and proteoglycans are the major noncollagenous structural proteins associated with elastic resistance to compression of this tissue. (*Cecil, Ch. 234*)

39.(A—True; B—True; C—False; D—True; E—True) *Discussion:* Phagocytes have on their plasma membrane receptors for C3b (CR1), which may function to clear circulating immune complexes and enhance phagocytosis. Activation of both complement pathways may lead to the generation of terminal components C6, C7, C8, and C9, which attach to the membrane and induce the formation of pores, with ultimate cell lysis. Recurrent sepsis with *Neisseria* species has been demonstrated in patients with deficiencies of the terminal components. C2 deficiency is by far the most common complement deficiency state, and this is usually associated with a low CH_{50}. Several rheumatic diseases, including SLE-like syndrome, vasculitis, and polymyositis, may occur in conjunction with C4 and C2 deficiencies. (*Cecil, Ch. 222*)

40.(A—True; B—True; C—True; D—False; E—True) *Discussion:* As noted in the answers, cytokines may have diverse or similar physiologic properties. They are all proteins with "hormone-like" properties having profound effects on inflammatory/immune cell function. (*Cecil, Ch. 221 and 235*)

41.(A—True; B—False, C—True; D—True; E—False) *Discussion:* Although the relative risk increases in individuals with a given disease associated with an HLA haplotype, a minority are afflicted with the disease. HLA-DR4 occurs in 75 to 80% of patients with rheumatoid arthritis. (*Cecil, Ch. 229 and 237*)

42.(A—False; B—True; C—True; D—False; E—False) *Discussion:* As noted in the text, rheumatic manifestations of HIV disease are being recognized with increased frequency. Musculoskeletal complaints are reported in 33 to 75% of HIV-infected patients and may present as a wide variety of rheumatologic disorders. Manifestations range from arthralgias, myalgias, and fever with acute seroconversion to polymyositis-like illness, Reiter's syndrome (indistinguishable from that in non–HIV-infected patients), Sjögren's syndrome, and a hepatitis B surface antigen–negative periarteritis nodosa syndrome. (*Cecil, Ch. 370*)

43.(A—False; B—True; C—False; D—False; E—False) *Discussion:* The pathology of polyarteritis consists of fibrinoid necrosis within small- and medium-sized vessels with a variable cellular infiltration, primarily neutrophils. Eosinophilia with lung involvement is not seen in patients with polyarteritis. Diminished total serum hemolytic complement with low C3 and C4 levels are seen in a small percentage of the patients. Subcutaneous nodules are infrequently found. (*Cecil, Ch. 244*)

44.(A—False; B—True; C—False; D—True; E—False) *Discussion:* Infiltration of various organs and vessels with cellular infiltrates consisting of atypical lymphoid and plasmacytoid cells is characteristic of lymphomatoid granulomatosis, not Wegener's granulomatosis. Hypersensitivity vasculitis is evidenced histologically by a small-vessel leukocytoclastic vasculitis and clinically by palpable purpura. Temporal arteritis usually involves extracranial elastic arteries. Takayasu's arteritis is a giant cell arteritis of the medium and large arteries, primarily of the aorta and vessels adjacent to it. Henoch-Schönlein purpura is usually a self-limited illness with prolonged renal insufficiency, with death being an uncommon outcome. (*Cecil, Ch. 243*)

45.(A—False; B—True; C—False; D—False; E—True) *Discussion:* Significant renal involvement in SLE occurs in approximately 50% of the patients. Although glomerular involvement is marked, renal tubular and interstitial disease is not uncommon. Neonatal lupus syndrome is associated with a placental transfer of maternal anti-Ro IgG antibodies to the fetus, sometimes causing congenital heart block in the fetus. Mothers do not have heart block, and it is thought that there are phase-specific antigens in the fetus that may be targeted by these antibodies. Vasculitic skin lesions are commonly seen in lupus and usually do not portend central nervous system vasculitis. Pleural fluid from patients with active SLE is usually transudative. (*Cecil, Ch. 240*)

46.(A—True; B—False; C—True; D—False; E—True) *Discussion:* Idiopathic midline granuloma is usually localized to the midline nasopharynx and is most appropriately treated with a combination of prednisone, cyclophosphamide, and radiation. Polymyalgia rheumatica is characterized by proximal upper and lower extremity muscle stiffness and soreness in patients older than 55 years but is not associated with an elevated creatine phosphokinase or myopathic electromyogram. In general, the alopecia associated with active lupus may improve with treatment of the disease except with discoid lesions, where there is follicular plugging and scarring that may result in permanent alopecia. A number of patients with end-stage renal disease caused by lupus have successfully received kidney transplants. (*Cecil, Chs. 240, 245, and 246*)

47.(A—True; B—True; C—False; D—False; E—False) *Discussion:* Nonspecific laboratory abnormalities such as neutrophilic leukocytosis and positive rheumatoid factor are often seen in patients with active Wegener's granulomatosis. An anticytoplasmic antibody directed to a 29-kD serine protease has been found in patients with active Wegener's granulomatosis. Idiopathic midline destructive disease is not a systemic vasculitis but is confined to the mid-paranasal sinuses. Lymphomatoid granulomatosis is an angiocentric immunoproliferative lesion with a tissue distribution that is very similar to Wegener's granulomatosis. It can be easily confused with Wegener's, but it is characterized by an angiocentric, inflammatory infiltrate of mononuclear cells with few granuloma. Necrotizing vasculitis involving the lungs and kidney is characteristic of Wegener's granulomatosis. However, limited forms of this disease without clinical renal or pulmonary involvement have been described. (*Cecil, Ch. 245*)

48.(A—False; B—True; C—False; D—False; E—True) *Discussion:* Erythema chronicum migrans is present in 75% of patients with Lyme disease and is manifest after an incubation period of 3 to 32 days. Approximately 60% of the patients develop frank arthritis. Antibodies to the specific IgM antibodies against the Lyme disease spirochete usually peak within 3 to 6 weeks; the specific IgG antibody titers rise more slowly and are present at the time of the arthritis weeks to months after infection. The decision to treat patients with antibiotics in an endemic area should be based not only on serologic but also on clinical features. (*Cecil, Ch. 321;* Primer)

49.(B); 50.(E); 51.(A); 52.(C) *Discussion:* The oxidation of homogentisic acid leads to the formation of an ochronotic brown pigment that is preferentially deposited in cartilage and tissue, which eventually leads to a degenerative arthropathy. Pigmented villonodular synovitis is characterized by synovial villous projections with a pleomorphic cellular infiltrate consisting of a variable number of lipid-laden and hemosiderin-laden macrophages, multinucleated giant cells, fibroblasts, and lymphocytes. Calcific deposits associated with calcium pyrophosphate deposition disease may occur not only in the articular and fibrocartilage but also in the joint capsule, ligaments, tendons, and synovial tissues. The calcium salts stain characteristic purple with hemaxtoxylin. The histologic features of rheumatoid arthritis are not specific but characteristically demonstrate synovial cell hyperplasia followed by infiltration of blood-borne lymphocytes and macrophages. (Primer)

53.(B); 54.(D); 55.(A); 56.(C) *Discussion:* Sudden painless loss of vision is a dreaded complication of temporal arteritis and is usually due to ischemic optic atrophy caused by involvement of the short posterior ciliary arteries and pial arterial network, which supply blood to the optic nerve and optic disc. Retinal vascular disease is a hallmark of eye involvement in SLE, usually with cotton wool spots (cytoid bodies) that are caused by distended and disrupted axons resulting from anoxia. In addition, hemorrhages are commonly observed in the retina. Eye manifestations of rheumatoid arthritis include sicca syndrome, with decreased tear formation as a result of secondary Sjögren's syndrome, and ''corneal melt'' with linear ulcerations usually at the limbus, leading to corneal perforation. Ankylosing spondylitis may be associated with an anterior uveitis, which is usually manifested by a painful red eye that demands attention. Failure to treat may lead to chronic iritis and blindness. (Primer)

57.(C); 58.(E); 59.(D); 60.(B) *Discussion:* Destruction of the tufts of the terminal phalanges is commonly seen in scleroderma, vinyl chloride disease, and secondary hyperparathyroidism. Acromegaly is characterized by premature or exaggerated osteoarthritis, including osteophyte formation. Punched-out erosions with overhanging bone around deposits of monosodium urate are characteristic of gout. Osteochondromatosis is characterized by the formation of multiple foci of metaplastic hyaline cartilage within the synovium. (Primer; *Resnick and Niwayama*)

61.(C); 62.(B); 63.(D); 64.(A) *Discussion:* A variety of musculoskeletal syndromes have been observed in patients on long-term (>8 to 10 years) chronic dialysis. Secondary hyperparathyroidism results from an elevated serum phosphorus level, which leads to increased release of parathyroid hormone, which in turn results in osteolysis of the pharyngeal tufts, demineralization of the bones of the appendicular and axial skeleton, and pathologic fractures. Deposition of beta$_2$-microglobulin amyloid within the carpal tunnel is associated with carpal tunnel syndrome, and deposition in the bone with subchondral cysts. Deposits of calcium salts in the skin and joints may lead to pruritus and periarthritis. Long-term use of aluminum-based antacids to bind phosphate has led to the syndrome of aluminum-related osteomalacia, characterized by muscle weakness and dementia. Some of these patients have been helped with desferoxamine. (*Cecil, Ch. 248;* Primer)

65.(A); 66.(D); 67.(E); 68.(C) *Discussion:* Many rheumatic syndromes have cutaneous manifestations. Erythema marginatum is a feature of rheumatic fever, seen in about 10 to 20% of afflicted children and rarely in adults. Nonthrombocytopenic purpura, usually involving the lower extremities, is one of the early manifestations of Henoch-Schönlein purpura, which histologically is a leukocytoclastic vasculitis. In addition, IgA may be found in the skin lesions. A variety of skin manifestations are part of the disseminated gonococcal arthritis syndrome. These include nonpainful, asymptomatic vesicles and vesiculopustular or hemorrhagic pustular lesions. Heliotrope rash with associated periorbital swelling and erythema is characteristic of dermatomyositis, both the childhood and adult forms. (Primer)

69.(C); 70.(A); 71.(B); 72.(D) *Discussion:* Acute gouty arthritis is the most frequent clinical manifestation of gout and occurs primarily in middle-aged and older men. Although the first MTP joint is characteristically involved, the first interphalangeal, ankle, and instep area are also commonly involved. The arthritis of Reiter's syndrome has an acute onset and consists of an asymmetric oligoarthritis primarily affecting the knees, ankles, and instep, and occurs most frequently in young men, presumably as a sexually acquired "reactive" arthritis. Rheumatoid arthritis is typically a symmetric polyarthritis predominantly involving the wrists, MCPs, PIPs, and MTP joints. The most common presentation pattern in children is a pauciarticular (four joints or less) arthritis. (*Cecil, Ch. 237, 238, and 251*)

73.(C); 74.(A); 75.(D); 76.(B) *Discussion:* One of the extra-articular manifestations that has been described in patients with ankylosing spondylitis is upper lobe lung fibrosis. Digital clubbing, periostitis, and painful swelling of bones and joints (hypertrophic osteoarthrophy) can develop in a wide variety of diseases such as lung malignancies and pulmonary infections. Acute arthritis, which is the most common rheumatic manifestation of sarcoidosis, affects the ankles and knees and less frequently the PIP joints of the hands, the wrists, and the elbows. Pleural effusions and pleuritis are often asymptomatic in rheumatoid arthritis patients, and the pleural fluid is typically exudative, with white blood cell counts rarely exceeding 5000 per cubic millimeter, with characteristically low glucose levels. (*Cecil, Ch. 237, 238, 256, and 257*)

77.(E); 78.(D); 79.(C); 80.(A) *Discussion:* Sudden painless loss of vision of the left eye associated with optic atrophy caused by occlusion of branches of the posterior ciliary artery is characteristic of temporal arteritis. Cauda equina syndrome can be seen in patients with longstanding ankylosing spondylitis. Bell's palsy, either unilateral or bilateral, may be a neurologic manifestation of Lyme arthritis. Deposits of beta$_2$-microglobulin in the carpal tunnel area may lead to motor weakness and atrophy of the muscles of the thenar eminence. (Primer)

81.(B); 82.(E); 83.(A); 84.(C) *Discussion:* Elevated levels of circulating parathyroid hormone leading to resorption of bone and vertebral body fractures have been described in primary and secondary hyperparathyroidism. Hypothyroidism can be associated with a proximal myopathy with an elevated creatine kinase level. This condition can easily be confused with polymyositis. Patients with acromegaly may have a transient Raynaud's-like illness. Patients with both adult and juvenile diabetes experience a painless limitation of joint mobility in the PIP and DIP joints called diabetic cheiropathy. (Primer)

85.(E); 86.(C); 87.(D); 88.(A) *Discussion:* A variety of rheumatic disease syndromes have been described in association with HIV infection. The most common relate to arthralgias and myalgias associated with acute seroconversion. Nemaline rods (thickened Z line seen in congenital myopathy, polymyositis, and secondary myopathies) may also be seen in HIV-related myopathy. Reiter's syndrome indistinguishable from that in non–HIV-infected patients may be seen. Several vasculitis syndromes have been reported, with the periarteritis nodosa type being the most common. This usually presents as a peripheral sensory or sensorimotor neuropathy. (*Cecil, Ch. 370*)

89.(D); 90.(A); 91.(C); 92.(B) *Discussion:* Palpable purpura is a primary skin feature of hypersensitivity vasculitis. Although multisystem involvement may occur in this small vessel vasculitis, involvement of the skin is the most common manifestation. Subcutaneous nodules occur in 20 to 25% of rheumatoid arthritis cases, may be freely moveable or fixed to the periosteum, and occur primarily in the pressure areas but may also be seen in the feet, hands, and scalp. They also occur in SLE and periarteritis nodosa, but this is very unusual. Gottron's papules are a pathognomic skin finding of dermatomyositis and are seen in one third of afflicted patients. They are manifested by flat-topped papules that overlie the dorsal surface of the MCP or PIP joints of the hands. Discoid lesions typically occur on the face, chest, or arms and may be either independent or associated with SLE, and may be associated with permanent scarring. (*Cecil, Ch. 237, 240, 243, and 247*)

93.(C); 94.(A); 95.(B); 96.(D) *Discussion:* C2 deficiency is associated with a SLE-like syndrome as well as vasculitis- and polymyositis-like syndromes. Clinically, it is characterized by a low CH$_{50}$ and may be diagnosed by quantitative C2 measurements. Antineutrophil cytoplasmic antibodies are directed against a 29-kD serine protease associated with the azurophil granules and have been found in many patients with Wegener's granulomatosis. The titer is thought to correlate with the severity of disease activity. The most common renal disorder associated with Sjögren's syndrome is renal tubular acidosis. The presence of glomerulonephritis has been described but is distinctly unusual in primary Sjögren's syndrome. Tender induration of the skin with retraction of subcutaneous tissue with eosinophilia is characteristic of diffuse fasciitis with eosinophilia, a syndrome primarily occurring in men, often following unaccustomed strenuous exercise. (*Cecil, Ch. 222, 242, and 245*)

97.(B); 98.(A); 99.(C); 100.(D) *Discussion:* Cytoid bodies, also called "retinal exudates," are actually degenerating neuronal elements that form as a response to anoxic tissue injury. They are not specific for lupus and may be seen in a variety of disorders, including leukemia and lymphoma. Mononeuritis multiplex, as evidenced by foot- or wristdrop or cranial nerve abnormalities, is characteristic of patients with polyarteritis nodosa but may also be seen in patients with a vasculitis secondary to SLE or Wegner's granulomatosis. Jaw claudication, a manifestation of ischemia to the lingual arteries, may be seen in patients with temporal arteritis. A variety of neurologic syndromes may occur in patients with Behçet's syndrome. Cerebellar, brain stem, and long tract signs with acute onset of headache and meningitis characterize the meningoencephalitis syndrome. (*Cecil, Ch. 240, 246, and 249*)

101.(A); 102.(B); 103.(C); 104.(D) *Discussion:* Recurrent fetal loss has been described in patients with minimal findings of lupus and has been found to be associated with the presence of anticardiolipin antibodies. Other features associated with the anticardiolipin antibody include premature strokes and recurrent arterial and venous thrombosis. Congenital heart block is one of the features of neonatal lupus and is thought to be mediated by the transplacental passage of IgG anti-SSA (Ro) antibody during the first trimester of pregnancy. Drug-induced lupus syndrome, most commonly associated with procainamide ingestion, may occur, with the ANAs including antibodies to antihistone components. Although only occurring in 20 to 30% of patients with lupus, the presence of anti-Smith antibodies is quite specific for this disorder. (*Cecil, Ch. 240*)

105.(D); 106.(A); 107.(B); 108.(C) *Discussion:* Churg-Strauss syndrome is a systemic necrotizing vasculitis that has clinical and pathologic manifestations similar to those of polyarteritis but differs with respect to the frequency of pulmonary involvement, eosinophilia, and allergic manifestations. Eosinophilia-myalgia syndrome, a recently described syndrome with protean manifestations, has been causally linked to contaminated preparations of L-tryptophan. Eosinophilic fasciitis is a scleroderma-like disorder characterized by symmetric sclerosis of the deep fascia, subcutis, and dermis. Fibromyalgia (fibrositis) is an extremely common disorder characterized by generalized pain and the presence of a large number of tender points. (*Cecil, Ch. 243; Schulman; Wolfe et al*)

BIBLIOGRAPHY

Bennett JC, Plum F (eds): Cecil Textbook of Medicine. 20th ed. Philadelphia, WB Saunders Company, 1996.

Fine MJ, Kapoor W, et al: Cholesterol crystal embolization: A review of 221 cases in the English literature. Angiology 38:769, 1987.

Lane NE, Mroczkowski PJ, et al: Prevention and management of glucocorticoid-induced osteoporosis. Bull Rheum Dis 44(5), 1995.

Primer on the Rheumatic Diseases. 10th ed. Atlanta, Arthritis Foundation, 1993.

Resnick D, Niwayama G: Diagnosis of Bone and Joint Disorders. 2nd ed. Philadelphia, WB Saunders Company, 1988.

Shulman LE: Editorial: The eosinophilia-myalgia syndrome associated with ingestion of L-tryptophan. Arthritis Rheum 33:913, 1990.

Weinblatt ME: Methotrexate. *In* Kelley WN, Harris ED Jr, Ruddy S, Sledge CB (eds): Textbook of Rheumatology. 4th ed. Philadelphia, WB Saunders Company, 1993.

Wolfe F, Smythe HA, et al: The American College of Rheumatology 1990 criteria for the classification of fibromyalgia. Arthritis Rheum 33:160, 1990.

PART 10

ENDOCRINE/REPRODUCTIVE DISEASES AND DISEASES OF BONE AND BONE MINERAL METABOLISM

Van B. Hayne, Jr. and Ayman A. Zayed

DIRECTIONS: For questions 1 to 42, choose the ONE BEST answer to each question.

1. A 5-year-old girl is referred to you after the mother noted early breast development with a finding of black terminal hair growth in the pubic area and a small of amount of bleeding from the vagina. On examination, you note Tanner stage 2 to 3 breast development and secondary sexual development with terminal hair growth in the genital area. There are a few terminal hairs noted in the axillae also. Magnetic resonance imaging (MRI) scan reveals a normal sella with a tumor apparent in the suprasellar region. All of the following statements are true regarding this condition EXCEPT

    A. This tumor is producing gonadotropin-releasing hormone (GnRH) and does so in a pulsatile manner not under normal prepubertal inhibitory influence.

    B. The lesion is likely a hypothalamic tumor known as a hamartoma.

    C. No therapy is necessary for the precocious puberty because it will resolve with time.

    D. Optimal therapy for the precocious puberty in this situation would be the use of the GnRH agonist to down-regulate pituitary GnRH receptors, diminishing gonadotropin secretion and suppressing bone growth.

    E. Hamartomas in the hypothalamus have also been associated with acromegaly, through production of growth hormone–releasing hormone (GHRH), and Cushing's syndrome, through production of corticotropin-releasing hormone.

2. A 32-year-old nurse comes to you because of a 3-month history of progressive nervousness, palpitations, and heat intolerance. She has lost 5 lb in the last month. Her past medical history is significant for a cesarean section with delivery of a live male infant 5 months ago. Physical examination reveals a pulse of 100 beats per minute, and the thyroid gland is not palpable, but her skin is hot and moist. The rest of the examination is normal. Her laboratory workup reveals a chemistry profile and complete blood count that are normal. Her total thyroxine (T_4) level is 16 μg per deciliter (normal: 5 to 12); triiodothyronine resin uptake (T_3RU) is 50% (normal: 30 to 40); and thyroid-stimulating hormone (TSH) level is less than 0.05 mIU per milliliter (normal 0.5

to 5.0). A ^{131}I thyroid uptake at 4 hours is 1% (normal: 5 to 10). The next best step in evaluation of this patient would be

    A. Start the patient on propranolol and methimazole

    B. Measure serum thyroglobulin

    C. Do a fine-needle thyroid biopsy

    D. Obtain total triiodothyronine (T_3) radioimmunoassay (RIA) measurement

    E. Reassure the patient that her condition is temporary and needs no further treatment or evaluation

3. A 64-year-old man is admitted through the emergency room to the intensive care unit after a 3- to 4-day history of abdominal pain, later developing fever along with nausea and vomiting. In the intensive care unit, he has a blood pressure of 80/50 mm Hg with a sodium level of 129 mEq per liter and potassium level of 5.5 mEq per liter. Past medical history is important in that the patient has been on anticoagulant therapy for the past 3 months after suffering a pulmonary thromboembolism. The patient has had appropriate cultures done and, despite aggressive fluid replacement, his blood pressure remains 90/60 mm Hg. A serum cortisol level drawn at 8:00 A.M. is 3 μg per deciliter. All of the following statements are true regarding this patient's condition EXCEPT

    A. The patient must have sepsis to explain his condition.

    B. Hyperpigmentation may or may not be present and would depend on the duration of the disease.

    C. Lymphocytosis and eosinophilia would be consistent with this patient's condition.

    D. Hypoglycemia may be present.

    E. Computed tomography (CT) scan of the abdomen might be expected to show evidence of blood and hemorrhage in both adrenal glands.

4. A 45-year-old woman consults with you because of the development of increasing hyperpigmentation and headache, and her state driver's licensing bureau refusing to renew her driver's license because of a loss of her peripheral vision on a screening exam. Important is the fact that the patient had Cushing's disease, with bilateral adrenalectomy done 3 years ago. She is on glucocorticoid and mineralocorticoid replacement. The patient most likely has

A. Addison's disease
B. Recurrent Cushing's disease
C. Schmidt's syndrome
D. Nelson syndrome
E. None of the above

5. All the following are causes of gynecomastia EXCEPT

A. Local chest trauma
B. Hepatic cirrhosis
C. Turner's syndrome
D. Testicular carcinoma
E. Leydig cell tumors of the testis

6. A 20-year-old woman comes to see you for help with secondary amenorrhea. The patient gives a history of menarche at age 14 with regular menses up until 18 months ago, when she had irregular periods for approximately 6 months and no periods for the past year. She has been sexually active and had been seen in the clinic with a negative pregnancy test on two separate occasions in the past year, the last time 1 month ago. The patient's past medical history is important because she has had vitiligo and recurrent candidiasis of the oral mucosa and has been on thyroid hormone for thyroid failure over the past 6 years. The normal values of luteinizing hormone (LH), follicle-stimulating hormone (FSN), and estradiol are as follows:

	LH (mIU/ml)	FSH (mIU/ml)	Estradiol (pg/ml)
Premenopausal		4–30	
Follicular phase	5–30		10–90
Midcycle peak	75–150	10–90	100–500
Luteal phase	3–40		50–240
Postmenopausal	30–200	40–250	10–30

The lab data that are most consistent with this patient's etiology for amenorrhea are:

A. FSH 5, LH 6, estradiol 80
B. LH 50, FSH 75, estradiol 15
C. LH 18, FSH 4, estradiol 60
D. LH 1, FSH 2, estradiol 10
E. LH 40, FSH 45, estradiol 100

7. The assessment of mutations in the *Ret* proto-oncogene may be important in the identification of all patients with the following EXCEPT

A. Familial medullary thyroid carcinoma
B. Medullary thyroid carcinoma as seen in multiple endocrine neoplasia (MEN) type IIA
C. Medullary thyroid carcinoma as seen in MEN type IIB
D. Papillary carcinoma of the thyroid

8. A 40-year-old woman comes to you because of generalized weakness, dizziness, and cold intolerance. A physical examination is positive for a mildly enlarged, firm, rubbery textured goiter. Her thyroid test reveals a free thyroxine

(FT$_4$) level of 0.5 μg per deciliter (normal: 0.7 to 1.85) with TSH level of 28 mIU per milliliter (normal: 0.3 to 5). The patient is begun on levothyroxine at 100 μg daily. Approximately 1 month later, she presents back to you with a 10-day history of generalized weakness, nausea, and vomiting and is noted to be hypotensive in the office. All the following are likely to be present in this patient EXCEPT

A. Positive antimicrosomal antibody titers
B. Eosinophilia
C. A.M. cortisol level of 3 μg per deciliter
D. History of transient hyperthyroidism a few months ago
E. Normal FT$_4$ level after 1 month on levothyroxine therapy

QUESTIONS 9 AND 10

A 40-year-old white man comes to see you about decreased libido and problems with erections dating back for 1 year. Otherwise, he denies complaints, shaves daily, and denies any psychological disturbances. He is on no medication. There is no history of any headache or any visual complaints. Physical examination is normal, including hair distribution, size of testes, and absence of any feminizing features. His lab tests reveal a total testosterone level of 100 ng per milliliter (normal: 400 to 1000) and LH level of 5 mIU per milliliter (normal: 2 to 10).

9. The next best step in evaluating this patient would be

A. Check prolactin level
B. Check TSH level
C. Start testosterone therapy
D. Do a karyotype analysis
E. Check a fasting blood sugar level

10. After carrying out the step above, your next step would be

A. Measure FSH
B. Measure free testosterone
C. Do a pituitary MRI scan
D. Do a testicular biopsy
E. Do a semen fluid analysis

11. All of the following are associated in the etiology of nephrogenic diabetes insipidus EXCEPT

A. Demeclocycline
B. Lithium
C. Cyclophosphamide
D. Methoxyflurane
E. Sarcoidosis

12. A 20-year-old woman presents because she has never had a period. She denies any health problems. Physical examination is basically normal, with a weight of 120 lb and height of 170 cm. Breast exam is normal, with Tanner stage 5. External genital examination reveals absence of pubic hair. Examination of the axillae reveals very scant and rare axillary hair. Pelvic examination reveals a short vagina with absent cervix. You may see all of the following EXCEPT

A. LH level of 2 mIU per milliliter (normal 2 to 10)
B. Total testosterone level of 990 mg per deciliter (normal for women: <100)

C. Estradiol level of 100 pg per milliliter (normal: 75 to 250)
D. Absent uterus by ultrasound of the pelvis
E. Karyotype of 46,XY

13. A 42-year-old white man comes in with a 5-month history of episodes associated with headaches, palpitations along with chest pain, and blurring of his vision. He had seen his family physician on several occasions with no abnormality noted on physical exam. However, he had one of the episodes when leaving his family physician's office on his last visit, and the nurse, who checked his blood pressure as he was about to leave, noted a blood pressure of 190/110 mm Hg, with his usual blood pressure being 130/78 mm Hg. His family physician referred him to you and told the patient that he had a "glandular disorder." The patient's physical examination is unremarkable, with a blood pressure of 126/85 mm Hg. Because he has been having one to two episodes a week, ambulatory blood pressure monitoring is done. During the next week he has one episode, revealing his blood pressure rising from approximately 140/80 to 220/130 mm Hg before returning to normal after the episode resolves. Six days after his last paroxysm, the patient has serum catecholamines properly collected, revealing a serum norepinephrine level of 200 pg per milliliter and an epinephrine level of 30 pg per milliliter (normal: norepinephrine <220 and epinephrine <35). Your best interpretation of the above test results in the context of this patient's symptoms and objective findings is

A. The above biochemical data exclude a pheochromocytoma.
B. The above biochemical data do not exclude pheochromocytoma because some patients with pheochromocytoma may have normal plasma catecholamine levels when they are asymptomatic and normotensive.
C. A 24-hour urine measure of vanillylmandelic acid (VMA), metanephrine, and catecholamine levels that is normal during an asymptomatic phase would absolutely exclude pheochromocytoma.
D. None of the above

14. A 56-year-old woman was referred to you for further evaluation of hypercalcemia. The patient was in to see her family physician and was noted to have a serum calcium level of 10.8 mg per deciliter (normal: 8.5 to 10.2) and an albumin level of 4 grams per deciliter to (normal: 3.5 to 4.5). The patient has had no symptoms of any type over the years and has been in good health. Two brothers, three sisters, and a mother are all living. She is unaware of any family history of calcium disorders but states, "my family never sees doctors." Laboratory testing done by you reveals

Serum Chemistries	Patient	Normal
Calcium (mg/dl)	10.9	8.5–10.2
Albumin (g/dl)	3.9	3.5–4.5
Phosphorus (mg/dl)	2.5	2.7–4.5
Magnesium (mEq/L)	2.2	1.3–2.1
Intact parathyroid hormone (PTH) (pg/ml)	40	15–65
Creatinine (mg/dl)	0.7	0.5–1.1

Her 24-hour urine calcium level with history of normal oral calcium intake was 40 mg (normal 100 to 300). The most appropriate next step in the evaluation/treatment of this patient is

A. Refer the patient to a surgeon for neck exploration.
B. Recommend no surgery for neck exploration now but recommend follow-up every 4 to 6 months, reassessing calcium, renal function, and parathyroid hormone levels for possible surgery to be done at a later time.
C. Place the patient on a low-calcium diet.
D. Advise the patient that she needs an evaluation for cancer to rule out hypercalcemia of malignancy.
E. Advise the patient to have her family members to come to see you for measurement of serum calcium to see if any of them have hypercalcemia.

15. All of the following are associated with Kallmann's syndrome EXCEPT

A. Anosmia or hyposmia
B. Testosterone level of 80 mg per deciliter (normal: 250 to 900); LH level of 50 mIU per milliliter (normal: 5 to 10); FSH level of 40 mIU per milliliter (normal: 5 to 10)
C. Color blindness
D. Short fourth metacarpal
E. Prolactin level of 10 ng per milliliter (normal for men: <20)

16. A 58-year-old man comes to see you because of rash and weight loss. He describes the rash as developing as redness of the skin that become swollen and developed blisters that broke and crusted over and after healing, leaving dark areas over the skin. He has noted this mainly over the face and along the lower abdomen, buttocks, and perineal areas as well as the upper legs. He gives a history of a 25-lb weight loss in the last 3 months, with the rash going on for about 6 weeks. On physical examination, the rash is as described by the patient and he has evidence of acute and recent weight loss. He also has evidence of glossitis and chelitis. His lab tests reveal a hematocrit and hemoglobin of 30% and 10 grams per deciliter, respectively, both of which are low. A fasting blood sugar measurement done on two occasions is 200 mg per deciliter on the first occasion and 220 mg per deciliter on the second. Renal function and liver function tests are normal. All of the following statements about this condition are true EXCEPT

A. The risk of malignancy in this condition is extremely low in 10% or fewer of patients.
B. Measure of glucagon in this patient is 1800 pg per deciliter (normal: 50 to 150).
C. Abdominal pain, diarrhea, nausea, and vomiting may occur.
D. Thromboembolic disease may occur.

17. All of the following statements about atrial natriuretic peptide (ANP) are true EXCEPT

A. ANP produces natriuresis.
B. ANP produces smooth muscle constriction.
C. ANP produces diuresis.
D. ANP inhibits renin and aldosterone secretion.
E. ANP is secreted primarily by the cardiac atria.

QUESTIONS 18 AND 19

A 32-year-old man is referred to you for evaluation of thyrotoxicosis. A referring physician noted, as you do from the history, that the patient has had increasing heat intolerance over the past 3 to 4 months, with a 10- to 15-lb weight loss, insomnia, tremor, and palpitations. The initial lab work done by the referring physician and sent to you revealed a FT_4 level of 0.6 μg per deciliter (normal: 0.5 to 1.85) and TSH level of less than 0.05 mIU per milliliter (normal: 0.32 to 5.0). A thyroid scan with uptake reveals essentially no visualization of the thyroid, and the 24-hour uptake was 1.5%. The patient denies any tenderness of the neck or any other symptoms except those noted. On examination, the patient has a normal blood pressure with a pulse of 110 beats per minute; warm, clammy skin; a fine tremor of his hands; velvety smooth skin; and small thyroid. He has no history of thyroid surgery. His repeated FT_4 and TSH tests confirm the findings by the referring physician.

18. The next best step to take in the evaluation of this patient would be

   A. Repeat his thyroid scan and uptake
   B. Measure TSH receptor antibodies
   C. Do a thyrotropin-releasing hormone (TRH) stimulation test
   D. Measure total serum T_3 level
   E. Place the patient on levothyroxine therapy and return him to his primary care physician

19. The proper test was done. Based on all the information you now have, the next best step to determine the etiology of this patient's problem would be

   A. Initiate therapy with thionamides
   B. Recommend subtotal thyroidectomy
   C. Recommend treatment with ^{131}I therapy
   D. Measure serum thyroid antibody titers
   E. Measure serum thyroglobulin level

20. In the nonthyroidal illness syndrome, the most frequently encountered combination of thyroid hormone values is

   A. Normal T_3 values, elevated T_4 values
   B. Low T_3 values, low T_4 values
   C. Low T_3 values, normal T_4 values
   D. Low T_3 values, elevated T_4 values
   E. Elevated T_3 values, elevated T_4 values

QUESTIONS 21 AND 22

A 22-year-old woman presents to your office with a 15-lb weight loss, tremors of the hands, heat intolerance, and a complaint of swelling in the neck noted over the last month or two. She has complained of palpitations and difficulty sleeping within the past 3 to 4 weeks. She has been on no medications and has had no previous symptoms as noted above. She does have a maternal grandmother who had thyroid surgery for "an overactive thyroid" many years ago. Examination reveals a diffusely enlarged thyroid that is nontender, with bilateral thyroid lobe bruits heard on auscultation. Her skin is velvety

smooth and she has a fine tremor noted in both hands when outstretched. Her pulse rate is 112 beats per minute. Your preliminary diagnosis is thyrotoxicosis caused by Graves' disease.

21. Based on this diagnosis, other features of thyrotoxicosis in Graves' disease that are possible in this patient include all of the following EXCEPT

   A. Oligomenorrhea or amenorrhea
   B. Menorrhagia
   C. Elevation in systolic blood pressure
   D. Elevation in alkaline phosphatase levels in a small percentage of patients
   E. Onycholysis

22. Features associated with Graves' disease include which of the following?

   A. Infiltrative ophthalmopathy
   B. Pretibial myxedema
   C. Thyroid acropachy
   D. Diffuse lymphadenopathy with splenomegaly
   E. All of the above

23. A 25-year-old woman in her eighth week of pregnancy is referred to you with an actual 3-lb weight loss during her pregnancy, palpitations, decreased appetite, tremor, and insomnia. Her obstetrician noted that her thyroid was enlarged to three times normal in a diffuse manner, and her thyroid test revealed a FT_4 level of 3.4 μg per deciliter (normal: 0.5 to 1.8) and TSH level of less than 0.05 mIU per milliliter (normal: 0.5 to 5.0). The patient has had no nausea or vomiting. Your physical examination reveals a diffusely enlarged, nontender thyroid, and she is noted to have bilateral proptosis, with a measurement by a Hertel exophthalmometer of 23 mm (normal: <20). Based on the findings and her laboratory data, you would recommend as the best therapy for her

   A. Initiation of propylthiouracil
   B. Initiation of methimazole
   C. Treatment only with propranolol, planning treatment throughout pregnancy
   D. Plan a referral to a surgeon during the second trimester of pregnancy for a subtotal thyroidectomy
   E. Recommend no treatment and simply follow thyroid function tests, because her hyperthyroid state is due to elevated human chorionic gonadotropin

QUESTIONS 24 AND 25

A 25-year-old woman presents to you with a complaint of lethargy and fatigue for 2 months. She delivered her first child approximately 6 months ago and had been doing well, and actually noted increased energy several months ago. Over the past 2 months, she has noticed a decrease in energy, feeling cold a good bit of the time, and having to wear a sweater in her home where just few months ago she had been staying hot. She now requires sleep of 10 to 12 hours per night, whereas before she was able to get by on 6 to 7 hours of sleep. Her skin has recently been more dry and her menses have been much heavier. She also has had problems with constipation, which she has never had in the past. Her examination reveals dry, coarse skin and a thyroid mildly enlarged in a diffuse manner, not tender, and somewhat firm without lymphadenopathy. Her deep tendon reflexes reveal delayed relaxation phase. She brings lab results showing a FT_4 level of 0.55 μg per deciliter (normal: 0.7 to 1.85) and TSH level of 45 mIU per milliliter (normal: 0.32 to 5). The patient had a radioactive iodine uptake test done 2 weeks ago by her primary care physician showing an uptake using ^{123}I of 40% (normal: 15 to 30). Her thyroid antibodies test is negative and there is no family history of any thyroid disease of which she is aware.

24. The most likely diagnosis for this patient based on all the above information is

    A. Chronic lymphocytic thyroiditis (Hashimoto's thyroiditis)
    B. Jodbasedow effect
    C. Hypothyroid phase of postpartum thyroiditis
    D. Hypothyroid phase of de Quervain's thyroiditis
    E. Reidel's thyroiditis

25. The elevated radioactive iodine uptake in this patient is best explained by

    A. An error made by the technician in the nuclear medicine lab
    B. Increased synthesis of thyroid hormone with repletion of the stores of hormone within the thyroid gland itself, as a result of elevation of TSH in the recovery phase of postpartum thyroiditis
    C. Thyroid receptor antibody that is elevated in patients with postpartum thyroiditis
    D. Iodine repletion in the diet, the treatment of choice in patients with postpartum thyroiditis
    E. Thyroid hormone replacement with levothyroxine in patients with postpartum thyroiditis

26. Which of the following may require a higher dosage of levothyroxine to be given to a hypothyroid patient?

    A. Cholestyramine
    B. Ferrous sulfate
    C. Rifampin
    D. Third-trimester pregnancy
    E. All of the above

27. A 45-year-old man presents to the emergency room with a history of 4 hours of aching substernal chest pain, radiating into the jaws and down the left arm, associated with shortness of breath and nausea. An electrocardiogram reveals inferior ischemic changes. He is admitted to the hospital, and cardiac enzyme measurements are done that rule out an acute mycardial infarction. Two days after admission, the patient undergoes coronary angiograms, which reveal a 95% occlusive lesion in the proximal portion of the right coronary artery. The cardiologist wants to do angioplasty of this lesion, but, in the course of taking further history and examining the patient, the cardiologist notes that his skin is dry, with a yellow appearance, and his hair is extremely brittle. On further history taking, the patient has noted cold intolerance for 8 months, along with increased drowsiness and constipation. The cardiologist obtains a cholesterol level of 280 mg per deciliter, FT_4 level of 0.65 per deciliter (nor-

mal: 0.7 to 1.85), and TSH level of 30 mIU per milliliter (normal: 0.32 to 5). With these data, the cardiologist wants an opinion as to when to do the angioplasty. Which of the following do you recommend to the cardiologist regarding the timing of the angioplasty, understanding that the cardiologist believes that it must be done during this hospitalization?

    A. Proceed with angioplasty the following day because the cardiologist plans to institute levothyroxine therapy at a low dose after angioplasty is completed and the patient is stable
    B. Postpone angioplasty until the patient can be normalized regarding his hypothyroid state, and initiate levothyroxine therapy at 12.5 μg daily
    C. Proceed with angioplasty the following day and give the patient levothyroxine 150 μg by mouth prior to angioplasty and continue this dose afterward
    D. Postpone angioplasty for 1 week and institute levothyroxine at 100 μg orally each day.
    E. Proceed with angioplasty the following day and explain to the cardiologist and patient that all of the patient's thyroid function abnormalities are due to nonthyroidal illness related to his unstable angina and recent angiograms

28. A 45-year-old woman is referred to you after a thyroid nodule was found on routine physical examination. The patient was not aware that she had a mass in her thyroid and has no history of any previous thyroid disease or thyroid nodule. There is no family history of thyroid disease or thyroid nodules. The patient has no history of radiation therapy of any type to the head or neck. The patient has no symptoms of hyper- or hypothyroidism. Lab tests reveal a TSH level of 1.5 mIU per milliliter (normal: 0.32 to 5), and the patient undergoes a fine-needle aspiration biospy of this nodule. The pathology report reveals a hypercellular lesion with no colloid, consistent with a "follicular lesion." Your next step in the evaluation of this patient's thyroid nodule, based on the laboratory and cytopathologic findings noted above, is

    A. Refer the patient to a surgeon specializing in thyroid surgery for thyroidectomy
    B. Initiate levothyroxine therapy to suppress the nodule
    C. Recommend follow-up with ultrasound in 6 months to see if the nodule is increasing in size
    D. Do a thyroid scan to determine if the nodule is "hot" versus "cold" or "warm"
    E. Advise the patient to have rebiopsy in 2 months

29. Which of the following thyroid cancers are responsive to ^{131}I therapy?

    A. Follicular cancer of the thyroid
    B. Medullary cancer of the thyroid
    C. Anaplastic thyroid cancer
    D. Primary lymphoma of the thyroid
    E. Both A and C

30. A 36-year-old white woman presents to you for evaluation of a 6-month history of polyuria, voiding 8 to 10 liters of urine mainly during the daytime hours. The patient states that she remains thirsty most of the time and drinks about 10 to 12 liters of different kinds of fluids every day. She has no family history of similar conditions. Her past medical history is significant for depression, for which she takes amitryptiline. Her physical examination is unremarkable. A random serum sodium level is 138 mEq per liter, potassium level is 3.9 mEq per liter calcium level is 9.1 mEq per liter, and albumin level is 3.8 grams per deciliter. A urine specific gravity was 1.003. The patient underwent a dehydration test and, after approximately 20 hours of dehydration, her plasma osmolality was 298 and her urine osmolality stabilized at 806. She was given 5 units of aqueous vasopressin subcutaneously, and 1 hour later her urine osmolality was 810. The most appropriate next step is

A. Initiate demeclocycline therapy
B. Encourage the patient to decrease her fluid intake
C. Initiate intranasal desmopressin acetate (DDAVP) therapy
D. Initiate oral chlorpropamide therapy
E. Initiate hydrochlorothiazide therapy

QUESTIONS 31 AND 32

A 47-year-old man presents to you because of a 2-year history of progressive erectile dysfunction. His work-up reveals a total testosterone level of 112 ng per milliliter (normal: 300 to 900), LH level of 2.5 mIU per milliliter (normal: 2 to 10), and FSH level of 3 mIU per milliliter (normal: 2 to 10). The patient is started on testosterone enanthate 200 mg intramuscularly every 2 weeks. He has a good response to this. However, 2 months later, the patient presents with progressive generalized weakness, malaise, anorexia, nausea, occasional vomiting, and a 10-lb weight loss. His blood pressure is 90/60 mm Hg, with a pulse that is 93 beats per minute (regular). His physical examination is otherwise unremarkable. Laboratory tests reveal

Serum electrolytes	
Sodium	139 mEq/L
Potassium	4.2 mEq/L
Chloride	102 mEq/L
Bicarbonate	25 mEq/L
Blood glucose	65 mg/dl
Hemoglobin	13.8 g/dl
Serum calcium	10.5 mEq/L
Albumin	3.8 g/dl

31. The most appropriate next step would be

A. Check thyroid function tests and treat accordingly
B. Synthetic adrenocorticotropic hormone (ACTH) stimulation test
C. Increase the testosterone dose
D. Measure somatomedin C level
E. Measure serum ACTH level

32. The proper test was ordered, and the patient was treated appropriately with significant improvement. Three days later, the patient starts to have 5 to 6 liters of polyuria with associated polydipsia. The following laboratory data were obtained:

Urine specific gravity	1.004
Serum chemistries	
Sodium	149 mEq/L
Potassium	3.5 mEq/L
Chloride	100 mEq/L
Bicarbonate	25 mEq/L
Calcium	10.1 mEq/L
Albumin	4.2 g/dl

The MOST likely explanation for his polyuria is

A. Hypokalemia
B. Hypercalcemia
C. Acquired diabetes mellitus precipitated by his new medication
D. Central diabetes insipidus unmasked by his new medication
E. None of the above

33. A 19-year-old female college student presents to you because she has never had a menstrual cycle. She is short of stature, with minimal breast development and scant axillary and pubic hair. The patient is also noted to have a webbed neck. All of the following are features of this disorder EXCEPT

A. Chromosome type of 45XO is the most common genotype
B. Low-set ears
C. Coarctation of the aorta
D. Short second metacarpals
E. Double eyelashes

34. A 19-year-old man comes to you for evaluation of sexual immaturity. The patient and family state that his development and growth were normal up until 13 to 14 years of age, and then he began to lag behind his peers, and he has noted very little axillary and pubic hair. It should be noted that he had a cleft palate that was repaired in the first few years after birth, and he and his family have noticed that he has decrease in his sensation of smell. Physical examination reveals an arm span greater than his height and a length from pubis to feet greater than the length from head to pubis. There are a few terminal hairs noted under the axillae and around the pubic area. It is noted that he has an extremely small penis and his testes are still prepubertal. All of the following could be expected to be found as part of this syndrome EXCEPT

A. Inheritance may be autosomal recessive
B. This condition occurs in males only
C. Short fourth metacarpals may occur
D. Serum testosterone, LH, and FSH levels are low
E. Most of the patients with this syndrome have either anosmia or hyposmia

35. McCune-Albright syndrome is associated with

A. Polyostotic fibrous dysplasia
B. Café-au-lait spots
C. Mutations in the alpha subunit of the Gs protein, a noninherited disorder
D. Endocrinopathies including precocious puberty, hyperthyroidism, and acromegaly
E. All of the above

36. In carcinoid syndrome, all of the following have been associated with triggering the flush that may be seen in patients with this disorder EXCEPT

    A. Serotonin
    B. Histamine
    C. Tachykinins
    D. Catecholamines

37. A 32-year-old male nurse, with a previous history of thyroid cancer with near-total thyroidectomy and radioactive iodine ablative therapy, developed hypocalcemia secondary to hypoparathyroidism. The patient was placed on calcium and vitamin D, taking approximately 1500 mg of calcium per day along with cholecalciferol (vitamin D) at 50,000 units per day. He presents to your office with malaise, anorexia, somnolence, and polyuria. His last calcium level check was 4 months ago and was normal. His present labs reveal a serum calcium level of 15.8 mg per deciliter with an albumin level of 4 grams per deciliter. The patient was supposed to be on 50,000 units of vitamin D per day, but he doubled the dose about 1 month ago because he felt some tingling in his hands. He has not notified you, nor did he reduce the dose with the onset of the present symptoms. Which of the following are the most likely diagnosis and the best treatment of the above patient's condition?

    A. The diagnosis is primary hyperparathyroidism, and best treatment is rehydration followed by surgery.
    B. The patient has underlying sarcoidosis and requires prednisone therapy.
    C. The patient most likely has hypervitaminosis D, and vitamin D and calcium should be stopped, with the patient rehydrated and administered glucocorticoids to lower the serum calcium level.
    D. The patient very likely has an underlying malignancy with humoral hypercalcemia of malignancy and needs treatment with rehydration and bisphosphonate therapy.
    E. The patient has hyperthyroidism caused by excess thyroid hormone replacement, which is causing hypercalcemia and needs treatment by reducing the thyroid hormone replacement level.

38. All of the following conditions can be associated with osteomalacia and low 25-hydroxy-vitamin D levels EXCEPT

    A. An 88-year-old woman who takes no milk products and has not been outside and exposed to the sunlight in 8 years
    B. A patient with vitamin D–dependent rickets, with elevated 1,25-dihydroxy-vitamin D levels who has been found to have decreased target organ responsiveness to 1,25-dihydroxy-vitamin D
    C. A patient with adult celiac disease

    D. A patient who has had a seizure disorder for 20 years and has been on phenytoin the entire time
    E. A patient with end-stage cirrhosis who has had poor intake for 8 months associated with anorexia and nausea

39. A 56-year-old man, who has been on hemodialysis for the past 3 years, has recently moved to town and comes to see you with a 4 to 5 month history of increasing bone pain. He has basically become bedridden in the last month. You order radiographs that reveal pathologic fractures in the bones of the lower extremities. He gives a history of using aluminum hydroxide as a phosphate binder over the past 3 years. The best treatment for this patient is

    A. Discontinue aluminum hydroxide, increase the calcium and phosphate intake in the diet
    B. Discontinue aluminum hydroxide, increase the frequency of dialysis
    C. Discontinue aluminum hydroxide agents and restrict vitamin D
    D. Discontinue aluminum hydroxide agents, restrict the phosphate in the diet, and give desferoxamine once weekly until the patient's clinical status improves
    E. Continue aluminum hydroxide and add calcium to the diet

40. All of the following conditions can lead to osteoporosis EXCEPT

    A. Anorexia nervosa
    B. Hyperthyroidism
    C. Primary biliary cirrhosis
    D. Acromegaly
    E. Homocystinuria

41. A 67-year-old man comes to see you for right hip pain. He saw an orthopedist, who took radiographs that revealed patchy osteolysis and osteosclerosis involving the right proximal femur, including the right hip and the right iliac crest. No fracture was seen. Which of the following problems could develop or be seen in this patient?

    A. Deafness and vertigo
    B. Cord or nerve root compression, especially involving the thoracic spine
    C. Heart failure
    D. Sarcoma arising from the abnormal bone
    E. All of the above

42. The most common tumors affecting the hypothalamus are

    A. Craniopharyngiomas
    B. Suprasellar dysgerminomas
    C. Pituitary adenomas
    D. Hypothalamic hamartomas
    E. None of the above

DIRECTIONS: Questions 43 to 77 are matching questions. For each numbered item, choose the most likely associated lettered item from those provided. Each numbered item has ONLY ONE answer. Within each set of questions, each answer may be used once, more than once, or not at all.

QUESTIONS 43–47

For each of the following patients, select the most likely thyroid values.

A. A 24-year-old nursing student who has lost 45 lb in the last 2 months and has noted jitterness, palpitations, and heat intolerance after seeing a diet physician and starting on a "diet pill"
B. A 20-year-old man who is asymptomatic, with a history of a brother and father with ^{131}I therapy given for elevated thyroid hormone levels despite a history that they also were asymptomatic
C. A 26-year-old woman with palpitations, insomnia, anxiety, and heat intolerance with a small, non-tender goiter who is 8 weeks postpartum
D. A 21-year-old football player on oral and systemic androgens
E. A 32-year-old woman with a small goiter, cold intolerance, dry skin, and weight gain for 3 months

	T_4 (*Normal: 5–11 μg/dl*)	T_3RU (*Normal: 25–35%*)	TSH (*Normal: 0.35–5 mIU/ml*)	24-hr ^{131}I Uptake (*Normal: 10–25%*)	Thyroglobulin (*Normal: 10–60 ng/mL*)
43.	4.3	45	1.88	18	18
44.	15.3	41	0	<1	88
45.	5.5	35	0	<1	<1
46.	16.5	37	0.89	12	36
47.	3.6	22	24.5	6	10

QUESTIONS 48–52

For each of the following patients, select the most likely lab values.

A. A 34-year-old woman on 100 mg of hydrocortisone per day for systemic lupus erythematosis
B. A 34-year-old man with weight gain, hypertension, facial plethora with centripetal obesity, and violaceous striae over the abdomen, who also has known MEN I syndrome with hypercalcemia with previous parathyroid surgery
C. A 36-year-old woman with hypertension, weight gain, hirsutism, and clitoromegaly, as well as male pattern hair loss and hypokalemia for the past 3 months, with an associated 8-cm left adrenal mass on CT scan
D. A 42-year-old man with a 2-month history of a 40-lb weight gain, hypertension, glucose intolerance with centripetal obesity, and a 2-cm right adrenal mass on CT scan
E. A 56-year-old man with a greater than 50-pack-year history of smoking with weight loss, darkening of the skin, hypokalemia, and peripheral edema with a 3-cm mass in the right lung on chest radiograph

		Overnight Dexamethasone Test			
	Fasting 8 A.M. Cortisol (*Normal: 5–25 μg/dl*)	*1-mg Low-Dose* (*Normal: <5 μg/dl*)	*8-mg High-Dose (Normal: <50% Baseline Fasting 8 A.M. Cortisol Level)*	**8 A.M. ACTH** (*Normal: 10–50 pg/ml*)	**8 A.M.DHEAS** (*Normal: 800–1600 ng/ml*)
48.	36	12	16	48	1425
49.	36	18	24	555	1580
50.	36	19	23	<1	3125
51.	36	17	21	<1	1375
52.	36	34	33	<1	250

QUESTIONS 53–57

Match the following syndromes with their characteristics.

A. Autoimmune polyglandular syndrome type I
B. Autoimmune polyglandular syndrome type II
C. Both
D. Neither

53. Mucocutaneous candidiasis is very common and is usually the very first manifestation

54. Hypoparathyroidism is rarely seen

55. Addison's disease is common

56. Inheritance is autosomal recessive

57. Vitiligo never occurs

QUESTIONS 58–62

Match the following disorders with their characteristics.

A. 21-Hydroxylase deficiency
B. 11-Beta-hydroxylase deficiency
C. Both
D. Neither

58. In its classic form, it may be associated with salt retention

59. It is usually associated with postnatal virilization

60. 17-Hydroxyprogestrone levels are typically significantly increased

61. Renin levels tend to be elevated

62. Cortisol levels are decreased

QUESTION 63–67

Match the following disorders with their associated conditions.

    A. Nephrogenic diabetes insipidus
    B. Hypothalamic or central diabetes insipidus
    C. Primary polydipsia
    D. None of the above

63. A 72-year-old with polyuria 4 days after removal of a large pituitary macroadenoma

64. In its familial form, the abnormal gene for the V_2 receptor is on the X chromosome, and females must be homozygous for symptoms to develop, whereas affected males have symptoms from birth

65. With the dehydration test, a further rise in urine osmolality is seen after giving aqueous vasopressin in the complete form of this disorder

66. These patients typically have serum sodium levels in the low 120s

67. A 34-year-old woman with a fluid intake of 25 liters per day with a long history of paranoid schizophrenia who basically never must get up at night to void

QUESTIONS 68–72

Match each of the following hormones with the substances acting on them.

    A. ACTH
    B. FSH
    C. Growth hormone
    D. TSH
    E. Prolactin

68. Insulin-like growth factor I can inhibit this anterior pituitary hormone.

69. Dopamine can inhibit this anterior pituitary hormone as well as inhibiting prolactin.

70. Vasopressin can act as a releasing factor for this anterior pituitary hormone.

71. Inhibin is known to inhibit the release of this anterior pituitary hormone.

72. TRH can stimulate the release of this anterior pituitary hormone as well as the release of TSH.

QUESTIONS 73–77

For each of the following conditions, select the most likely associated clinical situation.

    A. Increased thyroxine-binding globulin (TBG) concentration
    B. Decreased TBG concentration
    C. Drug interference with binding to normal TBG
    D. None of the above

73. A woman at the end of her first trimester of pregnancy

74. An acquired immunodeficiency syndrome (AIDS) patient with acute hepatitis

75. A 22-year-old epileptic on 400 mg of phenytoin daily

76. A 45-year-old woman with chronic renal insufficiency with 24-hour urine protein measurement of 12 grams.

77. A 52-year-old woman with rheumatoid arthritis on 4 grams of aspirin daily

DIRECTIONS: For questions 78 to 92, you are to decide whether EACH choice is true or false. Any combination of answers, from all true to all false, may occur.

78. A 44-year-old woman comes in for a routine exam and, in the course of evaluation, she is noted to have a 2-cm nodule in the right lobe of the thyroid. There is no previous history of irradiation and no symptoms of thyroid dysfunction. There is no family history of thyroid disease of any type. On further exam, no lymphadenopathy is noted in the neck. You advise her to have a fine-needle aspiration biopsy of the nodule, which is done, and the cytologic report reveals a hypercellular lesion with no colloid, consistent with a follicular neoplasm. The assessment and treatment of your patient would include which of the following?

   A. Initiation of levothyroxine as suppressive therapy with follow-up to see if the nodule decreases over the next 4 months

   B. Advise the patient to have an ultrasound of the thyroid to assess the size of the nodule and whether or not it has a cystic component

   C. Do a ^{123}I thyroid scan to determine if the nodule is ''hot,'' with suppression of the normal thyroid

   D. Refer the patient immediately to a surgeon skilled in thyroid surgery for a thyroid operation

   E. Reassure the patient that the nodule is benign and requires nothing more than yearly follow-up with neck exam

79. A 24-year-old woman entering into the third trimester of her first pregnancy, who has a history of autoimmune hypothyroidism, has been on levothyroxine for the last 3 years. The patient has had no problems with her pregnancy thus far and is followed regularly by her obstetrician. Thyroid function tests, including TSH, have been normal when last checked 2 months ago. Her physical exam is unremarkable and she appears to be euthyroid. Her labs reveal a free T_4 level of 0.88 μg per deciliter (normal: 0.7 to 1.85) and her TSH level is 12 mIU per milliter (normal: 0.32 to 5.0). She is on no other medications and denies missing any of her levothyroxine medication (0.125 mg of levothyroxine daily). Your recommendations would include which of the following?

   A. Because the patient is clinically euthyroid, it would be best simply to follow her and leave her on the same dose of levothyroxine.

   B. It is appropriate to increase the dose of levothyroxine, which may require a dosage increase by as much as 30 to 40% in the third trimester to normalize the TSH.

   C. The increase in levothyroxine that occurs in the latter part of pregnancy requires decreasing the dose to prevent overreplacement and iatrogenic hyperthyroidism after delivery.

   D. Women who are hypothyroid and inadequately replaced have an increased risk of fetal wastage.

   E. During the third trimester of pregnancy, it is more typical for patients who are adequately replaced with levothyroxine to require a lower dosage of levothyroxine replacement.

80. A 34-year-old white man gives a 1-year history of sudden onset of episodes of headache followed by palpitations and diaphoresis and a feeling of doom. These episodes initially were occurring about once every 2 weeks but now are occurring once every 3 to 4 days. They typically last 30 to 45 minutes. Recently, during an episode that led him to go to the emergency room, it was noted that his blood pressure was 190/130 mm Hg. He was given diazepam and, after the episode was over, his blood pressure was 140/96 mm Hg. In your office, exam reveals a blood pressure of 144/98 mm Hg without orthostatic drop and a pulse of 90 beats per minute (regular). Physical exam otherwise is unremarkable except for a 3-cm nodule in the left lobe of the thyroid, of which the patient was not aware. Which of the following statements is/are true with regard to this patient's history and clinical findings?

   A. A 24-hr urine for VMA, metanephrines, and catecholamines would be expected to be elevated in this patient, if done after a spell as described above.

   B. Family history of endocrine-related disorders, including pheochromocytoma, thyroid cancer, and/ or hyperparathyroidism, would be expected.

   C. The most likely explanation of the thyroid nodule in this patient with this presentation would be medullary cancer of the thyroid.

   D. Bilateral or extra-adrenal masses would be expected to be more frequent on CT scanning in relation to the symptoms and signs described above that are associated with his hypertension.

   E. Basal or stimulated serum calcitonin levels would be expected to be elevated in this patient.

81. A 34-year-old black woman presents to you for evaluation of enlargement of her hands and feet. She has noted, over the last several years, that she can no longer wear her rings and that her shoe size has increased by two sizes. She also notices excessive sweating. On physical exam she has frontal bossing, prognathism, increased spacing between the teeth, and enlargement of her tongue. Her hands are spadelike in appearance. Her skin is warm and moist. Laboratory tests reveal an 8:00 A.M. growth hormone level of 22 ng per milliliter. After a glucose tolerance test is done, the growth hormone level is 12 ng per milliliter. Which of the following statements is/are true with regard to this disorder?

   A. Arthralgias involving the hands, feet, hip, and knees are common and are caused by cartilage and synovial overgrowth

   B. Skin tags are common

   C. There is an increased incidence of colonic polyps

   D. Galactorrhea may be seen in women

   E. The increased mortality associated with acromegaly can be primarily attributed to cardiovascular and cerebrovascular diseases

82. Which of the following is/are associated with hypogonadotropic hypogonadism?

   A. Hyperprolactinemia

   B. Anorexia nervosa

C. A woman who is a world-class long distance runner and runs 10 to 15 miles every day in training
D. Turner's syndrome
E. Kallmann's syndrome

83. A 22-year-old woman presents to you with a weight loss of 10 lb in the last 3 months associated with increasing anxiety, increasing heat intolerance, and a complaint of palpitations. On physical examination, her pulse is noted to be 110 beats per minute resting, and she has a diffusely enlarged goiter approximately three times larger than normal with evidence of proptosis. She also has a fine tremor with warm moist palms. The thyroid function tests reveal a FT_4 level of 3.3 μg per deciliter (normal: 0.7 to 1.8) and a TSH level of 0 mIU per milliliter (normal: 0.32 to 5). Which of the following may also be seen in this patient with this problem?

A. Heavy menses that are irregular
B. Elevated systolic blood pressure with widened pulse pressure
C. Splenomegaly
D. Elevated alkaline phosphatase on laboratory testing
E. Renal tubular acidosis

84. A 44-year-old woman presents to you with a 1-year history of increasing dry skin, reduced scalp hair, marked cold intolerance that she has never had before, and difficulty with her memory, especially in the use of numbers (she is an accountant). She has noted that she requires 8 to 9 hours of sleep and still feels tired, despite always getting by with 6 hours of sleep in the past. Her family has noted that her voice seems to be lower pitched and her face has appeared puffy. Her lab tests reveal a FT_4 level of 0.4 μg per deciliter (normal: 0.7 to 1.85) and TSH level of 53 mIU per milliliter (normal: 0.32 to 5). Her thyroid antibodies test reveals an antimicrosominal antibody titer of 1:25,000 (normal: <1:100). An antithyroglobulin antibody titer is positive at 1:1200 (normal: 1:10). Which of the following statements is/are true of this patient's disorder?

A. A yellow skin complexion can be seen as a result of carotene accumulation.
B. Hypertension may occur in this patient and resolve with replacement therapy.
C. Hyponatremia may result from impairment of the kidneys to excrete a free water load and also from the syndrome of inappropriate antidiuretic hormone secretion (SIADH).
D. Hypocapnia is common.
E. Low-density lipoprotein (LDL) cholesterol is increased and high-density lipoprotein (HDL) cholesterol is decreased in this condition.

85. Familial pheochromocytomas can be seen in which of the following conditions?

A. MEN I
B. von Hippel–Lindau syndrome
C. MEN IIA
D. Hereditary neurofibromatosis (von Recklinghausen's disease)
E. MEN IIB

86. Licorice intoxication is a rare cause of hypertension. Which of the following statements is/are true with regard to licorice and licorice intoxication associated with hypertension?

A. It is a renin/angiotensin-dependent cause of mineralocorticoid excess.
B. Glycyrrhizic acid is the active ingredient in licorice and induces hypertension early in patients with licorice intoxication.
C. The most common source of licorice in the United States is chewing tobacco.
D. The mechanism of action of licorice through glycyrrhizic acid is that it is a competitive inhibitor of 17-hydroxylase and induces hypertension.
E. Glycyrrhizic acid is a competitive inhibitor of 11-beta-hydroxysteroid dehydrogenase, which prevents cortisol conversion to cortisone so that cortisol interacts with the mineralocorticoid receptor as an agonist.

87. A 32-year-old man presents with a complaint of fatigue over the last 4 to 6 months and, in the past 1 to 2 months, dizziness that is worse after standing or walking for a time. He has noted a 10- to 15-lb weight loss with loss of appetite and associated anorexia and nausea. He has noted low-grade fever and the need to eat salty foods for which he has had no desire in the past. He also has noted darkening of his skin, especially in the creases over the hands. An 8:00 A.M. cortisol level is 3 μg per deciliter (normal: 5 to 25) and an ACTH level is 170 pg per milliliter (normal: 0 to 90). A cortrosyn stimulation test reveals a baseline cortisol level of 3 with a 30-minute value of 5 and a 60 minute value of 7 μg per deciliter. Which of the following could be the cause of this patient's condition?

A. Bilateral adrenal hemorrhage seen on CT scan in individuals especially with chronic anticoagulation
B. Histoplasmosis involving the adrenal glands
C. AIDS with associated cytomegalovirus infection of the adrenal glands
D. Monilia
E. Lung cancer with metastases to the adrenal glands

88. Which of the following can be associated with diabetes mellitus?

A. VIPomas
B. Somatostatinomas
C. Glucagonomas
D. Gastrinomas
E. Nonfunctioning islet cell tumors

89. A 19-year-old woman presents to you with amenorrhea of 3 months. She gives a history of thelarche at age 13 with menses beginning at age 14. Over the last 4 years, she has had menses approximately every 30 days lasting 3 to 4 days each month. She has some mild dysmenorrhea during the first day or two of her menses. On examination, the patient is a fully developed female with Tanner stage 5 breast and sexual development. Which of the following could explain her amenorrhea?

A. Pregnancy
B. Hyperprolactinemia

C. Hyperthyroidism

D. Premature ovarian failure associated with hypoadrenalism, hypoparathyroidism, and mucocutaneous candidiasis

E. Oral contraceptive agents that were stopped 3 to 4 months ago

90. Which of the following statements regarding oral contraceptives is/are true?

A. The use of low-dose contraceptives increases the risk of fatal and nonfatal stroke in young women

B. Contraceptive steroids appear to be teratogenic

C. Women who use oral contraceptive agents are more likely to become hypertensive, especially when they are over 35 years of age

D. The risk of developing endometrial carcinoma is increased with the use of oral contraceptives

E. There appears to be an increased risk for the development of hepatocellular adenoma with combined oral contraceptives

91. A 32-year-old man presents to you for enlargement of his breasts. On physical examination, he is noted to have gynecomastia extending 2 to 3 cm beyond the areola of each breast. The breasts are mildly tender. There is no other obvious abnormality noted on physical examination. Which of the following is/are possible causes for this man's gynecomastia?

A. A 6-month use of ketoconazole

B. Regular and significant use of marijuana over the past year

C. Use of furosemide over the last 3 to 4 months

D. Ingestion of spironolactone for hypertension over the last 6 months

E. Use of cimetedine in doses of 400 to 600 mg per day over the last 4 to 6 months

92. Which of the following is/are characteristic of the carcinoid syndrome?

A. Telangiectasias may be a clinical manifestation occurring on the face and neck.

B. Although chronic diarrhea is common, malabsorption never occurs in the carcinoid syndrome.

C. Cardio-thickening of the valvular cusps and cardiac chambers occurs, primarily on the left side of the heart.

D. Carcinoid syndrome is a cause of sustained hypertension.

E. Bronchial constriction, which is usually most pronounced in flushing attacks, can occur and be severe.

ENDOCRINE/REPRODUCTIVE DISEASES AND DISEASES OF BONE AND BONE MINERAL METABOLISM

ANSWERS

1.(C) *Discussion:* Approximately one third of children with precocious puberty have hamartomas. These are hypothalamic tumors that can secrete GnRH in a pulsatile manner early in life, leading to the early development of puberty. Although specific therapy aimed at the hamartoma is usually not necessary because its course is benign, therapy of the precocious puberty is of importance for psychological reasons and for prevention of premature epiphyseal fusion and stunted growth. Treatment with long-acting progesterone or androgens to suppress gonadotropin response to GnRH has been used, but the best therapy is a GnRH agonist to down-regulate pituitary GnRH receptors and therefore diminish gonadotropin secretion. Hypothalamic hamartomas have been associated with acromegaly and growth hormone–secreting pituitary tumors, because they secrete GHRH, which can lead to growth hormone hypersecretion and somatotrope tumor formation. (*Cecil, Ch. 201; Stein*)

2.(B) *Discussion:* This patient has symptoms of thyrotoxicosis by examination and laboratory data along with a low ^{131}I uptake. The main possibilities for the etiology of this patient's condition would be silent or postpartum thyroiditis or factitious hyperthyroidism caused by ingestion of thyroid medications. Although the patient could have a low ^{131}I uptake because of recent ingestion of iodine or the use of contrast agents for certain radiographs, there is no history for this. These patients would not be specifically thyrotoxic on a routine basis from the ingestion of iodine or exposure to iodinated contrast agents. Of importance is the fact that this patient's thyroid gland is not palpable and, usually in patients with postpartum thyroiditis, the gland would be normal to slightly enlarged and firm. There is no evidence to suggest subacute thyroiditis because there has been no history of tenderness of the gland, and the patient has no evidence of leukocytosis. T_3 RIA measurement would not distinguish different etiologies of hyperthyroidism associated with a low ^{131}I uptake. Although patients with silent or postpartum thyroiditis typically will have resolution of symptoms over time, they sometimes may need propranolol therapy during the acute hyperthyroid stage. They may even need thyroid hormone replacement during the hypothyroid stage. Patients who have factitious hyperthyroidism because of the ingestion of thyroid medication typically will have a small, nonpalpable thyroid gland, and their thyroglobulin measurement will be suppressed, unlike patients with different forms of thyroiditis in which the thyroglobulin measurement during the acute phase is typically elevated. There is no evidence that this patient has Graves' disease or other conditions that lead to excess thyroid hormone production that would need

thionamide therapy, such as methimazole. Although a fine-needle biopsy to the thyroid certainly might differentiate thyroiditis from a normal thyroid gland, and even though it has low risk, it is nevertheless an invasive procedure and requires both a physician experienced in doing thyroid aspirations and an experienced pathologist to read thyroid cytologic specimens. Patients with postpartum or silent or painless thyroiditis may have positive thyroid antibodies of the antimicrosomal and antithyroglobulin type. (*Cecil, Ch. 203; Roti et al; Singer*)

3.(A) *Discussion:* This patient has what appears to be acute adrenal insufficiency, most likely acute primary adrenal insufficiency. The most common causes are sepsis and hemorrhage within the adrenal glands, especially in patients on anticoagulants. Fever is a common finding in acute adrenal insufficiency and does not require the presence of infection because it can occur simply as a result of the acute adrenal insufficiency. Although the patient may well have sepsis and might have positive cultures, this is not absolutely necessary because hemorrhage within the adrenal glands from anticoagulant therapy may well explain his acute adrenal insufficiency and clinical picture. (*Cecil, Ch. 204.1; Muir and Maclaren*)

4.(D) *Discussion:* This patient has features consistent with an enlarged pituitary gland, as can be seen in Cushing's disease when both adrenals have been removed and the ACTH-secreting pituitary adenoma has progressed. About one third of patients who have bilateral adrenalectomy will develop this disorder, and it is thought that this results from the lack of the cortisol feedback onto the pituitary when the bilateral adrenalectomy is done. Typically, these patients have ACTH levels in the thousands. The tumors are usually macroadenomas. There is nothing from the presentation to suggest recurrent Cushing's disease. The features of Addison's disease are not that typical of an expanding pituitary lesion with headache and visual field defect in the context of this patient on steroid replacement. Schmidt's syndrome is a disorder involving autoimmune thyroid disease and adrenal disease with adrenal insufficiency and sometimes type I diabetes mellitus. (*Cecil, Ch. 202.1; Schteingart; Klibanski and Zervas*)

5.(C) *Discussion:* Gynecomastia is a benign glandular enlargement of the male breast. All of the conditions listed can be associated with gynecomastia in the male except Turner's syndrome. In Turner's syndrome, the XO female may have breast tissue but is a female with hypoplastic ovaries. (*Cecil, Ch. 209.1; Braunstein*)

6.(B) *Discussion:* This patient has what appears to be the polyglandular autoimmune disorder, which can be associated with thyroiditis, hypoadrenalism with Addison's disease, hypoparathyroidism, diabetes mellitus (typically type I), vitiligo, mucocutaneous candidiasis, and pernicious anemia as well as associated primary ovarian failure. These patients typically have hypergonadotropic hypogonadism with amenorrhea. Treatment is with estrogen therapy. These patients do not have hypogonadotropic hypogonadism as in D. The other gonadotropin and estradiol levels may be present at different times of the normal menstrual cycle, including the follicular, midcycle, and luteal phases. (*Cecil, Ch. 210.1; Eisenbarth and Jacson*)

7.(D) *Discussion:* Mutations in the *Ret* proto-oncogenes have been identified in patients with medullary thyroid carcinoma as seen with familial forms for this cancer only as well as in MEN IIA and MEN IIB. There is no evidence that its identification in patients with papillary cancer of the thyroid is of any use. It is mainly used to identify patients at risk in families who have inherited the defective gene so they can be identified and have thyroid surgery prior to the development of medullary cancer of the thyroid (during the C-cell hyperplasia phase). Therefore, it serves a useful purpose in patients with a family history of medullary thyroid carcinoma. (*Cecil, Ch. 210.1; Mulligan et al; Thakker*)

8.(D) *Discussion:* This patient's presentation is very typical of hypothyroidism, with laboratory data consistent with this, and the most common cause of hypothyroidism in a middle-age female will be autoimmune disease, as seen with Hashimoto's thyroiditis with elevated antimicrosomal as well as antithyroglobulin antibodies. Patients with autoimmune hypothyroidism or Hashimoto's thyroiditis can sometimes have other associated autoimmune endocrine disorders, with the most common being adrenal insufficiency. Other autoimmune endocrine disorders that occur less commonly include hypoparathyrodism, gonadal failure, type I diabetes, and very rarely pituitary insufficiency. Some of these patients may have vitiligo and even vitamin B_{12} deficiency. There is a strong female predominance. These patients may not have obvious symptoms of hypoadrenalism until their hypothyroid condition is corrected. Once this occurs, adrenal insufficiency can be unmasked in these patients and is associated with weakness, nausea, vomiting, and hypotension as well as abdominal pain or even fever acutely, and over time even hyperpigmenation. This patient very likely has adrenal insufficiency that has been unmasked with treatment of her hypothyroid condition. All the possibilities listed are correct except for transient hyperthyroidism, which would be more suggestive of silent thyroiditis, which typically has a hyperthyroid phase followed by hypothyroid phase, but then typically normalization of the thyroid function occurs after a period of time elapses. In these patients with Schmidt's syndrome, hypothyroidism typically requires lifelong thyroid replacement. Eosinophilia would be expected in a patient with adrenal insufficiency, and a low morning cortisol level would be expected. Certainly with replacement with levothyroxine, the FT_4 level can normalize within a few weeks, although sometimes it can take the TSH level 6 to 8 weeks or longer to normalize. (*Cecil, Ch. 203; Rapoport*)

9.(A) *Discussion:* Men with hyperprolactinemia can present with low testosterone secondary to low gonadotropin levels, the latter suppressed by the elevated prolactin level. Patients with hyperprolactinemia typically have loss of libido, and men have inadequate erections or frank impotence. They also have features consistent with secondary hypogonadism, and, although some can have oligospermia when their androgen and gonadotropin levels are low, others who maintain their androgen and gonadotropin levels may have normal semen analysis. They typically do not have azoospermia. In this patient, there is nothing to suggest hypothyroidism. Starting testosterone therapy prior to determining the diagnosis of his secondary hypogonadism is not appropriate, especially with hyperprolactinemia, because testosterone therapy may not restore complete potency and libido if the prolactin level remains high and is not treated. There is nothing to suggest a genetic disorder requiring karyotyping, and a fasting blood sugar would not be useful in determining the etiology of this patient's secondary hypogonadism. (*Cecil, Ch. 202.1; Molitch, 1992*)

10.(C) *Discussion:* This patient has hyperprolactinemia, and the next step to determine the etiology is to do a pituitary MRI scan to assess for a pituitary microadenoma versus macroadenoma. Measurement of FSH would not be expected to add any useful information because the FSH level would be expected to be normal to low, as was the LH level. The free testosterone level would be expected to be low because the total testosterone level was quite low, and again it would add no useful information. There is nothing to suggest primary hypogonadism, and a testicular biopsy, which also is invasive, is not indicated. A semen analysis would not help in establishing the etiology of the hyperprolactinemia. (*Cecil, Ch. 202.1; Molitch, 1989*)

11.(C) *Discussion:* Lithium, methoxyflurane (an anesthetic agent), and demeclocycline all modify or inhibit the antidiuretic hormone (ADH) effect on the collecting ducts, thus causing nephrogenic diabetes insipidus. Sarcoidosis can also cause a vasopressin-resistant hyposthenuria and polyuria, as seen with nephrogenic diabetes insipidus. However, cyclophosphamide is a drug that can sometimes enhance the release of vasopressin and may lead to SIADH. (*Cecil, Ch. 202.2; Robinson and Verbalis; Miller et al*)

12.(A) *Discussion:* This patient has complete androgen insensitivity, otherwise known as testicular feminization. These are male pseudohermaphrodites who genetically are male and have a female phenotype because of an absence of the cytosol receptor for dihydrotestosterone, or qualitative abnormalities or postreceptor variance causing androgen insensitivity. These males therefore develop breasts and have a short vagina but do not have fallopian tubes, uterus, or the upper portion of the vagina because the testes produce müllerian inhibitory factor, which prevents the development of these structures. Testosterone levels are typically in the male high-normal range or higher. Estrogen levels typically are in the low-normal female range because of an increased production rate of estrone and estradiol believed to be testicular in origin. Because these individuals are males, they have a male genotype. Although FSH levels may be normal to elevated, LH levels are typically mildly to moderately elevated. (*Cecil, Ch. 210*)

13.(B) *Discussion:* This patient has typical symptoms and features of a pheochromocytoma. Although many patients with pheochromocytoma have elevated plasma catecholamines even during the asymptomatic phase and also will have elevated urinary catecholamines, including VMA and metanephrine values, there are a few patients during the normotensive phase between paroxysms who will have normal serum catecholamine levels and urinary measurements of VMA, metanephrines, and catecholamines. One must try to measure serum catecholamines or collect a 24-hour urine specimen during or immediately after a paroxysm to see elevations in the serum and urine catecholamine studies. Repeating this patient's serum catecholamine measurements immediately after a paroxysm or collecting a 24-hour urine specimen for VMA, metanephrine, and catecholamine measurement immediately after a paroxysm would be expected to show elevated findings consistent with a pheochromocytoma. (*Cecil, Ch. 204; Cryer*)

14.(E) *Discussion:* There are a number of causes of hypercalcemia, including familial hypocalciuric hypercalcemia, otherwise known as benign familial hypercalcemia. This condition is typically inherited as an autosomal dominant trait and is characterized by asymptomatic hypercalcemia, hypocalciuria, a tendency toward mild hypermagnesemia, and "normal intact PTH levels." Typically, the parathyroid glands in these patients are normal or may show some evidence of hyperplasia, but surgery is not indicated because it does not restore normal calcium levels in the serum. These patients are thought to have an increased response of nephrogenous cyclic AMP to PTH, which can lead to hypercalcemia. Typically, they will have urine calcium levels that are less than 100 mg per 24 hr, and they typically do not have the characteristic symptoms of primary hyperparathyroidism, including stones and osteitis fibrosa cystica. They require no surgery and simply require follow-up. Although there may be a family history of hypercalcemia, the best way to make the diagnosis is to document hypercalcemia in the immediate family of the patient. (*Cecil, Ch. 214*)

15.(B) *Discussion:* Patient's with Kallmann's syndrome have hypogonadotropic hypogonadism, so they have low testosterone, FSH, and LH levels. They typically have disorders of smell; midline defects, including cleft lip or palate, color blindness, renal agenesis, nerve deafness; and even skeletal abnormalities, including syndactyly, short fourth metacarpals, and craniofacial asymmetry. The other anterior pituitary hormone levels are normal. They may have micropenis and typically have aspermia. (*Cecil, Ch. 201*)

16.(A) *Discussion:* Patients with glucagonomas typically have a waxing and waning skin rash known as necrolytic migratory erythema and may have diabetes as well as hypoaminoacidemia, weight loss, and anemia. The rash is most prominent on the perineum, along the intertriginous folds, and around the mouth and nose. Glossitis, stomatitis, and chelitis may be present. Glucose intolerance or frank diabetes is seen in the majority of patients. Gastrointestinal symptoms such as abdominal pain, nausea, vomiting, and diarrhea can occur, and there are patients who have been described with thromboembolic disorders. Approximately 60% of these lesions are malignant. Surgery for cure, if the tumor

is confined to the pancreas, or for debulking followed by chemotherapy, is used for therapy. Somatostatin long-acting analogues will help in decreasing glucagon and help improve the rash, if the patient has metastatic disease. (*Cecil, Ch. 206.2; Vinik and Moattari*)

17.(B) *Discussion:* ANP is a peptide hormone secreted by the cardiac atria that produces natriuresis, diuresis, and the inhibition of renin and aldosterone secretion. Some major sites of actions include the cardiovascular, renal, and endocrine systems. It is thought that the stretch of the atria is the principle stimulus triggering the release of ANP, although all the exact mechanisms leading to its release are not known. ANP causes smooth muscle relaxation and not smooth muscle constriction. (*Cecil, Ch. 200.3; Cogan*)

18.(D) *Discussion:* The information given certainly suggests that this patient has thyrotoxicosis, but his FT_4 level is not elevated. This would suggest that some other hormone is causing his thyrotoxicosis, and the only other possibility would be T_3. At this point, there would be no reason to repeat the patient's scan and uptake study because this was just recently done. Measurement of TSH receptor antibodies may be positive in Graves' disease, but the scan and findings are not consistent with Graves' disease. A TRH stimulation test is very rarely needed now with the new-generation TSH assays, which can distinguish patients having hyperthyroidism from those having euthyroidism. Certainly, this patient with symptoms of thyrotoxicosis should under no circumstances be given levothyroxine simply because his FT_4 level is low, until it is clear what his serum T_3 level reveals. (*Cecil, Ch. 203, Roti et al*)

19.(E) *Discussion:* This patient has what appears to be hyperthyroidism caused by the ingestion of T_3 hormone based on the fact that the patient has symptoms of thyrotoxicosis, a low FT_4 level, suppressed TSH, and an elevated serum T_3 level (as determined by the test ordered in the preceding question). The major causes of thyrotoxicosis with a low radioactive iodine uptake are subacute thyroiditis; silent thyroiditis, including postpartum thyroiditis; and factitious hyperthyroidism caused by the ingestion of thyroid hormone. Rarely, iodine-induced hyperthyroidism may cause a low uptake. The latter is usually seen in the patient with an underlying multinodular goiter given iodine who then develops hyperthyroidism. This patient had a very small thyroid gland as per exam, and, in the other causes of low-uptake hyperthyroidism, patients usually have some enlargement of their thyroid. Patients with subacute thyroiditis almost always have a tender thyroid gland, and there are usually systemic symptoms and signs, including malaise, myalgia, and fever. This patient had no symptoms except for thyrotoxicosis. Treatment for subacute thyroiditis, silent thyroiditis, or factitious hyperthyroidism would not require thyroidectomy or radioactive iodine or thionamide therapy, because these therapies would be inappropriate in these conditions with release of preformed thyroid hormone from the gland. Because most preformed thyroid hormone is T_4, these conditions would be expected to be associated with a high FT_4 level, and this patient actually has a high T_3 value with a suppressed FT_4 level, as would be seen in the ingestion of T_3. The best next assessment to determine that this patient has factitious hyperthyroidism caused by the ingestion of T_3 will be a measure of serum thyroglobulin level. Serum thyroglobulin is typically in the high-normal to elevated range during the acute phase of thyroiditis caused by subacute or silent thyroiditis. This patient's thyroglobulin level would be expected to be suppressed and low, because the patient is ingesting T_3 hormone, suppressing TSH and thyroid hormone synthesis and therefore thyroglobulin release by the thyroid gland. Patients with factitious hyperthyroidism, who have an underlying normal thyroid otherwise, should have a low serum thyroglobulin level, allowing differentiation from other causes of thyroiditis that cause low uptake on the scans. (*Cecil, Ch. 203; Roti et al*)

20.(C) *Discussion:* In nonthyroidal illness syndrome, a number of illnesses, including severe systemic illnesses, physical trauma, and psychiatric disturbances, can alter thyroid hormone levels in patients without intrinsic thyroid disease. The most common combination of thyroid hormone values in those patients with nonthyroidal illness is a low T_3 level and normal T_4 value and typically a normal to low TSH value also. All of the other various combinations can be seen but are much less common. Elevated T_4 levels with normal T_3 levels can be seen in patients with acute liver disease, such as acute hepatitis; in some patients with AIDS; and in patients with psychiatric disorders, such as manic depressive disease and acute psychosis. Elevated T_3 and T_4 levels with suppressed TSH levels would be expected in patients with thyrotoxicosis. (*Cecil, Ch. 203*)

21.(B) *Discussion:* In patients with thyrotoxicosis, oligomeningorrhea or amenorrhea can occur, as can an elevation in systolic blood pressure with a widened pulse pressure. Also, patients can have an elevation in alkaline phosphatase as a result of increased bone turnover and have onycholysis, wherein the nail can loosen from the underlying nail bed of the fingers. Menorrhagia, or excessive and heavy menses, is not a feature of thyrotoxicosis but it may be a feature of hypothyroidism. (*Cecil, Ch. 203; McDougall*)

22.(E) *Discussion:* About 40% of patients with Graves' disease can have ophthalmopathy, and pretibial myxedema occurs in a very small number, usually at most 2 to 3%. Thyroid acropachy, which is a swelling of the distal part of the digits of the hands, can occur. Although rare, lymphadenopathy and splenomegaly also can occur related to Grave's disease specifically. (*Cecil, Ch. 203; McDougall*)

23.(A) *Discussion:* This patient appears to have Graves' disease not only because she has hyperthyroidism by laboratory data but also because she has a diffusely enlarged thyroid with proptosis, which is a unique feature of Graves' disease. Because this woman is 8 weeks pregnant, the best treatment will be propylthiouracil because it tends to cross the placenta to a lesser degree than methimazole and it also blocks T_4-to-T_3 conversion peripherally, which methimazole does not. Although beta blockers may be used as short-term therapy to control the adrenergic effects of hyperthyroidism, long-term treatment simply with a beta blocker in a patient who is pregnant and has Graves' disease would not be the best treatment because of complications that include low birth weight, postnatal bradycardia, and poor response to hypoxia that can occur in the newborns of mothers treated with long-term propranolol. In patients who cannot take thionamides because of side effects or who cannot be controlled with limited doses of thionamides, surgery during the second trimester can be considered but would not be considered the treatment of choice. Finally, treatment of a symptomatic woman during pregnancy should be done. Women who have hyperemesis gravidarum with very high human chorionic gonadotopin titers may present with elevated FT_4 levels and suppressed TSH that resolve later in pregnancy and may simply require the patient to be followed. However, this patient has typical features of Graves' disease, with a diffusely enlarged goiter and proptosis, the latter not being a feature of hyperemesis gravidarum. Also, this woman has had no vomiting, and a very typical feature in patients with underlying hyperemesis gravidarum is recurrent and profuse vomiting. (*Cecil, Ch. 203; Becks and Burrow*)

24.(C) *Discussion:* This patient most likely has postpartum thyroiditis because it usually will occur in the first few months after pregnancy, with an initial hyperthyroid phase followed by a hypothyroid phase, the latter lasting 2 to 4 months. Although the patient could have Hashimoto's thyroiditis, the thyroid antibody titers are normal and not elevated, which would be against this as a diagnosis. Jodbasedow phenomenon is due to the ingestion of iodine, typically in patients who are iodine deficient with goiters, or patients in this country with multinodular goiter with iodine ingestion inducing hyperthyroidism. This patient has hypothyroidism. In patients with the hypothyroid phase of subacute thyroiditis, one would expect a history of a tender thyroid gland preceding the hypothyroid phase, and there is no history of this in this patient. Finally, Reidel's thyroiditis is a very uncommon disorder, the etiology of which is not well understood, that can cause hypothyroidism, but it can occur anytime. This patient's thyroid problem appeared to occur at the time in which postpartum thyroiditis can occur, in the first 3 to 6 months after delivery. (*Cecil, Ch. 203; Singer*)

25.(B) *Discussion:* During the recovery phase of postpartum thyroiditis (as well as during the recovery phase of subacute thyroiditis and silent thyroiditis), once thyroid hormone is depleted from the gland and thyroid hormone levels become low, TSH rises and, as the gland recovers, the thyroid begins to synthesize T_4 and T_3, with repletion of the depleted stores of thyroid hormone within the thyroid gland. This ability to increase synthesis, even while the patient is still hypothyroid, can lead to a radioactive iodine uptake on scan that is actually elevated above normal. With time, serum thyroid hormone levels normalize and TSH becomes normal, with radioactive iodine uptake normalizing also. Although patients with postpartum thyroiditis are given levothyroxine if hypothyroid symptoms are severe enough, this would not explain the elevated radioactive iodine uptake. Patients with postpartum thyroiditis do not have TSH receptor antibodies, which are seen primarily in Graves' disease. Patients with postpartum thyroiditis are not iodine depleted from this disorder. (*Cecil, Ch. 203; Singer*)

26.(E) *Discussion:* Patients with hypothyroidism on levothyroxine may require higher doses of levothyroxine if they have malabsorption syndromes; if they are taking aluminum preparations such as antacids, cholestyramine, lovastatin, ferrous sulfate, and rifampin; and in pregnancy, especially during the third trimester, when thyroxine replacement needs may increase by 30%. (*Cecil, Ch. 203; Roti et al*)

27.(A) *Discussion:* There are a number of studies that show that patients can undergo coronary artery bypass grafting or angioplasty with mild to moderate hypothyroidism without significant increases in mortality or morbidity. Therefore, delaying angioplasty if the cardiologist believes that it is necessary to proceed immediately is not necessary in this patient because, despite this patient being hypothyroid, it appears to be mild to moderate in degree, and he should be able to undergo angioplasty and then receive thyroid replacement afterward. To delay the angioplasty and initiate even low-dose levothyroxine is not necessary. It is inappropriate to give the patient a full replacement dose of levothyroxine when he has had recent unstable angina or myocardial infarction because this may exacerbate the patient's symptoms of coronary artery disease. This patient clearly has clinical as well as laboratory evidence of primary hypothyroidism as a diagnosis, and there is nothing to point to nonthyroidal illness in this patient. (*Cecil, Ch. 203; Becker*)

28.(D) *Discussion:* This patient has what appears to be a follicular neoplasm, and fine-needle biopsy cannot distinguish between a well-differentiated follicular cancer and a follicular adenoma. To put the patient on suppressive therapy or to simply follow the patient or even rebiopsy after delaying for 2 months would be inappropriate, because there is a possibility that this lesion may be a follicular cancer. Although the patient may need surgery, the first step, prior to referring the patient to a surgeon, would be to do a thyroid scan to see if the nodule is "hot." "Hot" nodules that basically suppress uptake in the rest of the thyroid have a less than 1% chance of being malignant; if this nodule were "hot," then it would most likely represents a benign adenoma. If the nodule were "cold" (less radioactive uptake than the surrounding thyroid tissue) or "warm" (the same radioactive uptake as the surrounding thyroid tissue), then the patient would need to be referred to a surgeon, but only after the scan was done to assess the function of the nodule. (*Cecil, Ch. 203; Ridgeway*)

29.(A) *Discussion:* The only thyroid cancers that are responsive to ^{131}I therapy are papillary cancers of the thyroid and follicular cancers. No other thyroid cancers, including lymphomas, anaplastic cancers, and medullary cancer of the thyroid, are responsive to radioactive iodine, and radioactive iodine should not be used to treat these. (*Cecil, Ch. 203; Clark and Du; Mazzaferri*)

30.(B) *Discussion:* This patient appears to have primary polydipsia because she concentrates her urine with dehydration and, after given vasopressin, there is no further increase in her urine osmolality. Patients with partial pituitary or hypothalamic diabetes insipidus would be expected to have at least a further 10% increase in their urine osmolality after being given subcutaneous vasopressin. The patient has depression and is on amitryptiline, which is known to cause xerostomia and may be exacerbating the patient's thirst, leading her to drink large volumes of fluid. Because the polyuria occurs primarily during the day, when she is drinking large volumes of fluid, this also points to her problem

being primary polydipsia, rather than hypothalamic/pituitary or nephrogenic diabetes insipidus, in which case the patient would be expected to be having polyuria both day and night. Demeclocycline therapy is used in patients who have SIADH. DDAVP therapy or the use of chlorpropamide, which can enhance the effect of vasopressin at the renal tubule, may be useful in patients with partial hypothalamic/pituitary diabetes insipidus. The use of thiazide diuretics, which can cause sodium depletion and volume contraction and therefore decrease urine volume by increasing proximal tubular reabsorption of the glomeruli filtrate, would not be appropriate in a patient with primary polydipsia. Possibly changing to another antidepressant that does not cause xerostomia, and encouraging the patient to decrease her oral fluid intake, would be the most appropriate next step in this patient. (*Cecil, Ch. 202.2; Miller et al*)

31.(B) *Discussion:* This patient initially appeared to have hypogonadotropic hypogonadism. His gonadotropin levels were not elevated, as would be expected with primary hypogonadism, suggesting that his low testosterone level was due to a hypothalamic or pituitary disorder. He now has developed symptoms typical of adrenal insufficiency, and the best way to measure adrenal insufficiency is to do a baseline cortisol measurement followed by stimulation using synthetic ACTH to see if the serum cortisol level rises. Increasing the testosterone dose would not help with his present symptoms. Although his somatomedin C level possibly might be abnormal if the patient's growth hormone level was also low as a result of panhypopituitarism, it does not explain his present symptoms. Serum ACTH levels can be measured, but ACTH testing is not easily done and is not easily reproducible, and the range of normal is quite wide, making it less appropriate than doing a synthetic ACTH stimulation test and measuring cortisol levels. Giving this patient thyroid hormone replacement in the face of what appears to be adrenal insufficiency would exacerbate the patient's adrenal insufficiency and possibly induce adrenal crisis, and therefore would be inappropriate. (*Cecil, Ch. 202.1*)

32.(D) *Discussion:* This patient has what appears to be hypopituitarism, which could be due to a number of disorders involving either the hypothalamus or the pituitary. His polyuria is very likely related to central diabetes insipidus that has been unmasked by the replacement with glucocorticoids. Glucocorticoids are necessary for excretion of a free water load, and glucocorticoid insufficiency may mask vasopressin deficiency as seen in central diabetes insipidus until glucocorticoids are replaced. It is unlikely that, in a matter of 2 to 3 days, the patient has developed significant hyperglycemia, and he has no glycosuria. His potassium and calcium levels are not sufficient to explain the polyuria. (*Cecil, Ch. 202.2; Robinson and Verbalis*)

33.(D) *Discussion:* This patient has Turner's syndrome, with the cardinal features being a female phenotype, sexual infantilism, short stature, and sometimes the appearance of a webbed neck, low-set ears, multiple pigmented nevi, double eyelashes, micrognathia, epicanthal folds, shield-like chest with microthelia, an increased carrying angle to the arms, and sometimes cardiovascular defects, including coarctation of the aorta and aortic stenosis. The most common chromosome type is 45,XO. These patient also may have a short fourth metacarpal. They do not have a short second metacarpal. (*Cecil, Ch. 208.1; Rebar; Simpson and Rebar*)

34.(B) *Discussion:* This patient's problem is known as Kallmann's syndrome, which is a congenital disorder characterized by isolated hypogonadotropic hypogonadism, eunuchoidism, and usually anosmia or hyposmia. The gonadotropic deficiency is usually caused by deficiency of luteinizing hormone–releasing hormone (LHRH). Kallmann's syndrome is an inheritable disorder, and it may be expressed as an autosomal dominant, autosomal recessive, or X-linked recessive genetic disorder. These patients have eunuchoidal features and prepubertal testes with micropenis. Anosmia or hyposmia occurs in about 80%. Other midline defects such as cleft lip or palate, color blindness, renal agenesis, and nerve deafness can occur, as well as cryptorchidism and skeletal abnormalities such as syndactyly, short fourth metacarpals, and craniofacial asymmetry. These patients typically are aspermic and have low testosterone, LH, and FSH levels. However, this condition can occur in females, although not commonly. Treatment with androgen therapy in males leads to sexual maturation and helps to maintain sexual maturation. Spermatogenesis may be induced with gonadotropin or LHRH therapy. (*Cecil, Ch. 209.1; Plymate*)

35.(E) *Discussion:* McCune-Albright syndrome is a polyglandular disorder that can be associated with precocious puberty and is gonadotropin independent. Other features include hyperthyroidism caused by autonomous-functioning thyroid nodules, acromegaly caused by pituitary adenomas that produce growth hormone and usually prolactin, Cushing's syndrome associated with ACTH-independent adrenal adenomas, and hypophosphatemic rickets. McCune-Albright syndrome is associated with polyostotic fibrous dysplasia and café-au-lait spots. It is a noninherited disorder caused by point mutations in the alpha subunit of the Gs protein that lead to inappropriate activation of adenylate cyclase and increased levels of cyclic AMP that lead to cellular proliferation and increased hormone secretion, involving bone, skin, and endocrine tissues. (*Cecil, Ch. 210.1*)

36.(A) *Discussion:* Although most of the evidence points to tachykinins as mediators of the carcinoid flush, catecholamines may trigger flushing during exercise. In patients with gastric carcinoids, histamine can cause attacks of flushing. Serotonin, however, does not cause flushing in patients with carcinoid. (*Cecil, Ch. 210.2*)

37.(C) *Discussion:* This patient most likely has hypervitaminosis D with hypercalcemia that is related to the hypervitaminosis D and calcium replacement as a result of his increasing the dose of vitamin D in the treatment for hypoparathyroidism. There is nothing that suggests primary hyperparathyroidism, sarcoidosis, or a malignancy as the cause of his hypercalcemia, although all of these can certainly cause hypercalcemia. Although hyperthyroidism has been associated with hypercalcemia, it is usually mild. In patients with hypervitaminosis D and hypercalcemia, the treatment is to withdraw the calcium and vitamin D, rehydrate the patient, and give oral glucocorticoids to help normalize the serum calcium, the latter by inhibiting 1,25-dihydroxy-vitamin D production and inhibiting calcium absorption from the gastrointestinal tract. (*Cecil, Ch. 212; Reichel et al*)

38.(B) *Discussion:* All of the listed conditions are associated with decreased bioavailability of vitamin D as occurs in patients not exposed to sunlight or having inadequate nutritional intake of vitamin D or who have vitamin D malabsorption, as can occur with celiac disease or gastrectomy. Also, abnormal vitamin D metabolism can occur in patients with severe liver disease, which is usually also associated with nutritional deficiency. Drug-induced osteomalacia, in which circulating levels of 25-hydroxy-vitamin D are decreased as a result of increased metabolism secondary to drugs such as phenytoin or phenobarbital, also can occur. However, patients with vitamin D–dependent rickets typically have normal levels of 25-hydroxy-vitamin D and actually elevated 1,25-dihydroxy vitamin D levels but have decreased target organ responsiveness to 1,25-dihydroxy-vitamin D. (*Cecil, Ch. 213; Econs and Drezne*)

39.(D) *Discussion:* Patients with aluminum toxicity who are symptomatic with severe bone pain and pathologic fractures should have aluminum hydroxide, a phosphate binder, discontinued because aluminum toxicity can cause osteomalacia. It does this by being deposited in the interface between the osteotic tissue and the calcification front, where it is toxic to the osteoblast. These patients can be treated with desferoxamine to help reduce the aluminum toxicity, especially when they have severe pain and pathologic fractures. (*Cecil, Ch. 216*)

40.(D) *Discussion:* All of the conditions listed, except for acromegaly, can be secondary causes of osteoporosis. Anorexia nervosa does this by leading to hypogonadism with low sex hormone levels. Hyperthyroidism can cause increased bone resorption. Primary biliary cirrhosis can lead to low-turnover osteoporosis, and many of the connective tissue disorders can compromise peak adult bone mass. Acromegaly, however, does not cause osteoporosis. (*Cecil, Ch. 217; Christiansen; Riggs and Melton*)

41.(E) *Discussion:* This patient has what appears to be Paget's disease. Patients with this disease can have bone pain as well as fractures. They also can have neurologic complications, including deafness, vertigo, tinnitus, and cord and nerve root compression, as well as high-output failure, sarcomas, and sometimes benign and malignant giant cell tumors of the bone. Treatment is usually with calcitonin or bisphosphonates. (*Cecil, Ch. 218; Kanis*)

42.(C) *Discussion:* There are a number of tumors that affect the hypothalamus, but the most common are pituitary adenomas that have significant suprasellar extension. These tumors can cause hypopituitarism as well as diabetes insipidus and hyperprolactinemia by compressing the normal pituitary or the pituitary stalk and the mediobasal hypothalamus. Craniopharyngiomas are the next most common tumor affecting the hypothalamus. (*Cecil, Ch. 201*)

43.(D); 44.(C); 45.(A); 46.(B); 47.(E) *Discussion:* Some of these patients have true thyroid disease and some have TBG abnormalities or abnormal binding proteins. Patients with thyroiditis and thyrotoxicosis during the early phase (C) can be distinguished from patients who may be ingesting exogenous thyroid hormone (A). The difference can be determined by the suppression of thyroglobulin in patients taking exogenous thyroid hormone, with the levels normal to elevated in those with thyroiditis during the thyrotoxic phase. Patients who have abnormal binding globulins, such as dysalbuminemic hyperthyroidism (B) may have an elevated total T_4 level, but typically the free T_4 and T_3 levels are normal and these patients are euthyroid. Patients with suppressed TBG levels, such as those on androgens (D), can be distinguished from those patients with true primary hypothyroidism (E) by the elevated TSH levels in those with primary hypothyroidism. Those patients with low TBG levels typically have an elevated T_3RU so that the calculated free T_4 index in these patients will be normal, whereas it will be low because of the low T_3RU in patients with primary hypothyroidism. (*Cecil, Ch. 203; Nicoloff and Spencer*)

48.(B); 49.(E); 50.(C); 51.(D); 52.(A) *Discussion:* Cushing's syndrome can be associated with a pituitary adenoma with an inappropriately elevated ACTH level, with incomplete suppression with a low dose overnight dexamethasone suppression test and suppression greater than 50% with a high-dose dexamethasone suppression test (B). Other causes of Cushing's syndrome include adrenal adenomas, in which there is incomplete suppression with both low-dose and high-dose dexamethasone suppression tests, but ACTH levels would be expected to be suppressed (D). Cushing's syndrome associated with an adrenal cancer would have similar laboratory findings except that typically the dehydroepiandrosterone sulfate (DHEAS) level, which is a measure of androgen activity, is significantly elevated in patients with malignancy and women would be expected to have hirsutism and even possibly virilization (C). Cushing's syndrome can also be due to ectopic ACTH syndrome, as can be seen with malignancies, including malignancies of the lung, with significantly elevated ACTH levels and incomplete suppression with both low-dose and high-dose dexamethasone suppression tests (E). A patient ingesting glucocorticoids, and specifically hydrocortisone, which is measured primarily as cortisol (A), would be expected to have high measurable cortisol levels that did not suppress with low-dose and high-dose dexamethasone suppression, but to have low ACTH and DHEAS levels because the adrenal glands are suppressed by the exogenous steroids as a result of suppression of the hypothalamic-pituitary axis. (*Cecil, Ch. 204.1; Miller and Crapo*)

53.(A); 54.(B); 55.(C); 56.(A); 57.(D) *Discussion:* Autoimmune polyglandular syndromes are seen in childhood (type I) and during adulthood (type II). Mucocutaneous candidiasis is extremely common in polyglandular type I and is not seen in type II. Hypoparathyroidism, Addison's disease, primary hypogonadism, alopecia, keratopathy, and tympanic membrane calcification are common in type I. Addison's disease, autoimmune thyroid disease, and type I diabetes are common in type II polyglandular syndrome. Hypoparathyroidism rarely occurs and autoimmune hepatitis, keratopathy, and tympanic membrane calcification are not seen in type II polyglandular syndrome. Inheritance of type I syndrome is autosomal recessive, and type II has characteristic human leukocyte antigen associations, but this does not predict disease absolutely, and environmental factors are thought to play a role. Vitiligo is known to occur in both polyglandular type I and type II disorders. (*Cecil, Ch. 210.1; Eisenbarth and Jacson*)

58.(B); 59.(C); 60.(A); 61.(A); 62.(C) *Discussion:* The most common form of congenital adrenal hyperplasia is 21-hydroxylase deficiency, with 11-beta-hydroxylase deficiency being the second most common. Both can cause postnatal virilization. The classic form of 21-hydroxylase deficiency is known to cause salt wasting. It also can be associated with a high renin level, and typically 17-hydroxyprogesterone and androstenedione levels are elevated. In the 11-beta-hydroxylase deficiency, there is typically salt retention, and it is associated with low renin and elevated deoxycorticosterone and 11-deoxycortisol levels. Cortisol levels are diminished with both forms. (*Cecil, Ch. 210*)

63.(B); 64.(A); 65.(B); 66.(D); 67.(C) *Discussion:* Patients with hypothalamic or central diabetes insipidus typically have a loss of vasopressin release, which causes polyuria and polydipsia. In response to the dehydration test followed by giving aqueous vasopressin, there will be a further rise in the urine osmolality, not seen in the complete form of nephrogenic diabetes insipidus or in primary polydipsia with similar testing. Nephrogenic diabetes insipidus is associated with a congenital or acquired defect of the receptor for vasopressin at the collecting tubule, so that these patients have polyuria and polydipsia despite the presence of elevated levels of vasopressin. There is a familial form in which there is an abnormality of the gene for the V_2 receptor, which is located on the X chromosome, requiring the defect to be present on both X chromosomes in women for symptoms to develop, whereas men have the disorder if they receive the affected X chromosome from one parent. Nephrogenic diabetes insipidus can be acquired, and is associated with hypercalcemia and hypokalemia, the recovery phase of acute tubular necrosis and lithium therapy. Primary polydipsia is usually seen in patients with psychiatric disorders, although sometimes it is acquired after trauma in which a disorder of thirst develops. These patients typically have normal lab results, with their serum sodium levels in the low-normal range. They usually are imbibing large volumes of water, many times over 20 liters per day. Typically, patients with primary polydipsia do not imbibe fluid at night, and they have very little disruption of their sleep at night as a result of having to void, whereas those with hypothalamic and nephrogenic diabetes insipidus will have excessive urination day and night. None of the above problems cause markedly low serum sodium levels. This would be more likely in patients with SIADH. (*Cecil, Ch. 202.2; Robinson and Verbalis*)

68.(C); 69.(D); 70.(A); 71.(B); 72.(E) *Discussion:* The anterior pituitary hormones have more than one releasing factor and more than one inhibiting factor regulating many of them. TRH is known to act as a releasing factor for prolactin as well as TSH. Vasopressin can stimulate the release of ACTH. Dopamine can also inhibit the release of prolactin as well as TSH. Inhibin acts as an inhibitory factor for FSH. Insulin-like growth factor I can inhibit the release of growth hormone. (*Cecil, Ch. 202.1*)

73.(A); 74.(A); 75.(C); 76.(B); 77.(C) *Discussion:* There are a number of disorders as well as drugs that can increase and decrease TBG concentrations. Pregnancy and estrogen therapy, acute hepatitis, biliary cirrhosis, and acute intermittent porphyria, as well as drugs including tamoxifen, perphenazine, and clofibrate, can increase TBG concentrations. Other drugs, including pharmacologic doses of glucocorticoids, androgenic steroids, and asparaginase, along with systemic illnesses including nephrotic syndrome, chronic liver disease, and protein malnutrition, can decrease TBG concentrations. Drugs that interfere with binding to normal TBG include salicylates, diazepam, phenytoin, and furosemide; high levels of free fatty acids also interfere with binding. Congenital abnormalities are present in some families that cause both increased and decreased TBG concentrations. (*Cecil, Ch. 203*)

78.(A—False; B—False; C—True; D—False; E—False) *Discussion:* This patient has a follicular neoplasm by fine-needle aspiration biopsy, the only lesion in which malignancy cannot be determined simply by fine-needle aspiration and cytologic assessment. Because of the possibility of malignancy, giving the patient levothyroxine, doing an ultrasound, or attempting to reassure the patient at this stage would be inappropriate. Hypercellular or follicular lesions, however, may represent follicular adenomas, which are hot on a scan (suppressing the rest of the thyroid), and a hot nodule on the scan is rarely ever malignant. Therefore, the next best step would be to do a scan to see if this is a hot nodule; if it is, it would be appropriate to follow the patient. If the nodule is warm or cold, then the patient would need to have surgery to remove the nodule, because the risk of a follicular cancer would be significant. (*Cecil, Ch. 203; Clark and Du; Ridgeway*)

79.(A—False; B—True; C—True; D—True; E—False) *Discussion:* Women who have hypothyroidism of any cause require adequate replacement with levothyroxine to prevent fetal wastage if they become pregnant. It is known that hypothyroid women who are inadequately replaced with levothyroxine have a more difficult time conceiving. Even if the woman is adequately replaced with levothyroxine at the time of conception, there typically is an increase in dosage requirements of levothyroxine, especially during the third trimester, which can require an increase by as much as 30 to 50% over the previous dose to maintain a euthyroid state. Typically after birth and delivery, the dose of levothyroxine must be reduced to the preconception dosages to prevent over-replacement. It would be inappropriate to allow the patient to remain biochemically hypothyroid because of the negative impact, including the possibility of fetal wastage, that may occur. (*Cecil, Ch. 203; Becks and Burrow*)

80.(All are True) *Discussion:* This patient has the classic triad of pheochromocytoma, hypertension, and a thyroid nodule consistent with MEN type II disorders. Hyperparathyroidism can certainly be seen in the MEN IIA disorder. A thyroid nodule in a patient with a pheochromocytoma would raise a high concern that this represents a medullary cancer, which is associated with elevated calcitonin levels. A familial history of similar endocrine disorders would be expected to be found in the family, and a family history would be extremely important. In patients with familial pheochromocytomas, more of these are frequently bilateral and extra-adrenal, although they are less commonly malignant. (*Cecil, Ch. 204; Cryer; Ross and Aron*)

81.(All are True) *Discussion:* This patient has acromegaly, a disorder in which arthralgias in up to 75% of patients, carpal tunnel syndrome, skin changes including increased skin folds and skin tags, and increased sweating are all common findings. There is an increased incidence of colonic polyps, and galactorrhea may be seen in women, with some of them actually having an increase in their prolactin level. Acromegaly is associated with as much as two- to three-fold increase in mortality, with most of this increase attributed to cardiovascular and cerebrovascular diseases that may be related in part to hypertension and diabetes. There is some increase in cardiac hypertrophy, along with symptomatic heart disease consisting of coronary ischemia and congestive heart failure. (*Cecil, Ch. 202.1; Melmed*)

82.(A—True; B—True; C—True; D—False; E—True) *Discussion:* Hypogonadotropic hypogonadism can be related to Kallmann's syndrome, a congenital disorder causing a deficiency of GnRH. Secondary causes of hypogonadotropic hypogonadism include anorexia nervosa, stress, heavy exercise and associated weight loss, or severe illness. Other causes include hypothalamic lesions, central nervous system irradiation, and pituitary tumors. Hyperprolactinemia can suppress GnRH and reduce gonadotropin levels, causing hypogonadotropic hypogonadism. An acquired form of isolated gonadotropin deficiency can be encountered on occasion that has an autoimmune basis. Turner's syndrome is usually seen in XO females, who have gonadal streaks in place of their ovaries and actually have hypergonadotropic hypogonadism as a result of primary ovarian failure, causing a rise in gonadotropins in the face of hypogonadism. (*Cecil, Ch. 202.1; Vance*)

83.(A—False; B—True; C—True; D—True; E—True) *Discussion:* This patient has Graves' disease. Women with Graves' disease may have oligomenorrhea and amenorrhea but usually do not have heavy menses. Although true hypertension is not frequent in hyperthyroidism, a widened pulse pressure with an elevated systolic blood pressure does occur. Increase bone turnover with elevated calcium and increased alkaline phosphatase can also occur. Renal tubular acidosis and even immune complex nephritis have been reported. Both splenomegaly and lymphadenopathy were reported in some of the earliest descriptions of patients with Graves' disease. (*Cecil, Ch. 203; McDougall*)

84.(A—True; B—True; C—True; D—False; E—False) *Discussion:* This patient has hypothyroidism that appears to be caused by an autoimmune thyroid disease, most likely Hashimoto's thyroiditis. These patients may have the symptoms described in the case presentation and also may have a yellow complexion of the skin resulting from carotene accumulation. Approximately 10% may be hypertensive, and the hypertension may resolve after thyroid hormone replacement. Hyponatremia may occur as a result of the inability of the kidneys to excrete a free water load and of inappropriate ADH action. Patients with hypothyroidism typically have shallow, slow breathing and may have hypercapnia, but hypocapnia is not a typical finding. In patients with hypothyroidism, both LDL and HDL cholesterol levels are elevated, but the LDL is much more elevated in comparison to the HDL, increasing the risk of coronary artery disease over time. (*Cecil, Ch. 203; Rapoport*)

85.(A—False; B—True; C—True; D—True; E—True) *Discussion:* Familial pheochromocytomas constitute about 10% of all pheochromocytomas and may be seen in von Hippel–Lindau syndrome, an autosomal dominant disorder in which patients may have familial pheochromocytomas, retinal angiomas, cerebellar hemangioblastomas, renal cysts, and renal carcinomas as well as pancreatic cysts and epididymal cystadenomas. Patients with MEN IIA and MEN IIB both may have pheochromocytomas, and patients with hereditary neurofibromatosis, another autosomal dominant disorder, may have pheochromocytomas (seen in about 1% of these patients). MEN I is not usually associated with pheochromocytomas. (*Cecil, Ch. 204; Cryer*)

86.(A—False; B—True; C—True; D—False; E—True) *Discussion:* Licorice intoxication has been reported to cause hypertension and occurs through the action of glycyrrhizic acid, which inhibits 11-beta-hydroxysteroid dehydrogenase. This prevents the conversion of cortisol to cortisone, so that cortisol interacts with the mineralocorticoid receptor and assumes the role of aldosterone. Cortisone, the inactive metabolite, basically does not activate the mineralocorticoid receptor. Licorice intoxication thus represents a form of renin/angiotensin-independent mineralocorticoid excess and is not dependent on the renin/angiotensin system. The main source of licorice in the United States is chewing tobacco rather than candies. Although 17-alpha-hydroxylase deficiency can cause hypertension, licorice does not inhibit 17-hydroxylase. (*Cecil, Ch. 204.1*)

87.(A—True; B—True; C—True; D—False; E—True) *Discussion:* The primary adrenal insufficiency manifestations of this patient are most commonly due to an autoimmune process involving the adrenal glands. Tuberculosis can still cause primary adrenal insufficiency when it involves the adrenal glands. Fungal infections, including histoplasmosis, blastomycosis, coccidioidomycosis, and cryptococcosis, can cause adrenal insufficiency when they involve the adrenal glands. However, monilia does not cause adrenal destruction as the other fungi may. Adrenal hemorrhage, especially in patients on anticoagulation, with infection, or with some other illness, initially develops with back pain followed in a few days by symptoms and signs of adrenal insufficiency. Metastases to the adrenal by breast cancer, lung cancer, stomach cancer, colon cancer, melanoma, and some lymphomas can also cause adrenal insufficiency. In patients with AIDS, cytomegalovirus infection of the adrenal glands or *Mycobacterium avium-intracellulare* infections of the adrenal gland can cause primary adrenal insufficiency. (*Cecil, Ch. 204.1; Muir and Maclaren*)

88.(A—True; B—True; C—True; D—False; E—False) *Discussion:* Islet cell tumors can cause diabetes mellitus, and these include VIPomas, which secrete vasoactive intestinal polypeptide (VIP) and can cause diabetes or glucose intolerance as a result of either a glucagon-like effect of VIP or hypokalemia, which inhibits insulin secretion. Patients with glucagonomas also may have diabetes resulting from the counter-regulatory effect of glucagon on glucose synthesis and release, counteracting the effect of insulin. Somatostatinomas, by inhibiting insulin, sometimes can cause mild diabetes mellitus. Gastrinomas do not typically cause diabetes mellitus, nor do nonfunctioning islet cell tumors. (*Cecil, Ch. 206.2*)

89.(All are True) *Discussion:* This patient has secondary amenorrhea, and hyperprolactinemia is known to cause oligomenorrhea and also amenorrhea as a result of inhibition of GnRH and therefore gonadotropins. Hyperthyroidism can cause oligomenorrhea and amenorrhea. Pregnancy should always be excluded in a woman with secondary amenorrhea because it is the most common cause of this condition. Premature ovarian failure may occur in young women, especially those with polyglandular disorder type I, which is associated with hypoadrenalism, hypoparathyroidism, and mucocutaneous candidiasis. Finally, there are women on oral contraceptive agents who, after stopping these agents, do not resume menses within 3 months and are noted to have postpill amenorrhea. The prolonged amenorrhea in these patients is thought to be caused by underlying disorders unrelated to the oral contraceptive use. (*Cecil, Ch. 208.1; Rebar*)

90.(A—True; B—False; C—True; D—False; E—True) *Discussion:* The use of low-dose oral contraceptives approximately doubles the risk of fatal and nonfatal stroke in young women in the absence of smoking and hypertension. Oral contraceptive agents do not appear to be tetratogenic. Hypertension is more common in women using oral contraceptives, especially when they are over age 35, and smoking may contribute to the increased incidence of hypertension. Oral contraceptives appear to reduce the risk of developing endometrial carcinoma by about half and of developing ovarian carcinoma by about 40%. This protection is related to the duration of use of the oral contraceptives and persists for at least 10 years after stopping them. Oral contraceptives may increase the risk for development of hepatocellular adenomas, with the risk being greater in those who have used oral contraceptives for the longest duration. There is no evidence of any increased risk of liver cancer. However, hepatocellular adenomas may rarely rupture, hemorrhage, and cause death. (*Cecil, Ch. 208.1; Henzl*)

91.(A—True; B—True; C—False; D—True; E—True) *Discussion:* Gynecomastia can occur from a number of causes, including drug-related causes. Marijuana and digitalis can interact with the estrogen receptor, causing gynecomastia. Other drugs that can alter the androgen production, as well as its action at its receptor, include spironolactone, cimetidine, and ketoconazole. Furosemide does not cause gynecomastia. (*Cecil, Ch. 209.1; Braunstein*)

92.(A—True; B—False; C—False; D—False; E—True) *Discussion:* The carcinoid syndrome is known to cause cutaneous flushing; although a rise in blood pressure during flushing occurs rarely, carcinoid syndrome is not a cause of sustained hypertension. Telangiectasias on the face, neck, and malar areas can occur in some patients. These patients can have borborygmy, cramping, and explosive diarrhea. Chronic diarrhea is common, and malabsorption may occur. The plaque-like thickening of the endocardium of the valvular cusps and cardiac chambers occurs primarily on the right side of the heart and may involve the left side to a minimal degree. Although bronchial constriction is a less common feature of the carcinoid syndrome, it is most pronounced during the flushing attacks and may be severe. (*Cecil, Ch. 210.2*)

BIBLIOGRAPHY

Becker C: Hypothyroidism and atherosclerotic heart disease: Pathogenesis, medical management, and the role of coronary artery bypass surgery. Endocrinol Rev 6:432, 1985.

Becks GP, Burrow GN: Thyroid disease and pregnancy. Med Clin North Am 75:121, 1991.

Bennett JC, Plum F (eds): Cecil Textbook of Medicine. 20th ed. Philadelphia, WB Saunders Company, 1996.

Braunstein GD: Gynecomastia. N Engl J Med 328:490, 1993.

Christiansen CC (ed): Consensus Development Conference on Osteoporosis. Am J Med 95 (5A):1S, 1993.

Clark OH, Du Q-Y: Thyroid cancer. Med Clin North Am 75:211, 1991.

Cogan MG: Atrial natriuretic peptide. Kidney Int 37:1148, 1990.

Cryer PE: Pheochromocytoma. West J Med 156:399, 1992.

Econs MJ, Drezne, MK: Bone disease resulting from inherited disorders of renal tubule transport and vitamin D metabolism. In Coe FL, Favus MJ (eds): Disorders of Bone and Mineral Metabolism. New York, Raven Press, 1992, p. 935.

Eisenbarth GS, Jacson RA: The immunoendocrinopathy syndromes. In Wilson JD, Foster DW (eds): William's Textbook of Endocrinology. 8th ed. Philadelphia, WB Saunders Company, 1992, p. 1555.

Henzl MR: Contraceptive hormones and their clinical use. In Yen SSC, Jaffe RB (eds): Reproductive Endocrinology. 3rd ed. Philadelphia, WB Saunders Company, 1991, p. 807.

Kanis JA: Pathophysiology and Treatment of Paget's Disease of Bone. London, Martin Dunitz, 1991.

Klibanski A, Zervas NT: Diagnosis and management of hormone-secreting pituitary adenomas. N Engl J Med 324:8221, 1991.

Mazzaferri EL: Papillary thyroid carcinoma: Factors influencing prognosis and current therapy. Semin Oncol 14:315, 1987.

McDougall R: Graves disease. Med Clin North Am 75:79, 1991.

Melmed S: Acromegaly. N Engl J Med 322:966, 1990.

Miller J, Crapo L: The biochemical analysis of hypercortisolism. Endocrinologist 4:7, 1994.

Miller M, Dalakos T, Moses AM, et al: Recognition of partial defects in antidiuretic hormone secretion. Ann Intern Med 73:721, 1970.

Molitch ME: Management of prolactinomas. Annu Rev Med 40:225, 1989.

Molitch ME: Pathologic hyperprolactinemia. Endocrinol Metab Clin North Am 21:877, 1992.

Muir A, Maclaren NK: Autoimmune disease of the adrenal glands, parathyroid glands, gonads, and hypothalamic-pituitary axis. Endocrinol Metab Clin North Am 20:619, 1991.

Mulligan LM, Kwok JBJ, Healey CS, et al: Germ-line mutations of the RET proto-oncogene in multiple endocrine neoplasia type 2A. Nature 363:458, 1993.

Nicoloff JT, Spencer CA: The use and misuse of sensitive thyrotropin assays. J Clin Endocrinol Metab 71:493, 1990.

Plymate SR: Hypogonadism. Endocrinol Metab Clin North Am 23:749, 1994.

Rapoport B: Pathophysiology of Hashimoto's thyroiditis and hypothyroidism. Annu Rev Med 42:91, 1991.

Rebar RW: Premature ovarian failure. In Lobo RA (ed): Treatment of the Postmenopausal Woman: Basic and Clinical Aspects. New York, Raven Press, 1994, p. 25.

Reichel H, Koeffler HP, Norman AW: The role of the vitamin D endocrine system in health and disease. N Engl J Med 320:980, 1989.

Ridgeway EC: Clinician's evaluation of a solitary thyroid nodule. J Clin Endocrinol Metab 74:231, 1992.

Riggs BL, Melton LJ III: The prevention and treatment of osteoporosis. N Engl J Med 327:620, 1992.

Robinson AG, Verbalis JG: Diabetes insipidus. In Bardin CW (ed): Current Therapy in Endocrinology and Metabolism. 5th ed. St. Louis, CV Mosby, 1994, p. 1.

Ross NS, Aron DC: Hormonal evaluation of the patient with an incidentally discovered adrenal mass. N Engl J Med 323:1401, 1991.

Roti E, Minelli R, Gardini E, et al: The use and misuse of thyroid hormone. Endocrinol Rev 14:401, 1993.

Schteingart DE: Cushing's syndrome. Endocrinol Metab Clin North Am 18:311, 1989.

Simpson JL, Rebar RW: Normal and abnormal sexual differentiation and development. In Becker KL, et al (eds): Principles and Practice of Endocrinology and Metabolism. Philadelphia, JB Lippincott, 1990, p. 710.

Singer PA: Thyroiditis, acute, subacute, and chronic. Med Clin North Am 75:61, 1991.

Stein DT: New developments in the diagnosis and treatment of sexual precocity. Am J Med Sci 303:53, 1992.

Thakker RV: The molecular genetics of the multiple endocrine neoplasia syndromes. Clin Endocrinol 38:1, 1993.

Vance ML: Hypopituitarism. N Engl J Med 330:1651, 1994.

Vinik AI, Moattari AR: Treatment of endocrine tumors of the pancreas. Endocrinol Metab Clin North Am 18:483, 1989.

PART 11

DIABETES MELLITUS AND METABOLISM

Ayman A. Zayed and Stuart J. Frank

DIRECTIONS: For questions 1 to 40, choose the ONE BEST answer to each question.

QUESTIONS 1–5

A 36-year-old female nurse presents to the emergency room because of several hours of confusion, slurred speech, headache, and abnormal mentation. Her husband states that the patient has a history of mitral valve prolapse, depression, hypertension, peptic ulcer disease, and ethanol abuse. Her medications include propranolol, ranitidine, nifedipine, clonazepam, and quinine (for muscle cramps). Physical examination reveals a blood pressure of 110/70 mm Hg and a pulse of 110 beats per minute. The patient is lethargic but arousable, disoriented, and diaphoretic. Her skin is pale. An intravenous line is started and, after blood is drawn, 50 ml of 50% dextrose is given. Her acute manifestations resolve.

1. You would expect her plasma glucose level at the time of presentation to be

    A. 60 to 70 mg per deciliter
    B. 40 to 50 mg per deciliter
    C. Undetectable
    D. 70 to 80 mg per deciliter
    E. Within normal range

With further questioning, her husband reports that his wife did not take one of her medications for the last month.

2. Which medication is she likely not to have taken?

    A. Clonazepam
    B. Propranolol
    C. Nifedipine
    D. Quinine
    E. Ranitidine

Laboratory values are as follows:

Sodium	139 mEq/L
Potassium	4.3 mEq/L
Chloride	103 mEq/L
Bicarbonate	24 mEq/L
Creatinine	1.1 mg/dl
Blood urea nitrogen (BUN)	15 mg/dl
Plasma glucose	39 mg/dl
Urine ketones	Absent
Liver enzymes	Normal
Hemoglobin A_{1c} (normal: 4.0 to 6.0%)	5.2%

The patient is kept on intravenous 10% dextrose for 24 hours. On the second and third day her plasma glucose determinations are normal while eating regular meals and not receiving intravenous dextrose.

3. What is the most appropriate next step?

    A. Random insulin and C-peptide
    B. Adrenocorticotrophic hormone (ACTH) stimulation test
    C. Somatomedin C
    D. Five-hour oral glucose tolerance test
    E. None of the above

Other lab data (from the blood drawn at the time of presentation in the emergency room) show

	Patient	Normal
Insulin	7 mU/L	Fasting: 5–20 mU/L
C-peptide	3.0 ng/ml	0.5–2.0 ng/ml
Growth hormone (GH)	10 ng/ml	Response to provocative stimuli: >7 ng/ml
Cortisol	21 μg/dl	8:00 A.M.: 5–24 μg/dl

4. At this stage, the diagnostic test of choice would be

    A. Abdominal computed tomography (CT) scan
    B. Transhepatic sampling
    C. Insulin receptor antibodies assay
    D. Sulfonylurea measurement (on the admission serum samples)
    E. Ethanol measurement (on the admission serum samples)

5. The proper test was done and is positive. Your next step would be

    A. Screening laparotomy
    B. Psychiatric consultation
    C. Glucocorticoid therapy
    D. Plasmapheresis
    E. Refer the patient to an alcohol rehabilitation program

QUESTIONS 6 AND 7

A 72-year-old white woman presents to you for evaluation of 9 months' history of loose, foul-smelling diarrhea, four to five times a day, which has been associated with a 6.0-kg weight loss, generalized weakness, and decreased appetite. Her son reports that she has become forgetful in the last 6 months. Physical examination reveals an elderly lady without apparent distress. Her pulse is 70 beats per minute (regular) and blood pressure is 140/70 mm Hg. Head and neck examination reveals a red tongue with wide fissures. Heart, chest, abdomen, and lower limb examination is normal. Skin examination reveals dark scaling and cracking skin lesions over the forearms and neck. Her neurologic examination is normal apart from impairment of short-term memory.

6. All of the following conditions may produce or aggravate her disease EXCEPT

A. 6-Mercaptopurine therapy
B. Isoniazid therapy
C. Alcoholism
D. Malignant carcinoid tumor
E. Hypothyroidism

7. Her diagnosis can be established by

A. Measuring urinary 5-hydroxyindoleacetic acid
B. Measuring serum nicotinamide adenine dinucleotide (NAD)
C. ACTH stimulation test
D. Thyroid function tests
E. Measuring urinary N-methylnicotinamide

QUESTIONS 8 AND 9

An 18-year-old single woman is brought in by her parents because they are concerned about her weight. They report that she has lost about 70 lb (32 kg) over the last 2 years and has had a very poor appetite. On questioning, the patient says that she is not concerned about her weight and would like to lose more weight. However, she reports a 3-year history of constipation, cold intolerance, and dry skin. The patient denies weakness, polyuria, polydypsia, and cardiac, respiratory, or urinary symptoms. Her last menstrual period was 9 months ago. Physical examination shows a tense, young, thin patient with a weight of 110 lb (50 kg), height of 175 cm, pulse of 62 beats per minute, blood pressure of 100/60 mm Hg and temperature of 36.9°C. Her skin is cold and dry. The head, neck, chest, heart, and abdomen examinations are normal. Reflex testing shows delayed relaxation of the ankle reflex.

8. The most likely diagnosis is

A. Adrenal insufficiency
B. Hypothyroidism
C. Type I diabetes mellitus
D. Bulimia
E. None of the above

9. You would expect to see all of the following EXCEPT

A. Decreased triiodothyronine (T_3)
B. Elevated GH
C. Elevated somatomedin C
D. Elevated cortisol
E. Decreased follicle-stimulating hormone (FSH)

10. All of the following, when present, can independently increase the risk of macrovascular complications of diabetes mellitus EXCEPT

A. Hypertension
B. Cigarette smoking
C. Hyperglycemia
D. Dyslipidemia

11. Which of the following patients should have the greatest glycemic control?

A. A 21-year-old man with type I diabetes mellitus without evidence of microvascular complications. His hemoglobin A_{1c} level is 10.2% (normal: 4.0 to 6.0).
B. A 31-year-old man with type I diabetes mellitus complicated by peripheral neuropathy and background diabetic retinopathy. His hemoglobin A_{1c} level is 11%.
C. A 29-year-old diabetic pregnant woman with a fasting plasma glucose level of 123 mg per deciliter.
D. A 38-year-old diabetic obese woman who is maintained on 220 units of insulin per day.
E. A 62-year-old man with type II diabetes mellitus and coronary artery disease (CAD).

QUESTIONS 12–14

A 27-year-old woman with a 5-year history of diabetes mellitus is maintained on 8 to 12 units Regular insulin before each meal and 20 units neutral protamine Hagedorn insulin (NPH) at bedtime. In the last 6 months, the patient started progressively to reduce her insulin dose because of frequent episodes of hypoglycemia. Currently she takes 2 to 3 units Regular insulin before each meal and 6 units NPH at bedtime. Her hemoglobin A_{1c} level 1 week ago was 6.1% (normal: 4.0 to 6.0). The patient presents to the emergency room today with a few days' history of progressive generalized weakness, malaise, and nausea. However, there has been no vomiting. Her blood pressure is 80/50 mm Hg and her pulse is 94 beats per minute (regular). Random finger stick blood glucose level is 69 mg per deciliter.

12. The most appropriate next step is

A. Administration of 50 ml of 50% dextrose intravenously
B. Intravenous normal saline
C. Intravenous hydrocortisone after ACTH stimulation test
D. A and B
E. B and C

The patient was treated successfully with the appropriate treatment. Three months later she presents with a 10-lb weight gain over the last 3 months, general weakness, constipation, and thinning of her hair. In addition, she complains of hot flashes and dyspareunia.

13. You would expect to see all of the following EXCEPT

A. High thyroid-stimulating hormone (TSH) level
B. Positive antimicrosomal antibodies test
C. Hypocalcemia with low parathyroid hormone (PTH) level
D. High FSH level
E. Hypopigmented skin lesions consistent with vitiligo

14. Which of the following statements is true about this patient?

A. Her history of mucocutaneous candidiasis is consistent with the diagnosis.

B. Pernicious anemia is a frequent complication of her disease.
C. Her diagnosis is polyglandular autoimmune syndrome type I.
D. Her disorder is human leukocyte antigen (HLA) DR3 and DR4 associated.
E. C and D

QUESTIONS 15–20

A 21-year-old man with no past medical history presents to the emergency room with a 3-day history of generalized malaise, anorexia, nausea, abdominal pain, and watery, nonbloody diarrhea three to four times per day. Physical examination reveals a lethargic young man with dry mucous membranes. His blood pressure is 100/60 mm Hg, pulse is 100 beats per minute, and respiration is 22 per minute (deep). Head, neck, and chest examination is normal. Cardiovascular examination reveals tachycardia without murmurs. The central abdomen is mildly tender. Stool is hemoccult negative. His lab data show

Hemoglobin	15.2 g/dl
White blood cell (WBC) count	12,000/μl
Sodium	138 mEq/L
Potassium	4.8 mEq/L
Cloride	108 mEq/L
CO_2	10 mEq/L
BUN	25 mg/dl
Creatinine	2.5 mg/dl
Plasma glucose	308 mg/dl
Serum nitroprusside reaction	Weakly positive
pH	7.25
P_{CO_2}	24 mm Hg

15. All of the following statements about this patient are true EXCEPT

A. The predominant energy source for his non–central nervous system tissues is circulating free fatty acids.
B. His hepatic gluconeogenesis is increased.
C. The only source of energy for his brain is glucose.
D. His serum epinephrine level is increased.
E. His lipoprotein lipase activity is impaired.

16. The acid-base disturbance in this patient is

A. Pure high anion-gap metabolic acidosis
B. Mixed high anion-gap and normal anion-gap metabolic acidosis
C. Mixed high anion-gap metabolic acidosis and metabolic alkalosis
D. Mixed high anion-gap metabolic acidosis and respiratory alkalosis
E. None of the above

17. You would expect to see all of the following during the first 24 hours of management EXCEPT

A. Decreased creatinine level
B. Increased nitroprusside reaction
C. Increased sodium level
D. Increased potassium level
E. Increased chloride level

18. All of the following are indicated during his management EXCEPT

A. Normal saline
B. Dextrose 5%
C. Intravenous potassium
D. Intravenous phosphate
E. Intravenous bicarbonate

19. Which one of the following might you expect to find on admission lab tests?

A. Low low-density lipoprotein (LDL) cholesterol level
B. Low very-low-density lipoprotein (VLDL) cholesterol level
C. Low chylomicron level
D. High high-density lipoprotein (HDL) cholesterol level
E. A and B

20. The least likely gene associated with the patient's disease is

A. HLA-DR3
B. HLA-DR4
C. HLA-DR15
D. HLA-B8
E. HLA-B15

QUESTIONS 21–27

A 52-year-old man with a history of hypertension and type II diabetes mellitus for the last 5 years presents to you with acute abdominal pain and vomiting of 2 days' duration in addition to bilateral hand numbness. His medications include glyburide, hydrochlorothiazide, and nifedipine. His physical examination reveals a stressed patient in pain, with blood pressure of 130/95 mm Hg, pulse of 100 beats per minute, and temperature of 37.4°C. The patient is oriented but his recent memory is impaired. His retinal vessels have a salmon-pink color. There is upper abdominal tenderness with positive rebound. Stool hemoccult is negative. Skin lesions (see Figure 1) are apparent.

Figure 1

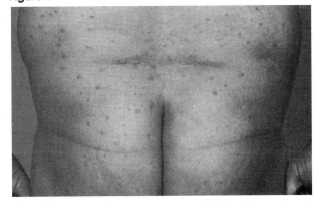

(From Gotto AM Jr.: Sandoz Pharmaceuticals Dyslipoproteinemia Education Program: Clinical Manuals, p. 33. London, Science Press, Ltd., 1991, with permission.)

21. Which one of the following is directly responsible for his manifestations?

   A. Total cholesterol level of 1000 mg per deciliter
   B. Triglyceride level of 5200 mg per deciliter
   C. HDL cholesterol level of 10 mg per deciliter
   D. LDL cholesterol level of 560 mg per deciliter
   E. Blood glucose level of 630 mg per deciliter

22. You would expect to see all of the following EXCEPT

   A. Amylase level of 100 U per liter
   B. Milky plasma
   C. Hemoglobin A_{1c} level of 14.2%
   D. Splenomegaly on abdominal CT scan
   E. Triglyceride level of 1200 mg per deciliter

23. In the first 24 hours, the most effective way to correct the underlying abnormality leading to his symptoms is

   A. No oral intake
   B. Insulin therapy
   C. Gemfibrozil therapy
   D. Niacin therapy
   E. Intravenous fluid

The patient received the appropriate management. Three days later his fasting lab data show the following: plasma glucose level of 129 mg per deciliter, triglyceride level of 1120 mg per deciliter, total cholesterol level of 270 mg per deciliter, and HDL cholesterol level of 27 mg per deciliter.

24. The drug of choice for his hyperlipidemia is

   A. Niacin
   B. Gemfibrozil
   C. Lovastatin
   D. Cholestyramine
   E. Gemfibrozil and lovastatin

25. Which one of the following statements about his lipid profile is true?

   A. His calculated LDL cholesterol level is 28 mg per deciliter.
   B. His calculated LDL cholesterol level is 55 mg per deciliter.
   C. His LDL cholesterol level cannot be calculated.
   D. A small to moderate amount of alcohol is indicated to raise his HDL cholesterol level.
   E. C and D

26. His lipid profile is consistent with which type of hyperlipedemia?

   A. Type IIa
   B. Type IIb
   C. Type III
   D. Type IV
   E. Type V

27. Which of the following statements is true about the skin lesions of the patient?

   A. They are extremely pruritic.
   B. The patient has had them since the onset of his diabetes.

   C. They are completely reversible in response to the treatment of the underlying disorder.
   D. Cholesterol is the chief constituent of these skin lesions.
   E. They are drug induced.

QUESTIONS 28–34

A 57-year-old male patient presents to you for evaluation of his diabetes mellitus, CAD, which was diagnosed 8 years ago. His past medical history is significant for hypertension, CAD, gouty arthritis, and irritable bowel syndrome with manifestations of bloating and constipation. He takes human insulin: 22 units NPH and 10 units Regular before breakfast; 12 units NPH and 6 units Regular before dinner. Other medications include allopurinol, aspirin, isosorbide dinitrate, and hydrochlorothiazide. His blood glucose pattern (in milligrams per deciliter) as determined by self-monitoring is

7:00 A.M.	11:00 A.M.	4:00 P.M.	9:00 P.M.
216	110	140	122
242	116	129	105

28. Which of the following insulin dose adjustments would be the most appropriate?

   A. Increase A.M. NPH insulin
   B. Increase P.M. NPH insulin
   C. Increase P.M. Regular insulin
   D. Increase P.M. Regular and NPH insulin
   E. Decrease P.M. NPH insulin

The appropriate insulin adjustment is made. His blood glucose pattern becomes as follows:

7:00 A.M.	11:00 A.M.	4:00 P.M.	9:00 P.M.
132	112	139	125
125	121	119	112

The patient's wife reports that, on the new insulin regimen, her husband gets sweaty between 2:00 A.M. and 3:00 A.M., with a blood glucose level of 60 to 70 mg per deciliter.

29. The most appropriate insulin dose adjustment at this stage would be

   A. Decrease P.M. NPH insulin
   B. Decrease P.M. Regular insulin
   C. Administer the evening NPH insulin at 9:00 P.M. rather than before dinner
   D. Change back to his original regimen
   E. Do not change the insulin regimen

His physical examination shows him to be in fair general condition, with blood pressure of 138/98 mm Hg, pulse of 82 beats per minute (regular), weight of 176 lb (80 kg), and height of 68 inches (170 cm). There is xanthelasma on the right lower eyelid. An ejection systolic murmur, grade II/VI, is noted. The chest is clear. Ophthalmologic examination reveals mild background diabetic retinopathy. The rest of his examination is within normal limits. Initial laboratory studies show

Sodium	134 mEq/L
Potassium	5.5 mEq/L
Chloride	105 mEq/L
Bicarbonate	20 mEq/L
BUN	25 mg/dl
Creatinine	1.4 mg/dl
Liver enzymes	Normal
Fasting lipid profile	
Total cholesterol	310 mg/dl
Triglycerides	220 mg/dl
HDL cholesterol	40 mg/dl
Hemoglobin A_{1c} (normal: 4.0 to 6.0%)	8.2%
24-Hour urine albumin	212 mg

30. The drug of choice for his hypertension would be

    A. Captopril
    B. Nifedipine
    C. Diltiazem
    D. Propranolol
    E. Continue on hydrochlorothiazide

31. Which one of the following (if present) would explain his electrolyte pattern?

    A. An A.M. cortisol level of 12 μg per deciliter
    B. A P.M. cortisol level of 4 μg per deciliter
    C. Plasma renin activity of 0.1 ng per milliliter per hour (standing position) (normal: 0.2 to 3.6)
    D. Calcium level of 10.2 mg per deciliter with intact PTH level of 60 pg per milliliter (normal: 10 to 65).
    E. An 8:00 A.M. cortisol level of 1.2 μg per deciliter after 1 mg of dexamethasone at 11:00 P.M. the prior evening.

32. All of the following drugs may give similar electrolyte patterns EXCEPT

    A. Clonidine
    B. Propranolol
    C. Indomethacin
    D. Cyclosporine
    E. Ranitidine

The patient was started on a low-fat, low-cholesterol diet. Six months later, his fasting total cholesterol level is 295 mg per deciliter, triglyceride level is 192 mg per deciliter, and HDL cholesterol level is 41 mg per deciliter.

33. The cholesterol-lowering agent of choice would be

    A. Gemfibrozil
    B. Niacin
    C. Lovastatin
    D. Cholestyramine
    E. Six months of low-fat, low-cholesterol diet

34. All of the following can cause similar cholesterol levels EXCEPT

    A. Hypothyroidism
    B. Nephrotic syndrome

    C. Obstructive liver disease
    D. Lack of exercise
    E. Thiazides

35. A 42-year-old female patient with diabetes mellitus for the last 25 years is maintained on 12 units Regular insulin plus 30 units NPH insulin before breakfast (8:00 A.M.) and 8 units Regular insulin plus 20 units NPH before dinner (5:00 P.M.). She occasionally wakes up with early morning headaches and nightmares. Her blood glucose pattern (in milligrams per deciliter) for the last 2 months is as follows:

7:30 A.M.	11:00 A.M.	4:00 P.M.	9:00 P.M.
230–272	140–161	134–152	105–123

The most appropriate next step is

    A. Trial of late-evening administration of octreotide
    B. Check her blood glucose level at 3:00 to 4:00 A.M.
    C. Increase her evening NPH insulin dose
    D. Increase her evening Regular insulin dose
    E. Refer her to a neurologist

QUESTIONS 36 AND 37

A 43-year-old woman with diabetes mellitus for the last 23 years presents with a 2-week history of progressive painless swelling of the anterior part of the right foot. The patient denies a history of trauma. Physical examination reveals an afebrile patient with erythema and increased localized temperature but no tenderness. The dorsalis pedis is bounding. Knee and ankle reflexes are absent. Pain sensation is decreased in both feet. Lab results are as follows:

Hemoglobin	13.2 g/dl
WBC count	8900/μl
Neutrophils	65%
Lymphocytes	28%
Monocytes	5%
Eosinophils	3%
Platelets	Adequate
Electrolytes	Normal
Serum uric acid (normal: 2.5 to 8.0 mg/dl)	7.9 mg/dl

A right foot radiograph shows a well-demarcated marked osteopenia in the metatarsal bones surrounded by a normally mineralized bone. There is no evidence of fracture and there are no signs of soft tissue swelling, calcification, periosteal thickening, or elevation.

36. The most likely diagnosis is

    A. Charcot joint
    B. Osteomyelitis
    C. Cellulitis
    D. Reflex sympathetic dystrophy
    E. Pseudogout

37. The treatment of choice of this patient's problem is

    A. Absolute non–weight bearing and cast immobilization of the right foot

B. Intravenous culture-directed antibiotics
C. Oral antibiotics
D. Glucocorticoids
E. Nonsteroidal anti-inflammatory drugs

38. A 37-year-old white man with type I diabetes mellitus presented with fissuring about the heels of 3 months' duration. You would expect to see all of the following EXCEPT

A. Dry feet
B. Cold feet
C. Charcot joint
D. Osteopenia of the feet bones
E. Distended dorsal veins of the feet

QUESTIONS 39 AND 40

A 62-year-old man with a history of type II diabetes mellitus diagnosed 1 year ago, maintained on glyburide 5 mg twice per day presents with sudden right-sided headache and diplopia of 2 days' duration. Nevertheless, his visual acuity has been normal and stable. There is no history of feet or hand numbness, diarrhea, constipation, or vomiting. He states that he has normal sexual function. Physical examination shows a blood pressure of 140/85 mm Hg with a pulse of 72 beats per minute (regular). There are no orthostatic changes. His right eye is deviated inferiorly and temporally, with partial ptosis. He is unable to turn his right eye upward, downward, and inward. The right pupil is dilated and does not respond to direct or consensual stimulation, whereas the left pupil is normal and responds to both direct and consensual stimulation.

39. Which of the following nerves is/are affected?

A. Right oculomotor nerve
B. Right trochlear nerve
C. Right abducens nerve
D. Right oculomotor and right optic nerves
E. Right oculomotor and left optic nerves

40. Which one of the following makes diabetes unlikely as a cause for his ocular neuropathy?

A. Sudden onset
B. Unilateral headache
C. Mydriasis
D. Absence of diffuse neuropathy
E. None of the above

DIRECTIONS: For questions 41 to 63, decide whether each choice is true or false. Any combination of answers, from all true to all false, may occur.

QUESTIONS 41–52

A 32-year-old man presents to you for evaluation of his diabetes mellitus, which was diagnosed 15 years ago. Currently he takes 10 units Regular insulin plus 22 units NPH insulin every morning and 7 units Regular insulin plus 18 units NPH insulin before dinner. His diabetic notebook shows that his blood glucose level is unstable, ranging from 25 to 432 mg per deciliter. His hypoglycemic episodes are frequent, occur at no specific time of day, and are manifested by loss of consciousness without warning. He checks his blood sugar twice a day. His hospital records show a history of diabetic ketoacidosis (DKA) three times in the last 5 years. He reports a progressive bilateral burning sensation in the legs and bilateral hand numbness for the last 8 years. He says that the rubbing of bedclothes against his legs evokes a severe burning sensation, so he usually leaves his legs uncovered. In addition, he reports early satiety and postprandial upper abdominal discomfort with nausea and occasional vomiting. His bowel habits have been normal until 4 years ago, when he started to have watery diarrhea, which is worse at night and associated occasionally with fecal incontinence. There is no history of blood, undigested food, or greasy material in the stool. The patient has been married for the last 9 years and has one child, who is 8 years old. On questioning, he admits that he has been impotent for the last 7 years. His impotence started gradually and currently he only occasionally gets weak morning erections. His libido is normal. His hemoglobin A_{1c} level 1 week ago was 12.9% (normal: 4.0 to 6.0), and his retinal examination 1 month ago is shown in Figure 2.

Figure 2

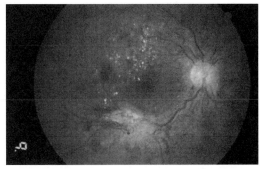

41. Which of the following is/are possible causes of his hypoglycemic episodes?

  A. Gastroparesis
  B. Deficiency of glucagon secretion
  C. Marked increase in physical activity
  D. Decrease in food intake
  E. Faulty injection technique

42. Which of the following measures is/are indicated in the management of his hypoglycemic episodes?

  A. The patient's partner should be instructed about the use of intramuscular glucagon in the event of hypoglycemia.
  B. The patient should carry identification noting his diabetes status.
  C. Measurement of ACTH-stimulated cortisol level should be done.
  D. A Metoclopramide therapy trial should be instituted.
  E. The patient should be instructed to use a nonexercised injection site prior to exercising.

43. What would you do to help the patient regulate his blood sugar?

  A. Provide dietary consultation
  B. Order gastric scintigraphy
  C. Suggest frequent self-monitoring of blood sugar at least four times per day
  D. Suggest injections of insulin immediately before eating

44. His hypoglycemia unawareness may reflect

  A. Adrenal medullary dysfunction
  B. Peripheral sympathetic dysfunction
  C. Glucagon deficiency
  D. Rapid decline of blood glucose concentration
  E. Adrenocortical insufficiency

45. The patient wishes to have an insulin pump to regulate his blood sugar. Which of the following may contraindicate the use of insulin pump therapy?

  A. He is not willing to perform frequent self-monitoring of blood glucose
  B. The presence of significant neuropathy
  C. His psychological status is inadequate to manage intensive therapy
  D. The presence of retinopathy
  E. The history of hypoglycemia episodes

46. Which of the following complications will you expect to see if an insulin pump is used?

  A. Increased risk for DKA
  B. Increased frequency of localized skin infections
  C. Increased risk for hypoglycemia compared to intensive insulin therapy using multiple insulin injections per day
  D. Increased weight gain compared with conventional insulin therapy
  E. Possible transient worsening of retinopathy

47. Which of the following statements is/are true about the burning sensation in the patient's legs?

  A. It worsens at night.
  B. You would expect his vibratory sensation to be absent.

C. You would expect his ankle jerk reflex to be absent.

D. Ambulation may result in a transient clinical improvement.

E. Charcot joint is a possible complication.

48. The burning in his legs may be treated with

A. Topical 0.075% capsacin
B. Amitriptyline
C. Carbamazepine
D. Codeine sulfate
E. Mexiletine

49. Which of the following would you expect to see in this patient?

A. Heart rate of 52 beats per minute
B. Postural decrease of 15 mm Hg in diastolic blood pressure
C. Decreased RR variation on electrocardiogram in relative to respiration
D. Absence of post-Valsalva bradycardia
E. Failure of stimulation of plasma renin release on standing

50. Which of the following is/are true statements about his diarrhea?

A. The worsening of his diarrhea at night makes diabetes unlikely as the underlying etiology.
B. The use of pancreatic enzymes is usually helpful in the management of his diarrhea.
C. Tetracycline therapy may cause improvement in his diarrhea.
D. The use of cisapride may provide symptomatic relief.
E. Celiac disease is more common in this patient than in the general population.

51. Which of the following is/are true statements about his impotence?

A. Tight diabetes control will result in significant improvement in his erectile dysfunction.
B. Testosterone therapy would be beneficial.
C. His tests are most likely small and soft.
D. His luteinizing hormone level is most likely elevated.
E. The occurrence of his impotence prior to any other autonomic dysfunction argues against diabetes being the main responsible factor.

52. Which of the following would be effective in the treatment of his retinal changes?

A. Photocoagulation
B. Epalrestat (an aldose reductase inhibitor)
C. Blood glucose control
D. Aspirin
E. Blood pressure control

QUESTIONS 53–55

A 42-year-old man with a history of type I diabetes mellitus for the last 18 years is maintained on insulin. His clinical evaluation reveals a blood pressure of 142/95 mm Hg and a pulse of 82 beats per minute (regular). Fundoscopic examination shows microaneurysms, soft and hard exudates, and small hemorrhages. The rest of his examination is within normal limits. His initial lab tests show

Plasma glucose (2 hr postprandial)	240 mg/dl
Hemoglobin A_{1c}	14.2%
Creatinine	1.8 mg/dl
Serum albumin	3.7 g/dl
24-Hour urine protein	3.19 g

53. Which of the following statements is/are true?

A. The patient most likely will develop end-stage renal disease within 10 years.
B. His serum renin level most likely is high.
C. A kidney biopsy should be done.
D. Diffuse thinning of the glomerular basement membrane will be noted if kidney biopsy is performed.
E. The patient would have had his kidney disease at an earlier age if he had type II diabetes mellitus.

54. Which of the following would be effective in the management of his kidney disease?

A. Blood pressure control.
B. Keeping his hemoglobin A_{1c} in the 7 to 8% range.
C. Low protein intake at 0.6 to 0.8 grams per kilogram of body weight per day.
D. Renal transplantation when renal failure develops.

55. Which of the following statements is/are true in regard to his retinal findings?

A. The patient has proliferative diabetic retinopathy.
B. Tight blood glucose control most likely will slow the progression of eye disease.
C. Ophthalmologic examination is recommended every 5 years.
D. The soft exudates are lipid-containing fluid that has leaked from surrounding capillaries.
E. Normal visual acuity would not be consistent with his retinal findings.

QUESTIONS 56 AND 57

A 46-year-old diabetic man is maintained on insulin. His average range of blood glucose values (in milligrams per deciliter) in the last 2 months is

7:00 A.M.	11:00 A.M.	4:00 P.M.	9:00 P.M.
200–231	220–231	180–231	191–212

His hemoglobin A_{1c} level 2 days ago was 8.2% (normal: 4.0 to 6.0%).

56. The discrepancy between his hemoglobin A_{1c} level and his blood glucose pattern can be due to

A. Thalassemia
B. Sickle cell disease
C. Hemoglobin C

D. Large doses of aspirin
E. Inaccurate blood glucose measurements

57. Which of the following statements is/are true about glycohemoglobin?

A. It is influenced by acute changes in blood glucose.
B. It provides an index of glycemic control during the preceding 4 months.
C. It can determine specific changes in the insulin regimen.
D. It is a sensitive test for the diagnosis of diabetes mellitus.
E. Glycohemoglobin ranges for nondiabetics may vary from lab to lab.

58. A 32-year-old white man presents to you complaining of anginal chest pain. Examination of his eyes is significant for bilateral corneal arcus. His feet are shown in Figure 3. Which of the following statements about this patient is/are true?

Figure 3

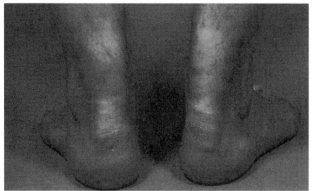

(From Gotto AM Jr.: Sandoz Pharmaceuticals Dyslipoproteinemia Education Program: Clinical Manuals, p. 30. London, Science Press, Ltd., 1991, with permission.)

A. You would expect his total cholesterol concentration to be 400 mg per deciliter and his triglyceride level to be normal.
B. The patient may present (secondary to his disease) with exercise-related Achilles tendinitis.
C. His disease is inherited as an autosomal recessive trait.
D. His disease results from defects in the gene encoding the hepatic LDL receptors.

59. A 52-year-old obese woman is referred to you because of changes in her hands as shown in Figure 4. Her laboratory evaluation reveal normal renal, liver, and thyroid function. Which of the following statements about this patient is/are true?

A. The patient has type IV hyperlipidemia.
B. You would expect to see tuberoeruptive xanthomas on the knees.
C. You would expect to see a total cholesterol level of 210 mg per deciliter and triglyceride level of 900 mg per deciliter.

Figure 4

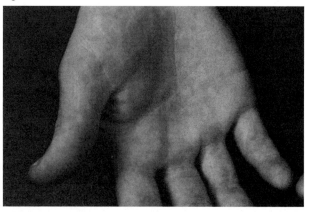

(From Gotto AM Jr.: Sandoz Pharmaceuticals Dyslipoproteinemia Education Program: Clinical Manuals, p. 33. London, Science Press, Ltd., 1991, with permission.)

D. Her disorder predisposes her to premature atherosclerosis.
E. Her disease is characterized by an autosomal recessive defect in apoprotein E.

QUESTIONS 60 AND 61

A 52-year-old man presents with weakness, thirst, polyuria, blood pressure of 100/60 mm Hg, plasma glucose level of 1200 mg per deciliter, sodium level of 142 mEq per liter, potassium level of 4.2 mEq per liter, and bicarbonate level of 21 mEq per liter.

60. Which of the following statements is/are true?

A. You would expect his serum insulin level to be undetectable.
B. The presence of aphasia would be inconsistent with his presentation.
C. His condition could be precipitated by phenytoin therapy.
D. His calculated effective osmolality is 357 mOsm per liter.
E. The normal serum sodium level indicates that the patient is dehydrated.

61. Which of the following is/are true statements about his management?

A. The most urgent therapy is insulin.
B. Initial volume expansion with one-quarter normal saline should be started to establish circulatory integrity.
C. The patient may require 5% dextrose solution.
D. With careful therapy, the outcome of such a disorder is usually good.

62. Which of the following may be associated with the skin lesions shown in Figure 5?

A. Obesity
B. Acromegaly
C. Cushing's disease
D. Circulating anti–insulin receptor antibodies
E. Gastric adenocarcinoma

Figure 5

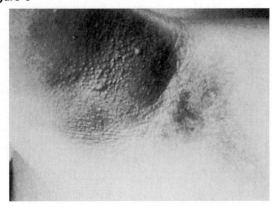

63. In which of the following patients is/are sulfonylurea drugs contraindicated in treating diabetes mellitus?

A. A 45-year-old diabetic man secondary to total pancreatectomy

B. A 28-year-old pregnant woman with fasting blood glucose level of 130 to 142 mg per deciliter

C. A 21-year-old diabetic obese man with undetectable serum C-peptide level

D. A 56-year-old obese woman with a 5-year history of diabetes whose hemoglobin A_{1c} level is 10.2% on a 1500-calorie American Diabetes Association diet

E. A 42-year-old female patient with a few months' history of episodic palpations, headache, and sweating whose fasting blood glucose range is 142 to 153 mg per deciliter

DIRECTIONS: Questions 64 to 95 are matching questions. For each numbered item, choose the most likely associated lettered item from those provided. Each numbered item has ONLY ONE answer. Within each set of questions, each answer may be used once, more than once, or not at all.

QUESTIONS 64–70

Match the following clinical effects with the most likely associated therapeutic agent.

    A. Chlorpropamide
    B. Tolbutamide
    C. Phenformin
    D. Metformin
    E. Glyburide

64. Can cause significant hyponatremia

65. The sulfonylurea agent with the shortest duration of action

66. The sulfonylurea agent with the longest duration of action

67. Associated with the development of an intensive flush after the consumption of alcohol

68. Can be used in the treatment of partial central diabetes insipidus

69. Most common inducer of lactic acidosis in a diabetic patient

70. The most potent sulfonylurea agent

QUESTIONS 71–77

For each of the patients described below, select the most likely vitamin or mineral deficiency.

    A. Vitamin B_1 deficiency
    B. Vitamin E deficiency
    C. Vitamin A deficiency
    D. Vitamin K deficiency
    E. Vitamin C deficiency
    F. Zinc deficiency
    G. Niacin deficiency
    H. Selenium deficiency
    I. Chromium deficiency

71. A 32-year-alcoholic man with human immunodeficiency virus (HIV) infection who presents with several weeks' history of diarrhea, depression, hyposmia, and skin rash over the face, perineum, and extremities

72. A 45-year-old man with ulcerative colitis receiving parenteral nutrition who starts to develop muscle pains with tenderness and heart failure

73. A 62-year-old woman who has been on total parenteral nutrition for 5 years who recently developed diabetes mellitus, peripheral neuropathy, ataxia, and confusion

74. A 29-year-old man with Crohn's disease who develops ophthalmoplegia, ataxia, decreased proprioception, areflexia, and anemia

75. A 50-year-old alcoholic woman with night blindness, dryness of the cornea, and loss of taste

76. A 76-year-old woman with leg pains and appearance of petechiae over the arm after the application of a sphygmomanometer

77. A 42-year-old alcoholic man who presents to the emergency room with vomiting, confusion, and fever and is found to have horizontal nystagmus, ophthalmoplegia, and ataxia

QUESTIONS 78–84

For each of the clinical and lab findings described below, select the most likely diagnosis.

    A. Vermer-Morrison syndrome (vasoactive intestinal peptide [VIP]-secreting tumor or VIPoma)
    B. Glucagonoma
    C. Somatostatinoma
    D. Insulinoma
    E. Hepatoma

78. Serum bicarbonate level of 14 mEq per liter, serum potassium level of 2.8 mEq per liter, watery diarrhea (4.0 liters per day)

79. Onycholysis

80. Necrolytic migratory erythema

81. Marked elevation of serum calcitonin

82. Serum calcium level of 10.8 mg per deciliter, albumin level of 3.3 g per deciliter, intact PTH level of 10 pg per milliliter (normal: 10 to 65)

83. Cholelithiasis

84. Elevated levels of insulin-like growth factor II (IGF-II)

QUESTIONS 85–90

For each of the family members of diabetic patients described below, select the most likely lifelong risk of developing diabetes.

    A. 6%
    B. 33%
    C. 95%
    D. 15%
    E. 0.4%

85. Diabetes in a monozygotic twin of a type I diabetes mellitus patient

86. Diabetes in a monozygotic twin of a type II diabetes mellitus patient

87. Type I diabetes mellitus in a son of a type I diabetes mellitus patient

88. Type I diabetes mellitus in an HLA-identical brother of a type I diabetes mellitus patient

89. Type II diabetes mellitus in a brother of a type II diabetes mellitus patient

90. Diabetes in a son of a patient with type II diabetes mellitus

QUESTIONS 91–95

For each patient described below, select the most likely laboratory values during hypoglycemia.

	Serum Insulin	Serum C-peptide	Sulfonyl-ureas	Antibodies
A.	Elevated	Low	0	0
B.	Elevated	Elevated	0	0
C.	Elevated	Low	0	+ Insulin receptor
D.	Undetectable	Very low	0	0

91. A 30-year-old homosexual man with acquired immunodeficiency syndrome (AIDS) who presents with an acute episode of weakness, diaphoresis, and lethargy and a blood pressure of 80/50 mm Hg. Lab tests show

Plasma glucose	42 mg/dl
Sodium	133 mEq/L
Potassium	5.5 mEq/L
Chloride	108 mEq/L
Bicarbonate	20 mEq/L
Calcium	10.0 mg/dl
Albumin	3.2 g/dl
Intact PTH	10 pg/ml

His acute episode resolves with intravenous glucose.

92. A 9-year-old boy with short stature who presents with a symptomatic episode of hypoglycemia. His plasma glucose level is 45 mg per deciliter and creatinine level is 0.7 mg per deciliter. His acute episode resolves with intravenous glucose.

93. A 36-year-old woman with a history of Hashimoto's thyroiditis and vitiligo who presents with an acute episode of palpitations, diaphoresis, and hand tremors. Physical examination reveals a pulse of 110 beats per minute, blood pressure of 110/70 mm Hg, vitiligo on the hands, and acanthosis nigricans on the posterior aspect of the neck. Her plasma glucose level is 43 mg per deciliter. Her acute episode resolves with intravenous glucose. Medical records show four previous similar episodes. The patient is put on glucocorticoid therapy with good response in regard to the development of hypoglycemia.

94. A 32-year-old obese woman who presents with a 1-year history of frequent episodes of blurred vision, sweating, palpitations, and weakness with occasional confusion and abnormal behavior 5 to 6 hours after meals. Her symptoms are relieved with eating. The patient denies other complaints except for irregular menses and frequent frontal headaches. Her last menstrual period was 8 months ago. Her last medical history is significant for a right kidney stone 2 years ago. Blood chemistries done 2 hours after eating reveal

Glucose	80 mg/dl
Sodium	144 mEq/L
Potassium	3.5 mEq/L
Chloride	95 mEq/L
Bicarbonate	33 mEq/L
Calcium	10.5 mg/dl
Albumin	4.1 g/dl
Phosphorus	2.1 mg/dl

95. A 29-year-old female lab technician with a history of depression who presents to the emergency room with a symptomatic episode of hypoglycemia (plasma glucose level of 36 mg per deciliter) which resolves with intravenous glucose. Blood ethanol, ketone bodies, and lactate are undetectable. The patient is admitted and continuously administered a 10% dextrose solution intravenously for 16 hours, during which she is completely normal. She then undergoes a prolonged supervised fast for 72 hours, during which she is asymptomatic and her plasma glucose level is 65 mg per deciliter at its lowest. Medical records show two previous similar episodes. She has a sister with type I diabetes mellitus.

DIABETES MELLITUS AND METABOLISM

ANSWERS

1.(B); 2.(B) *Discussion:* The presentation of the patient described is consistent with hypoglycemia. The diagnosis of hypoglycemia is made if Whipple's triad is present. The components of this triad include (1) symptoms consistent with hypoglycemia; (2) documentation of a low plasma glucose level, below the level at which symptoms are expected to occur (usually below 45 mg per deciliter, although levels between 45 and 70 mg per deciliter are suspicious); and (3) a satisfactory response of symptoms to glucose administration. All of these criteria should be met before labeling a patient as having hypoglycemia.

The clinical manifestations of hypoglycemia have been classified into two major categories: neurogenic and neuroglucopenic. Neurogenic manifestations are caused by increased activity of the autonomic nervous system (catecholamines and acetylcholine release) and are usually recognized at plasma glucose levels of approximately 60 mg per deciliter. (Tightly controlled diabetics may have decreased sensitivity to hypoglycemia.) These manifestations include anxiety, tremulousness, irritability, perspiration, tachycardia, palpitations, tingling of mouth and fingers, hunger, and rarely nausea and vomiting. Neuroglucopenic manifestations are caused by decreased activity of the central nervous system and include headache, inability to concentrate, confusion, amnesia, seizures, and coma. These kinds of manifestations usually appear at plasma glucose levels of approximately 50 mg per deciliter.

Although neurogenic manifestations usually precede overt neuroglucopenic symptoms, this is not always the case. Some patients may manifest only neuroglucopenic symptoms. This may occur (1) if plasma glucose concentrations fall slowly enough not to activate the autonomic nervous system, and (2) in diabetics with hypoglycemia unawareness resulting from impaired glucagon, epinephrine, and autonomic nervous system responses.

The patient described here has both neurogenic and neuroglucopenic manifestations of hypoglycemia, indicating that her plasma glucose level would likely be approximately 50 mg per deciliter or less. Although low, her plasma glucose level would be detectable. The presence of tachycardia during her hypoglycemic episode indicates adequate adrenergic nervous system response without endogenous or exogenous impairment (e.g., beta-adrenergic blockers). (*Service, 1995; Lavin, Ch. 34*)

3.(E); 4.(D); 5.(B) *Discussion:* Hypoglycemia is not a diagnosis but a marker for an underlying disorder. Therefore, its cause must be determined. According to its relation to food intake, hypoglycemia has been divided into two major categories: spontaneous (fasting) and reactive (postprandial). Patients with spontaneous hypoglycemia may have their symptoms in the fasting state and/or after meals, whereas reactive hypoglycemia occurs only within 5 hours after meals. The differential diagnosis of hypoglycemia in adults is described in the table below.

At minimum, laboratory evaluation of a patient with hypoglycemia should include measurement of plasma concentrations of *glucose, insulin,* and *C-peptide,* as well as a screen for the presence of sulfonylureas in either blood or urine, at the time of occurrence of Whipple's triad. Further evaluation may require assessment during hypoglycemia of plasma concentrations of proinsulin, beta-hydroxybutyrate, cortisol, and

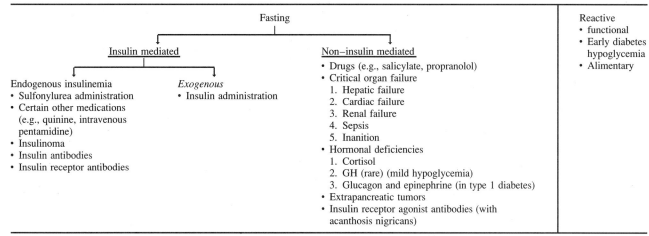

DIFFERENTIAL DIAGNOSIS OF HYPOGLYCEMIA IN ADULTS

Fasting

Insulin mediated

Endogenous insulinemia
- Sulfonylurea administration
- Certain other medications (e.g., quinine, intravenous pentamidine)
- Insulinoma
- Insulin antibodies
- Insulin receptor antibodies

Exogenous
- Insulin administration

Non–insulin mediated
- Drugs (e.g., salicylate, propranolol)
- Critical organ failure
  1. Hepatic failure
  2. Cardiac failure
  3. Renal failure
  4. Sepsis
  5. Inanition
- Hormonal deficiencies
  1. Cortisol
  2. GH (rare) (mild hypoglycemia)
  3. Glucagon and epinephrine (in type 1 diabetes)
- Extrapancreatic tumors
- Insulin receptor agonist antibodies (with acanthosis nigricans)

Reactive
- functional
- Early diabetes hypoglycemia
- Alimentary

DIFFERENTIAL DIAGNOSIS OF INSULIN-MEDIATED HYPOGLYCEMIA

Diagnosis	Insulin	C-peptide	Sulfonylurea	Antibodies
Exogenous insulin	Elevated	Suppressed	Absent	Absent*
Insulinoma	Elevated	Elevated	Absent	Absent†
Sulfonylurea-induced hypoglycemia	Elevated	Elevated	Detectable	Absent
Insulin antibodies	Elevated	Variable	Absent	Detectable (insulin)
Insulin receptor antibodies	Elevated	Suppressed	Absent	Detectable (insulin receptor)

* Insulin antibodies may be detectable with animal insulin.
† Insulin antibodies can be detectable in rare instances.

GH. If a spontaneous episode does not occur under observation, hypoglycemia can be provoked with a 72-hour fast. Blood for determination of insulin antibodies and insulin receptor antibodies can be drawn during hypoglycemic or euglycemic states.

In evaluating the cause of hypoglycemia, two questions should be answered. First, is the hypoglycemia insulin mediated (hyperinsulinemic hypoglycemia) or non–insulin mediated (hypoinsulinemic hypoglycemia)? Causes of spontaneous insulin-mediated hypoglycemia include exogenous insulin administration, sulfonylurea administration, hypoglycemia induced by certain other drugs (e.g., quinine, intravenous pentamidine), insulinomas, and insulin antibody–induced hypoglycemia. Insulin-mediated hypoglycemia is characterized by elevated plasma insulin concentration (>6 μU per milliliter) and suppressed concentrations of beta-hydroxybutyrate in the face of hypoglycemia. Ratios of glucose and insulin have not been proven reproducibly useful in discriminating endogenous from exogenous insulin-mediated hypoglycemia.

Second, if hypoglycemia is insulin-mediated, is insulinemia endogenous or exogenous? The plasma concentration of C-peptide—the connecting peptide deleted in the posttranslational processing of insulin—can indicate if the insulinemia is endogenous or exogenous. Suppressed C-peptide concentrations indicate exogenous insulin administration, because commercial insulin preparations do not contain C-peptide. Endogenous hyperinsulinemic hypoglycemia is characterized by an elevated C-peptide level (except for insulin receptor antibody–mediated hypoglycemia) because insulin and C-peptide are secreted in equimolar amounts from beta cells. Discrimination among the causes of endogenous hyperinsulinemic hypoglycemia (insulinomas, sulfonylurea-induced hypoglycemia, and autoimmune hypoglycemia caused by autoantibodies to insulin or to the insulin receptor) also requires screening for the presence of sulfonylurea in either blood or urine and determination of the presence of insulin receptor antibodies and insulin antibodies in the plasma. The table *above* shows the diagnostic laboratory evaluation of each cause.

The plasma proinsulin/insulin percentage is elevated ($>20\%$) in most but not all insulinomas because of defective post-translational processing of proinsulin to insulin. The 5-hour oral glucose tolerance test has no role in evaluating spontaneous hypoglycemia. The laboratory data of the patient described are consistent with endogenous insulin-mediated hypoglycemia. Measurement of the sulfonylurea level (on the admission serum) should be the next step.

Drug-induced hypoglycemia is the most common type of hypoglycemia, and insulin and sulfonylurea are the most common causative drugs. Other drugs that can cause hypoglycemia include salicylates, intravenous pentamidine, beta blockers, quinine, monoamine oxidase inhibitors, disopyramide, and oxytetracycline. Drug-induced hypoglycemia is most commonly observed in emotionally disturbed women in health-related occupations or in relatives of diabetic patients. Psychiatric evaluation is important to avoid recurrent episodes. (*Service, 1995; Lavin, Ch. 34; Cryer et al*)

6.(E); 7.(E) *Discussion:* The patient described has pellagra, a disease that results from niacin deficiency. Pellagra is a chronic progressive disease, typically associated with *d*ermatitis, *d*iarrhea, and *d*ementia (the three Ds). Death (the fourth D) may result and is usually due to secondary complications. Dermatitis is characterized by dark, scaling and cracking skin lesions that appear prominently in sites exposed to sunlight. In addition to dementia and diarrhea, patients with pellagra may exhibit other nonspecific symptoms, including weight loss, stomatitis, glossitis, and generalized weakness. Niacin deficiency may arise as a result of several factors: (1) dietary deficiency, because normally about 1.5% of dietary tryptophan is converted to niacin (e.g., diet dependent mainly on corn, the tryptophan content of which is low); (2) alcoholism, in which the absorption and metabolism of niacin may be impaired; (3) vitamin B_6 and riboflavin deficiencies, which decrease conversion of tryptophan to niacin because these vitamins regulate this metabolic pathway; (4) certain drugs that may interfere with niacin metabolism, leading to deficiency state (e.g., isoniazid and 6-mercaptopurine); (5) malignant carcinoid syndrome, because of diversion of dietary tryptophan to serotonin; and (6) Hartnup's disease, in which several amino acids, including tryptophan, are poorly absorbed. Although hypothyroidism may cause dementia, it does not cause or aggravate niacin deficiency. The diagnosis of pellagra can usually be suspected on clinical grounds and confirmed by measuring urinary *N*-methylnicotinamide using high-performance liquid chromatograph. Blood levels of NAD and NAD phosphate are reduced, but they are not specific for niacin deficiency. (*Cecil, Ch. 192*)

8.(E); 9.(C) *Discussion:* The history of constipation, cold intolerance, dry cold skin, secondary amenorrhea, bradycardia, and delayed relaxation of the reflexes are suggestive of hypothyroidism. Nevertheless, the history of significant weight loss and the patient being tense make hypothyroidism unlikely. Although type I diabetes mellitus and adrenal insufficiency can be associated with weight loss, the patient described lacks the other manifestation of these disorders. Bulimia is also unlikely given the absence of the characteristic binge-purge cycles and the history of profound weight loss (bulimics usually have normal body weight). The key point is not only that the patient is not concerned about her profound weight loss but that she also wishes to lose more weight in spite of being underweight. This is a typical feature of patients with anorexia nervosa. Anorexia nervosa is a chronic disorder characterized by body image disturbance and self-induced weight loss to achieve an unrealistic degree of weight loss. This is usually accomplished through exercise and dietary restriction, with or without self-induced vomiting. In spite of profound weight loss, anorectics insist that they are too fat.

Anorexia nervosa is associated with various kinds of physical, metabolic, and endocrine abnormalities, the severity of which correlates with the nutritional state. Anorectics may exhibit bradycardia, hypothermia, hypotension, and some of the clinical features of hypothyroidism (e.g., dry skin, constipation, cold intolerance, and delayed relaxation of the deep tendon reflexes). Total T_3 levels can be low, with increase in reverse T_3 indicating impairment of thyroxine (T_4)-to-T_3 peripheral conversion. However, total T_4 and free T_4 levels and the TSH response to thyrotropin-releasing hormone are normal. Other endocrine findings include low serum FSH and luteinizing hormone levels and normal or slightly elevated serum cortisol level with normal or increased response to ACTH stimulation. The serum GH levels are normal or slightly elevated, with low somatomedin C levels. (*Cecil, Ch. 195*)

10.(C) *Discussion:* There is an increased risk for macrovascular disease as a result of accelerated atherosclerosis in both type I and type II diabetes. This is reflected clinically by a two- to threefold increase in the likelihood of cardiovascular events and cerebrovascular disease and an 8- to 12-fold increase in peripheral vascular disease as compared with nondiabetic individuals. The coexistence with diabetes of known macrovascular risk factors such as dyslipedemia and hypertension may account for some of this increased risk. However, these factors cannot account for the entire risk, suggesting an independent risk for diabetes. Abnormalities induced by or related to diabetes that could be responsible for this increased risk include hyperinsulinemia and its associated metabolic effects, increased platelet aggregation, hyperviscosity, endothelial cell dysfunction, and increased levels of clotting factors and fibrinogen. Although it is the main risk factor for the microvascular complications of diabetes, hyperglycemia itself is not an independent risk factor for diabetic macrovascular disease. Glycemic control has been shown to delay the onset and slow the progression of microvascular complications unequivocally in type I diabetes mellitus (Diabetes Control and Complications Trial [DCCT]) and probably in type II diabetes mellitus. In contrast, there are no studies yet available to indicate that glycemic control will delay or slow the risk for macrovascular complications. (*Cecil, Ch. 205; Mazzaferri, pp. 219–239*)

11.(C) *Discussion:* Intensive glycemic control is indicated in most diabetic patients, including those with microvascular complications (B) and insulin resistance (D). Its benefits include delay of the onset and retardation of the progression of retinopathy, neuropathy, and nephropathy in type I diabetics (DCCT) (and probably in other types of diabetes mellitus), improved psychological well-being, improved plasma lipid profiles, decreased platelet aggregation, and avoidance of the symptoms and acute complications of hyperglycemia. Because it is associated with increased risk of hypoglycemia, intensive glycemic control should be compromised in patients with hypoglycemia unawareness or cardiac disease (E). In contrast, pregnant diabetic women (C) require the most intensive glycemic control to minimize the incidence of fetal mortality and morbidity, which may complicate a diabetic pregnancy. The most important fetal complication of diabetic pregnancy is the increased incidence of congenital anomalies involving the heart and the nervous and skeletal systems. Because such complications occur as a result of poor glycemic control early in gestation, intensive metabolic control should be initiated before conception. The cornerstones of tight control of diabetes during pregnancy include strict dietary control and insulin therapy. Target plasma glucose concentrations are 60 to 100 mg per deciliter during fasting and 100 to 120 mg per deciliter in the postprandial state. As in other situations, hypoglycemia should be avoided. (*Hirsch et al; Felig, Ch. 19*)

12.(E) *Discussion:* The history of frequent episodes of hypoglycemia requiring significant reduction in insulin dose, generalized weakness, malaise, nausea, and hypotension in a type I diabetic patient suggests adrenal insufficiency. The simplest reliable test for diagnosing adrenal insufficiency is the rapid ACTH stimulation test (cosyntropin test). Patients with presentations suggestive of acute adrenal insufficiency should receive intravenous hydrocortisone after a rapid ACTH stimulation test is done. An intravascular expanding fluid is added (e.g., normal saline) to correct associated hypotension (as in the patient described). A 50-ml bolus of 50% dextrose can be given, but it is unlikely that the patient's presentation is a result of symptomatic hypoglycemia, because the blood glucose level is 69 mg per deciliter. The priority in the management of this patient is to take care of her possible adrenal crisis. (*Cecil, Ch. 204; Felig, Ch. 12*)

13.(C); 14.(D) *Discussion:* The symptoms of weight gain, general weakness, constipation, and thinning of the hair are suggestive of hypothyroidism. Patients with hypothyroidism who have concomitant adrenal insufficiency may not manifest overt hypothyroidism unless corticosteroids are replaced (as in the patient described). This is because corticosteroid deficiency may decrease the metabolism of thyroid hormones and thus mask a borderline hypothyroidism. With replacement, corticosteroids will accelerate thyroid hormone metabolism, unmasking the borderline thyroid status and leading to overt hypothyroidism. The hot flashes and dyspareunia are indicative of estrogen deficiency (ovarian failure). Putting these together, the patient described has type I diabetes mellitus, adrenal insufficiency, hypothyroidism, and ovarian failure. Each can be a result of an autoimmunity, indicating an autoimmune polyglandular failure. There are two polyglandular autoimmune syndromes (types I and II). Type II (Schmidt's syndrome) is familial in about 50% of patients, and HLA-DR3 and -DR4 associated. Its classic manifestations are adrenal insufficiency, autoimmune thyroid disease, and type I diabetes mellitus. Other manifestations include vitiligo (5%) and gonadal failure in about 5 to 50% of patients (rare in men). Hypoparathyroidism (C in question 13), mucocutaneous candidiasis (A in question 14), and pernicious anemia (B in question 14) are part of the polyglandular autoimmune syndrome type I, not type II. Other manifestations of type I include adrenal insufficiency, gonadal failure, and autoimmune thyroid disease. Type I diabetes mellitus is rare in polyglandular autoimmune syndrome type I. (*Felig, Ch. 12*)

15.(C) *Discussion:* The presentation of this patient is typical for DKA. Pathophysiologically, DKA represents an acute insulin deficiency state combined with increased counter-regulatory hormones (epinephrine, glucagon, cortisol, and GH). The synergistic effects of these two factors lead to hyperglycemia (diabetic), hyperketonemia (keto-), and metabolic acidosis (acidosis)—the cardinal biochemical features of DKA. The hyperglycemia is due to increased hepatic gluconeogenesis, increased glycogenolysis, and decreased peripheral glucose uptake. It results in osmotic diuresis, which leads to volume and electrolyte depletion. Hyperketonemia results from overproduction and underutilization of free fatty acid–derived ketone bodies (beta-hydroxybutyrate, acetone, acetoacetate) in the liver. The increase in production of ketone bodies causes consumption of bicarbonate in the process of buffering and leads to development of metabolic acidosis. Another effect of insulin deficiency is impairment of lipoprotein lipase, an enzyme that is normally stimulated by insulin. Such impairment leads to accumulation of triglyceride-rich particles (chylomicrons and VLDL) the main lipid abnormality found in DKA and uncontrolled diabetes mellitus.

In DKA, in which there is a marked decrease in glucose metabolism by insulin-sensitive tissues, the predominant energy source for non–central nervous system (CNS) tissues is circulating free fatty acids. Because CNS glucose uptake is not insulin dependent, hepatically produced glucose from amino acids continues to serve as a source of energy for CNS cells. In addition, ketone bodies can be utilized by the CNS and muscle for energy, sparing critical body proteins. (*Cecil, Ch. 205*)

16.(B) *Discussion:* Metabolic acidosis is a characteristic finding in DKA. It is caused by consumption of bicarbonate in the process of buffering the overproduced ketone bodies. At presentation, patients with DKA have a "classic" high anion-gap metabolic acidosis, a mixed hyperchloremic (normal anion gap) acidosis, or a predominantly hyperchloremic metabolic acidosis. Two factors determine the presence of hyperchloremic acidosis at presentation in a DKA patient. The first is the adequacy of intravascular volume and glomerular filtration rate (GFR). Patients who maintain adequate volume and GFR are able to exchange ketoacid anions for chloride, leading to hyperchloremia. The second factor is the coexistence of other conditions that can cause hyperchloremic metabolic acidosis (e.g., diarrhea as in the patient described).

A low pH of 7.25 and a low measured bicarbonate level (venous CO_2) of 10 mEq per liter indicate metabolic acidosis. The patient's anion gap $Na^+ - (Cl^- + HCO_3^-)$ is high at 20 mEq per liter (average normal is 12 mEq per liter), indicating a high anion-gap metabolic acidosis. Is this high anion-gap metabolic acidosis pure or mixed with other acid-base disturbances? In general, a high anion-gap acidosis is pure if the following two criteria are present:

1. The decrease in P_{CO_2} (ΔP_{CO_2}), the normal compensatory change, is appropriate to the decrease in HCO_3^- (ΔHCO_3^-), the primary change. This can be known by applying different equations (e.g., $P_{CO_2} = 1.5 (HCO_3^-) + 8 \pm 2$). A discrepancy between these changes (ΔP_{CO_2} and ΔHCO_3^-) suggests coexistent respiratory alkalosis or respiratory acidosis.

2. The reduction in HCO_3^- (ΔHCO_3^-) equals the increase in the anion gap (ΔAG). If ΔAG is greater than ΔHCO_3^-, this suggests coexistent metabolic alkalosis or respiratory acidosis in a patient with hypochloremia. On the other hand, if ΔHCO_3^- is greater than ΔAG, this suggests a coexistent normal anion-gap metabolic acidosis in a patient with hyperchloremia.

In the patient described, there is an appropriate decrease in P_{CO_2} with regard to the decrease in HCO_3^-, eliminating the possibility of respiratory alkalosis or respiratory acidosis. However, the reduction in the patient's HCO_3^- (24 − measured HCO_3^- = 14 mEq per liter) is greater than the increase in AG (calculated AG − 12 = 8 mEq per liter), suggesting a coexistent normal anion-gap hyperchloremic metabolic acidosis. (*Cecil, Ch. 205; Androgue et al*)

17.(D) *Discussion:* In addition to the cardinal biochemical features of DKA—hyperglycemia, hyperketonemia, and metabolic acidosis—other laboratory abnormalities in DKA include the following:

1. Hyponatremia caused by sodium depletion and a shift of intracellular water to the extracellular space as a result of hyperglycemia and hyperosmolality (true hyponatremia). For each 100-mg per deciliter increase in glucose, there is a reduction in sodium of 1.5 to 2.0 mEq per liter. The presence of hypertriglyceridemia can also spuriously contribute to lowered serum sodium (1.5 to 2.0 mEq per liter for each 1000 mg triglycerides per deciliter). With reduction of hyperglycemia and restoration of vascular volume, the lowered sodium starts to increase.

2. At presentation, serum potassium levels can be low, normal, or elevated. However, patients usually have total body deficits of potassium of about 3 to 5 mEq per kilogram of body weight. Appropriate potassium replacement is therefore necessary even if the serum potassium level is normal or borderline elevated. Doses and adjustments of potassium supplementation should be based on the initial potassium level, renal function, and electrocardiographic findings. An initially low potassium level is ominous and necessitates aggressive management. Potassium replacement should be given cautiously to patients with compromised renal function. Once intravenous fluid and insulin are started, serum potassium level falls as a result of correction of acidosis, dilution, urinary excretion, and increased cellular uptake by insulin.

3. Although serum phosphate levels can be normal at presentation, patients with DKA have substantial phosphate depletion (1.0 mmol per kilogram of body weight). Replacement therapy is probably not necessary and even may be complicated by hypocalcemia unless magnesium supplementation is provided.

4. Hypomagnesemia. Replacement is not necessary unless DKA is associated with chronic wasting, diarrhea, or large doses of administered phosphate.

5. At presentation, chloride can be low, normal, or high. With administration of intravenous normal saline, chloride is invariably overcorrected.

6. Prerenal azotemia.

7. Serum creatinine may be spuriously increased, independent of decrease in GFR, as a result of acetoacetic acid and acetone

interference with chemical determination. Once these ketone bodies are reduced and cleared, serum creatinine decreases.

8. Hyperamylasemia, which is usually of nonpancreatic origin. Acidemia (pH <7.32) may also spuriously elevate serum amylase.

9. Leukocytosis (15,000 to 20,000 WBC per microliter) can be caused by DKA even without evidence of infection.

Hyperketonemia (excesses of beta-hydroxybutyrate, acetoacetate, and acetone) is usually assessed in clinical practice qualitatively using standard nitroprusside reagents (e.g., Acetestat, Ketostix). These reagents react most strongly with acetoacetate, weakly with acetone, and not at all with beta-hydroxybutyrate. Because beta-hydroxybutyrate is usually the most abundant ketone body in patients with DKA, a weak nitroprusside reaction does not necessarily imply that DKA is minimal or absent. During the course of treatment, beta-hydroxybutyrate is converted to acetoacetate, producing a more positive nitroprusside reaction. This may give the false impression of a worsening of the DKA. (*Cecil, Ch. 205; Lavin, Ch. 40*)

18.(E) *Discussion:* The keystones in management of a patient with DKA are as follows:

1. Hydration and restoration of vascular volume, usually by intravenous administration of normal saline.

2. Correction of hyperglycemia by prompt use of intravenous Regular insulin. Glucose should be added to avoid hypoglycemia when the glucose level reaches 250 to 300 mg per deciliter.

3. Correction of electrolyte imbalances. Potassium replacement is crucial. Phosphate therapy can be given with magnesium, although its addition does not affect outcome (see the discussion of question 17)

4. Treatment of underlying precipitating events (e.g., omission of insulin; emotional stress; medical illnesses such as infections, myocardial infarctions, cerebrovascular accidents). DKA occurs in about 20% of patients not previously known to have diabetes (as in the patient described).

5. Patient education after recovery to avoid recurrent episodes.

What about the routine use of bicarbonate in DKA? Acidosis is associated with adverse effects such as impairment of myocardial contractility, predisposition to arrhythmia, and vasodilation. Nevertheless, the routine use of bicarbonate is not usually recommended because it can potentiate hypokalemia, decrease peripheral oxygen delivery, cause paradoxical cerebral acidosis, aggrevate high serum osmolality, and overcorrect acidosis, leading to alkalosis because ketone bodies are metabolized to bicarbonate. However, most authorities agree that in DKA the use of bicarbonate may be justified in the following situations: (1) severe acidosis (pH < 7.0), (2) life-threatening hyperkalemia, and (3) significant lactic acidosis. If it is given, bicarbonate therapy should be administrated slowly (44 mEq per hour) and discontinued when pH rises to 7.1. (*Cecil, Ch. 205; Lavin, Ch. 40*)

19.(A) *Discussion:* The lipid abnormalities associated with untreated DKA are elevated triglyceride-rich lipoprotein concentrations (chylomicrons and VLDL) and low LDL and HDL cholesterol concentrations. Physiologically, insulin increases the activity of liproprotein lipase, an enzyme that results in lipolysis of chylomicrons and VLDL. With severe insulin deficiency (as in DKA), lipoprotein lipase activity decreases, which leads to decreased clearance of chylomi-

crons and VLDL. As a result of this, triglyceride-rich lipoproteins accumulate while LDL and HDL cholesterol concentrations decrease. These abnormalities are reversible with therapy of the DKA. (*Mazzaferri, pp. 219–239*)

20.(C) *Discussion:* The patient described most likely has type I diabetes mellitus, an autoimmune disease that results from an interplay of genetic and environmental factors. Genetic susceptibility to type I diabetes mellitus has been ascribed to genes located on the short arm of chromosome 6 encoding certain HLA haplotype antigens. These high-risk antigens include HLA-DR3, -DR4, -DR1, -DR8, -DR16, -B8, and -B15. Genes other than HLA genes associated with a predisposition to type I diabetes mellitus include a gene on the short arm of chromosome 11 in the region of the genes for insulin and IGF-II, and the TAP gene. TAP (transporter involved in antigen presentation) is an intracellular protein that transports antigenic peptides into the endoplasmic reticulum. Conversely, there are certain other genes that have a negative association with type I diabetes mellitus (protect against it), such as HLA-DR11, -DR5, and -DR2. (*Cecil, Ch. 205; Atkinson and Maclaren*)

21.(B); 22.(E) *Discussion:* The patient described has chylomicronemia syndrome complicated most likely by acute pancreatitis. The chylomicronemia syndrome is characterized by marked chylomicron excess, with plasma triglycerides usually greater than 2000 mg per deciliter. The manifestations of the chylomicronemia syndrome include abdominal pain and/or pancreatitis, chest pain, recent memory impairment, paresthesias of the extremities, hepatomegaly, splenomegaly, eruptive xanthomas, lipemia retinalis, and milky plasma. The marked hypertriglyceridemia usually reflects coexistence of the genetic and acquired forms of hypertriglyceridemia. Untreated diabetes mellitus, alcoholism, hypothyroidism, uremia, estrogens, diuretics, beta-adrenergic blockers, and glucocorticoids frequently cause chylomicronemia when they are present in the setting of familial hypertriglyceridemia. Although triglyceride concentrations of 1000 mg per deciliter or above are associated with an increased risk for acute pancreatitis, triglyceride levels in excess of 2000 mg per deciliter are required for a classic presentation of the chylomicronemia syndrome. In acute pancreatitis associated with hypertriglyceridemia, serum amylase levels are often spuriously normal. (*Cecil, Ch. 173*)

23.(A); 24.(B) *Discussion:* Discontinuation of oral intake is the most effect *initial* measure to decrease triglyceride levels in patients with the chylomicronemia syndrome. Other measures in the management of such patients include a low-fat and low-cholesterol diet, weight loss, increased physical activity, diabetes mellitus control, avoidance of alcohol intake, and avoidance of drugs that may increase triglyceride levels (e.g., estrogens, beta-adrenergic blockers, and diuretics). The importance of a low-saturated-fat, low-cholesterol diet cannot be overemphasized. Diet therapy (National Cholesterol Education Program guidelines) should be tried for at least 6 months before initiating pharmacologic therapy. If diet therapy has been unsuccessful after 6 months (as in the patient described), drug therapy may be initiated.

The drugs of choice for lowering elevated triglyceride levels (chylomicrons or VLDL) are gemfibrozil or clofibrate.

These fibric acid–derivative drugs increase lipoprotein lipase activity and promote VLDL clearance. Gemfibrozil also decreases VLDL production. With fibric acid therapy, cholesterol levels are usually decreased; however, they may rise especially in some patients with low or normal cholesterol levels. If cholesterol levels fail to respond or rise with fibric acid therapy, a bile acid resin (e.g., cholestyramine) can be added. Nictotinic acid (niacin) can effectively lower elevated triglyceride levels by inhibiting the secretion of VLDL from the liver. Because it may produce insulin resistance and thus worsening of glucose tolerance, niacin is not recommended to be used in diabetic patients (as in the patient described). Hydroxymethylglutaryl coenzyme A (HMG CoA) reductase inhibitors (e.g., lovastatin) lower mainly LDL cholesterol and to less extent triglyceride levels. Because of the increased rise of myositis, it is recommended not to use HMG CoA reductase inhibitors with gemfibrozil or niacin. Bile acid resins (e.g., cholestyramine) may increase triglycerides by increasing hepatic VLDL production. Their main use is to treat hypercholesterolemia. (*Cecil, Ch. 173*)

25.(C) *Discussion:* The LDL cholesterol level is calculated as follows:

LDL cholesterol =

$$\text{total cholesterol} - \text{HDL cholesterol} - \frac{\text{triglycerides}}{5}$$

This equation is valid only if triglyceride levels are <400 mg per deciliter. Therefore, because triglyceride levels are >400 mg per deciliter in the patient described, LDL cholesterol estimates are not accurate. The patient described has low levels of HDL cholesterol, most likely secondary to hypertriglyceridemia and type II diabetes mellitus. A low level of HDL cholesterol is associated with an increased incidence of coronary heart disease, as has been shown by a number of epidemiologic studies. Because alcohol consumption increases hypertriglyceridemia, its use is not recommended in patients with hypertriglyceridemia, especially if they have a history of pancreatitis (as in the patient described). Even though alcohol use is not recommended in patients with isolated deficiency of HDL cholesterol, it has been suggested (in some studies) that consumption of alcohol may increase HDL cholesterol levels. The reasons for that are beyond the scope of this discussion. Instead of alcohol consumption, other measures can be used to raise HDL cholesterol concentrations. These include diet, weight loss, cessation of cigarette smoking, exercise, and correcting hypertriglyceridemia if present. (*Cecil, Ch. 173*)

26.(E) *Discussion:* Blood lipids are found in the serum as lipoproteins, which are spherical macromolecular complexes that consist of a nonpolar lipid core (cholesterol ester and triglycerides) surrounded by a coat of phospholipids and apoproteins. There are five major types of lipoproteins in the plasma: chylomicrons, VLDL, intermediate-density lipoprotein (IDL), LDL, and HDL. Each has different components and function. Fredrickson classified six types of lipoprotein disorders according to the predominant type(s) of lipoprotein particle(s) in the patient's serum, as shown in the table *below*.

This patient's markedly elevated triglyceride level of 1120 mg per deciliter and moderately elevated cholesterol level (270 mg per deciliter) are consistent with type V (VLDL and chylomicrons) rather than type IV hyperlipidemia. Triglyceride levels of >500 mg per deciliter are rarely found in type IV hyperlipidemia. This is because the normal clearance mechanisms of triglyceride concentrations in excess of 500 mg per deciliter are impaired, leading to hyperchylomicronemia and elevated VLDL (type V hyperlipedemia). In uncontrolled type II diabetes mellitus without an underlying lipid disorder, triglyceride elevations in the range of 200 to 500 mg per deciliter, which are more modest than in the patient described, are seen. (*Cecil, Ch. 173; Felig, Ch. 22*)

27.(C) *Discussion:* The skin lesions shown in the accompanying figure are typical of eruptive xanthomas, which imply severe hyperchylomicronemia as seen in type I or type V hyperlipidemias. These triglyceride-containing lesions are nonpruritic, small (1 to 5 mm), yellowish papules surrounded by an erythematous base that appear predominantly on the buttocks, thighs, trunk, and extensor surfaces of the arms over a period of several weeks. With treatment of the under-

CLASSIFICATION OF HYPERLIPIDEMIAS BASED ON LIPOPROTEIN CONCENTRATIONS

Lipoprotein Abnormality	Type	Lipid Profile*	Typical Values (mg/dl)
Chylomicrons	I	TG: elevated (in thousands)	4000
		Chol: moderately elevated	320
VLDL	IV	TG: moderately elevated	400
		Chol: normal or slightly elevated	200
Chylomicrons + VLDL	V	TG: elevated (in thousands)	5000
		Chol: markedly elevated	700
IDL	III	TG: ⎱ equally	700
		Chol: ⎰ elevated	500
LDL	IIa	TG: normal	90
		Chol: moderately to markedly elevated	370
LDL + VLDL	IIb	TG: ⎱ elevated in	400
		Chol: ⎰ various proportions	350

Modified from Illingworth DR, Duell PB, Conner WE: Disorders of lipid metabolism. In Felig P, et al. (eds): Endocrinology and Metabolism. 3rd ed. New York, McGraw-Hill, 1995; reprinted with permission.
* TG, triglycerides; Chol, cholesterol.

lying hyperlipidemia, they are reversible and gradually disappear over several weeks. (*Cecil, Ch. 173; Felig, Ch. 22*)

28.(B) *Discussion:* The patient's blood glucose pattern shows morning hyperglycemia. *The most common cause* of such hyperglycemia is dissipation of insulin action. Because the peak effect of Regular insulin occurs after 2 to 4 hours and that of NPH insulin occurs after 6 to 14 hours, a larger evening dose of NPH insulin is needed to lower the patient's morning hyperglycemia to an acceptable level. The fasting blood glucose target levels are approximately 100 to 130 mg per deciliter without episodes of hypoglycemia. Other possible causes of morning hyperglycemia include rebound hyperglycemia (Somogyi phenomenon) and the dawn phenomenon, but there is no clinical evidence of such possibilities in the patient described. (*Felig, Ch. 19*)

29.(C) *Discussion:* The increase in P.M. NPH insulin led to correction of the patient's morning hyperglycemia but at the expense of symptomatic hypoglycemia at 2:00 to 3:00 A.M. This is because the peak effect of the 6-P.M. administered NPH insulin is at 12 midnight to 8:00 A.M. (6 to 14 hours later). Because patients with CAD (such as the patient described) are at more risk of hypoglycemia complications, glycemia control in such patients should not be as tight as in other patients. To avoid midnight and very early morning hypoglycemia and to keep fasting blood glucose levels in a reasonable range, the evening NPH insulin dose may be administered at bedtime (9:00 to 10:00 P.M.) rather than before dinner. Decreasing P.M. Regular insulin most likely will not achieve these goals because its peak effect is after 2 to 4 hours. Furthermore, decreasing this dose may worsen hyperglycemia at bedtime. (*Cecil, Ch. 205*)

30.(C) *Discussion:* The excretion of urine albumin in the microalbuminurea range (20 to 200 μg per minute) in a diabetic patient indicates early diabetic nephropathy. This is supported by the presence of background diabetic retinopathy in the patient described. The keystones to the prevention of diabetic nephropathy and/or retardation of its progression are intensive glycemic control, control of hypertension, restricted protein intake (0.6 to 0.8 gram per kilogram of body weight per day) and the use of angiotensin-converting enzyme (ACE) inhibitors, such as captopril. ACE inhibitors are the treatment of choice for hypertension in diabetic patients with or without nephropathy. This is not only because of their blood pressure–lowering effects but also because of their ability to lower intraglomerular pressure and preserve renal function. Even in *normotensive diabetic* patients, there is evidence that ACE inhibitors have a protective role in decreasing proteinuria and in retardation of the rate of progression to gross proteinuria.

Diltiazem and nicardipine also have a protective role in diabetic patients with nephropathy more than other calcium channel blockers. They decrease glomerular pressure and thus albuminuria by increasing efferent arteriolar dilation. They should be considered first for the control of hypertension in diabetic patients when ACE inhibitors are contraindicated (e.g., hyperkalemia as in the patient described). Thiazides may worsen glucose control, may cause or exacerbate impotence, and may contribute to CAD. Because of those possible adverse effects, these agents are not recommended for use in diabetic patients. (*Cecil, Ch. 205; Felig et al*)

31.(C); 32.(E) *Discussion:* The blood chemistry profile of the patient described shows borderline hyponatremia, mild hyperkalemia, and a normal anion-gap metabolic acidosis. This pattern usually results from hypoaldosteronism, which can be isolated renal tubular acidosis [type IV (RTA)] or associated with cortisol deficiency (Addison's disease). The simplest reliable diagnostic test for Addison's disease is the rapid ACTH stimulation test (cosyntropin test). However, a random cortisol level is not reliable for diagnosing Addison's disease because of the diurnal variation in serum cortisol. The exceptions for this are (1) a random cortisol value >20 μg per deciliter at any time, which rules out Addison's disease; and (2) a morning cortisol value <3 μg per deciliter, which indicates adrenal insufficiency. Therefore, a morning cortisol level of 12 μg per deciliter (A) or an evening cortisol level of 4 μg per deciliter (B) can be consistent with *normal* adrenal function, and neither necessarily indicates adrenal insufficiency. The 1-mg overnight dexamethasone suppression test (E) is a screening test for Cushing's syndrome and is not indicated in patients suspected of having adrenal insufficiency or isolated hypoaldosteronism. Primary hyperparathyroidism (D) can be associated with classic distal RTA type I (hypokalemic metabolic acidosis with urinary pH >5.5), but not RTA type IV (hyporeninemic hypoaldosteronism).

Isolated hypoaldosteronism can result from problems with renin production and release (hyporeninemic hypoaldosteronism), conversion of angiotensin I to angiotensin II or aldosterone production (hyper-reninemic hypoaldosteronism), or renal tubular insensitivity to aldosterone (pseudohypoaldosteronism). Hyporeninemic hypoaldosteronism is characterized by hyperkalemia and normal anion-gap metabolic acidosis. It is usually seen in patients with diabetes mellitus, especially with diabetic neuropathy. Other causes include renal parenchymal disease, Liddle's syndrome, and certain drugs (e.g., nonsteroidal anti-inflammatory agents, beta-adrenergic blockers, cyclosporine, clonidine). Ranitidine is not associated with this disorder. Patients with hyporeninemic hypoaldosteronism have low plasma renin activity (PRA) and low plasma aldosterone concentration (PA) with a normal PA/PRS ratio. Upright posture will not provoke a significant increase in PRA (C). (*Cecil, Ch. 204; Jagger*)

33.(C); 34.(D) *Discussion:* The lipid profile of the patient described shows hypercholesterolemia, normal triglycerides, and normal HDL. This is consistent with hyperlipoproteinemia Type IIa. The current guidelines are that the therapeutic goal in patients with CAD is lowering of the plasma LDL concentration to less than 100 mg per deciliter. The lowering of LDL cholesterol is believed to slow the progression and, in some cases, to induce regression of atherosclerosis in patients with CAD (secondary prevention). These effects are associated with reductions in CAD events, cardiovascular mortality, and overall mortality, as has been shown in secondary prevention trials.

The patient's (calculated) LDL cholesterol concentration is still significantly elevated at 206 mg deciliter in spite of 6 months of treatment with a low-fat, low-cholesterol diet. This indicates that more aggressive therapy is necessary. The drugs of choice for lowering elevated cholesterol levels include HMG CoA reductase inhibitors (e.g., lovastatin), niacin, and bile acid resins (e.g., cholestyramine). Cholestyramine and niacin are not the cholesterol-lowering agents of choice for the patient described because of their possible side effects. Cholestyramine may cause bloating and constipation, about which the patient already complains, and niacin may increase his glucose intolerance. Gemfibrozil would not be indicated because its main effect is to lower elevated triglyceride levels and its effects on cholesterol concentrations are variable.

Common causes of secondary hypercholesterolemia include hypothyroidism, obstructive liver disease, nephrotic syndrome, and certain drugs (e.g., thiazides but not furosemide, progestins). The main effects of lack of exercise on serum lipids are hypertriglyceridemia and decreased HDL levels, not hypercholesterolemia. (*Cecil, Ch. 173*)

35.(B) *Discussion:* The blood glucose pattern of the patient described shows fasting hyperglycemia. Causes of fasting hyperglycemia include dissipation of insulin action (the most common cause), the Somogyi phenomenon, and the dawn phenomenon. The Somogyi phenomenon is characterized by an exaggerated rebound hyperglycemia that results from the release of counter-regulatory hormones (catecholamines, cortisol, and GH) in response to acute hypoglycemia in the early morning hours. Clinically, patients with the Somogyi phenomenon usually present with signs of hypoglycemia in early morning (e.g., waking up with headaches and nightmares, as in the patient described) and morning (rebound) hyperglycemia.

The morning hyperglycemia of the dawn phenomenon, in contrast, does not occur in response to early morning hypoglycemia. Rather, it is likely due to a nocturnal increase in GH secretion in some patients. The differentiation between these possible causes of fasting hyperglycemia is important from a therapeutic point of view. Fasting hyperglycemia caused by dissipation of insulin action or the dawn phenomenon might require an increase in the evening dose of intermediate-acting insulin, whereas rebound hyperglycemia (Somogyi phenomenon) should prompt a decreased evening dose. Theoretically, the administration of octreotide (a long-acting somatostatin analogue) to prevent a nocturnal increase in GH secretion, may improve the fasting hyperglycemia found in the setting of the dawn phenomenon. However, the clinical role of octreotide in such a situation has not been established.

The history of symptoms and signs of hypoglycemia in the early morning suggests Somogyi hyperglycemia. However, before any therapeutic intervention, it is important to check blood glucose levels at 3:00 to 4:00 A.M. Low values at that time suggest the Somogyi phenomenon, whereas high values might indicate dissipation of insulin action or possibly the dawn phenomenon. (*Felig, Ch. 19*)

36.(A); 37.(A) *Discussion:* The clinical presentation described is consistent with neuropathic osteoarthropathy, or what is commonly called a Charcot joint. Charcot joint simply implies that a neurologic disease has led to an arthropathy. The most common cause of such arthropathy is diabetes mellitus, even though the disorder occur in only 5 to 10% of people with diabetes. Other common causes include tabes dorsalis, syringomyelia, and spinal cord injury. Diabetic neuropathy produces abnormal motor function of the intrinsic

muscles of the foot and abnormal proprioception, thereby altering weight distribution on the foot, which can result in repeated painless fractures (because of lack of sensation) and displacement of normal joint surfaces, producing a Charcot joint. In addition, an alteration in the sympathetic control of bone blood flow leads to active bone resorption and hyperemia, which may give a false clinical impression of cellulitis and osteomyelitis. The presentation is usually painless or moderately painful swelling of the foot with erythema, increased skin temperature, and bounding pedal pulses but without fever or leukocytosis. A well-demarcated bone demineralization is characteristic. Progressive deformity of the affected joint(s) may be present. Other joints (e.g., ankle, knee, spine, arm) may be affected. When a Charcot joint is suspected, osteomyelitis and other conditions with more or less similar presentation should be ruled out. The treatment of choice for an acute Charcot joint is immediate and absolute non–weight bearing in addition to cast immobilization until skin temperature and edema equal those of the contralateral limb. The importance of glycemic control and standard foot care measures, including therapeutic shoes, cannot be overemphasized. (*Cecil, Ch. 205; Bardin, pp. 446–452*)

38.(B) *Discussion:* Fissuring about the heel of a diabetic patient is usually caused by anhidrosis secondary to autonomic neuropathy. Fissuring and dryness is treated with hydrocortisone cream (1%) applied after soaking the foot for about 20 minutes in comfortably warm water. It is important that the patient wears stockings and shoes that fit well and eliminates all types of footwear that slap against the bottom of the heel when walking. Another foot manifestation of autonomic neuropathy is vascular denervation, which results in arteriovenous shunting with excessive bone resorption, distended dorsal veins, and an increase in blood flow to the foot. With the increased flow of blood, the temperature of the foot increases, giving a false clinical impression of cellulitis or osteomyelitis. Stress painless fractures develop secondary to osteopenia and, with continuous weight bearing, damage to the joints of the foot and ankle can occur (Charcot joint). (*Bardin, pp. 446–452*)

39.(A); 40.(C) *Discussion:* The presentation is typical for a third nerve palsy. The pupil on the affected side is usually dilated and does not respond to direct or consensual stimulation because of the involvement of the parasympathic fibers that travel along with the third nerve. However, typically (but not always), third nerve lesions caused by vascular disease (including diabetes mellitus) spare the pupil. Other common causes of an isolated third nerve palsy in an adult include neoplasm, trauma, aneurysms (internal carotid artery or posterior communicating artery aneurysms), and brain herniation. Diabetic third nerve palsy is the most common diabetic cranial mononeuropathy. It is usually of sudden onset, self-limited and most commonly observed in older patients. Recovery within several weeks is the rule. It may be recurrent and/or bilateral and may occur in the absence of diffuse neuropathy. It is believed that isolated mononeuropathy in diabetics has a vascular basis. (*Cecil, Ch. 448*)

41.(A—True; B—False; C—True; D—True; E—True); 42.(All are True); 43.(A—True; B—True; C—True; D—False) *Discussion:* The patient described has type I diabetes mellitus with a notably unstable blood glucose, leading to frequent episodes of hypoglycemia and hypoglycemia unawareness. His long-term complications include proliferative retinopathy as shown in the accompanying figure, symptomatic peripheral and autonomic neuropathy as evidenced by the presence of diarrhea, erectile impotence, and possible gastroparesis.

Hypoglycemia is one of the most common and serious complications encountered in insulin-treated diabetic patients. Factors that predispose to the development of such hypoglycemia include: (1) faulty injection technique, such as errors in the preparation of an insulin mixture or accidental injection into muscles or sites where insulin absorption is irregular; (2) decreased food intake; (3) increased physical exertion; (4) combined deficiencies of both glucagon and epinephrine (counter-regulatory insufficiency; however, a deficiency of glucagon only does not of itself predispose to hypoglycemia); (5) onset of adrenal or pituitary insufficiency; (6) onset of pregnancy; (7) renal failure leading to a decrease in insulin turnover; and (8) gastroparesis.

Gastroparesis may lead to hypoglycemia in diabetics as a result of discrepancies between the onset of glucose-lowering agent action and the absorption of food from the small intestine. Gastroparesis usually presents with early satiety, abdominal distention, nausea, and vomiting as in the patient described. Nevertheless, the predictive value of such symptoms is relatively poor. Although it is caused by irreversible autonomic nerve dysfunction, gastroparesis also cannot be predicted merely by evidence of other autonomic neuropathy. The diagnosis is best accomplished, at present, by gastric scintigraphy. Other methods of assessing gastric motor function, such as a barium meal and ultrasonography, are less accurate. Before diagnosing a patient as having diabetic gastroparesis, other causes of delayed gastric emptying, such as duodenal obstruction, significant hypokalemia, anorexia nervosa, cigarette smoking, hypothyroidism, and drugs (e.g., anticholinergics, narcotics, antidepressants and beta-adrenergic agonists), should be excluded. Likewise, it is important to consider other conditions that may present with similar gastrointestinal symptoms, such as peptic ulcer disease and Addison's disease.

Treatments of diabetic gastroparesis include diet therapy in the form of low-fat and frequent small meals, attempts to avoid hyperglycemia (if possible), and pharmacologic therapy to improve the delay in gastric emptying. It is not clear, however, whether such pharmacologic therapy results in better glycemic control. Metoclopramide, erythromycin, or cisapride may result in some improvement in the gastric emptying. Patients who are refractory to medical therapy may benefit from enteral nutrition through a jejunostomy tube.

The approach to the type I diabetic patient with unstable blood glucose and frequent hypoglycemia must also involve instructions with regard to various aspects of diabetes. It is crucial to emphasize the importance of frequent self-monitoring of blood glucose and issues related to insulin therapy, such as timing of premeal insulin, selection of injection sites, and mixing insulin. For example, the patient should be instructed to administer insulin 30 to 40 minutes prior rather than immediately before meals and to use a nonexercised injection site. The patient and his or her partner should be instructed about the symptoms of hypoglycemia and the use of intramuscular glucagon in the event of hypoglycemia. Carrying identification noting the patient's diabetes status cannot be overemphasized. (*Felig, Ch. 19; Mazzaferri, pp. 81–114*)

44.(A—True; B—True; C—False; D—False; E—False) *Discussion:* Regarding hypoglycemia in diabetics, it is important to remember that diabetic patients may have an altered threshold for hypoglycemic symptoms. Thus, in chronically hyperglycemic diabetic patients, hypoglycemic symptoms may occur when plasma glucose concentration rapidly declines to even normal range (e.g., 100 mg per deciliter). In contrast, tightly controlled diabetic patients may have a low plasma glucose threshold for symptoms, with hypoglycemia symptoms occurring at a low plasma glucose concentration (40 to 50 mg per deciliter).

Hypoglycemia unawareness refers to the patient's experience of neuroglucopenic manifestations without the usual adrenergic warning signs and symptoms of hypoglycemia. It is usually caused by impaired glucagon, epinephrine, and autonomic nervous system responses to hypoglycemia. Patients with type I diabetes mellitus for more than 5 years usually have an impaired glucagon response to hypoglycemia. However, this attenuated glucagon response alone does not predispose the patient to hypoglycemia or hypoglycemia unawareness. As the duration of diabetes increases, patients may respond to hypoglycemia with impaired catecholamine responses as a result of autoimmune neuropathy, adrenal medullary dysfunction, and adaptation to normal glucose levels achieved by intensive therapy. Combined deficiency of the glucagon and epinephrine responses to hypoglycemia is usually associated with hypoglycemia unawareness and impaired recovery from hypoglycemia. In this situation, plasma glucose goals should be compromised for safety. Adrenal insufficiency may cause hypoglycemia; however, it does not result in hypoglycemia unawareness. (*Felig, Ch. 19; Lavin, Ch. 34*)

45.(A—True; B—False; C—True; D—False; E—False); 46.(A—True; B—True; C—False; D—True; E—True) *Discussion:* Continuous subcutaneous insulin infusion using insulin pumps is one method to achieve meticulous glycemic control in a type I diabetes. However, it is not clear whether insulin pump therapy is superior to multiple insulin injection therapy in achieving glycemic control. Other advantages of insulin pump therapy include improvement in psychological functioning and the quality of life. Because of its adjustable programmability, the insulin pump allows flexibility in meal timing, physical activity, and achievement of the required plasma glucose goals. The most important factor in the success of insulin pump therapy is patient selection. Criteria for selection include patient motivation to pursue intensive therapy, ability and willingness to perform frequent-self monitoring of blood glucose, compliance with diabetic diet, sufficient education and technical ability to take care of the insulin pump, and adequate psychological stability. Patients who do not meet these criteria are not candidates for insulin pump therapy. Additionally, children and patients in the honeymoon period are not good candidates. The wide swings of glucose levels, as in the patient described, make insulin pump therapy a good solution because it delivers regular insulin at a low basal rate and can deliver adequate increments of insulin before meals. This better mimics normal physiology and may achieve a more stable glycemic control. A history of hypoglycemic episodes with unawareness does not preclude the use of insulin pump therapy. However, plasma glucose goals must be raised to a level at which hypoglycemia will be avoided.

Intensive glycemic control (with insulin pump or multiple insulin injections) effectively delays the onset and slows the progression of early diabetic retinopathy, early nephropathy, and early neuropathy in patients with type I diabetes mellitus (DCCT). Although no study to date has shown an improvement in advanced retinopathy, nephropathy, or neuropathy with intensive glycemic control, the presence of these advanced complications does not preclude intensive glycemic control or the use of insulin pump therapy. However, because of potential transient worsening of retinopathy associated with rapid introduction of glycemic control, close ophthalmologic evaluation is necessary. Slower introduction of tight glycemic control may avoid this potential complication. Insulin pump therapy is not free of risks or disadvantages. These include the following:

1. An increase in the incidence of DKA in the case of pump malfunction because of a lack of subcutaneous depot insulin.

2. Increased frequency of needle site abscesses and allergic skin reactions to tape.

3. Increased frequency of severe hypoglycemia as a result of tight glycemic control *rather than as a result of insulin pump therapy itself.* In the DCCT tight control group, there was no difference in the incidence of severe hypoglycemia between insulin pump users and those who used multiple injection therapy.

4. Transient worsening of retinopathy because of rapid correction of chronic hyperglycemia, rather than because of insulin pump therapy per se. This is believed to be a consequence of retinal ischemia caused by a decrease in retinal blood flow.

5. Weight gain. This is again due to hyperinsulinemia, not to insulin pump therapy per se.

6. High expense, the major disadvantage of insulin pump therapy (initially $4000 plus $300 per month for the cost of supplies).

(*Bell; Hirsch et al*)

47.(All are True); 48.(A—True; B—True; C—True; D—False; E—True) *Discussion:* The burning sensation in the legs of the patient described is consistent with symmetric peripheral diabetic polyneuropathy, which is the most common form of diabetic neuropathy. It is characterized by numbness, tingling, and ultimately paresthesias in the extremities, especially the feet. Involvement of the hands and motor loss are less frequently observed. Symptoms characteristically worsen at night, and ambulation may result in a transient clinical improvement. Physical examination demonstrates loss of vibratory sensation, absence of the ankle jerk reflex, symmetrical loss of sensation distally, and occasionally wasting of the intrinsic muscles of the feet and hands. Foot ulceration and Charcot joint (neuropathic osteoarthropathy) are possible complications (see the discussion of questions 36 and 37). The diagnosis is usually made on clinical grounds. However, other conditions of similar presentation (e.g., alcohol abuse, heavy metal toxicity, uremia, amyloidosis) must be excluded. Treatment of diabetic painful peripheral neuropathy is symptomatic. Current therapies include tricyclic antidepressants (e.g., amitriptyline),

phenytoin, carbamazepine, and topical capsaicin. It is recommended not to use narcotic agents, if possible, because of their high potential for abuse. As yet, the role of aldose reductase inhibitors (e.g., sorbinil, tolrestat) is limited. (*Cecil, Ch. 205; Clarke and Lee; Felig, Ch. 19*)

49.(A—False; B—True; C—True; D—True; E—True); 50.(A—False; B—False; C—True; D—False; E—True); 51.(All are False) *Discussion:* Diabetic autonomic neuropathy is usually associated with other chronic complications of diabetes and often complicates symmetric peripheral polyneuropathy (as in the patient described). Therefore, the finding of isolated autonomic neuropathy in a diabetic patient should suggest other disorders. Diabetic autonomic neuropathy can affect cardiovascular system, sudomotor, gastrointestinal tract, urinary bladder, and sexual function. Involvement of one system or organ is usually associated with widespread subclinical autonomic dysfunction. An exception to this rule is that diabetic impotence may occur as an isolated finding.

Cardiovascular autonomic neuropathy manifests initially with signs of impairment of cardiac parasympathetic function, and later with cardiac and peripheral sympathetic dysfunction. Cardiac parasympathetic dysfunction is reflected clinically by (1) a resting tachycardia (>100 beats per minute) and a decrease in the normal sleep bradycardia; and (2) loss of RR variation relative to respiration. The latter can be tested clinically by measuring the response of heart rate to deep breathing or the Valsalva maneuver. Normally, heart rate increases during Valsalva such that the ratio of the longest RR interval after release to the shortest RR interval during Valsalva is >1.2. In cardiac parasympathetic dysfunction, the ratio is <1.1. RR variability relative to respiration can be assessed more accurately using computerized electrocardiographic techniques. Cardiac sympathetic dysfunction interferes with normal cardiovascular response to exercise and stress. Patients with cardiovascular autonomic neuropathy have an increased rate of silent myocardial ischemia or infarctions and abnormal prolongation of the QT interval. Additionally, cardiorespiratory arrest and sudden death have been reported. The most disabling cardiovascular effect is orthostatic hypotension (a decrease of 10 mm Hg or more in diastolic blood pressure). This results from impairment of the sympathetic vasoconstrictor response and failure of stimulation of plasma renin release. Treatment of orthostatic hypotension is usually difficult, and includes increased salt intake, stocking supports, sleeping with the head of the bed elevated, and the use of fludrocortisone.

Gastrointestinal autonomic neuropathy is characterized by esophageal dysmotility, gastroparesis (see discussion of questions 41 to 43), diarrhea, and constipation. The diarrhea is often nocturnal and may be associated with fecal incontinence. It is usually caused by hypermotility resulting from impaired sympathetic inhibition. Other causes include bacterial overgrowth, pancreatic insufficiency, and a spruelike syndrome. Tetracycline may cause improvement in some patients with or without bacterial overgrowth, whereas the use of pancreatic enzymes is usually not helpful unless there is pancreatic insufficiency. If tetracycline is ineffective, diarrhea may respond to diphenoxylate, imodium, clonidine, cholestyramine, or octreotide. Cisapride, which acts by enhancement of the release of acetylcholine from the myenteric plexus of the gut, is used in the treatment of gastroparesis, not diarrhea. Of interest, celiac disease is more common in type I diabetics than in the general population.

Genitourinary autonomic neuropathy produces bladder dysfunction leading to recurrent urinary tract infections, retrograde ejaculation leading to infertility, and erectile impotence, which is present in about 40 to 50% of diabetic males. As mentioned earlier, erectile impotence can present as an isolated autonomic neuropathic finding. Its cause is multifactorial, including neuropathic and vascular abnormalities. However, other causes of impotence, such as hypogonadism, medications, alcohol, and psychogenic causes, should be excluded. Diabetic impotence is usually associated with normal testicular examination and function. Testosterone and gonadotropin concentrations therefore are normal. It is rarely reversed by testosterone therapy or glycemic control. However, patients with diabetic impotence may benefit from vacuum erectile aids, intracorporal papaverine or phentolamine injections, or penile prosthetic implants. (*Cecil, Ch. 205; Felig, Ch. 19; Harrison, Ch. 337; Green et al*)

52.(A—True; B—False; C—False; D—False; E—True) *Discussion:* Diabetic retinopathy is divided into two main categories: background retinopathy and proliferative retinopathy. Background retinopathy will be discussed in detail in question 55. The figure accompanying questions 41 to 52 shows retinal changes consistent with proliferative diabetic retinopathy (PDR). The main features of PDR are new blood vessel formation (neovascularization) and the development of fibrous tissue. Both pathologic processes may extend into the vitreous, leading to hemorrhages and retinal detachment, the main contributors to blindness. Although glycemic control effectively delays the onset and slows the progression of diabetic background retinopathy (DCCT), it is not beneficial once proliferative retinopathy develops. However, the treatment of choice of proliferative retinopathy is photocoagulation, which has been associated with significant reduction in the risk of visual loss. Aggressive treatment of hypertension is indicated because this may modify the development of retinopathy. Vitrectomy may be required in patients with massive vitreous hemorrhage, extensive scarring, or muscular detachments. There is no proven benefit provided by treatment of PDR with aspirin, other antiplatelet agents, or aldose reductase inhibitors (e.g., epalrestat). Moreover, aspirin and other antiplatelet agents should be avoided in patients at high risk for the development of vitreous hemorrhage. Although hypophysectomy has been associated with some improvement of diabetic retinopathy, it should be abandoned because its risks outweigh its benefits in the management of this situation. (*Cecil, Ch. 205; Felig, Ch. 19; Clark and Lee*)

53.(A—True; B—False; C—False; D—False; E—False); 54.(A—True; B—False; C—True; D—True) *Discussion:* This type I diabetic patient has background retinopathy and diabetic nephropathy, manifested by gross albuminuria and renal impairment. In early type I diabetes mellitus, hyperglycemia causes generalized hypertrophy of glomeruli, intraglomerular hypertension, and renal hyperperfusion. This is reflected clinically by increased GFR and microalbuminuria. The latter is defined as an albumin production rate of 20 to 200 μg per minute (30 to 300 mg per 24 hr), detected by radioimmunoassay (but undetectable by most standard dipsticks). Microalbuminuria has a significant predictive value (80%) for the development of renal insufficiency and is associated with an increased risk for cardiovascular disease. However, it can be stabilized or reversed by intensive glycemic control and the use of ACE inhibitors.

As the duration of diabetes increases, some patients develop gross proteinuria (>0.3 gram of albumin per 24 hr), usually approximately 15 years after the diagnosis of diabetes mellitus. This is often associated with hypertension. Nevertheless, renal function remains normal at this stage. After gross proteinuria occurs, GFR decreases and serum creatinine level increases. At this stage, intensive glycemic control has no significant role in amelioration of this advanced nephropathy. Once azotemia has appeared, most patients develop end-stage renal disease within 10 years. It should be noted that the course of diabetic nephropathy is highly variable. This is true especially in type II diabetes mellitus, in which progression of microalbuminuria to gross proteinuria is usually slower than in type I diabetes mellitus.

The earliest histopathologic markers of diabetic nephropathy are thickening of the glomerular capillary basement membrane and the expansion of extracellular matrix material within the mesangial region. These features characterize diabetic glomerulosclerosis. The diagnosis of diabetic nephropathy is usually made on clinical grounds. The presence of retinopathy and gross proteinuria, with or without azotemia, in a patient with longstanding diabetes (as in the patient described) strongly suggest the presence of diabetic nephropathy. Such a presentation is so characteristic that renal biopsy is rarely necessary.

The cornerstones of the treatment of clinically overt diabetic nephropathy include meticulous control of hypertension, dietary protein restriction (0.6 to 0.8 gram per kilogram of body weight per day), and avoidance of nephrotoxic drugs and dyes. ACE inhibitors and certain calcium channel blockers (diltiazem and nicardipine) are the treatment of choice for hypertension in patients with diabetic nephropathy (see the discussion of question 30). ACE inhibition should be avoided in patients with hyperkalemia, which is commonly seen with the hyporeninemic hypoaldosteronism (type IV RTA) associated with diabetic nephropathy. As noted earlier, intensive glycemic control has no significant value in the treatment of clinically overt diabetic nephropathy. For patients with end-stage renal disease, renal transplantation or dialysis should be considered. Transplantation is the treatment of choice for most young type I diabetics, whereas most type II patients are offered dialysis. (*Cecil, Ch. 205; Felig, Ch. 19; Clark and Lee*)

55.(A—False; B—True; C—False; D—False; E—False) *Discussion:* Background diabetic retinopathy is characterized by microaneurysms, hard and soft exudates, dot-and-blot hemorrhages, and retinal edema. Hard exudates are lipid-containing fluid that has leaked from surrounding capillaries, whereas soft exudates (cotton wool) represent areas of microinfarction of the superficial nerve fiber layer. Background retinopathy is usually associated with normal visual acuity unless there is macular hemorrhage, retinal edema, or a plaque of hard exudate. Although intensive gly-cemic control can be associated with transient worsening of background retinopathy, it can effectively delay its onset and slow its progression in the long term. *Annual* retinal examinations by ophthalmologists are recommended after the onset of type II diabetes mellitus and after 5 years in type I diabetes mellitus. Patients with significant retinopathy (e.g., proliferative retinopathy), pregnant diabetic women, and patients who are beginning intensive therapy may re-quire more frequent ophthalmologic examinations. (*Cecil, Ch. 205; Felig, Ch. 19; Clark and Lee*)

56.(A—False; B—True; C—True; D—False; E—True); 57.(A—False; B—False; C—False; D—False; E—True) *Discussion:* Glycohemoglobin is formed when glucose reacts nonenzymatically with the he-moglobin A molecule. Glycohemoglobin has several constit-uents, the major one being hemoglobin A_{1c}. Because the life span of the red blood cell is about 15 to 17 weeks, glycohemoglobin concentration (expressed as the percentage of total hemoglobin) provides an index of glycemic control over a 6- to 12-week period (the average of the life span of all red blood cells). Therefore, glycohemoglobin is not influenced by acute changes in blood glucose and cannot replace blood glucose measurements to adjust the insulin regimen of a patient. Although glycohemoglobin concentra-tion depends mainly on the concentration of blood glucose, other factors may increase or decrease it. Factors that may increase glycohemoglobin concentration include increased hemoglobin F (e.g., thalassemia, myeloproliferative disor-ders) and large doses of aspirin. Factors that may decrease glycohemoglobin concentration include pregnancy, sickle cell disease or trait, hemoglobins C and D, and other hemo-lytic anemias. These conditions, in addition to inaccurate self-measurement of blood glucose, can explain discrepan-cies between glycohemoglobin concentration and self-mea-surement glucose level. There is a lack of available standards for the different glycohemoglobin assay methods. Because of this, clinicians must become familiar with the assays used in their own labs and the nondiabetic reference range. Al-though glycohemoglobin has a specificity of >99% in the diagnosis of diabetes mellitus, its sensitivity is <50%. Thus, a normal glycohemoglobin concentration does not exclude the diagnosis of diabetes mellitus. (*Cecil, Ch. 205*)

58.(A—True; B—True; C—False; D—True) *Discus-sion:* Normally about two thirds of LDL is removed from plasma by hepatic and extrahepatic LDL receptors, and the removal of the remaining one third is non–receptor me-diated. The LDL receptor pathway depends on a complex interaction between the apolipoprotein B component of LDL and the LDL receptor. A defect in the LDL receptor or in apolipoprotein B will result in significant elevation in LDL cholesterol. This characterizes familial hypercholesterol-emia (type IIa hyperlipidemia), a common autosomal domi-nant lipid disorder. Most patients with familial hypercholes-terolemia have one abnormal allele for the LDL receptor (heterozygous familial hypercholesterolemia); a defect in both alleles (homozygous familial hypercholesterolemia) is very rare (only 1 in 1 million people).

Clinically, patients with heterozygous familial hypercho-lesterolemia present with

1. Clearly elevated total cholesterol (generally in the range of 300 to 500 mg per deciliter) and LDL cholesterol levels, usually with normal triglyceride and HDL concentrations.
2. Characteristic xanthomas in the Achilles tendons (as shown in the figure accompanying question 58) and the extensor ten-dons of the hands. Recurrent Achilles tendinitis may occur, which is usually exercise related.
3. Corneal arcus, a nonspecific finding for familial hypercho-lesterolemia. Nevertheless, it is considered diagnostic in white patients under 35 years of age.
4. Xanthelasma, which occurs in about 20% of cases but it is not specific for familial hypercholesterolemia.
5. Increased risk for CAD, peripheral vascular disease, and cerebrovascular disease. (*Cecil, Ch. 173, Molitch, pp. 216–226; Gotto et al*)

59.(A—False; B—True; C—False; D—True; E—True) *Discussion:* The figure accompanying question 59 shows a yellow-orange discoloration of the palmer creases of the hand. This is consistent with palmar xantho-mas, or what is called xanthoma striatum palmare. These skin lesions are highly characteristic of type III hyperlipid-emia (betalipoproteinemia) and are considered diagnostic in the absence of obstructive liver disease and hypothyroidism. Type III hyperlipidemia is an inherited disorder character-ized by elevated plasma concentrations of IDL and chylomi-cron and VLDL remnants. It results from an interaction be-tween genetic and environmental factors. The primary genetic factor is an autosomal recessive defect in apoprotein E, resulting in diminished removal of IDL and remnant parti-cles. Normally, VLDL is converted into VLDL remnants and IDL particles containing apolipoproteins E and B. VLDL remnants and IDL are removed from plasma by the liver through an interaction with the LDL receptor and the rem-nant receptor, which is specific for apolipoprotein E. In addi-tion, a significant fraction of IDL is converted into LDL.

Apolipoprotein E is essential for both the direct removal of IDL particles and their conversion to LDL. There are three isoforms of apolipoprotein E (E2, E3, and E4), each with a different binding affinity for the remnant receptor. Individuals who are homozygous for the apolipoprotein E isoform that has a low affinity for the remnant receptor (E2) may have diminished IDL and remnant catabolism. How-ever, this genetic defect alone is not enough for the pheno-typic expression of the disorder. Other conditions character-ized by overproduction of VLDL, such as obesity, hypothyroidism, and diabetes mellitus, are typically present.

In addition to palmar xanthomas, clinical manifestations of type III hyperlipidemia include tuberoeruptive xanthomas of the elbows, knees, or buttocks; parallel elevations of cho-lesterol and triglycerides [typical values: cholesterol level of 500 mg per deciliter and triglyceride level of 700 m per deciliter); and increased risk for premature CAD and periph-eral vascular disease. (*Cecil, Ch. 173; Felig, Ch. 22; Molitch, pp. 216–226*)

60.(A—False; B—False; C—True; D—True; E—True); 61.(A—False; B—False; C—True; D—False) *Discussion:* The laboratory data of the patient described show profound hyperglycemia, slightly decreased bicarbonate concentration, and an apparently normal serum sodium level. These are consistent with hyperosmolar hyper-glycemic nonketotic syndrome (HHNS). HHNS is character-ized by

1. Profound hyperglycemia, usually >600 mg per deciliter. The severity of hyperglycemia is probably related to polyuria, impaired thirst, and coexistent impairment of renal function.

2. Hyperosmolality (>320 mOsm per liter). Effective osmolality can be calculated using the following formula:

Effective osmolality (mOsm/L)
$$= 2[Na^+ + K^+ (mEq/L)] + \text{plasma glucose (mg/dl)}/18$$

This formula does not take into account the urea concentration, which it has little influence on osmolality because it is freely diffusible throughout the body.

3. Intravascular volume depletion and dehydration. Because water is usually lost in excess of solute, hypernatremia may develop. However, because of a shift of intracellular water to the extracellular space caused by hyperglycemia, the serum sodium level may be normal or even low (for each 100-mg per deciliter increase in glucose, there is a reduction of serum sodium of 1.5 to 2.0 mEq per liter). Therefore, a normal serum sodium level in the face of profound hyperglycemia implies severe volume depletion.

4. Absence of severe acidosis and ketosis. This is possible because of residual circulating free insulin sufficient to prevent lipolysis and ketogenesis but insufficient to prevent hyperglycemia.

In contrast to DKA, which usually occurs in type I diabetics, HHNS generally presents in older patients with mild or undiagnosed type II diabetes. Clinical manifestations include weakness, thirst, polyuria, signs of mental obtundation (10% of patients present with coma), and a variety of reversible neurologic abnormalities (e.g., seizures, aphasia, extensor plantar reflex, motor deficits).

Patients with HHNS urgently require correction of the severe volume depletion and restoration of vascular volume. This is best accomplished *initially* by isotonic normal saline (0.9% NaCl solution) or one-half normal saline according to the degree of the hyperosmolality, the serum sodium level, and the presence of hypotension, oliguria, or underlying cardiovascular disease. The type of intravenous fluid and the rate of infusion must be adjusted depending on the response to fluid replacement and the clinical status of the patient. It must be remembered that serum sodium will increase as the glucose level decreases. If serum sodium increases to >150 mg per deciliter, a more hypotonic fluid should be used. Insulin therapy is important to reverse the hyperglycemia. In spite of the marked hyperglycemia encountered in HHNS, only modest amounts of insulin are usually required. Five per cent dextrose may be required once plasma glucose declines to approximately 250 mg per deciliter to prevent hypoglycemia. Other aspects of treatment include electrolyte correction and identification of the predisposing factor(s) for HHNS. These include infections, cerebrovascular events, pancreatitis, myocardial infarction, and drugs such as steroids, phenytoin, thiazides, and propranolol. In spite of even the best therapy, HHNS carries high mortality (10 to 40%) and morbidity. Death is usually due to associated medical problems rather than to hyperosmolality. (*Cecil, Ch. 205; Lavin, Ch. 40*)

62.(All are True) *Discussion:* The skin lesion shown in the figure accompanying question 62 is consistent with acanthosis nigricans. Acanthosis nigricans is characterized by a soft, velvety brown hyperpigmented skin lesion occurring in the body folds, especially those of the neck and axillae and under the breasts and upper thighs. Most cases of acanthosis nigricans in individuals under 40 years of age are associated with insulin-resistant states such as obesity, type II diabetes mellitus, GH excess, glucocorticoid excess, and type A and type B extreme insulin resistance syndromes. Type A syndrome is due to a decrease in insulin receptor numbers and can be associated with polycystic ovary syndrome and virilization. Type B syndrome, in contrast, is associated with the presence of circulatory anti–insulin receptor antibodies interfering with insulin binding. When it occurs in individuals over 40 years of age, acanthosis nigricans may signal the presence of an occult malignancy, most often adenocarcinoma of the gastrointestinal tract (in particular, the stomach) and uterus. (*Cecil, Ch. 475; Felig, Ch. 19*)

63.(A—True; B—True; C—True; D—False; E—False) *Discussion:* Sulfonylureas act mainly by enhancing insulin release and by increasing sensitivity to insulin. Appreciable endogenous insulin secretion is necessary for a clinically significant effect of these drugs. Therefore, sulfonylurea drugs are totally ineffective in type I diabetes (C) or in diabetes secondary to total pancreatectomy (A). Other circumstances that preclude their use include pregnancy (because of possible teratogenic effects), allergy to the particular drug, significant liver disease, and end-stage renal disease. Sulfonylureas are generally indicated in patients with type II diabetes mellitus in whom diet and exercise fail to achieve treatment goals (D), and in some secondary diabetic conditions [e.g., pheochromocytoma (E)]. (*Cecil, Ch. 205*)

64.(A); 65.(B); 66.(A); 67.(A); 68.(A); 69.(C); 70.(E) *Discussion:* There are two classes of oral glucose-lowering agents: the sulfonylureas and biguanide compounds. Sulfonylureas include tolbutamide, chlorpropamide, acetohexamide, and tolazamide (first-generation agents) and glipizide and glyburide (second-generation agents). The various sulfonylurea agents differ with respect to potency, metabolism, side effects, and duration of action. Tolbutamide has the shortest duration of action (6 to 10 hours), and therefore it is to be taken two to three times per day. Chlorpropamide has the longest duration of action (24 to 72 hours) and therefore requires only once-per-day dosing. The most common and important side effect for all sulfonylureas is hypoglycemia, which should be carefully monitored. Because of its ability to enhance the action of antidiuretic hormone, chlorpropamide can cause significant hyponatremia (especially in the elderly when they are taking diuretics) and can be used in the treatment of partial central diabetes insipidus. In some patients, chlorpropamide administration is associated with the development of an intensive flush after consumption of alcohol ("disulfiram effect"). The second-generation sulfonylurea agents glyburide and glipizide differ from the first-generation agents in structure and potency. Because glyburide is the most potent, prolonged hypoglycemia can occur with its use.

Biguanide compounds include phenformin and metformin. They are antidiabetic rather than hypoglycemic agents, so they do not cause hypoglycemia in nondiabetic individuals. Phenformin is capable of inducing lactic acidosis in diabetic patients. Because of this, the U.S. Food and Drug Administration has withdrawn it from the market. Metformin, in comparison, very rarely causes lactic acidosis and has recently become available in the United States. (*Cecil, Ch. 205; Felig, Ch. 19*)

71.(F); 72.(H); 73.(I); 74.(B); 75.(C); 76.(E); 77.(A) *Discussion:* Vitamin and mineral deficiencies may be caused by a number of conditions, including drugs, alcoholism, malnutrition, malabsorption, total parenteral nutrition, hemodialysis, and certain inborn errors of metabolism. In general, the diagnosis of vitamin or mineral deficiencies can be accomplished by recognition of their clinical manifestations, determination of decreased body content of the specific vitamin or mineral involved, and demonstration of a response to replacement therapy. It is important to recognize the clinical manifestations of vitamin and mineral deficiencies for early diagnosis and treatment.

The presentation of the 32-year-old alcoholic man with HIV infection (71) is consistent with zinc deficiency. Clinical manifestations of zinc deficiency include diarrhea; mental disturbances; depression; growth retardation; hypogonadism; reduced taste; hyposmia; crusting skin lesions of the face, perineum, limbs, and skin folds (acrodermatitis); alopecia; impaired immune function; and hypercholesterolemia. Zinc deficiency may complicate alcoholism, inflammatory bowel disease, AIDS, diabetes, cirrhosis, and malabsorption. An autosomal recessive inherited disorder of zinc metabolism, known as acrodermatitis enterohepatica, is associated with a chronic form of zinc deficiency.

Selenium deficiency (72) may result in peripheral painful myopathies and cardiomyopathy. It is endemic in the Keshan province in China (Keshan disease), probably because of low soil selenium content. Replacement therapy with selomethionine is associated with reversal of its clinical manifestations. Selenium deficiency has been reported in patients with inflammatory bowel disease, chronic total parenteral nutrition administration, malignant disease, and occasionally myocardial infarction.

Chromium deficiency can be associated with diabetes mellitus, peripheral neuropathy, and encephalopathy as seen in the patient described in question 73. Other manifestations include weight loss. It usually complicates chronic total parenteral nutrition administration. Chromium plays a significant role in normal glucose homeostasis. It is postulated that chromium glucose tolerance factor facilitates insulin receptor activity. Therefore, its deficiency may cause impairment of insulin activity.

The 29-year-old man with Crohn's disease, ophthalmoplegia, areflexia, ataxia, decreased proprioception, and anemia has classic features of vitamin E deficiency (74). Other causes include (1) abetalipoproteinemia, a genetic disorder in which there is failure of intestinal absorption and serum transport of vitamin E; and (2) familial isolated vitamin E deficiency caused by failure of incorporation of dietary vitamin E into VLDL, resulting in very rapid clearance from plasma. Premature infants are at increased risk for vitamin E deficiency. It is important to replace vitamin E in premature infants because its deficiency can lead to serious complications such as intraventricular cerebral hemorrhage, bronchopulmonary dysplasia, hemolytic anemia, and edema.

Vitamin A deficiency (75) presents with night blindness followed by degenerative changes in the retina, dryness and ulceration of the cornea leading to its perforation (keratomalacia), dryness and hyperkeratosis of skin, and taste loss. Vitamin A deficiency also increases the frequency and severity of infectious diseases (e.g., measles). It is usually encountered in the setting of inadequate intake, malabsorption, alcoholism, protein-calorie malnutrition, liver disease, proteinuria, and chronic use of mineral oil, and after prolonged use of certain drugs such as bile acid resins, cholchicine, and neomycin. The diagnosis of vitamin A deficiency is based on the clinical presentation and demonstration of abnormal dark adaptation rather than on determination of low plasma vitamin A concentration. The reason for this is that plasma vitamin A levels do not reliably correlate with body stores of the vitamin.

Vitamin C plays a significant role in collagen synthesis. It is required for hydroxylation of proline residues in the collagen molecule. Therefore, deficiency of this vitamin can cause impairment of collagen synthesis, leading to unstable nonhydroxylated collagen. It is believed that this defect in collagen synthesis is the basis for many of the manifestations of vitamin C deficiency (scurvy), including poor wound healing and capillary fragility leading to hemorrhagic complications. Such complications include pain in bones and joints resulting from hemorrhage below the periosteum; swollen, bleeding gums; petechiae that may appear over the arm after the application of a sphygmomanometer (Rumpel-Leed test) (as in the patient described in question 76; and perifollicular hemorrhages. Anemia may result because of prolonged bleeding and/or associated folic acid deficiency. In severe vitamin C deficiency, intracerebral hemorrhage, oliguria, edema, and neuropathy may occur. Vitamin C deficiency is usually encountered in a setting of low dietary intake of the vitamin. Alcoholics, elderly individuals following a "tea and toast" diet, and children fed only with cow's mild for the first year of life are at increased risk for scurvy.

Thiamine (vitamin B_1) deficiency is characterized by high-output heart failure with sodium retention and edema (wet beriberi), and/or Wernicke-Korsakoff syndrome (dry beriberi). The Wernicke encephalopathy (as described in question 77) can be followed by the Korsakoff component of the syndrome, which is characterized by retrograde amnesia and confabulation. The most common cause of thiamine deficiency in the United States is alcoholism. Other less common causes include a poor diet, diabetes, cancer, hemodialysis, refeeding after starvation, and administration of glucose to asymptomatic but thiamine-depleted patients. (*Cecil, Ch. 192; Harrison, Ch. 77*)

78.(A); 79.(B); 80.(B); 81.(C); 82.(A); 83.(C); 84.(E) *Discussion:* The pancreatic islets of Langerhans contain different kinds of cells, each of which produces a single hormone. These cells include glucagon-secreting cells (A cells), insulin-secreting cells (B cells), somatostatin- and gastrin-secreting cells (D cells), pancreatic polypeptide–secreting cells (F cells), and vasoactive intestinal polypeptide (VIP)–secreting cells. The clinical presentation of such tumors usually reflects the effects of the hormone produced and/or the mass effects of local or metastatic spread. In addition, these tumors may be part of the multiple endocrine neoplasia type I (MEN I) syndrome.

Glucagonoma, a tumor that arises from A cells, is characterized by diabetes mellitus, weight loss, anemia, glossitis, and the characteristic waxing and waning skin rash. The skin rash, known as necrolytic migratory erythema, is erythymatous with raised superficial central blistering. It ultimately crusts and may heal with hyperpigmentation. It is located usually on the perineum, abdomen, face, and distal extremities. Other manifestations include onycholysis, brittle nails, diarrhea, and thromboembolic disease. Somatostatinoma, a tumor arising from D cells, is associated with a syndrome of diabetes mellitus, cholelithiasis, steatorrhea, and weight loss. Cholelithiasis, steatorrhea, and diabetes mellitus may result from chronic use of octreotide, a synthetic somatostatin analogue used as adjuvant therapy in the treatment of acromegaly. Somatostatinomas may secrete additional hormones such as ACTH, causing Cushing's syndrome, and calcitonin, causing watery diarrhea.

VIPoma (Vermer-Morrison syndrome) is also called pancreatic cholera and WDHA (watery diarrhea, hypokalemia, achlorhydria). The most striking feature is the secretory diarrhea, with peak volumes exceeding 3 liters per day. This is in contrast to the other endocrine causes of secretory diarrhea (gastrinoma, carcinoid, and somatostatinoma), which rarely exceed 3 liters per day. The severe watery diarrhea leads to hypokalemia and metabolic acidosis secondary to loss of potassium and bicarbonate, respectively. Additional features of VIPoma include non–PTH-dependent hypercalcemia, which remits with VIPoma resection.

Insulinoma, a well-known cause of hypoglycemia, is the most common islet cell tumor. It is characterized by elevated serum insulin and C-peptide levels in the face of symptomatic hypoglycemia. Non–beta cell tumors (e.g., hepatoma

RISK OF DEVELOPING DIABETES MELLITUS

Group	Risk (%)	
	Type I	Type II
Prevalence in U.S. population	0.4	5
Risk in relatives		
Parent	3	
Offspring	6	10–15
With affected father	8	
With affected mother	3	
Sibling	5	10–15
Identical twin	33 (30–50)	95
HLA-identical sibling	15	
HLA haplo-identical sibling	5	
No HLA identity	1	

Data from Cecil, Ch. 205; Atkinson and Maclaren.

and mesenchymal tumors) also may cause hypoglycemia, which could be related to the elevated levels of IGF-I and IGF-II associated with such tumors. (*Cecil, Ch. 159*)

85.(B); 86.(C); 87.(A); 88.(D); 89.(D); 90.(D) *Discussion:* Susceptibility to diabetes mellitus is determined by genetic and environmental factors. Genetic susceptibility to type I diabetes mellitus is associated with certain HLA haplotype antigens (e.g., DR3/X, DR4/X, DR3/DR4) that can allow an autoimmune insulitis following a certain environmental event such as viral illness (e.g., coxsackievirus B). The role of genetic factors in type II diabetes mellitus is more prominent than in type I, as is evident by the higher

concordance rate in monozygotic twins. However, the identity of genetic components for type II diabetes mellitus remains largely obscure. The lifelong risk for a family member to develop diabetes mellitus depends on the familial relationship with the diabetic patient see the table *bottom left.* (*Cecil, Ch. 205; Atkinson and Maclaren*).

91.(D); 92.(D) *Discussion:* Hypoglycemia may sometimes complicate certain endocrine deficiency states, such as (1) cortisol (as in question 91); (2) GH in children (as in question 92); and (3) both glucagon and epinephrine in type I diabetes mellitus. The presentation of the patient described in question 91 is consistent with acute primary adrenal insufficiency, most likely due to AIDS. A few percent of patients with AIDS have adrenal insufficiency resulting from adrenal infections (e.g., cytomegalovirus, mycobacterial, fungal) and/or adrenal involvement with Kapsosi's sarcoma or lymphoma. Hypoglycemia in a 9-year-old boy with short stature and normal renal function (as in the patient described in question 92) is most likely due to GH deficiency. Whereas cortisol deficiency may cause hypoglycemia as a result of decreased hepatic gluconeogenesis in both adults and children, GH deficiency may cause symptomatic hypoglycemia only in children. However, adults with isolated GH deficiency may manifest mild hypoglycemia after prolonged fasting. During hypoglycemia caused by one of these hormonal deficiencies, plasma insulin and C-peptide concentrations are suppressed. (*Cecil, Ch. 206; Felig, Ch. 20*)

93.(C) *Discussion:* The patient described has the following clinical findings: (1) autoimmune diseases (Hashimoto's thyroiditis and vitiligo); (2) insulin resistance manifested as acanthosis nigricans; and (3) hypoglycemia episodes with good response to glucocorticoid therapy. These clinical features characterize autoimmune insulin receptor hypoglycemia, in which patients have autoantibodies to the insulin receptor. Such patients usually have insulin resistance with or without diabetes mellitus and evidence for autoimmune diseases prior to the development of hypoglycemia. Hypoglycemia may occur because of the insulinomimetic effect of the antibodies and reduced insulin clearance from plasma. During hypoglycemia, plasma insulin concentrations are elevated while C-peptide levels are suppressed. Antibodies to the insulin receptor are positive. Long-term treatment of hypoglycemia consists of glucocorticoid therapy or methylpalmoxinate (an inhibitor of free fatty acid oxidation). (*Cecil, Ch. 206; Felig, Ch. 20*)

94.(B) *Discussion:* The main features of the patient's presentation are (1) frequent episodes as described that are indicative of hypoglycemia, (2) secondary amenorrhea and frequent frontal headaches, (3) borderline hypoglycemia and elevated bicarbonate concentration, and (4) hypercalcemia, hypophosphatemia, and a history of a right kidney stone, all suggestive of primary hyperparathyroidism, the most common cause of outpatient hypercalcemia. How can these features be put together to reach a diagnosis?

Hypoglycemia and hypercalcemia can be manifestations of familial multiple endocrine neoplasia (MEN) type I syndrome. MEN I is inherited in an autosomal dominant fashion and includes primary hyperparathyroidism (usually caused by *p*arathyroid hyperplasia), *p*ancreatic islet cell tumors, and pituitary tumors (the three Ps). The history of secondary amenorrhea and frequent frontal headaches can be due to a pituitary tumor leading to secondary hypogonadism. The most common pancreatic tumors in MEN I are gastrinomas, leading to Zollinger-Ellison syndrome. However, in one third of patients with islet cell tumors insulinomas may be found, leading to hypoglycemia that can be fasting and/or reactive. Insulinomas may secrete additional hormones such as ACTH, glucagon, gastrin, and somatostatin, modifying the clinical presentation. ACTH secretion may lead to hypokalemia, elevated bicarbonate concentration (as in the patient described), or other features of Cushing's syndrome. The diagnosis of insulinoma is established by demonstrating elevated plasma insulin and C-peptide concentrations at the time of occurrence of Whipple's triad. Proinsulin levels are elevated in most but not all insulinomas because of defective post-translational processing of proinsulin to insulin.

Conditions with similar biochemical findings should be excluded (e.g., sulfonylurea-induced hypoglycemia and insulin autoimmune hypoglycemia). Critical to management of a patient with insulinoma is localization of the tumor, which is best accomplished by intraoperative ultrasonography and careful palpation by an experienced surgeon. Successful surgical removal is associated with a normal life expectancy. Medical therapy, if indicated, may include diazoxide, verapamil, phenytoin, propranolol, or octreodide. (*Favus et al; Service, 1995*)

95.(A) *Discussion:* Because the supervised 72-hour fast did not provoke an episode of hypoglycemia in the patient described, this indicates that her presenting hypoglycemic episode was self-limited and probably induced. Self-limited induced hypoglycemia is usually caused by drugs or alcohol. The most likely cause of the hypoglycemia of the patient described is exogenous insulin administration. This is supported by a family history of type I diabetes mellitus in her sister. Sulfonylurea-induced hypoglycemia is unlikely because of the short duration of hypoglycemic effects in the patient described (<16 hr); such hypoglycemia usually lasts longer and may relapse. Hypoglycemia induced by other drugs (other than insulin) is also unlikely given the lack of other manifestations that are usually associated with these drugs. Alcohol abuse can cause hypoglycemia even in the absence of detectable blood ethanol levels or signs of acute inebriation. However, it is unlikely as a cause of hypoglycemia in the patient described, as evidenced by the lack of ketonemia and increased plasma lactate, which are usually associated with alcohol-induced hypoglycemia. Exogenous insulin-induced hypoglycemia is characterized by elevated plasma insulin and suppressed C-peptide concentrations. Insulin antibodies can be found when animal insulin is used but usually not with human insulin. Psychiatric evaluation is necessary to prevent recurrent episodes. (*Felig et al; Service, 1993*)

BIBLIOGRAPHY

Androgue HJ, Wilson H, Boyd AE, et al: Plasma acid-base patterns in diabetic ketoacidosis. N Engl J Med 307:1603, 1982.

Atkinson MA, Maclaren NK: The pathogenesis of insulin-dependent diabetes mellitus. N Engl J Med 331:1428, 1994.

Bardin CW (ed): Current Therapy in Endocrinology and Metabolism. 5th ed. St. Louis, Mosby-Year Book, 1994.

Bell DSH: Insulin pump therapy for the 90s. Endocrinologist 4:270, 1994.

Bennett JC, Plum F (eds): Cecil Textbook of Medicine. 20th ed. Philadelphia, WB Saunders Company, 1996.

Clark CM Jr, Lee DA: Prevention and treatment of the complications of diabetes mellitus. N Engl J Med 332:1210, 1995.

Cryer PE, Fisher JN, Shamoon H: Hypoglycemia. Diabetes Care 17:734, 1994.

Favus MJ: Primer on the Metabolic Bone Diseases and Disorders of Mineral Metabolism. 2nd ed. New York, Raven Press, 1996.

Felig P, Baxter JD, Frohman LA (eds): Endocrinology and Metabolism. 3rd ed. New York, McGraw-Hill, 1995.

Gotto AM Jr (ed): Dyslipoproteinemia Education Program (Clinician's Manual). London, Science Press Ltd, Sandoz Pharmaceutical, 1991.

Green DA, Sima AAF, Pfeifer, et al: Diabetic neuropathy. Annu Rev Med 41:303, 1990.

Hirsch IB, Farkas-Hirsch, Skyler JS: Intensive insulin therapy for treatment of type I diabetes. Diabetes Care 13:1265, 1990.

Isselbacher KJ, Braunwald E, Wilson JD, et al. (eds): Harrison's Principles of Internal Medicine, 13th ed. New York, McGraw-Hill, 1994.

Jagger PI: Hypoaldosteronism. Endocrinologist 5:23, 1995.

Lavin N (ed): Manual of Endocrinology and Metabolism. 2nd ed. Boston, Little, Brown and Co. 1994.

Mazzaferri EL, Bar RS, Kreisberg RA (eds): Advances in Endocrinology and Metabolism. Vol. 4: St. Louis, Mosby-Year Book, 1993.

Molitch ME (ed): Medical Knowledge Self-Assessment Program in the Subspecialty of Endocrinology and Metabolism. Philadelphia, American College of Physicians, 1995.

Service FJ: Hypoglycemias. J Clin Endocrinol Metab 76:269, 1993.

Service FJ: Hypoglycemic disorders. N Engl J Med 332:1144, 1995.

PART 12

NEUROLOGY

Gwendolyn C. Claussen

DIRECTIONS: For questions 1 to 29, choose the ONE BEST answer to each question.

1. A 23-year-old patient is brought to the emergency room by a friend who found him unconscious at home. Examination demonstrates small pinpoint pupils, slow irregular respiration, hypotension, and hypothermia. After stabilizing him, what diagnostic test would you perform first?

    A. Electroencephalogram (EEG)
    B. Cranial computed tomography (CT) scan
    C. Administration of naloxone
    D. Serum drug screen
    E. Lumbar puncture

2. The neuromuscular transmission defect in myasthenia gravis is due to which of the following?

    A. Presynaptic disorder caused by inadequate release of acetylcholine
    B. Presynaptic disorder secondary to an antibody against the voltage-gated calcium channel
    C. Postsynaptic disorder caused by an antibody against the acetylcholine receptor
    D. Nondepolarizing blockade of the acetylcholine receptor
    E. Delayed degradation of acetylcholinesterase

Figure 1

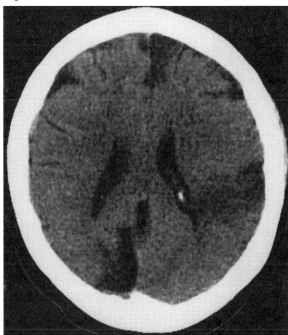

3. A 28-year-old woman is admitted to the hospital with acute onset of right hemiparesis, hemisensory loss, and mild expressive aphasia. A cranial CT scan without contrast is performed and reveals multiple abnormalities, as shown in Figure 1. What diagnostic test will most likely give the greatest yield in evaluation of the etiology?

    A. Urine drug screen
    B. Carotid ultrasound
    C. Lumbar puncture
    D. Echocardiogram
    E. Antiphospholipid antibodies

4. A 55-year-old man is brought to the emergency room after complaining of a severe headache followed by progressive obtundation. Ocular fundoscopic examination reveals subhyaloid hemorrhage. The most likely diagnosis is

    A. Bacterial meningitis
    B. Brain stem infarction
    C. Intracerebral hematoma
    D. Subarachnoid hemorrhage (SAH)
    E. Glioblastoma multiforme

5. A 63-year-old man is brought to the hospital by his family, who report that he became confused for 4 hours and was unable to remember where he was. During the episode, he knew who he was and had normal speech and reasoning power. Examination now is normal except the patient is amnestic for the last 12 hours. What is the most likely diagnosis?

    A. Complex partial seizure
    B. Vertebrobasilar insufficiency
    C. Korsakoff's amnesia
    D. Transient global amnesia
    E. Alzheimer's disease

6. What type of aphasia is characterized by fluent speech with some articulatory deficits and intact comprehension but inability to repeat a phrase?

    A. Wernicke's (sensory)
    B. Broca's (motor)
    C. Transcortical motor
    D. Transcortical sensory
    E. Conductive

7. If a cranial CT scan is normal in a patient with a history of severe headache followed by progressive obtundation, what test should be performed next?

    A. Lumbar puncture
    B. EEG

C. Tensilon test
D. Angiogram
E. CT with contrast

8. A 70-year-old man is brought to the hospital because of sudden onset of confusion. On examination, he talks with jargon-like phrases. He speaks fluently but selects the wrong words. He is unable to answer your questions but follows visually cued directions well. The exam is otherwise normal. Where is the cerebral lesion most likely located?

A. Dominant temporal lobe
B. Dominant frontal lobe
C. Thalamus
D. Dominant supramarginal gyrus
E. Diffuse cortical dysfunction

9. Which one of the following medications has shown the most benefit in the treatment of Alzheimer's disease?

A. Ticlopidene
B. Vitamin E
C. Pyridostigmine
D. Sinemet
E. Tacrine

10. A 56-year-old woman complains of several weeks of brief, lightning-like pain in the midface area on the left that is brought on by eating. Her neurologic examination is normal. The drug of choice for treatment is

A. Lorazepam
B. Haloperidol
C. Phenytoin
D. Carbamazepine
E. Valproic acid

11. A 14-year-old patient twisted her ankle during a soccer game. Initial examination and roentgenograms were normal. Two weeks later, the patient complains of severe burning pain in her foot. The foot is somewhat cold to the touch and discolored, although pedal pulses are intact. Another evaluation, including repeat roentgenograms, vascular stud-

ies, and electrophysiologic studies, is unrevealing. The most likely etiology is which of the following?

A. Vasculitis
B. Small fiber neuropathy
C. Fibromyalgia
D. Reflex sympathetic dystrophy
E. Peroneal neuropathy

12. What is the best treatment for a solitary non–small cell lung metatasis to the brain?

A. Local irradiation
B. Whole brain radiation
C. Chemotherapy with intra-arterial *cis*-platinum
D. Resection of the tumor
E. Glucocorticoids alone

13. A 65-year-old patient presented initially with focal motor seizures. A cranial magnetic resonance imaging (MRI) scan with gadolinium was obtained (Figure 2). What tumor is most likely?

A. Glioblastoma multiforme
B. Meningioma
C. Oligodendroglioma
D. Primary central nervous system (CNS) lymphoma
E. Ependymoma

14. A state of sustained loss of cognition with intact sleep/wake cycles and autonomic functions is known as

A. Stupor
B. Delirium
C. Vegetative state
D. Coma
E. Locked-in state

15. Clinical fluctuations (on-off effect) in a patient on carbidopa/levodopa for Parkinson's disease can be treated with all of the following EXCEPT

A. Use of Sinemet CR (long-acting formulation)
B. Addition of bromocriptine

Figure 2

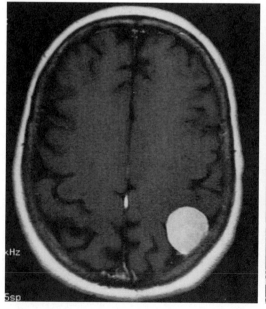
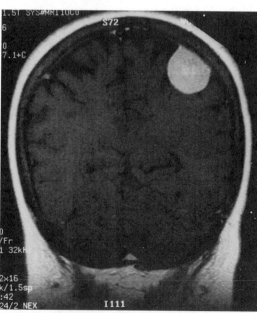

C. Addition of pergolide

D. Increasing dose and interval between doses of Sinemet (carbidopa/levodopa)

E. Decreasing dose and interval between doses of Sinemet (carbidopa/levodopa)

16. A 24-year-old woman is brought to the hospital after being found unresponsive. Examination reveals no withdrawal in response to pain, but all brain stem reflexes are present. An EEG is obtained and is normal. The most likely etiology is

A. Phenobarbital overdose

B. Brain stem stroke

C. SAH

D. Psychogenic state

E. Alpha rhythm coma

17. A 65-year-old man presents with sudden onset of right leg weakness. Examination reveals right hemiparesis and hemisensory loss with the leg most affected. Which vascular distribution is most likely involved if he has suffered a stroke?

A. Anterior cerebral artery

B. Middle cerebral artery (MCA)

C. Posterior cerebral artery

D. Lenticulostriate artery

E. Basilar artery

18. Temporal arteritis is best treated initially with

A. Cyclophosphamide

B. Prednisone, 20 mg per day

C. Prednisone, 80 mg per day

D. Nonsteroidal anti-inflammatory agents

E. Carbamazepine

Figure 3

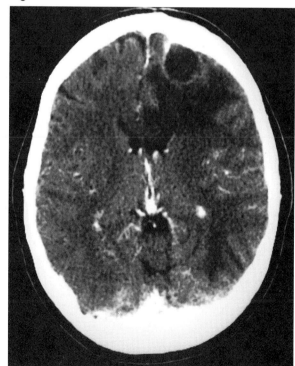

19. After reviewing the cranial CT scan with contrast shown in Figure 3, what is the most likely cause of this patient's focal seizure?

A. Acute stroke

B. Remote stroke

C. Intracerebral hemorrhage

D. Cerebral metastasis

E. Herpes simplex encephalitis

20. A 60-year-old man with alcohol on his breath is brought to the emergency room and examination reveals ophthalmoplegia, gait difficulties, and confusion. Treatment should include which of the following?

A. Folate

B. Phenytoin

C. Pyridoxine

D. Thiamine

E. Benzodiazepine

21. A 27-year-old man is evaluated for gait difficulties. Examination reveals increased tone and reflexes in the lower extremities and extensor Babinski toe sign. His gait is stiff and spastic. Upper extremities reveal normal strength, reflexes, and tone. The most important initial diagnostic test should be which of the following?

A. MRI of the lumbosacral spine

B. Cranial MRI

C. Nerve conduction and needle electromyography (EMG) studies

D. Thoracic MRI

E. Lumbar puncture for multiple sclerosis

22. A 64-year-old man presents with painless weakness in his arms. Examination reveals weakness, atrophy, and fasciculations of multiple muscles in his arms, and slight weakness of his right anterior tibialis muscle. Sensation is normal. Deep tendon reflexes are brisk. Electrophysiologic studies reveal diffuse denervation of multiple muscles with normal sensory nerve conduction studies. The most likely diagnosis is which of the following?

A. Adult-onset spinal muscular atrophy

B. Lambert-Eaton myasthenic syndrome

C. Fascioscapulohumeral muscular dystrophy

D. Amyotrophic lateral sclerosis

E. Multifocal motor neuropathy

23. Injection of botulinum toxin has been proven most useful in which one of the following disorders?

A. Cervical dystonia/torticollis

B. Myasthenia gravis

C. Hemidystonia caused by cerebral palsy

D. Essential tremor

E. Myoclonus

24. A 32-year-old man with a history of severe neck trauma several years ago presents with a suspended sensory level with loss of pain and temperature in the lower cervical and upper thoracic dermatomes, and wasting of muscles in the hands. Proprioception and light touch sensation are intact. A cervical MRI scan is shown in Figure 4. The most likely diagnosis is which of the following?

Figure 4

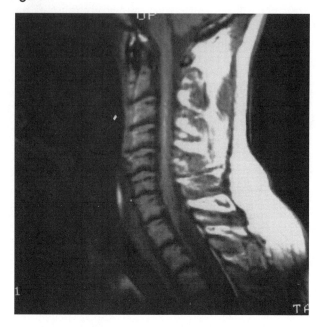

A. Cervical spondylosis
B. Cervical syringomyelia
C. Amyotrophic lateral sclerosis
D. Transverse myelitis
E. Multiple sclerosis

25. Which of the following tests is most useful in the initial evaluation of polyneuropathy?

A. Needle EMG
B. Nerve conduction studies
C. Somatosensory evoked potentials
D. Repetitive nerve stimulation test
E. None of the above

26. A 54-year-old woman reports a 6-month history of difficulty getting out of a chair and difficulty holding her arms overhead. Her serum creatine phosphokinase level is elevated at 350 IU per liter. The most likely etiology of this acquired myopathy is which one of the following?

A. Inclusion body myopathy
B. Polymyositis
C. Minicore myopathy
D. Mitochondrial myopathy
E. Limb-Girdle muscular dystrophy

27. What serious complication is associated with the use of ticlopidine in cerebrovascular disease?

A. Marked elevation of liver transaminases
B. Renal insufficiency
C. Aplastic anemia
D. Neutropenia
E. Pulmonary fibrosis

28. A 35-year-old woman reports a 3-week history of left-sided weakness, hyperreflexia, and Babinski sign. Four years ago she had transient loss of vision in the right eye for several weeks. A cranial MRI scan is performed (see Figures 5A and 5B). What is the most likely diagnosis?

A. CNS toxoplasmosis
B. Venous thrombosis
C. Multiple sclerosis
D. CNS vasculitis
E. Microangiopathy

29. A 68-year-old man with diabetes and hypertension presents with a 2-day history of left retro-orbital pain, followed by ptosis and inability to adduct the eye. Examination reveals left eye ptosis, opthalmoparesis in all directions except abduction, and normal pupillary response. The most likely etiology is which of the following?

A. Aneurysm
B. Retro-orbital tumor
C. Myasthenia gravis
D. Hyperthyroid eye disease
E. Diabetic oculomotor neuropathy

Figure 5A   **5B**

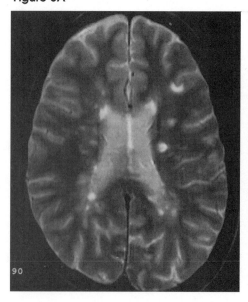
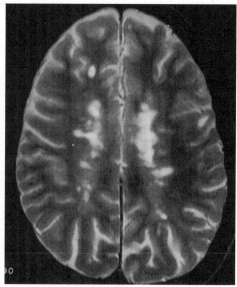

DIRECTIONS: Questions 30 to 68 are matching questions. For each numbered item, choose the most likely associated lettered item from those provided. Each numbered item has ONLY ONE answer. Within each set of questions, each answer may be used once, more than once, or not at all.

QUESTIONS 30–34

Match the following common types of headache with the appropriate descriptions.

    A. Classic migraine
    B. Cluster headache
    C. Tension headache
    D. Cranial arteritis
    E. Common migraine

30. Head pain in the fronto-temporal region; tenderness on palpation; jaw claudication; elderly patient

31. Visual fortification spectra followed by unilateral throbbing pain; associated with nausea, vomiting, and photophobia

32. Sharp, ice pick–like pain lasting 30 to 60 minutes located behind the eye, occurring primarily at night; patient paces relentlessly; most frequent in men

33. Tight, bandlike pain around the head of a moderate degree that can occur every day

34. Severe, unilateral throbbing pain associated with nausea, photophobia, vomiting; no preceding aura

QUESTIONS 35–38

Match the following CNS infections with the appropriate clinical syndrome.

    A. Tropical spastic paraparesis
    B. Poliomyelitis
    C. Jakob-Creutzfeldt disease
    D. Progressive multifocal leukoencephalopathy
    E. Subacute sclerosing panencephalitis

35. Progressive loss of cognitive function and motor dysfunction leading to spastic quadriparesis and death; associated with measles virus

36. Associated with JC virus (papovavirus); results in progressive focal neurologic deficits (hemiparesis, hemisensory loss, homonymous hemianopsia) in immunocompromised patients

37. Infection of the anterior horn cells that leads to flaccid paralysis in the involved regions

38. Associated with human T-cell lymphotropic virus type I (HTLV-I) infection

QUESTIONS 39–43

Match the following antiepileptic medications with the most appropriate seizure type.

    A. Carbamazepine
    B. Valproate
    C. Ethosuximide
    D. Intravenous phenytoin
    E. None

39. Complex partial seizure

40. Simple absence seizure (no tonic-clonic seizures)

41. Myoclonic seizure

42. Generalized tonic-clonic seizure

43. Status epilepticus

QUESTIONS 44–46

Match the following specific lumbosacral root lesion with the appropriate symptoms.

    A. L3 nerve root
    B. L4 nerve root
    C. L5 nerve root
    D. S1 nerve root
    E. S2 nerve root

44. Pain radiating from the low back into posterior thigh and into the foot; weakness of the big toe extensors; numbness of the big toe

45. Pain radiating from the low back into the lateral aspect of the thigh, with weakness of the quadriceps and loss of the patella reflex

46. Pain radiating from the low back into the posterior thigh and lateral aspect of foot; weakness of the ankle and foot flexors; loss of the Achilles tendon reflex

QUESTIONS 47–51

Match the following anatomic lesion locations with the visual field deficit noted on exam.

    A. Optic nerve
    B. Optic chiasm
    C. Temporal loop of optic radiation
    D. Parietal-occipital optic radiation
    E. Parietal projection of optic radiation

47. Homonymous superior quadrantanopia

48. Unilateral amaurosis

49. Congruous homonymous hemianopsia

50. Bitemporal hemianopsia

51. Homonymous inferior quadrantanopia

QUESTIONS 52–54

Match the following clinical syndromes with the appropriate disorder.

    A. Tuberous sclerosis
    B. Neurofibromatosis
    C. Sturge-Weber syndrome
    D. Ataxia-telangiectasia

52. Disorder characterized by facial angioma (port-wine stain), seizures, and mental deficiency

53. Disorder characterized by mental deficiency, seizure disorder, facial adenoma sebaceum, hypopigmented spots, and hamartomas

54. Disorder characterized by café au lait spots, axillary freckles, cutaneous and subcutaneous fibromas

QUESTIONS 55–60

Match the following cerebrospinal fluid (CSF) findings with the most appropriate disorder.

- A. Opening pressure 180 mm CSF, 100 white blood cells (WBCs) (90% lymphocytes), 5 red blood cells (RBCs), protein 90 mg per deciliter, glucose 40 mg per deciliter
- B. Opening pressure 350 mm CSF, 2 WBCs, 0 RBCs, protein 34 mg per deciliter, glucose 52 mg per deciliter
- C. Opening pressure 150 mm CSF, 3 WBCs, 0 RBCs, protein 134 mg per deciliter, glucose 62 mg per deciliter
- D. Opening pressure 120 mm CSF, 5 WBCs (100% lymphocytes), protein 60 mg per deciliter, glucose 62, mg per deciliter, immunoglobulin (Ig)G index 1.2, 3 oligoclonal bands, increased myelin basic protein
- E. Opening pressure 250 mm CSF, 740 WBCs (84% polynuclear), 4 RBCs, protein 215 mg per deciliter, glucose 15 mg per deciliter
- F. Opening pressure 200 mm CSF, 150 WBCs (94% lymphocytes), 2 RBCs, protein 100 mg per deciliter, glucose 10 mg per deciliter

55. Pneumococcal meningitis

56. Neurosyphilis

57. Multiple sclerosis

58. Tuberculosis meningitis

59. Guillian-Barré syndrome

60. Pseudotumor cerebri

QUESTIONS 61–64

Match the following brain tumors to the appropriate descriptions.

- A. Oligodendroglioma
- B. Glioblastoma multiforme
- C. Medulloblastoma
- D. Meningioma
- E. Ganglioglioma

61. Most common and most aggressive glial tumor

62. Benign tumor that is extra-axial in location

63. Tumor frequently associated with flecks of calcium on cranial imaging

64. Benign tumor frequently seen in the temporal lobes associated with complex partial seizures

QUESTIONS 65–68

Match the following extrapyramidal disorders with the appropriate clinical descriptions.

- A. Shy-Drager syndrome
- B. Progressive supranuclear palsy
- C. Parkinson's disease
- D. Olivopontocerebellar degeneration

65. Postural instability, unsteady gait, external ophthalmoparesis, axial rigidity, no tremor

66. Resting tremor, postural instability, bradykinesia, cogwheel rigidity

67. Rigidity, bradykinesia, prominent dysautonomia

68. Bradykinesia, ataxia

DIRECTIONS: For questions 69 to 81, decide whether EACH choice is true or false. Any combination of answers, from all true to all false, may occur.

69. Medications useful for benign essential tremor include which of the following?

- A. Propranolol
- B. Lisinopril
- C. Lithium
- D. Valproic acid
- E. Primidone

70. Which of the following administration route(s) of phenytoin is/are contraindicated in a patient in status epilepticus?

- A. Intramuscular
- B. Intravenous in 5% dextrose in water
- C. Oral load of 300 mg
- D. Intravenous in normal saline

71. Which of the following characteristics is/are typical of narcolepsy?

- A. Cataplexy
- B. Hypnagogic hallucinations
- C. Nocturnal breath cessation
- D. Delayed-onset rapid eye movement sleep

72. A 64-year-old man complains of a 1-month history of tremor, slowness of movement, and rigidity. Medications that can result in this syndrome include which of the following?

- A. Atenolol
- B. Haldol
- C. Metoclopramide
- D. Levodopa

73. CNS infections that can initially present with dementia include which of the following?

- A. Cryptococcal meningitis
- B. Syphilis
- C. Human immunodeficiency virus
- D. Jakob-Creutzfeldt

74. Mandatory criteria for brain death include which of the following?

- A. Absent pupillary response to light
- B. Absent gag reflex
- C. Absent oculovestibular response to cold water caloric testing
- D. Absent spinal reflexes

75. Tumors that commonly have cerebral metastasis include which of the following?

- A. Lung
- B. Melanoma
- C. Prostate
- D. Breast

76. Glossopharyngeal neuralgia can be characterized by which of the following?

- A. Lancinating pain in the posterior pharynx
- B. Association with head and neck tumors
- C. Pain triggered by touching posterior auricular area
- D. Can be associated with cardiac arrest
- E. Does not usually respond to carbamazepine

77. Frequent presenting signs of Alzheimer's disease include which of the following in addition to memory loss?

- A. Disorder of gaze
- B. Paranoia or suspiciousness
- C. Visual field deficits
- D. Anomia

78. A 16-year-old girl presents with a brief spell characterized by a sudden onset of staring and smacking movements of the mouth. Which of the following seizure disorders can be described like this?

- A. Generalized tonic-clonic seizure
- B. Absence seizure
- C. Myoclonic seizure
- D. Complex partial seizure

79. A 34-year-old patient is admitted with acute Guillian-Barré syndrome. Which of the following statements is/are true concerning this syndrome?

- A. Autonomic instability is a frequent cause of mortality
- B. Respiratory failure rarely occurs
- C. Patients are usually areflexic
- D. Nerve conduction studies typically demonstrate an axonal neuropathy

80. Concerning treatment of focal brain ischemia, which of the following statements is/are true?

- A. A patient with a blood pressure of 190/100 mm Hg who presents with an acute stroke should be treated aggressively with an antihypertensive medication.
- B. Embolic strokes are more likely to become hemorrhagic than thrombotic strokes.
- C. Carotid endarterectomy has been proven more useful than medical therapy in a patient with recent transient ischemic attack and 80% ipsilateral carotid stenosis.

81. Carpal tunnel syndrome is characterized by which of the following?

- A. Pain in the hand and wrist that frequently awakens the patient at night
- B. Ulnar neuropathy on nerve conduction studies

ANSWERS

1.(C) *Discussion:* All of these tests are useful in the evaluation of the unconscious patient in different situations. This patient has signs frequently seen in severe opiate toxicity, and a naloxone reversal test can be performed quickly to confirm this. If there is no response to two doses of naloxone, 0.4 mg intravenously or intramuscularly (separated by a 15-min interval), then another cause of coma should be suspected. (*Cecil, Ch. 394*)

2.(C) *Discussion:* Myasthenia gravis is a disorder of weakness secondary to a defect of neuromuscular transmission that occurs because of autoantibodies that induce acetylcholine receptor depletion at the motor end-plate. It presents with fatigable weakness of the voluntary muscles. The eye muscles are the most frequently involved, but the proximal limb and bulbar muscles are also affected in many patients. The diagnosis is confirmed by demonstrating an increased titer of acetylcholine receptor antibody, by demonstrating an abnormal decremental response to repetitive nerve stimulation, and by demonstrating increased strength with anticholinesterase medications (Tensilon test). (*Cecil, Ch. 459*)

3.(D) *Discussion:* This cranial CT scan demonstrates an acute left MCA distribution stroke and an old ischemic lesion in the right occipital region. Multiple strokes in different arterial distributions in a young adult would be most suggestive of a cardiac embolic source of stroke. Cardiac emboli are the most frequent cause of stroke in the young adult. Therefore, the echocardiogram has the greatest diagnostic yield. (*Cecil, Ch. 419*)

4.(D) *Discussion:* Subarachnoid hemorrhage frequently presents with severe headache followed by progressive obtundation and neck stiffness. Subhyaloid hemorrhages are retinal hemorrhages that are frequently associated with subarachnoid hemorrhage. Other ocular signs seen include preretinal hemorrhages and papillaedema. (*Cecil, Ch. 420*)

5.(D) *Discussion:* Transient global amnesia is a self-limited, isolated memory disorder in which reasoning, attention, and language are unaffected. The patient is disoriented and distressed, and frequently asks what is going on. These episodes typically last several hours, leave no impairment, and generally do not reoccur. The etiology is unclear, but they may be secondary to transient vascular insufficiency. The differential diagnosis includes complex partial seizures, but patients with seizures usually have an alteration of attention. (*Cecil, Ch. 399*)

6.(E) *Discussion:* Conductive aphasia occurs with a lesion in the dominant supramarginal gyrus and is characterized by a deficit in repetition without a loss in fluency or understanding. Wernicke's or sensory aphasia is characterized by fluent speech with deficits in comprehension and repetition. Broca's or motor aphasia is characterized by a loss of fluency and repetition but intact comprehension. Transcortical motor and sensory aphasis are similar to motor and sensory aphasis but repetition is spared. (*Cecil, Ch. 399*)

7.(A) *Discussion:* If the cranial CT scan is normal in an obtunded patient, including no signs of brain swelling, a lumbar puncture should be performed next for evaluation of meningitis and SAH. SAH can be missed on cranial CT scan in a small percentage of patients. CSF evaluation should include testing of WBCs, RBCs, glucose, protein, cultures, serology, and xanthochromia. In SAH, the RBCs begin to hemolyze after a few hours, giving rise to a yellow supernatant; this is called xanthochromia. (*Cecil, Ch. 420*)

8.(A) *Discussion:* This patient most likely suffers from Wernicke's aphasia, which is a fluent aphasia with loss of comprehension. Although speech is fluent, the patient's well-formed verbal messages are not intelligible. This is frequently interpreted as "confusion." Because of the loss of verbal comprehension, the patient does not realize the deficit. This aphasia occurs with lesions of the posterior and superior temporal lobe. Wernike's aphasia frequently presents without other neurologic signs, unlike Broca's aphasia (dominant frontal lobe), which is frequently associated with contralateral hemiparesis. (*Cecil, Ch. 398 and 399*)

9.(E) *Discussion:* Tacrine is a central cholinesterase inhibitor that has been shown to result in a small functional improvement, as well as a small improvement in scores on the Alzheimer Disease Assessment Scale, in a select group of patients. Most of these patients had mild disease and their improvement was modest. Tacrine frequently results in nausea and vomiting. Liver function studies increase in up to 40% of patients and therefore must be monitored closely during administration. (*Cecil, Ch. 400*)

10.(D) *Discussion:* This patient most likely suffers from trigeminal neuralgia, which is a facial pain that is brief, intense, and lancinating. The pain is located in one of the trigeminal nerve branch distributions and can be triggered by touch, talking, or eating. In the ideopathic type, the neurologic exam is normal. Treatment options include carbamazepine (drug of choice), liorisal, phenytoin (less responsive than carbamazepine), and surgery, including gasserian ganglion lesioning. If sensory loss or other abnormality is noted on exam, a search for a structural lesion in the brain stem or along the nerve should be performed. (*Cecil, Ch. 405*)

11.(D) *Discussion:* Reflex sympathetic dystrophy is a pain disorder characterized by burning, hyperpathic pain associated with autonomic changes, vasomotor instability, and osteoporosis. It frequently follows a trivial trauma and, unless associated with a nerve lesion, the routine electrophysiologic studies are normal. It is believed to be secondary to dysfunction in the autonomic nervous system. It is best treated with sympathetic blockade. (*Cecil, Ch. 405*)

12.(D) *Discussion:* Studies have shown that resection of the tumor is the best treatment for most patients with a solitary cerebral metastasis, especially in non–small cell lung cancer. This has resulted in protracted remission for many patients, especially if the lung cancer is resected as well. (*Cecil, Ch. 435*)

13.(B) *Discussion:* Meningiomas are formed from fibroblast-like cells of the dura that are typically attached to the dura of the sphenoid sinus, sagittal sinus, or cerebral convexities. An enhancing lesion attached to the dura is shown on the cranial MRI in the accompanying figure. The tumors are usually benign and slow growing. (*Cecil, Ch. 392.6 and 435*)

14.(C) *Discussion:* A vegetative state is a condition of altered consciousness in which autonomic function remains intact, including the sleep/wake cycle, but there is complete loss of cognition. This condition can occur with acute, severe bilateral cerebral damage or can develop as the end stage of a dementia. (*Cecil, Ch. 393 and 394*)

15.(D) *Discussion:* Motor fluctuations are one of the most common side effects of long-term treatment in Parkinson's disease. This can present as either a wearing off effect at the end of the dosing interval or as abnormal movements during peak drug levels of carbidopa/levodopa. This complication can be improved by maintaining as steady a drug level as possible, which can be accomplished by giving less drug more often or by using the long-acting formulation, Sinemet CR. The addition of other dopamine agents such as bromocriptine and pergolide has also proven useful. Increasing the dose and interval between doses of Sinemet could result in more motor fluctuations.

16.(D) *Discussion:* A completely normal EEG in an unconscious patient rules out organic causes of unresponsiveness. (*Cecil, Ch. 394*)

17.(A) *Discussion:* The anterior cerebral artery supplies the midline cortex and subcortical structures, where the foot and leg motor areas are localized. In a MCA stroke, the face, arm, and hand are frequently the most severely involved. (*Cecil, Ch. 419*)

18.(C) *Discussion:* The best initial treatment for biopsy-proven temporal arteritis is high-dose prednisone. Failure to treat can result in blindness secondary to occlusion of the retinal arteries. (*Cecil, Ch. 405*)

19.(D) *Discussion:* The contrast cranial CT scan demonstrates vasogenic edema in the left frontal and parital-occipital regions, midline shift, and distortion of the frontal horn of the left lateral ventricle. There is the suggestion of a ring enhancing lesion within the left frontal region. This appearance would be most suggestive of a tumor, but other etiologies, such as abscess, may also have this appearance. (*Cecil, Ch. 392*)

20.(D) *Discussion:* Wernicke-Korsakoff syndrome is characterized by the classic triad of ophthalmoplegia, gait disorder, and confusion; it occurs as a result of thiamine (vitamin B_1) deficiency. Thiamine deficiency is frequently found in alcoholics. (*Cecil, Ch. 406*)

21.(D) *Discussion:* The examination suggests a diagnosis of spastic paraparesis, which is frequently caused by dysfunction within the spinal cord. Because of upper motor neuron signs in the legs, the lesion is above the lumbosacral root level and most likely involves the thoracic or cervical regions. Because the examination is normal in the arms, the cervical region may be spared. Initially, spinal cord compression must be excluded with a MRI scan of the thoracic and cervical regions. If this is unrevealing, evaluation for other etiologies, such as HTLV-I, multiple sclerosis, acute transverse myelitis, vitamin E deficiency, and hereditary spastic paraparesis, must be performed. (*Cecil, Ch. 392.6, 414, and 428*)

22.(D) *Discussion:* Amyotrophic lateral sclerosis is a degenerative disorder characterized by progressive motor neuron loss. Both upper and lower motor neurons are affected, giving a mixed clinical picture of fasciculations and atrophy (lower motor neuron loss) with increased reflexes and Babinski response (upper motor neuron loss). Electrophysiologic studies reveal no abnormalities in the sensory nerves, no significant nerve conduction slowing as seen in neuropathies, and diffuse denervation on needle EMG. (*Cecil, Ch. 415*)

23.(A) *Discussion:* Botulinum toxin results in muscle weakness as a result of a presynaptic block of the neuromuscular junction. It has been used quite successfully with focal dystonias such as hemifacial spasm, spasmodic dysphonia, and cervical dystonia (torticollis). It is not useful in the generalized dystonias and is not used for essential tremor or myoclonus. Because of neuromuscular blockade, botulinum toxin is contraindicated in most patients with myasthenia gravis. The toxin works by temporarily paralyzing a portion of an overactive muscle. (*Cecil, Ch. 410*)

24.(B) *Discussion:* This patient most likely suffers from a cervical syringomyelia, which is a progressive enlargement of a fluid-filled cavity within the central spinal cord or medulla. Most are congenital and associated with an Arnold-Chiari malformation; others are associated with intraspinal tumor or trauma. Clinically the patients have a suspended sensory level from involvement of the crossing spinothalamic tracts at the level of the syrinx. As the central canal increases, anterior horn cells become affected and weakness and atrophy develop. The dorsal columns are usually spared, and therefore proprioception and light touch are frequently not affected. (*Cecil, Ch. 416*)

25.(B) *Discussion:* Nerve conduction studies are the most useful in the initial evaluation of neuropathy. The study evaluates the conduction velocity and amplitude response (approximate number of nerve fibers) in the motor and sensory nerves. Nerve conduction studies can differentiate axonal from demyelinating abnormalities. (*Cecil, Ch. 392.5*)

26.(B) *Discussion:* The most common etiology of acquired myopathy during adulthood is inflammatory myopathy (polymyositis, dermatomyositis, inclusion body myopathy). Of these, inclusion body myopathy is extremely rare. It presents with progressive weakness and atrophy with a predilection for the forearm and quadriceps muscles and is poorly responsive to therapy. Polymyositis presents with proximal weakness and in some patients produces myalgias. Dermatomyositis presents like polymyositis but is accompanied by a characteristic rash. Diagnostic evaluation should include electrophysiologic studies, which will reveal small-amplitude and short-duration motor unit potentials as seen in myopathy. Muscle biopsy reveals perivascular and endomysial collections of inflammatory cells and muscle fiber necrosis. (*Cecil, Ch. 456*)

27.(D) *Discussion:* Ticlopidine is an antiplatelet agent that inhibits platelet aggregation and prolongs bleeding time. Ticlopidine is indicated to reduce the occurrence of thrombotic strokes in patients with a previous history of thrombotic stroke or transient ischemic attack. It has been associated with neutropenia, which can be life threatening. Severe neutropenia, when it occurs, does so in the first 3 months of treatment. The current recommendations are that a complete blood count with differential be performed every 2 weeks during the first 3 months of therapy. (*Cecil, Ch. 419; Physicians' Desk Reference*)

28.(C) *Discussion:* Multiple sclerosis is a disorder of central demyelination of unknown etiology but is likely immune mediated. Patients are generally 20 to 45 years old at disease onset and develop relapsing and remitting or chronic progressive focal neurologic signs. Cranial MRI reveals multiple, hyperintense white matter lesions with a predilection for the periventricular regions and corpus callosum. The MRI findings are not specific for the diagnosis, but, given the age of the patient, the clinical scenario, and the previous history of what was most likely optic neuritis, the most likely diagnosis for this patient is multiple sclerosis. (*Cecil, Ch. 432*)

29.(E) *Discussion:* Diabetes can lead to vascular injury of the third cranial nerve. Clinically the patient presents with acute incomplete third nerve lesion with localized pain. Typically the pupil is not involved because the pupillary fibers are located superficially in the nerve bundle and therefore are less susceptible to ischemia. With compressive lesions (tumor, aneurysm), the pupil is frequently involved. (*Cecil, Ch. 449*)

30.(D); 31.(A); 32.(B); 33.(C); 34.(E) *Discussion:* Common and classic migraine result in pain that is frequently unilateral, throbbing in nature, and associated with nausea, vomiting, photophobia, and occasional focal neurologic deficits. Classic migraine has an aura, whereas common migraine does not. Both have a familial tendency. Cluster headache is a brief lancinating pain that is frequently located behind the eye or nostril and is associated with tearing, rhinorrhea, and Horner's syndrome. Clusters of headaches occur for several weeks at a time and then resolve for several weeks; they are more frequent in men. Tension headache can occur daily and begins with a dull pressure on the top of the head the spreads to involve the entire head in a vicelike manner. Rarely is tension headache associated with nausea or vomiting. Cranial arteritis is a serious head pain that occurs in patients over 50 years of age as a result of vasculitis in the temporal artery. The temporal area is tender and may demonstrate thickening of the artery on palpation. The pain

is aggravated by chewing (jaw claudication). The sedimentation rate is usually elevated. Diagnosis is confirmed by temporal artery biopsy. (*Cecil, Ch. 405*)

35.(E); 36.(D); 37.(B); 38.(A) *Discussion:* Tropical spastic paraparesis is due to infection with the HTLV-I virus. It is characterized by slowly progressive spastic paraparesis with features typical of myelopathy on examination. Infection is prevalent in the Caribbean, Japan, and parts of the southeastern United States. Poliomyelitis is caused by an enterovirus that attacks the anterior horn cells and results in multifocal flaccid weakness. Subacute sclerosing panencephalitis is a rare disease seen most frequently in adolescents; most have a history of measles infection during early childhood. It is characterized by progressive cognitive and motor decline that leads to death. Progressive multifocal leukoencephalopathy results from papovavirus infection in an immunocompromised patient. Progressive focal neurologic deficits associated with multifocal white matter loss characterize the disorder. (*Cecil, Ch. 425, 428, and 429*)

39.(A); 40.(C); 41.(B); 42.(B); 43.(D) *Discussion:* Antiepileptic medications most useful for partial-onset seizures include carbamazepine and phenytoin as first-line agents. Second-line medications include valproate, gabapentin, lamotrigene, and primidone. Valproate is the drug of choice for primary generalized seizures, and carbamazepine and phenytoin are second-line medications. Myoclonic seizures respond best to valproate or clonazepam. In absence seizures, ethosuximide is useful for absence alone but, if the patient also has generalized tonic-clonic seizures, valproate should be used. Status epilepticus is a neurologic emergency and should be treated with intravenous lorazepam and phenytoin. (*Cecil, Ch. 433*)

44.(C); 45.(B); 46.(D) *Discussion:* Radiculopathy results in pain in the distribution of the involved nerve root. A L4 lesion presents with pain in the lateral thigh; weakness in L4-innervated muscles, including the quadriceps; numbness in the lateral thigh; and loss of the patella reflex. L5 lesions result in weakness and numbness of the big toe extensors and weakness of ankle extensors (dorsiflexion). S1 lesions result in weakness of ankle and toe plantar flexion, numbness on the lateral aspect of the foot and posterior calf, and loss of the ankle deep tendon reflex. (*Cecil, Ch. 405*)

47.(C); 48.(A); 49.(D); 50.(B); 51.(E) *Discussion:* Monocular vision loss occurs with a lesion of either the retina or optic nerve. A lesion of the central optic chiasm results in interruption of the crossing nasal retinal fibers from both eyes, which clinically results in a bitemporal hemianopsia. Postchiasmal lesions result in homonymous deficits (loss of vision in corresponding halves or quadrants of the visual fields in each eye). Lesions affecting the temporal radiations affect the superior visual field quadrants and lesions of the parietal radiations affect the inferior visual field quadrants. Lesions near the visual cortex that affect the parieto-occipital radiations result in a congruous homonymous hemianopsia. (*Cecil, Ch. 403*)

52.(C); 53.(A); 54.(B) *Discussion:* The neurocutaneous syndromes are congenital disorders characterized by disordered growth of the ectodermal tissues resulting in skin lesions and tumors of the nervous system. Sturge-Weber syn-

COMMON CSF FINDINGS IN MENINGITIS

Type	Pressure	Cells*	Protein (mg/dl)	Glucose
Acute bacterial	Increased	>300 poly	100–500	Decreased
Tuberculous	Increased	25–100 lymph†	100–200	Decreased
Viral	Increased/normal	5–300 lymph†	<100/normal	Normal
Herpes simplex viral	Increased/normal	5–300 lymph†	50–250	Normal
Syphilitic	Increased	500 lymph	100	Normal
Fungal	Increased	0–800 lymph	20–500	Reduced

* Poly, polynuclear; lymph, lymphocytes.
† Initially may have polynuclear pleocytosis.

drome is characterized by facial angioma, seizures, and mental deficiency. The facial angioma is usually unilateral and in the distribution of the trigeminal nerve. Tuberous sclerosis is an autosomal dominant disorder characterized by mental deficiency, epilepsy, facial eruption known as adenoma sebaceum, and retinal and intracranial hamartomas. In addition to the facial lesions, patients also have numerous hypopigmented skin patches. In neurofibromatosis, multiple café au lait spots, axillary freckles, and peripheral nerve tumors (swannomas and neurofibromas) occur. The less frequent neurofibromatosis type II is also characterized by intracranial tumors, including acoustic neuromas and meningiomas. (*Cecil, Ch. 417*)

55.(E); 56.(A); 57.(D); 58.(F); 59.(C); 60.(B) *Discussion:* The table *above* reviews the common CSF findings in meningitis. The multiple sclerosis CSF profile typically reveals 0 to 30 WBCs, protein is normal or slightly increased, and CSF IgG synthesis is increased, with the production of oligoclonal bands and increased myelin basic protein. In pseudotumor cerebri, the opening pressure is elevated but other findings are normal. In Guillian-Barré syndrome, the CSF protein is typically elevated and the WBC count is normal. (*Cecil, Ch. 422, 424, and 426*)

61.(B); 62.(D); 63.(A); 64.(E) *Discussion:* Glioblastoma multiforme is a very aggressive glioma that accounts for more than 50% of all brain tumors. Patients present acutely with headache, seizures, and focal neurologic symptoms. Survival is usually less than 1 year even with aggressive surgery, radiation, and chemotherapy. Oligodendrogliomas are more benign glial tumors. They frequently present with focal seizures and have a predilection for the frontal lobes. Many contain calcium, which can be seen on neuroimaging. Meningiomas are fibroblast derivatives that attach to dural surfaces; they are extra-axial in location. These tumors are very slow growing and benign. Some patients can be cured with surgical resection. Gangliogliomas are rare tumors formed of neoplastic astrocytes and neurons that are very slow growing and have a predilection for the temporal lobes. These tumors can present with complex partial seizures. (*Cecil, Ch. 435*)

65.(B); 66.(C); 67.(A); 68.(D) *Discussion:* Parkinsonism is a clinical syndrome characterized by resting tremor, bradykinesia (slowness of movement), rigidity, and postural instability. It can occur in a primary form with degeneration of the substantia nigra (Parkinson's disease), or can occur secondary to dopamine-blocking drugs, toxins (MPTP), en-

cephalitis, vascular insufficiency, or repeated head trauma. Other extrapyramidal disorders that share features of parkinsonism include Shy-Drager syndrome, which has prominent dysautonomia; progressive supranuclear palsy, which has supranuclear loss of eye movements; and olivopontocerebellar degeneration, which has prominent ataxia. (*Cecil, Ch. 407 and 408*)

69.(A—True; B—False; C—False; D—False; E—True) *Discussion:* Benign essential tremor is characterized by flexion-extension oscillations of the hands at the wrists when the arms are outstretched. The tremor's amplitude increases with sustained posture and with action. It is the most frequent form of tremor and is inherited in an autosomal dominant pattern. Treatment includes beta blockers, primidone, and lorazepam. Both valproic acid and lithium frequently result in a drug-induced tremor. Lisinopril has no effect on the tremor. Alcohol will also improve the tremor but is not a useful treatment option. (*Cecil, Ch. 409*)

70.(A—True; B—True; C—True; D—False) *Discussion:* In status epilepticus, phenytoin should be given intravenously in normal saline or one-half normal saline. Administration in 5% dextrose in water results in precipitation of the drug, and intramuscular administration results in muscle necrosis. Oral loading can be performed by administering 300 mg every 8 hours for 24 hours, but this should not be performed in status epilepticus because of inability to obtain adequate drug levels quickly. (*Cecil, Ch. 433*)

71.(A—True; B—True; C—False; D—False) *Discussion:* Narcolepsy is a disorder characterized by excessive daytime sleepiness with sleep attacks, and is associated with cataplexy (sudden loss of muscle tone), sleep paralysis (inability to move on initial awakening), and hypnagogic hallucinations (vivid hallucinations that occur during transition from wakefulness to sleep). Sleep studies reveal sleep-onset rapid eye movement and shortened sleep latency. (*Cecil, Ch. 397*)

72.(A—False; B—True; C—True; D—False) *Discussion:* Medications that have antidopaminergic properties can result in extrapyramidal disorders, including parkinsonism; these medications include the phenothiazines and many of the antinausea medications (metoclopramide, compazine, promethazine), as well as reserpine, which works through dopaminergic antagonist. Levadopa, a dominergic agent, and atenolol, a beta blocker, have not been associated with drug-induced parkinsonism. (*Cecil, Ch. 408*)

73.(All are True) *Discussion:* Any patient who presents with a subacute or atypical dementia should be evaluated for chronic infections. Evaluation should include lumbar puncture. Cryptococcal meningitis, syphilis, human immunodeficiency virus, and Jakob-Creutzfeldt disease can all present with dementia. (*Cecil, Ch. 422 and 428*)

74.(A—True; B—True; C—True; D—False) *Discussion:* Brain death requires the absence of all cerebral and brain stem function, including the presence of fixed pupils, absent gag reflex, absent oculovestibular response to cold water calorics, presence of apnea off the ventilator for 10 minutes, and no behavioral response to noxious stimuli above the foramen magnum. Pure spinal reflexes can be seen. The nature and duration of coma must also be known to exclude a possible reversible cause (i.e., hypothermia, drug intoxication). (*Cecil, Ch. 395*)

75.(A—True; B—True; C—False; D—True) *Discussion:* All systemic tumors are capable of metastasizing to the brain, although some do it more frequently; these include lung, breast, renal cell, and melanoma. Prostate cancer infrequently metastasizes to the brain. (*Cecil, Ch. 435*)

76.(A—True; B—True; C—False; D—True; E—False) *Discussion:* Glossopharyngeal neuralgia is characterized by a sharp, lancinating pain in the posterior pharynx with radiation toward the jaw or ear, triggered by eating or swallowing. It can be symptomatic of a tumor or other lesion in the posterior pharynx. Because of vagal involvement, some patients have bradycardia and even cardiac arrest associated with an episode. Many patients respond to carbamazepine and liorisal. Others may require transection of the glossopharyngeal nerve roots. (*Cecil, Ch. 405*)

77.(A—False; B—True; C—False; D—True) *Discussion:* Alzheimer's disease is a degenerative disorder characterized by progressive cognitive dysfunction that primarily affects memory. Other presenting symptoms include early aphasia, typically beginning with progressive anomia (inability to name), and behavior abnormalities, including paranoia and delusional thoughts. Early presentation of seizures, gaze abnormalities, focal motor or sensory signs, or visual field deficits are extremely rare and should prompt a search for another diagnosis. About 25% of patients with Alzheimer's disease have an affected relative. The primary pathology seen on brain biopsy is the presence of neurofibrillary tangles and amyloid plaques. (*Cecil, Ch. 400*)

78.(A—False; B—True; C—False; D—True) *Discussion:* Both complex partial and absence seizures can present with staring spells and automatic behaviors such as lip smacking. The typical complex partial seizure of temporal lobe origin consists of a stare associated with an alteration of consciousness followed by automatisms, which are repetitive purposeless complex movements. Typical seizures last 1 to 2 minutes. In absence seizures, there is a sudden lapse of awareness; most seizures last less than 30 seconds. Longer absence seizures are associated with automatisms. Most absence seizures occur in children. Unlike complex partial seizures, patients with absence seizures do not have a postictal state. (*Cecil, Ch. 433*)

79.(A—True; B—False; C—True; D—False) *Discussion:* Guillian-Barré syndrome is an acute inflammatory demyelinating polyneuropathy that frequently follows a viral illness. It has been associated with *Camyplobactor jejuni* infection. Clinically it is characterized by progressive motor loss and areflexia caused by peripheral nerve demyelination. CSF protein is increased, and nerve conduction studies typically demonstrate demyelination of the peripheral nerves. Cranial nerves can also be affected, leading to severe facial weakness and dysphagia. Dysautonomia is common and is a frequent contributor to morbidity and mortality. Respiratory failure is the other leading cause of morbidity, resulting from involvement of the phrenic nerve. (*Cecil, Ch. 447*)

80.(A—False; B—True; C—True) *Discussion:* Because cerebral autoregulation is lost in ischemic brain, cerebral blood flow will decrease with aggressive treatment of blood pressure. If hypertension is severe (>200/120 mm Hg), blood pressure should be lowered very slowly and in a stepwise approach. Overaggressive treatment can result in stroke progression. Although all strokes can become hemorrhagic, embolic strokes are more likely to do so than thrombotic events. Many experts advocate anticoagulation for embolic strokes, but this must be done with caution and is frequently delayed 48 to 72 hours after an embolic stroke to decrease the risk of hemorrhagic conversion. Indications for carotid endarterectomy include recent transient ischemic attack or small stroke, ipsilateral carotid stenosis of 70 to 99%, and low surgical risk. Indications for carotid endarterectomy in asymptomatic patients are still being evaluated at the time. (*Cecil, Ch. 419*)

81.(A—True; B—False) *Discussion:* Carpel tunnel syndrome is an entrapment neuropathy of the median nerve at the wrist. It is the most common entrapment neuropathy and frequently presents with pain in the hand and wrist at night, loss of grip strength, tingling numbness in the first three digits, and a Tinnel's sign at the wrist (shooting electrical pain on tapping of the nerve at the site of entrapment). Nerve conduction studies reveal evidence of a median neuropathy distal to the wrist.

BIBLIOGRAPHY

Bennett JC, Plum F (eds): Cecil Textbook of Medicine. 20th ed. Philadelphia, WB Saunders Company, 1996.

Physicians' Desk Reference. 49th ed. Montvale, NJ, Medical Economics, 1995.

PART 13

DERMATOLOGY

Ann M. Lindgren and W. Mitchell Sams

DIRECTIONS: For questions 1 to 14, choose the ONE BEST answer to each question.

1. Functions of the epidermis include

   A. Protective barrier
   B. Thermal regulation
   C. Immunoregulation
   D. Protection from ultraviolet radiation
   E. All of the above

2. A patient comes to the office with a severe reaction to poison ivy. The cell in the skin responsible for generating this delayed-type hypersensitivity reaction is the

   A. Melanocyte
   B. Granular cell layer
   C. Langerhans' cell
   D. Basal cell layer

3. Generalized pruritus without evidence of a rash may be attributed to

   A. Lymphoma
   B. Uremia
   C. Stress
   D. Obstructive biliary disease
   E. All of the above

4. An 80-year-old man with a long history of psoriasis and reduced cardiac output resulting from a history of myocardial infarctions in the past presents with fever, chills, and erythroderma. He appears to be in high-output failure. This is because

   A. The patient is septic.
   B. His psoriasis has not been appropriately treated.
   C. The tremendous cutaneous vasodilation of erythroderma diverts 10 to 20% of his cardiac output to the skin.
   D. He has vancomycin red man syndrome.

5. A 23-year-old man presents with a keloid on his chest at the site of an injury that required stitches in the past. He wants to have the keloid cut off because it itches, and he also wants to have a mole removed from his right upper arm at the same time. You counsel him

   A. To see a plastic surgeon to achieve the best possible result from both procedures
   B. That keloids typically recur after excision and that he may develop a keloid after any surgical procedure, particularly on the upper chest, upper back, and shoulder region
   C. To schedule a surgical appointment with you so that you can cut both lesions out

   D. That the keloid is benign and to do nothing

6. A patient comes in for a follow-up after a punch biopsy of a generalized rash. All around the biopsy site are erythematous papules, and the patient complains that the site is quite itchy. She has been applying Neosporin to the biopsy site, as the postbiopsy directions stated. Which of the following is the most appropriate recommendation?

   A. That she switch from Neosporin to Mycitracin
   B. A short course of systemic antibiotics for infection
   C. That she use bacitracin on the site instead of Neosporin
   D. Intralesional steroid injections

7. A 4-year-old presents to the office with an abrasion injury on the knee. On physical examination, you notice some honey-colored crusts forming. You recommend which of the following for topical treatment?

   A. Neosporin/Polysporin ointment
   B. Polysporin/bacitracin ointment
   C. Mupirocin ointment
   D. Acyclovir ointment

8. A 3-year-old presents to the emergency room with a pruritic rash. Close examination reveals erythematous papules on the forearms and trunk, with papules in the axillae and groin. A burrow is seen in the interdigital web space and a scabies prep is positive. A medical resident recommends lindane as topical therapy. You recommend which of the following?

   A. Agree and recommend treatment for everyone at home
   B. Suggest permethrin for the patient and lindane for the adults at home
   C. Only recommend treatment for the patient
   D. Suggest better hygiene for the patient

9. A patient with extensive psoriasis has heard about phototherapy (PUVA) and wants to try it. You recommend

   A. Referral to a dermatologist's office where phototherapy is done for information regarding ultraviolet B (UVB) versus PUVA therapy.
   B. Prescribe psoralens and have the patient go to the beach
   C. Prescribe psoralens and have the patient go to a local tanning salon
   D. Have the patient go to the tanning salon without taking psoralens

10. Lichen planus
    A. Usually affects elbows and knees
    B. Has a delicate collarette around the edge of the lesions
    C. Presents with a unique flat-topped polygonal purple papule
    D. Never affects the mucous membranes

11. A patient presents with pruritic, almost vesicular-appearing papules and pustules on the trunk, some of which appear to surround a hair follicle. The previous weekend she had been on a ski trip and was in a swimming pool and a hot tub in the evening. The likely explanation for these findings is
    A. Intertrigo caused by friction from her ski clothes
    B. Folliculitis caused by *Pseudomonas aeruginosa*
    C. Superficial candidiasis
    D. Multiple *Staphylococcus aureus* carbuncles

12. A patient presents with a mole that has recently begun itching. Which of the following is the best approach to the patient's complaint?

    A. Recommend treatment with a topical steroid
    B. Prescribe an antihistamine
    C. Perform an excisional biopsy
    D. Recommend sunscreen

13. A 2-month-old girl presents with a rapidly growing, bright red, 1.5-cm nodule on the upper trunk. Which of the following is most appropriate?
    A. Recommend immediate excision
    B. Recommend no treatment
    C. Discuss laser therapy with the parents
    D. Recommend hospitalization

14. A patient with a history of ulcerative colitis presents with an enlarging necrotic-appearing ulcer on the lower leg. A surgeon carefully debrides the necrotic tissue and is shocked when the lesion doubles in size. The most likely diagnosis is
    A. Venous insufficiency
    B. Arterial occlusion
    C. Ecthyma gangrenosum
    D. Pyoderma gangrenosum

DIRECTIONS: Questions 15 to 92 are matching questions. For each numbered item, choose the most likely associated lettered item from those provided. Each numbered item has ONLY ONE answer. Within each set of questions, each answer may be used once, more than once, or not at all.

QUESTIONS 15–18

Match the following skin types with the appropriate descriptions.

   A. Black skin
   B. White skin
   C. Neither
   D. Both

15. Contains more melanocytes

16. Has more melanin dispersed within melanocytes and keratinocytes

17. Has the same number of melanocytes

18. Has the same amount of melanin dispersed within melanocytes and keratinocytes

QUESTIONS 19–23

As the skin ages, many structures and functions change. For which of the following structures or functions is presence/activity increased and decreased?

   A. Increased
   B. Decreased

19. Cross-linking of collagen and elastin

20. Epidermal cell turnover

21. Function of sebaceous glands and sweat glands

22. Melanocyte activity

23. Seborrheic keratosis, skin tags, and cherry angiomata

QUESTIONS 24–28

Match the following dermatologic terms with the best description.

   A. Raised circumscribed area greater than 1.0 cm
   B. Solid elevation of 1.0 cm or less in size
   C. Red, raised, edematous area that may change position
   D. Flat lesion
   E. Area of indentation
   F. Fluid-filled lesion 0.5 cm or larger

   24. Wheal

   25. Macule

   26. Plaque

   27. Bullae

   28. Papule

QUESTIONS 29–34

Specific diagnostic signs can help make a diagnosis for particular disorders. Match the following diseases with their appropriate diagnostic signs.

   A. Darier's sign
   B. Pathergy
   C. Koebner phenomenon
   D. Nikolsky's sign
   E. Diascopy
   F. Wood's light

29. Psoriasis

30. Toxic epidermal necrolysis

31. Urticaria pigmentosa

32. Lichen planus

33. Pyoderma gangrenosum

34. Sarcoidosis

QUESTIONS 35–39

Microscopic examination of skin conditions may reveal diagnostic findings. Match each disease with the appropriate diagnostic test.

   A. Tzanck smear
   B. Potassium hydroxide (KOH)
   C. Gram's stain
   D. Periodic acid–Schiff (PAS) stain

35. Tinea pedis

36. Cold sore

37. Tinea versicolor

38. Shingles

39. Chickenpox

QUESTIONS 40–43

Match each of the following therapeutic uses with the appropriate drug.

   A. Griseofulvin
   B. Ketoconazole
   C. Both
   D. Neither

40. Effective against superficial dermatophyte infections

41. Effective against tinea versicolor and superficial *Candida* infections

42. Associated with hepatotoxicity

43. Treatment for tinea capitis

QUESTIONS 44–48

Match each of the following skin reactions with the appropriate type of dermatitis.

   A. Allergic contact dermatitis
   B. Irritant contact dermatitis

44. Pruritic erythematous papules occurring under a patient's wedding band, but not under his/her metal watch band

45. Pruritic erythematous papules on both earlobes when patient wears earrings

46. Linear, erythematous papules and vesicles on the forearms and thighs

47. Delayed-type hypersensitivity response occurring after sensitization

48. Direct toxic affect on the skin

QUESTIONS 49–53

Eczematous dermatitis is typical of a variety of cutaneous disorders and is characterized by the presence of pruritic erythematous papules and vesicles. Often the distribution or other diagnostic clues may help differentiate between these disorders. Match the following diagnostic clues with the appropriate diagnosis.

A. Atopic dermatitis
B. Stasis dermatitis
C. Nummular dermatitis
D. Eczema craquelé
E. Dyshidrotic eczema

49. Involves lower one third of the legs secondary to venous insufficiency, often brown or hyperpigmented

50. Pruritic tiny vesicles on the palms and soles

51. Associated with a family history of allergies, asthma, Dennie-Morgan fold, and flexural distribution

52. Coin-shaped patches, often on extensor surfaces of arms and legs

53. Fissuring of the lower legs, more common in winter time as a result to xerosis

QUESTIONS 54–58

Match each of the following sets of clinical findings with the appropriate disease.

A. Seborrheic dermatitis
B. Lichen simplex chronicus
C. Tinea corporis
D. Candidiasis
E. Tinea versicolor

54. Annular, erythematous plaques with peripheral scale on the trunk

55. Yellow greasy scales, often in the central face, nasolabial folds, and eyebrows

56. Bright red erythema of the intertriginous area with satellite pustules

57. Very common hyperpigmented to scaly white patches over central trunk, back, and upper arms

58. Pruritic, lichenified, eczematous eruption often found on the posterior neck folds, legs, or groin as a result of repeated rubbing (often a nervous habit)

QUESTIONS 59–62

Viral exanthems are often similar in appearance, usually morbilliform. Certain clinical clues may aid in the appropriate diagnosis. Match each of the following diseases with the appropriate clinical findings.

A. Koplik's spots
B. Rash appearing following the administration of ampicillin
C. Fever, redness, and swelling of palms and soles, conjunctivitis, strawberry tongue, and cervical adenopathy
D. Slapped cheek appearance

59. Kawasaki's syndrome

60. Erythema infectiosum (fifth disease)

61. Measles

62. Infectious mononucleosis

QUESTIONS 63–66

Match each of the following clinical conditions with the appropriate etiology.

A. Papillomavirus
B. Pox virus
C. Streptococcus erythrogenic toxin
D. *Staphylococcus aureus* toxin
E. Unknown etiology

63. Molluscum contagiosum

64. Toxic shock syndrome

65. Verruca vulgaris

66. Scarlet fever

QUESTIONS 67–71

Match each of the following skin conditions with the appropriate finding.

A. Autosomal dominant
B. Symmetric papules or vesicles on elbows, knees, and buttocks
C. Large tense blisters
D. Painful erosions of the oral mucosa are typical
E. Scarring of the conjunctiva that leads to blindness
F. Occurs during pregnancy

67. Pemphigus vulgaris

68. Familial benign pemphigus

69. Bullous pemphigoid

70. Herpes gestationis

71. Cicatricial pemphigoid

QUESTIONS 72–75

Match each of the following benign lesions with the appropriate description.

A. Firm nodule, often with central enlarged pore filled with white cheesy material

B.   Soft, fleshy, protruding nodule that can be invaginated into the skin
C.   Annular yellow papules with a central pore, usually on the face
D.   Firm, rubbery nodule with normal epidermis
E.   Rapidly growing nodule with central keratin-filled crater

72. Sebaceous hyperplasia

73. Epidermal inclusion cyst

74. Keratoacanthoma

75. Neurofibroma

QUESTIONS 76–78

Match each of the following descriptions with the correct diagnosis.

A.   Squamous cell carcinoma
B.   Basal cell carcinoma
C.   Actinic keratosis
D.   Melanoma

76. Pearly papule with telangiectasia; may be locally destructive but rarely metastasizes

77. Rough, scaly, slightly erythematous patch; precancerous

78. Red scaly plaques that may be locally invasive and may metastasize

QUESTIONS 79–82

Match each of the following diagnoses with the correct description.

A.   Flat, light brown, well-circumscribed, 4-mm macule
B.   Irregular edges, asymmetric shape, dark black/purple color, usually greater than 6 mm in size
C.   Dark brown firm nodule with a positive dimple sign
D.   Waxy, brown to black, greasy-appearing plaque
E.   Bright red 2-mm flat to slightly raised papule

79. Dermatofibroma

80. Seborrheic keratosis

81. Junctional nevus

82. Melanoma

QUESTIONS 83–88

Match each of the following skin diseases with the appropriate description.

A.   Hyperpigmentation, usually on the face of women
B.   Diffuse brown hyperpigmentation, especially increased in the palmar creases
C.   Associated with neurofibromatosis
D.   Associated with atopic dermatitis
E.   Associated with diabetes, thyroid disease, and pernicious anemia
F.   Autosomal dominant; depigmented macules on the trunk
G.   Autosomal recessive; hypomelanosis of the skin, hair and eyes

83. Vitiligo

84. Melasma

85. Albinism

86. Addison's disease

87. Tuberous sclerosis

88. Café au lait spots

QUESTIONS 89–92

Match each of the following hair disorders with the appropriate description.

A.   Self-induced, with broken hairs of different lengths
B.   Transient, diffuse hair loss, often occurring several months following a severe illness or childbirth
C.   Round patch of nonscarring hair loss with "exclamation point" hairs
D.   Conversion of terminal hairs to vellus hairs
E.   Moth-eaten alopecia

89. Alopecia areata

90. Trichotillomania

91. Secondary syphilis

92. Telogen effluvium

DIRECTIONS: For questions 93 to 106, decide whether EACH statement is true or false. Any combination of answers, from all true to all false, may occur.

93. Which of the following statements is/are true regarding Langerhans' cells?

A. Langerhans' cells are the most important immunologic cell in the epidermis
B. Langerhans' cells are dendritic, like melanocytes
C. Langerhans' cells contain Birbeck granules
D. Langerhans' cells are important in graft-versus-host reactions, skin graft rejections, and contact dermatitis

94. Topical steroids are often the mainstay of dermatologic treatment. Which of the following statements regarding the use of topical steroids is/are true?

A. Topical steroids may be applied every 4 hours throughout the day
B. Ointment forms of topical steroids are the least effective because the occlusive nature interferes with permeability through the stratum corneum.
C. The side effects of topical steroids are least likely to occur in the intertriginous areas, when occluded by dressings or wraps, or on the face.
D. Fluorinated steroids can be used on the face to treat perioral dermatitis.
E. Topical steroids reduce the redness and itchiness of fungal infections of the skin, making them a useful therapeutic agent.

95. Retinoids are very useful therapies for several dermatologic conditions. Which of the following statements is/are true regarding retinoids?

A. Etretinate is useful in severe psoriasis and ichthyosis.
B. Pustular and erythrodermic psoriasis respond better to isotretinoin than etretinate.
C. Severe cystic acne responds to isotretinoin.
D. Small doses of isotretinoin can be used to treat severe acne and avoid some of the side affects.
E. Side effects of isotretinoin include cheilitis, conjunctivitis, dry skin, birth defects, bone spurs, night blindness, and elevated triglyceride and cholesterol levels.
F. Retinoids inhibit sebaceous gland activity and decrease epidermal cell proliferation and keratinization.

96. Acyclovir is useful in the treatment of which of the following conditions?

A. Neonatal herpes simplex
B. Shingles
C. Primary genital herpes simplex virus (HSV)
D. Eczema herpeticum
E. Recurrent herpes simplex

97. Which of the following statements regarding phototherapy is/are true?

A. Phototherapy may be useful in the treatment of psoriasis, vitiligo, atopic dermatitis, pityriasis rosea, mycosis fungoides, and uremic pruritus.

B. UVB phototherapy may cause a sunburn.
C. PUVA therapy stands for psoralen (topical or systemic) and UVA light.
D. Side effects of PUVA include squamous cell carcinoma and cataracts.

98. A patient with a known history of allergic reaction to poison ivy returns from a trip to Hawaii with a severe pruritic papulovesicular eruption around the mouth. Which of the following is/are the likely explanations to her findings?

A. She was exposed to poison ivy.
B. She was eating mangos.
C. She was eating cashews.
D. She was eating bananas.

99. Nonpalpable purpura is associated with which of the following?

A. Schamberg's disease
B. Meningococcemia
C. Rocky Mountain spotted fever
D. Henoch-Schönlein syndrome
E. Bacterial endocarditis

100. Psoriasis is a genetic hyperproliferative disease of the skin. Which of the following statements is/are true?

A. Psoriasis may be limited to the extensor surfaces, such as the elbows and knees, or may appear in an area such as the axillary or groin folds.
B. Psoriasis may run a self-limited, approximately 6-week course.
C. Trauma to the skin, such as a surgical excision or scratching, may induce the appearance of new psoriasis lesions.
D. Following a streptococcal infection, the sudden appearance of numerous small psoriasiform papules may appear.
E. Palms, soles, nails, scalp, and the intergluteal cleft are spared in psoriasis.
F. Certain medications such as lithium or beta blockers are known triggers for psoriasis.
G. Treatment for psoriasis includes topical creams, steroids, vitamin D analogues, tar, phototherapy (either UVB or PUVA), and systemic therapy with methotrexate, cyclosporin, or etretinate.

101. Which of the following is/are true regarding pityriasis rosea?

A. Typically involves the palms and soles
B. May appear in a Christmas tree pattern, with lesions appearing along skin form lines on the back
C. May be preceded by a herald patch
D. Aggressive treatment may be needed

102. Which of the following is/are true regarding ichthyosis vulgaris?

A. May be inherited in an autosomal dominant fashion

B. Appears at birth

C. Appears as fishlike scales on the extensor surface of the extremities

D. Is a result of an enzyme deficiency

103. Which of the following is/are true regarding rosacea?

A. Is an acne-related condition usually affecting older individuals

B. Consists of papules, pustules, erythema, and telangiectasias over the nose and cheeks

C. May be accompanied by recurrent flushing

D. Long-term effects include ocular involvement and development of rhinophyma

104. Which of the following is/are causes of urticaria?

A. Sinusitis

B. Aspirin

C. Strawberries

D. Exercise

E. Sunlight

105. Which of the following statements is/are true with regard to Kaposi's sarcoma?

A. It is associated with acquired immunodeficiency syndrome (AIDS) and may pursue an aggressive course, with mucosal membrane, visceral, or lung tumors in addition to cutaneous lesions.

B. A typical patient with Kaposi's sarcoma may be an elderly man, usually of Mediterranean descent.

C. With the lower legs involved, it usually runs an indolent course.

D. It may occur in patients being treated with immunosuppressive medications.

106. Which of the following statements is/are true regarding the immunocompromised host?

A. Skin cancer is more common in transplant patients than expected.

B. In the immunocompromised patient, skin biopsy should be avoided if possible.

C. Human immunodeficiency virus (HIV) infection may be associated with giant molluscum, chronic herpes simplex, or widespread psoriasis.

D. Characteristic diseases of AIDS include Kaposi's sarcoma, oral hairy leukoplakia, bacillary angiomatosis, and eosinophilic folliculitis.

ANSWERS

1.(E) *Discussion:* The cornified cells of the stratum corneum form an impermeable barrier to both outward loss of fluids and inward penetration of chemicals and microorganisms. The cutaneous vasculature and eccrine (sweat) glands are the major mechanisms of thermal regulation for the body. The Langerhans' cells are immunocompetent cells that monitor the skin for the presence of external antigens. In response to UV radiation, melanocytes produce melanin and the epidermis thickens to protect the body from penetration of carcinogenic UV radiation. (*Cecil, Ch. 472*)

2.(C) *Discussion:* The Langerhans' cells are the immunocompetent cells of the skin with surface receptors for immunoglobulins, complement, and Ia antigens. The Rhus antigen (from poison ivy) will be processed and presented by Langerhans' cells in the skin to sensitized T cells, which in turn initiate the delayed-type hypersensitivity response. (*Cecil, Ch. 472*)

3.(E) *Discussion:* Generalized pruritus without primary skin disease may be a sign of internal disease. Lymphoma (Hodgkin's disease), uremia, obstructive biliary disease, myeloproliferative disorders, endocrine disorders, and visceral malignancies may all produce pruritus. Psychiatric disorders, including stress, may also be a cause. (*Cecil, Ch. 472*)

4.(C) *Discussion:* Erythroderma may be caused by a variety of conditions, including psoriasis. The cutaneous vasculature vasodilates and up to 20% of the cardiac output can be diverted to the skin. Fever and chills are common because the thermoregulatory mechanism of the body is altered by the cutaneous inflammation. Patients usually need supportive care to rule out sepsis and aggressive skin care and biopsies to determine the etiology. (*Cecil, Ch. 472*)

5.(B) *Discussion:* Keloids are scar tissue that overzealously expands into the normal tissue beyond the original injury. The most common sites of keloid formation include the anterior chest, the upper back, and deltoid regions. Keloids rarely regress but commonly recur after excision. Patients must be educated as to the nature of keloids and the risk of developing a keloid after any procedure in keloid-prone sites. (*Cecil, Ch. 472*)

6.(C) *Discussion:* Topical antibiotics are often used on biopsy sites to prevent superficial infection. All topical antibiotics have the potential to sensitize, but neomycin in particular is a frequent cause. Neosporin contains polymyxin and neomycin. Mycitracin also contains neomycin. Polysporin contains polymyxin as well as bacitracin. A patient who reacts to both Neosporin and Polysporin may be having allergic reaction to the polymyxin present in both preparations. Bacitracin contains no other active ingredients. Intralesional steroid injections are useful for acne cysts, keloids, or localized areas of alopecia areata, granuloma annulare, discoid lupus erythematosus, or psoriasis, which may be unresponsive to topical therapy. (*Cecil, Ch. 474*)

7.(C) *Discussion:* Impetigo is a superficial cellulitis of the skin, most commonly caused by staphylococcal and streptococcal organisms. Bactroban (mupirocin) is an effective topical therapy when used three times a day for superficial infections caused by these organisms. Intranasal use of mupirocin can decrease nasal carriage of *S. aureus*. Acyclovir ointment can decrease viral shedding from lesions of herpes simplex. (*Cecil, Ch. 474*)

8.(B) *Discussion:* Scabies is well treated topically with lindane or permethrin. However, lindane is not recommended for children less than 6 years old or for pregnant or lactating women. Treating the patient with permethrin and the adults with lindane or permethrin would be adequate. If the child is infected, it is likely that the parents have been exposed and may be infected as well. If the entire family is not treated, recurrent infections typically occur. (*Cecil, Ch. 474*)

9.(A) *Discussion:* Phototherapy must be administered by appropriate equipment and trained staff capable of monitoring and recording the patient's dose of UVB or UVA. Systemic psoralens make the entire body photosensitive, and severe burns and fatality may occur if the patient receives excessive UV radiation. The beach, where exposure to both UVB and UVA occurs, is especially dangerous. UVB is 1000 times more penetrating than UVA. Use of psoralens and tanning salons is not recommended because too much UVA may be administered, resulting in a burn. UVA alone, as in the tanning bed, is not strong enough to improve psoriasis without systemic or topical psoralen. (*Cecil, Ch. 474*)

10.(C) *Discussion:* Lichen planus is an idiopathic condition with a unique papule that is flat topped and polygonal with a purple hue. Characteristically, the papules have reticulate white lines on their surface known as Wickham's striae. The distribution of lichen planus includes ankles, wrists, genitalia, and mucous membranes. Like psoriasis, trauma may induce lesions (the Koebner phenomenon). Psoriasis tends to affect elbows and knees. Pityriasis rosea has a typical collarette and scale. (*Cecil, Ch. 475*)

11.(B) *Discussion:* Hot tub folliculitis is a pruritic folliculitis caused by *Pseudomonas aeruginosa* from infected hot tubs or swimming pools. It may appear almost vesicular or pustular on the trunk and extremities but spares the head and neck. It may resolve without treatment. Intertrigo usually occurs in areas where the skin becomes macerated, such as under the breasts or in the inguinal folds. Candidiasis is beefy red with peripheral pustules. Carbuncles are multiple, draining, deep-infected follicles that require systemic antibiotics. (*Cecil, Ch. 475*)

12.(C) *Discussion:* One third of melanomas may arise within a pre-existing nevus. Typically signs or symptoms of a changing nevus include an alteration in size, shape, or color or the development of itching. Any suspicious pigmented lesion should be biopsied, preferably with an excisional biopsy so that the depth of malignant cells may be adequately assessed. (*Cecil, Ch. 475*)

13.(B) *Discussion:* Strawberry hemangiomas are benign proliferations of small superficial vessels. Characteristically they develop shortly after birth and rapidly grow during the first year or two. No treatment is necessary because they usually improve on their own, by the time the patient reaches school age. It is important to avoid procedures that would leave a scar, especially when nature does a good job on its own. (*Cecil, Ch. 475*)

14.(D) *Discussion:* Pyoderma gangrenosum is an unusual form of ulceration that presents with an enlarging deep necrotic ulcer with an undermined violaceous border. These lesions demonstrate pathergy, in which trauma, such as surgical debridement, will stimulate their growth. The best treatment is with systemic corticosteroids. They are associated with inflammatory bowel disease, rheumatoid arthritis, dysproteinemias, and leukemia or lymphoma. Venous insufficiency usually presents with malleolar ulcers, brawny edema, and hyperpigmentation of the lower legs. Arterial occlusion usually presents with sudden pain, numbness, and the development of an ulceration. Ecthyma gangrenosum typically presents with ulcers of the body folds caused by *Pseudomonas* septicemia. (*Cecil, Ch. 475*)

15.(C); 16.(A); 17.(D); 18.(C) *Discussion:* Black skin contains the same number of melanocytes as white skin, but there is more melanin synthesis, which is distributed from the melanocytes to the keratinocytes. (*Cecil, Ch. 472*)

19.(A); 20.(B); 21.(B); 22.(B); 23.(A) *Discussion:* Many structural, physiologic, and biochemical changes take place as the skin ages. Specifically, epidermal cell turnover decreases by 50% between the third and seventh decade. Crosslinking of collagen and elastin increase, which makes the dermis more rigid and more easily torn by shearing forces. There is a decrease in sebaceous and sweat gland function, which causes xerosis and impaired thermoregulation. Melanocyte enzyme activity decreases 10 to 20% per decade, causing pigmentary changes in the skin and gray hair. Skin tags, cherry angiomata, seborrheic keratosis, lentigines, and lesions of sebaceous hyperplasia all increase. (*Cecil, Ch. 472*)

24.(C); 25.(D); 26.(A); 27.(F); 28.(B) *Discussion:* Appropriate descriptions of a "rash" will help establish a differential diagnosis. A wheal, typical of urticaria, is usually an erythematous, edematous, annular plaque that typically changes location. A macule is a flat discoloration of the skin, either white as in vitiligo or brown as in a freckle. A plaque is a circumscribed raised area typically greater than 1.0 cm, seen in diseases such as a plaque of psoriasis. Bullae are fluid-filled blisters greater than 0.5 cm, as seen in herpes

zoster and with the immunoblistering diseases such as bullous pemphigoid. A papule is a raised area less than 1.0 cm (smaller than a plaque), as seen in eczema or drug eruptions. Atrophy of the skin, as seen in lupus or other scarring processes, will usually leave an area of indentation. (*Cecil, Ch. 473*)

29.(C); 30.(D); 31.(A); 32.(C); 33.(B); 34.(E) *Discussion:* Psoriasis and lichen planus both exhibit the Koebner phenomenon, in which new skin lesions develop in areas that are traumatized. Toxic epidermal necrolysis is a superficial blistering condition of the skin, and pressure on these blisters will make the blister expand, a positive Nikolsky's sign. Urticaria pigmentosa has collections of mast cells in the skin that, when rubbed, will release histamine, making the skin lesion red and raised, a positive Darier's sign. Pyoderma gangrenosum may develop at sites of injury, particularly at needle puncture sites, which is typical of pathergy. Sarcoidosis and other granulomatous diseases will give an apple-jelly color when pressed with a glass slide (diascopy). A Wood's light, which is long-wave UVA light, allows appreciation of subtle pigmentary changes in the skin, as in the ash leaf macules of tuberous sclerosis. (*Cecil, Ch. 473*)

35.(B); 36.(A); 37.(B); 38.(A); 39.(A) *Discussion:* Dermatophyte infections of the skin may be diagnosed by a KOH exam. KOH is added to the scale from the patient on a microscope slide and heated to dissolve the keratin. Dermatophytes, which cause tinea pedis and other tinea infections, may be seen as branching hyphae. Tinea versicolor is caused by the yeast *Pityrosporum ovale*. On KOH exam, one may see hyphae and spores. A Tzanck smear is useful for detecting the presence of a herpesvirus, such as HSV or varicella zoster virus (chicken pox). A vesicle base is scraped and allowed to air dry on the slide prior to staining with Giemsa or Wright's stain, which will demonstrate multinucleated giant cells. Gram's stain may reveal bacteria, and a PAS stain is performed on pathologic sections from skin biopsies to look for fungal and yeast elements. (*Cecil, Ch. 473*)

40.(C); 41.(B); 42.(B); 43.(A) *Discussion:* Griseofulvin and ketoconazole are both systemic antifungal agents effective against extensive superficial dermatophyte infections. Ketoconazole has the added advantage of being effective as well against the yeasts of tinea versicolor and superficial *Candida* infections. However, ketoconazole has been associated with fatal hepatotoxicity, and liver function tests should be used to monitor its use. Griseofulvin is the choice for tinea capitis, onychomycosis, and extensive tinea corporis. (*Cecil, Ch. 474*)

44.(B); 45.(A); 46.(A); 47.(A); 48.(B) *Discussion:* Contact dermatitis may be either allergic or irritant in nature. Allergic contact dermatitis is a delayed-type hypersensitivity reaction requiring sensitization. Irritant contact dermatitis is the result of a direct toxic or irritant reaction on the skin. Dermatitis under a ring, but not from other metal jewelry, is most likely an irritant dermatitis from soap and water becoming trapped under the ring. Allergic contact dermatitis can occur on both earlobes from nickel hypersensitivity present in earrings. Poison ivy or poison oak, causes of allergic contact dermatitis, cause papular vesicular eruptions in a linear array where the plant brushes across the skin. (*Cecil, Ch. 475*)

49.(B); 50.(E); 51.(A); 52.(C); 53.(D) *Discussion:* Stasis dermatitis is an eczematous dermatitis of the lower one third of the legs caused by venous insufficiency. Acutely there would be weeping, and more chronically one may see edema, brawny discoloration, or hyperpigmented plaques with scale. Eczema craquelé often involves the lower legs, although actual fissuring of the skin is seen as a result of excessive dryness. Atopic dermatitis is often familial, occurring in association with asthma, allergic rhinitis, and atopic eczema. Distribution characteristically involves the antecubital and popliteal fossae and the flexural areas. The Dennie-Morgan fold is a redundant crease below the lower eyelid, present in many atopics. Nummular dermatitis refers to coin-shaped eczematous patches on extensor surfaces. (*Cecil, Ch. 475*)

54.(C); 55.(A); 56.(D); 57.(E); 58.(B) *Discussion:* Tinea corporis can be caused by a variety of dermatophyte species with the similar appearance of an annular, raised, erythematous, scaly edge with central clearing that can occur anywhere on the body. A KOH exam of the scale will reveal hyphae. Seborrheic dermatitis typically occurs in the areas of skin with a high concentration of sebaceous glands, such as the central face, eyebrows, nasolabial folds, presternal area, and even the groin. Typically, greasy yellow scales are seen with some erythema. Candidiasis often occurs in the intertriginous areas of the groin and inframammary and axillary areas, with bright red erythema with erosions and small satellite pustules. KOH scraping of the scale will reveal pseudohyphae and spores. Tinea versicolor, a superficial infection caused by *Pityrosporum orbiculare,* may have a variety of colors from hypopigmented to white, red, or brown, typically with scale distributed over the upper back, chest, and arms. KOH reveals hyphae and spores, also known as spaghetti and meatballs. Lichen simplex chronicus, or neurodermatitis, is a result of repeated scratching and itching in one area, often a nervous habit. Typical sites of predilection include the neck, nape, lower legs, or groin, all areas easily reached. (*Cecil, Ch. 475*)

59.(C); 60.(D); 61.(A); 62.(B) *Discussion:* Kawasaki's syndrome, or mucocutaneous lymph node syndrome, causes a scarlatiniform eruption with fever, mucous membrane inflammation with conjunctivitis and strawberry tongue, edema and erythema of palms and soles, and asymmetric cervical adenopathy. Approximately 2 weeks after the fever, desquamation occurs on the palms and soles. There is a risk of coronary artery aneurysms and myocardial infarction in 1 to 2% of the patients. Erythema infectiosum (fifth disease) is one of the childhood viral exanthems, with a typical ''slapped cheek appearance'' of erythema on the face and a reticulate lacy rash on the extremities. Measles may be preceded by the appearance of Koplik's spots, gray-white papules with surrounding erythema on the buccal mucosa across from the molars. These appear very early in the course of the disease. Infectious mononucleosis occasionally presents with a viral exanthem; however, close to 100% of these patients treated with ampicillin will develop a maculopapular eruption. (*Cecil, Ch. 475*)

63.(B); 64.(D); 65.(A); 66.(C) *Discussion:* Molluscum contagiosum is caused by a DNA pox virus that produces translucent umbilicated small papules, typically in small children. Toxic shock syndrome has occurred in menstruating women using tampons and in postsurgical patients. The disease is mediated by a toxin elaborated by *Staphylococcus aureus,* and is characterized by fever, strawberry tongue, hypotension, vomiting, renal insufficiency, and a diffuse maculopapular eruption. Desquamation of palms and soles occurs later. Common warts (verruca vulgaris) are due to papillomavirus. Scarlet fever is due to an erythrogenic toxin produced by a streptococcal infection. A rough, sandpaper-like eruption begins on the neck and upper chest and spreads distally. A flushed face, with circumoral pallor, and strawberry tongue are seen, and desquamation occurs later. (*Cecil, Ch. 475*)

67.(D); 68.(A); 69.(C); 70.(F); 71.(E) *Discussion:* The vesiculobullous diseases may be differentiated by the level of the blister formation in the skin. Superficial, or intraepidermal, blisters are characterized by a positive Nikosky sign, in which the blister spreads easily and the cutaneous lesions may appear only as superficial erosions. The pemphigus family of disorders is a group of autoimmune blistering diseases that are intraepidermal. Pemphigus vulgaris usually presents with painful oral mucosal erosions and superficial bullae erosions on the skin, especially at sites of pressure or friction. Familial benign pemphigus, also known as Hailey-Hailey disease, is not an autoimmune disorder but is inherited in autosomal dominant fashion. Superficial blisters and erosions typically occur in the flexural areas of the neck, axillae, and groin. The mouth is spared. Heat and superficial infections will contribute to flares.

The subepidermal blistering diseases typically have tense blisters with a negative Nikosky sign. Bullous pemphigoid, an autoimmune disease of the elderly, presents with large tense blisters. Herpes gestationis, which has no association with the herpesvirus, is an autoimmune blistering disease that typically occurs during pregnancy and resolves postpartum. It may recur with menstrual periods, the use of oral contraceptives, or subsequent pregnancies. There may be an association with fetal mortality and prematurity. Cicatricial pemphigoid typically affects the mucous membranes and conjunctiva and can lead to blindness resulting from scarring. Symmetric papules and vesicles of the buttocks, elbows, and knees are seen in dermatitis herpetiformis. (*Cecil, Ch. 475*)

72.(C); 73.(A); 74.(E); 75.(B) *Discussion:* Sebaceous hyperplasia is typically found on the faces of older individuals, and may be confused with basal cell carcinoma because of the presence of telangiectasia. However, the annular yellow papules with a central pore help differentiate it. Epidermal inclusion cysts are firm nodules that may have a central enlarged pore. Squeezing the cyst will extrude a white, cheesy, foul-smelling keratin and sebum mixture. Keratoacanthomas have a characteristic rapid growth history over 6 to 8 weeks and a central keratin-filled crater. These lesions may spontaneously regress; however, excision may be best because keratoacanthoma may be difficult to differentiate from squamous cell carcinoma. Neurofibromas are soft, fleshy, protruding nodules that may be invaginated (the buttonhole sign). Multiple neurofibromas are associated with von Recklinghausen's disease. (*Cecil, Ch. 475*)

76.(B); 77.(C); 78.(A) *Discussion:* Basal cell carcinomas typically appear on sun-exposed surfaces and demonstrate a pearly papule with telangiectasia and a rolled border. With time, these cancers can be very destructive locally but rarely metastasize. Actinic keratoses are considered precancerous because they may evolve into a squamous cell carcinoma. These appear as red patches and papules with scale. Squamous cell carcinoma may be both locally invasive and metastatic. Clinically it may appear as red scaly crusted friable plaques that may also form cutaneous horns. (*Cecil, Ch. 475*)

79.(C); 80.(D); 81.(A); 82.(B) *Discussion:* Dermatofibromas are benign growths of focal dermal fibrosis. They may be brown in color and firm, and with lateral pressure they demonstrate a central dimple known as the "dimple sign." Seborrheic keratoses are also benign and may be dark in color but have a greasy, waxy, verrucous surface. A junctional nevus is usually flat with a light brown color. Melanoma, by contrast, is usually larger than other nevi (greater than 6 mm), with asymmetric shape, irregular border, and dark black or purple color. Cherry angiomas are benign, small, red papules. (*Cecil, Ch. 475*)

83.(E), 84.(A); 85.(G); 86.(B); 87.(F); 88.(C) *Discussion:* Melasma is usually a symmetric hyperpigmentation on the face, typically of the malar eminences, forehead, and upper lip, caused by hormonal simulation of the melanocytes, usually by oral contraceptives or pregnancy. Café au lait macules are light-colored macules; if six or more are present and greater than 1.5 cm in size, the diagnosis of neurofibromatosis can be made. Addison's disease, with increased melanocyte-stimulating hormone and adrenocorticotrophil hormone secretions, produces a generalized hyperpigmentation with accentuation of pigment in the body creases, such as the palmar crease. Vitiligo is a circumscribed area of hypomelanosis caused by absent melanocytes. Vitiligo occurs in families and is associated with thyroiditis, diabetes, pernicious anemia, and Addison's disease. Albinism is a group of autosomal recessive traits resulting in hypomelanosis of the skin, with white hair and translucent irides. Tuberous sclerosis is an autosomal dominant condition with depigmented macules, often in an ash leaf configuration on the trunk, that appear early in life. Other symptoms include seizures, mental retardation, phakomas, renal hamartomas, Shagreen patch, adenoma sebaceum, and ungual fibromas. (*Cecil, Ch. 475*)

89.(C); 90.(A); 91.(E); 92.(B) *Discussion:* Alopecia areata is a well-circumscribed patch of nonscarring alopecia. Typically, the quarter-sized areas will have "exclamation point" hairs, which have tapered shafts. Trichotillomania is a self-induced area of alopecia caused by compulsive twisting or pulling, resulting in broken hairs of different lengths. Secondary syphilis can cause a spotty hair loss described as "moth eaten." Telogen effluvium is a transient or self-limited phase of diffuse hair loss caused by a change in the hair cycle, usually after extreme stress, severe illness, surgery, childbirth, or by a medication. Male pattern alopecia occurs when terminal hairs are converted to fine, nonpigmented vellus hairs. (*Cecil, Ch. 475*)

93.(All are True) *Discussion:* Langerhans' cells are derived from the bone marrow and contain a tennis racquet–shaped organelle, the Birbeck granule, visible on electron microscopy. Langerhans' cells are the most important immunologic cell in the epidermis and reside in the suprabasal layer of the epidermis. These cells express Ia antigens, process and present foreign antigens to sensitized T cells, and mediate graft-versus-host reactions, skin graft rejection, and contact dermatitis, such as the poison ivy reaction. (*Cecil, Ch. 472*)

94.(All are False) *Discussion:* Topical steroids are usually applied twice a day. The stratum corneum acts as a reservoir and continues to release the medication throughout the day. Additional applications do not increase absorption. The ointment forms are the most effective because the steroids are more soluble in the ointment vehicles. The ointment vehicle allows greater permeability through the stratum corneum. Side effects of topical steroids are seen most often with the intermediate and high potency preparations when used on the face and intertriginous areas and when occluded. Fluorination of steroids increases their potency and, when used on the face, fluorinated steroids may cause perioral dermatitis with scale, papules, and pustules. Although topical steroids might initially reduce the erythema and/or pruritus associated with a superficial dermatophyte or candidal infection, they typically worsen or predispose to these infections. Their use may alter the physical characteristics of the infection, causing delay in appropriate diagnosis and therapy. (*Cecil, Ch. 473*)

95.(A—True; B—False; C—True; D—False; E—True; F—False) *Discussion:* Retinoids have a variety of systemic effects, including decreasing epidermal cell proliferation, keratinization, and inhibition of sebaceous gland activity. Etretinate is useful in ichthyosis and severe psoriasis, including the pustular and erythrodermic forms. Isotretinoin has been useful in severe cystic acne. All patients treated with retinoids will experience side effects. These include cheilitis, conjunctivitis, dry skin, congenital malformations, osteophytic growths, night blindness, and elevation of very-low-density and low-density lipoprotein levels. Isotretinoin is usually given for a 20-week course, and appropriate dosing at 1 mg per kilogram daily is necessary to avoid treatment failures and the need for repeat therapy in the future. Because the retinoids have many systemic side effects, one must be familiar with the use of the medication and the necessity of patient monitoring before prescribing these medications. (*Cecil, Ch. 474*)

96.(All are True) *Discussion:* Acyclovir is phosphorylated by HSV thymidine kinase, and the active triphosphate state inhibits the viral DNA synthesis. Acyclovir is useful against HSV and varicella zoster virus. HSV infections, such as neonatal herpes, primary genital and recurrent herpes, and eczema herpeticum, respond to 200 mg of acyclovir five times a day. Herpes zoster infections, such as shingles, require higher dosing, 800 mg five times a day for 7 to 10 days. (*Cecil, Ch. 339 and 474*)

97.(All are True) *Discussion:* Phototherapy is useful for treating a variety of disorders, including psoriasis, vitiligo, eczema, pityriasis rosea, and mycosis fungoides. UVB is 1000 times stronger than UVA light and can cause a sunburn. UVA is usually used in conjunction with topical or systemic psoralens, which bind to DNA. This binding lasts for 24 hours, so the patient must protect the corneas and genitalia from UV radiation, because cataracts and squamous cell carcinomas are known long-term side effects of PUVA therapy. Patients must wear special UV-protective glasses, and regular eye exams are required. (*Cecil, Ch. 474*)

98.(A—False; B—True; C—True; D—False) *Discussion:* The allergen responsible for allergic contact dermatitis from poison ivy or sumac is pentadecylcatechol. This allergen is also present in mangos, cashews, and ginkgo trees. The contact dermatitis from mangos and cashews can occur around the mouth when contact with the offending agent occurs. (*Cecil, Ch. 475*)

99.(A—True; B—True; C—True; D—False; E—True) *Discussion:* Nonpalpable purpura refers to the presence of petechiae or purpura in the skin that is macular (flat). Schamberg's disease, an idiopathic capillaritis, produces petechiae that look like Cayenne pepper. Meningococcemia may produce petechiae and purpura that may become confluent, with central necrosis. Rocky Mountain spotted fever may begin acrally on the hands or feet with petechiae or purpura and spread to the extremities and trunk. Henoch-Schönlein syndrome is associated with a leukocytoclastic vasculitis that typically produces palpable purpura. Endocarditis also produces petechiae on conjunctiva, buccal mucosa, and extremities. (*Cecil, Ch. 475*)

100.(A—True; B—False; C—True; D—True; E—False, F—True; G—True) *Discussion:* Psoriasis typically affects the elbows and knees but it may also involve the trunk, scalp, intergluteal cleft, and umbilicus. Palms and soles may be involved with erythema and scale. Nail pitting is common, and onycholysis with oil spots is characteristic of psoriasis. Inverse psoriasis occurs in the intertriginous folds of the body, such as the axilla or groin, as a result of excess moisture and maceration. The Koebner phenomenon, in which trauma to the skin induces the appearance of new lesions, is typical of psoriasis. Being a genetic disease, psoriasis is chronic with flares and remissions. Pityriasis rosea, another papulosquamous disorder, may run a self-limited course in 6 to 8 weeks. Known aggravating factors for psoriasis include streptococcal pharyngitis, stress, and medications such as lithium and beta blockers. One to 3 weeks following the streptococcal infection, guttate psoriasis may appear, with a showering of small psoriatic lesions over the trunk. Psoriatic treatments include topical steroids of various strengths, topical tars, and recently a vitamin D analogue, calcipotriene. Psoriasis is often responsive to sunlight and UVB or psoralens with UVA (PUVA). Severe psoriasis may require systemic treatment with methotrexate, cyclosporin, etretinate, or hydroxyurea. These systemic medications require follow-up and laboratory monitoring. (*Cecil, Ch. 475*)

101.(A—False; B—True; C—True, D—False) *Discussion:* Pityriasis rosea usually begins with a herald patch, a large solitary lesion that precedes the generalized eruption. A generalized rash consists of oval patches with a collarette of scale that follows the skin cleavage lines, creating a Christmas tree–like pattern, especially on the back. Palms and soles are typically spared; however, the differential diagnosis includes secondary syphilis and, if palmar or sole lesions are noted, a rapid plasma reagin test should be performed. Pruritus is a common symptom, but no specific treatment is necessary. Topical steroids, antihistamines, and UVB or sunlight may provide some relief. (*Cecil, Ch. 475*)

102.(A—True; B—False; C—True; D—False) *Discussion:* Ichthyosis vulgaris is an autosomal dominantly inherited disease characterized by fishlike scales on the extensor surfaces of the extremities. Typically it appears in childhood. Treatment consists of emollients and keratolytics. Other ichthyoses may present at birth, such as lamellar ichthyosis, which presents as a collodion baby. (*Cecil, Ch. 475*)

103.(All are True) *Discussion:* Rosacea is a common disease of middle-aged people, with the development of papules, pustules, erythema, and telangiectasias of the central face. Flushing is a common complaint and may be triggered by alcohol, caffeine, or spicy foods. Complications of rosacea include rhinophyma, a red bulbous nose, and ocular involvement such as blepharitis, chalazion, conjunctivitis, or keratosis. Treatment includes long-term systemic tetracyclines and topical antibiotics. (*Cecil, Ch. 475*)

104.(All are True) *Discussion:* Acute urticaria presents with wheals, or hives, in the skin resulting from a type I IgE hypersensitivity reaction. Drugs such as aspirin, infections such as sinusitis or toothaches, and food, particularly berries and shellfish, are common causes. Physical modalities such as sunlight, cold, heat, pressure, or exercise can induce hives. Skin lesions move from area to area. Acute urticaria usually resolves in approximately 6 weeks. In chronic urticaria, which lasts longer than 6 weeks, it is more difficult to find an offending agent. (*Cecil, Ch. 475*)

105.(All are True) *Discussion:* Kaposi's sarcoma was originally described in elderly men of Mediterranean descent, and usually affects the lower legs and runs an indolent course, with development of chronic lymphedema. Kaposi's sarcoma has been noted to appear in patients treated with immunosuppressive medications, such as lupus patients, or in renal transplant patients. In the AIDS patient, Kaposi's sarcoma may be aggressive, affecting young men and typically occurring in the mucous membranes, viscera, and lungs as well as the skin. (*Cecil, Ch. 475*)

106.(A—True; B—False; C—True; D—True) *Discussion:* Immunosuppressive therapy has been correlated with a higher frequency of skin cancer than expected. Transplant patients have a seven times greater risk of developing skin cancer. Appropriate counseling about the use of sunscreen and sun protection is crucial because survival times continue to lengthen. In the immunosuppressed patient, skin lesions must be promptly evaluated. Clinical morphologies may be altered and pathologic diagnosis is often necessary. In addition, unusual opportunistic infections can occur. Prompt biopsy for pathology as well as bacterial and fungal cultures may provide a rapid diagnosis and guide appropriate therapy. In HIV infection, common diagnoses may appear atypical. Molluscum contagiosum, tiny umbilicated papules in children, may present as large (1- to 2-cm) nodules, typically on the face in HIV patients. Herpes simplex may persist as large chronic ulcers. Psoriasis in HIV-infected patients may be widespread. Diseases characteristic of AIDS include Kaposi's sarcoma, with firm violaceous papules and plaques. Oral hairy leukoplakia presents with white-appearing plaques on the edges of the tongue. Bacillary angiomatosis presents as red papules with a slightly scaly base. Eosinophilic folliculitis is a pruritic follicular-based papular eruption seen on the trunk in patients with AIDS. (*Cecil, Ch. 475*)